AF251678

ADVANCES IN NEURO-ONCOLOGY

edited by

Paul L. Kornblith, M.D.

Professor and Chairman
Leo M. Davidoff Department of Neurological Surgery
Albert Einstein College of Medicine
and Montefiore Medical Center
Bronx, New York

and

Michael D. Walker, M.D.

Director of Stroke and Trauma Program
National Institutes of Health
Bethesda, Maryland

With a Preface by
Paul C. Bucy, M.D.

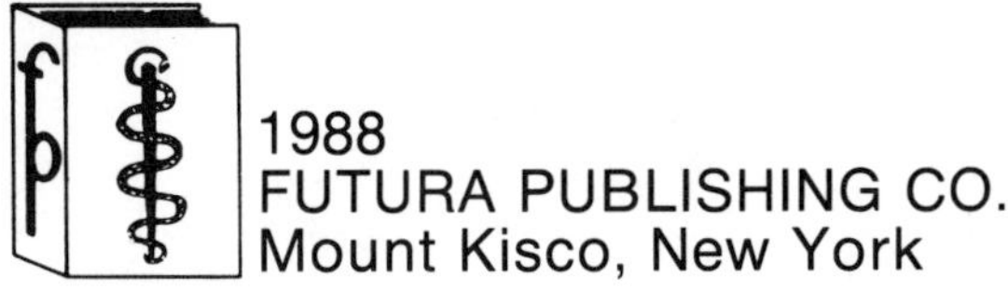

1988
FUTURA PUBLISHING CO.
Mount Kisco, New York

Library of Congress Cataloging-in-Publication Data
Main entry under title

Advances in neuro-oncology / edited by Paul L. Kornblith, Michael D.
   Walker.
      p.   cm.
   Includes bibliographies and index.
   ISBN 0-87993-275-9
   1. Brain—Tumors.   I. Kornblith, Paul L.   II. Walker, Michael D.
   [DNLM: 1. Brain Neoplasms.   WL 358 A244]
RC280.B7A29   1988
616.99′281—dc19
DNLM/DLC
for Library of Congress   88-11191
                                  CIP

Copyright 1988
Futura Publishing Company, Inc.

Published by
Futura Publishing Company, Inc.
295 Main Street, P.O. Box 330
Mount Kisco, New York 10549

L.C. no.: 88-11191
ISBN no.: 0-87993-275-9

Printed in the United States of America.

Contributors

Michael L. J. Apuzzo, M.D.
Professor of Neurosurgery, Department of Neurological Surgery, University of Southern California, School of Medicine, Los Angeles, California

Judith L. Bader, M.D.
Senior Investigator, Radiation Oncology Branch, National Cancer Institute, Bethesda, Maryland

J. Behnke, M.D.
Neurosurgical Service, CHUV, Lausanne, Switzerland

Deborah Benzil, M.D.
National Institutes of Health, Surgical Neurology Branch, NINCDS, Bethesda, Maryland

Peter McL. Black, M.D., Ph.D.
Neurosurgeon-in-Chief, Brigham and Women's Hospital, Boston, Massachusetts

Harold Brem, M.D.
Resident in Surgery, Ohio State University, Columbus, Ohio

Henry Brem, M.D.
Assistant Professor of Neurosurgery, Ophthalmology, and Oncology, Director, Adult Neurosurgical Oncology, The Johns Hopkins Hospital, Department of Neurosurgery, Baltimore, Maryland

Steven S. Brem, M.D.
Chief of Neurosurgery, Jewish General Hospital, Associate Professor of Neurosurgery, McGill University, Montreal, Canada

Joseph Bressler, M.D.
National Institutes of Health, Surgical Neurology Branch, NINCDS, Bethesda, Maryland

S. Carrel, M.D.
Ludwig Institute for Cancer Research, Epalinges, Switzerland

Terence L. Chen, M.D.
Resident, Section of Neurosurgery, Yale University School of Medicine, New Haven, Connecticut

Hugh B. Coakham, M.D.
Department of Neurosurgery, Brain Cancer Research Fund, Frenchay Hospital, Bristol, England

Dierdre Cohen, M.D.
Assistant Professor of Clinical Radiation Oncology, Department of Radiation Oncology, University of Southern California, School of Medicine, Los Angeles, California

Craig J. Cummins, M.D.
Surgical Neurology Branch, National Institutes of Health, Bethesda, Maryland

John L. Darling, M.Sc., Ph.D.
Neuro-Oncology Section, Gough-Cooper Department of Neurological Surgery, Institute of Neurology, National Hospital, London, England

Nicholas de Tribolet, M.D.
Professor and Chairman, Service de Neurochirurgie, Centre Hospitalier Universitaire Vaudois, Lausanne, Switzerland

Daniel L. Dexter, Ph.D.
Research Associate, Du Pont Company, Glenolden Laboratory, Glenolden, Pennsylvania

George J. Dohrmann, III, M.D., Ph.D.
Associate Professor of Surgery (Neurosurgery), Surgery Brain Research Institute, University of Chicago, Chicago, Illinois

James Ellis, Ph.D.
National Institutes of Health, Biomedical Engineering and Instrumentation Branch, DRS, Bethesda, Maryland

Duncan K. Fischer, M.D., Ph.D.
Resident, Department of Neurosurgery, Baylor College of Medicine, Houston, Texas

Anthony L. Gard, Ph.D.
Department of Microbiology, University of Connecticut Medical School, Farmington, Connecticut

Carter Gibson, M.D.
National Institutes of Health, Biomedical Engineering and Instrumentation Branch, DRS, Bethesda, Maryland

Eli Glatstein, M.D.
Chief, Radiation Oncology Branch, Clinical Oncology Program, Division of Cancer Treatment, National Cancer Institute, Bethesda, Maryland

Elizabeth Ann Grimm, Ph.D.
Senior Investigator, Chief of Cellular Immunology Unit, Surgical Neurology Branch, NINCDS, National Institutes of Health, Bethesda, Maryland

Janet L. Gross, Ph.D.
Cancer Chemotherapy Program, Pharmaceuticals Division, Biomedical Products Department, E. I. Du Pont de Nemours and Co., Inc., Wilmington, Delaware

Christopher Guerin, M.D.
Resident, The Johns Hopkins Hospital, Department of Neurosurgery, Baltimore, Maryland

M. Peter Heilbrun, M.D.
Professor and Head, Division of Neurosurgery, University of Utah, School of Medicine, Salt Lake City, Utah

Robert Highsmith, Ph.D.
Associate Professor of Physiology and Biophysics, Department of Physiology and Biophysics, University of Cincinnati Medical Center, Cincinnati, Ohio

Alan Hirschfeld, M.D.
Director of Neurosurgery, Bronx Municipal Hospital Center, and Assistant Professor, Albert Einstein College of Medicine and Montefiore Medical Center, Bronx, New York

Joanne H. Jepson, M.D.
Associate Professor of Clinical Radiation Oncology, and Head of Radiation Physics Division, Department of Radiation Oncology, University of Southern California, School of Medicine, Los Angeles, California

James D. Kolker, M.D.
Instructor, Center for Radiation Therapy, University of Chicago Medical Center, Chicago, Illinois

Kurt W. Kohn, M.D.
Laboratory of Molecular Pharmacology, Developmental Therapeutics Program, Division of Cancer Treatment, National Cancer Institute, Bethesda, Maryland

Paul L. Kornblith, M.D.
Professor and Chairman, Leo M. Davidoff Department of Neurological Surgery, Albert Einstein College of Medicine and Montefiore Medical Center, Bronx, New York

Patrick A. LaSala, M.D.
Assistant Professor of Neurosurgery, Albert Einstein College of Medicine and Montefiore Medical Center, Bronx, New York

Gary Luxton, M.D.
Professor of Neurosurgery, Department of Neurological Surgery, University of Southern California, School of Medicine, Los Angeles, California

J. P. Mach, M.D.
Ludwig Institute for Cancer Research, Epalinges, Switzerland

Marius Maxwell, MB.BChir
Research Fellow, Neurosurgical Service, Massachusetts General Hospital, and Department of Surgery, Harvard Medical School, Boston, Massachusetts

Paul E. McKeever, M.D., Ph.D.
Chief, Section of Neuropathology, Department of Pathology, University of Michigan Medical School, Ann Arbor, Michigan

William D. Moore, M.D.
Neuroradiologist, Division of Neuroradiology, Georgetown University Hospital, Washington, DC

Raj K. Narayan, M.D.
Assistant Professor, Department of Neurosurgery, Baylor College of Medicine, Houston, Texas

Mary Ann Oberc-Greenwood, M.D.
Surgical Neurology Branch, National Institute of Neurological and Communicative Disorders and Strokes, National Institutes of Health, Bethesda, Maryland

Nicholas J. Patronas, M.D.
Professor of Neuroradiology, Division of Neuroradiology, Georgetown University Hospital, Washington, DC

Zbigniew Petrovich, M.D.
Albert Soiland Professor and Chairman, Department of Radiation Oncology, University of Southern California, School of Medicine, Los Angeles, California

Steven E. Pfeiffer, Ph.D.
Professor, Department of Microbiology, University of Connecticut Medical School, Farmington, Connecticut

Jacob R. Rachlin, M.D.
Resident, Department of Neurological Surgery, University of California, San Francisco, California

Raymond Sawaya, M.D.
Director, Division of Neuro-Oncology, Assistant Professor, Department of Neurosurgery, University of Cincinnati Medical Center; Chief of Neurosurgical Service, Veteran's Administration Medical Center, Cincinnati, Ohio

D. R. Schellinger, M.D.
Professor of Neuroradiology, Division of Neuroradiology, Georgetown University Hospital, Washington, DC

Barry H. Smith, M.D., Ph.D.
Medical and Scientific Director, Dreyfus Medical Foundation, New York, New York

Rafael J. Tamargo, M.D.
Resident, The Johns Hopkins Hospital, Department of Neurosurgery, Baltimore, Maryland

David G. T. Thomas, M.D.
Chairman of Radiotherapy, University of Chicago, Chicago, Illnois

Michael D. Walker, M.D.
Director, Stroke and Trauma Program, NINCDS, National Institutes of Health, Bethesda, Maryland

Ralph R. Weichselbaum, M.D.
Department of Radiation Therapy, University of Chicago Medical Center, Chicago, Illinois

John Zovickian, M.D.
Chief Resident, Neurological Surgery, Division of Neurological Surgery, San Diego, California

Acknowledgments

The editors wish to acknowledge a continued excellent support from Rose Giannotto whose assistance was invaluable in the coordination and preparation of the material.

We would also like to thank Steven Korn, publisher, and Linda Shaw, editor, at Futura Publishing Company who made the difficult task of preparing this book a pleasure. A special thanks accrues to Mr. Korn whose personal support and infinite patience were remarkable.

Paul L. Kornblith, M.D.
Michael D. Walker, M.D.

Preface

A little more than 100 years ago (1879), modern neurological surgery was born. William Macewen (later Sir William) was the first neurological surgeon. Working in Glasgow, Scotland, a backwater city from a medical standpoint, he performed the first operation upon the brain. Such a procedure was delayed until that time awaiting the development of general anesthesia, of aseptic surgery, and of knowledge about localization of function in the brain.

In 1879, Macewen was 31 years old. (Neurological surgery has always been a young man's game.) Knowledge of localization of function had begun in 1861 with Broca, who demonstrated that small lesions in the postero-inferior part of the left frontal lobe could render the patient speechless. This demonstration was soon followed by the experimental work of Fritsch and Hitzig in Germany and David Ferrier in England. These men experimentally produced movement in the extremities by electrical stimulation of the motor areas of the brain in dogs and in subhuman primates.

In 1884, five years later, Rickman Godlee in London performed the first surgical removal of a brain tumor in England but did not pursue a neurosurgical career. Two years later, Sir Victor Horsley began his illustrious career in neurosurgery at the National Hospital at Queen Square in London.

Harvey Cushing had decided upon becoming a brain surgeon and went to England at the turn of the century to learn from Horsley. He was so greatly disappointed by the crude surgery which he observed that he practically gave up his desire to engage in that field. Furthermore, the high surgical mortality and poor results of brain surgery were such that operations upon the brain were losing the support of the medical profession in general. Cushing went to Berne, Switzerland, to study with the famous general surgeon, Kocher. There, however, he was directed into the physiological laboratories of Professor Kronecker. Here he performed his famous studies on the effects of increased intracranial pressure upon the respiration, the pulse, and the blood pressure.

When Cushing returned to The Johns Hopkins Hospital after his sojourn in Europe, he began doing brain surgery. His aim then and later was to reduce the appalling surgical mortality which he had found in Europe, which was sometimes as high as 65%. In this he succeeded and by 1930 his surgical mortality was only 10%, an almost unbelievable figure at that time. Surgical approach to brain tumors with the aim of curing the patient, however, was the aim of Walter Dandy, Cushing's pupil and his successor at The Johns Hopkins Medical School. Since Dandy's time further progress in curing the patient with a brain tumor has been attained but principally with the less aggressive, slower-growing tumors such as meningiomas and acoustic neuromas. Except for a few gliomas, notably the astrocytomas of the cerebellum, it is still uncommon for a patient with a glioma to be cured of his tumor. Nevertheless, this should be our aim and can be attained. This is the purpose of this book. Anyone interested in gliomas, their treatment, and their cure will find this book both intriguing and stimulating.

There are many questions concerned with the occurrence of a cerebral glioma which remain to be answered and which all thinking neurosurgeons must recognize. What stimulates normal glial cells to become neoplastic? Certainly there must be an etiological factor or perhaps more than one. Is this factor a chemical one, something in the environment, a viral one, or what? What are the factors that cause these gliomas to continue to grow? What stimulates them to cause new blood vessels to form and to continue to form as the tumor grows? Why do some tumors commonly become cystic as compared with other tumors? Why do some tumors invade and destroy normal brain whereas others seem to merely push normal brain aside? It seems likely that the answers to these questions will probably be different for the astrocytomas as compared with the glioblastomas.

In any consideration of brain tumors, it is important to constantly bear in mind the realization that gliomas of the central nervous system differ in many respects from tumors in other parts of the body. This is true regardless of whether one is considering etiology, growth, or therapy. Although it is common to falsely refer to some gliomas as "malignant," they are not malignant in the sense that carcinomas or sarcomas are malignant. They do not metastasize. They do not invade the normal brain tissue for any considerable distance. They arise in one place and they stay confined to that region even though they continue to increase in size.

One must be impressed from a review of the publications cited in this book that the studies in this field are largely the work of the past 10 to 15 years. In other words, this is a new and rapidly expanding field of investigation. At the same time one must be impressed by the fact that this book contains no final answers. This is an ongoing field of investigation that promises much but as yet delivers little as to the final effective treatment of tumors of the nervous system, particularly of the gliomas.

Paul C. Bucy, M.D.

Introduction

The recent decades have seen remarkable advances in the management of patients with many forms of cancer and also in the surgical treatment of many types of CNS disease. When one looks at cancer and the nervous system, great strides forward are not so easy to discern. The management of benign tumors of the CNS has improved with the development of modern microsurgery, but in the malignant tumors we are still at the most primeval stage. It is hard to believe but the justification for significant resections of malignant brain tumors is just now being obtained. The value of radiotherapy was statistically proven just a little over a decade ago and the current modalities of chemotherapy have only slightly shifted the balance in favor of the patient.

With this background, the field of neuro-oncology has become one of the most challenging albeit frustrating areas for cancer treatment. These challenges have led to an outpouring of all types of efforts at the basic science level, in diagnosis and in therapy aimed at solving these complex problems. In this book, certain selected topics in each of these areas that represent exciting, often promising or at least intriguing glimpses into the future have been chosen for presentation.

The topics in some cases are updates on well-established approaches, and in other instances they are new and as yet untried insights into the biology or potential therapy of these tumors.

The focus of this book is primarily on the primary tumors of the brain. Many of the biological observations apply to tumors of the spinal cord and some of the therapeutic information does relate to secondary (metastatic) tumors of the brain and spinal cord.

Of the primary tumors, the most common and deadliest type is the malignant astrocytoma, which in its most aggressive form is called glioblastoma multiforme. This tumor is the major target of much of the research effort in neuro-oncology and is therefore the primary focus of this book. This tumor is locally invasive, kills patients in about 15 weeks after diagnosis with surgery as the only treatment, and the best we can currently do is to extend life to a median survival of about 1 year.

This tumor type is also tantalizing in that it rarely metastasizes, it often involves young otherwise healthy individuals, and detection with CT scanning is now straightforward. Yet it challenges the therapist because the brain cannot be aggressively encroached upon by any modality of therapy without potentially unacceptable neurological sequelae. The therapeutic ratio is thus very narrow. The modality which will kill the tumor is also likely to kill essential functional brain.

Furthermore, the brain has a blood-brain barrier which variably blocks access of large molecules into its substance, limiting therapeutic modalities from reaching the tumor. Diagnosis is not difficult but defining tumor margins is not precise. Responses to therapy are also difficult to monitor.

It is this complex series of obstacles to effective management that makes this tumor type so challenging. It is also this challenge that makes it essential to review some of the most important advances in the various aspects of the field in order to stimulate further efforts and to make clear the complexity of the problem.

It is therefore the goal of this book to bring together the work of a range of basic and clinical scientists who are approaching these tumors from a variety of directions. It is our hope that reading about this series of advances will help to provide the substrate for continued efforts in attacking this tremendously difficult and complex problem.

Paul L. Kornblith, M.D.
Michael D. Walker, M.D.

Contents

Section I
Basic Studies in Brain Tumor Biology

Introduction to Basic Studies

It is clear that no simple solution currently exists for successful therapy of the malignant primary brain tumor. The remarkably distinctive features of the neuroectodermal cells which give rise to these tumors has therefore been a major focus for investigative work as the nature and biology of these enigmatic cells are studied.

In the first section of this book, some of these distinctive features are described. The biochemical and molecular cell-specific markers define the prototypical cells giving rise to these tumors. The ways in which these phenotypic characteristics can be modulated give insight into the significance of molecular parameters in tumor differentiation. The recent advances in two-dimensional gel electrophoresis have made a careful analysis of specific protein patterns possible and this technique thus allows for profiling of antigens in specific brain tumors. The exciting discovery that tumors produce a substance which causes vascular proliferation has found particular importance in the field of brain tumor research as these tumor angiogenesis factors are at the highest levels in brain tumors.

A very recent observation involves the fibrinolytic system and brain tumors. It is well known that clotting disorders are very common in brain tumor patients and the biochemical correlates have now been found to study this clinical phenomenon at the basic level.

Oncogenes and viruses in cancer have created much recent interest and these new approaches have been shown to be applicable to the study of brain tumors.

It is apparent that these two areas are only a small portion of the entire spectrum of the investigative background in brain tumor biology. They serve as what we feel is a useful sampler of some of the most intriguing and promising leads in our understanding of brain tumor biology.

1

Biochemical, Immunological, and Molecular Cell-Type Specific Markers of the Central Nervous System

S.E. Pfeiffer and A.L. Gard

Introduction

Cellular studies of the central nervous system (CNS) in both its normal and diseased state have historically proceeded largely through the use of empirically developed fixatives, staining procedures, microscopic techniques, and above all, the ingenuity and insight of the investigators who have taken these images and made some sense of them. However, during development, in disease, and in tissue culture, morphology *alone* is frequently unreliable as a sole criterion for establishing a cell's identity, a point previously made by drawing on three insightful comments found in the literature.[1]

"Certain identification of neuroglial cells as either astrocytes or oligodendroglia is at least as difficult in tissue culture as it is in fixed and stained material when viewed through the light or electron microscope."[2] "The difficulty is not with cells which are morphologically similar to those described in classical anatomy, but, rather, with

From: Kornblith PL, Walker MD (editors). Advances in Neuro-Oncology. Futura Publishing Company, Inc., Mount Kisco, NY, © 1988.
Acknowledgments: Supported in part by a grant from the National Institutes of Health, NS10861-13. The word processing help of Ms. Janice Seagren is gratefully acknowledged.

the many intermediate forms present."[3] "It would be difficult to overestimate the value of specific markers for identifying and quantitating the different cell types present in heterogeneous cultures and for studying the properties of individual cells."[4]

Only in recent years has the use of specific biochemical, immunological, and molecular parameters for identifying specific CNS cell types and for probing the state of gene expression attained prominence. This chapter attempts to summarize the range of available central nervous system markers, and to look briefly at the impact that cell-type specific markers are making on the field of neuro-oncology. Examples are drawn from biochemical assays, immunological probes, and molecular probes for the transcription of specific genes. While not a comprehensive catalogue of all available markers, an attempt has been made to present enough examples to give a sense of the range of possibilities.

The choice of markers is broad, for in principle, any component of the CNS that has some degree of cellular specificity can be used as a cell-type marker, either alone or as part of a panel of markers. Neurotransmitters and the enzymes that catalyze their synthesis or degradation, receptors, transport molecules, neuropeptides and growth factors, cell adhesion molecules, structural lipids and proteins, cytoskeletal components, and soluble and membrane-bound proteins of currently unknown function are all potential candidates. Examples of each of these categories are found in the literature.

Cell-Type Specific Markers

Histochemical and Biochemical Markers

A large number of CNS markers can be visualized by histochemical, fluorescence, and autoradiographic techniques,[5] although these approaches will not be the primary focus in this chapter. Examples include colorimetric, radiolabel, or histochemical assays for neurotransmitter enzymes such as choline acetyltransferase,[6] acetylcholinesterase,[7,8] or cytochrome oxidase;[9,10] histofluorescence for catecholamines;[11] radiolabeled neurotransmitter uptake;[12–15] and radioligand receptor binding.[16,17]

Immunological Markers

The development of immunological probes and methods has had a major impact on diverse areas of neurobiology (see ref. 18–20 for

Table 1
Immunologically Identifiable Neuronal Markers

Cytoskeleton
  Neurofilaments (24–29)
  Microtubule-associated proteins
    (MAPs) (30–32)
Neurotransmitters
  GABA (33–35)
  Glutamic acid (33)
  Serotonin (36–38)
Neurotransmitter enzymes
  Adenine deaminase (14, 39)
  Acetylcholinesterase (20)
  Choline acetyl transferase (41, 42)
  Cysteine-sulfinic acid decarboxylase
    (43)
  Dopamine-β-hydroxylase (44)
  Glutamate decarboxylase (GAD) (35,
    45–47)
  Glutaminase (48)
  Histidine decarboxylase (14, 39)
  Phenylethanolamine-N-methyl
    transferase (49–51)
  Tyrosine hydroxylase (44, 47, 50–52B)
Neuropeptides (20, 52–55)
  ACTH (56)
  Met-enkephalin (57–59)
  Neurophysin (35)
  Oxytocin (56)
  Somatostatin (57)
  Substance P (38, 58–65)
  Vasopressin (66)
Cell adhesion and migration molecules
  Neuronal cell adhesion molecule
    (N-CAM = D2 = BSP-2) (67–74A)
  Neuron-glial cell adhesion molecule
    (Ng-CAM = L1 = NILE) (73, 75–80)
  G4; F11 (81, 82)
Pumps and channels
  Sodium channel (reviewed in ref. 19,
    20)
  Na^+, K^+-ATPase exchange pump (82,
    83)
  Ca^{2+} pumps (84, 85)

Receptors
  α-adrenergic receptor (86)
  β-adrenergic receptor (87)
  GABA/benzodiazepine receptor (88–
    90)
  Glycine receptor (91)
  Muscarinic acetylcholine receptor (86)
  Nicotinic acetylcholine receptor (19,
    20, 92, 93)
  Nerve growth factor receptor (94)
Lipids
  A_2B_5, GQ ganglioside (95–99)
  Chol-1 (100)
  Tetanous toxin receptor, gangliosides
    GD_{1b} and GT_1 (101–103)
Other enzymes and antigens (20)
  Neuron specific enolase (NSE) (104–
    107)
  Calcineruin (108, 109)
  Calmodulin-dependent protein kinase
    II (110)
  CAT 301 (111)
  CNS surface antigen (112)
  Drosophila/human cross-reacting
    antigens (113)
  Fodrin (114–117)
  Neuron-specific mitochondrial protein
    (118)
  Protein kinase C (119)
  Retinal membrane antigens (22, 120,
    121)
  Sensory neuron subpopulations (122)
  Synapsin I (123)
  Synaptic vesicle proteins (124)
  Thy-1 (125–129)
  Visual cortex neurons (130)

Numbers in parentheses are reference numbers.

recent reviews). One index of the rapid progress in this area is the steady expansion of identified markers.[21–23] Both polyclonal and monoclonal antibodies to essentially all molecular classes of antigens are available. In fact, the variety of markers seems to be limited only by the biochemical diversity of the neurons and glia themselves. Many of the markers for which antibodies are available are summarized in Tables 1, 2, and 3.

Antisera to many of the markers cross-react with human material and are currently being studied in human neurotumors (below). Not all markers are completely cell-type specific. Some, such as neuron-specific enolase, appear to be general markers for all neurons, while

---

Table 2
Immunologically Identifiable Glial Markers

General Glial
  Non-neuronal enolase (107, 131)
Astrocytes
  α_2-glycoprotein (132)
  Adhesion molecule on glia (AMOG) (133)
  Apolipoprotein E (134, 135)
  Glial fibrillary acidic protein (GFAP) (4, 136–140)
  Glutamine synthetase (141, 142)
  M1, C1 (143, 144)
  Ran-2 (145)
  S100 (104, 105, 137, 146–148)
  Stage-specific embryonic antigen (SSEA-1) (149, 150)
  Thy-1 (151; but see also Table 1)
  Vimentin (24, 25, 152–155)
Oligodendrocytes (1, 156, 157)
  Galactosylcerebroside (GC) (4, 158–167)
  1A9 (217)
  Carbonic anhydrase (168–171)
  2′,3′-cyclic nucleotide 3′-phosphohydrolase (CNP) (170, 172–178)
  Ganglioside GD_3 (179–181)
  Glycerol-3-phosphate dehydrogenase (GPdH) (L169, 170, 182–184)
  GM_4 (179, 185–187)
  Lactate dehydrogenase (LDH) (169, 170, 184)
  Myelin associated glycoprotein (MAG) (73, 177, 188)
  Myelin basic protein (MBP) (4, 177, 189–193)
  Proteolipid protein (PLP) (177, 191–195)
  Sulfatide (161, 162, 167)
  Transferrin receptor (196)

Numbers in parentheses are reference numbers.

Table 3
Immunologically Identifiable Markers of Other
Cell Types

Ependymal cells
  Ran-2 (145)
  Vimentin (155)
Endothelial Cells
  Factor VIII antigen (197)
  γ-glutamyl transpeptide (198)
  MESA-1 (199)
Microglia (200)
  MAC-1, MAC-3
  Acetylated low density lipoprotein receptors

Numbers in parentheses are reference numbers.

others define subclasses of neurons in a specific changing developmental pattern (e.g., Thy-1,[129]). Others cross-react among the major CNS cell types, neurons, glia, and fibroblasts, sometimes in a developmentally specified fashion. For example, the tetanus toxin receptor (primarily gangliosides GD_{1b}/GT_{1b}) was originally thought to be a neuron-specific marker.[101–103] More recent experiments have shown that it is also transiently present on rodent progenitor cells for astrocytes and oligodendrocytes,[201] but can be used as a neuronal marker in cultures of human brain.[187] A similar story has developed for monoclonal antibody (mAb) A_2B_5 that recognizes ganglioside GQ_{1c}.[95,98] Ganglioside GD_3[179] is expressed on the plasma membrane of immature neuronal and glial neuroectodermal cells;[181] it has been used in culture, however, as a marker for human, rat, and bovine oligodendrocytes.[180,187] Therefore, in many cases, positive cell-type identification is made with a panel of markers, the sum of which defines a particular cell-type.[126,202,203] It should be noted that cross-reactivity can also prove useful, as in the shared antigenic determinants found on human hematopoietic and brain cells. For example, the mAbs anti-LEU-7 (HNK-1), anti-LEU-M1, and anti-LEU-11 have proven useful in neuropathological analyses (discussed in ref. 204–205).

Techniques[207–209]

Many of the immunological techniques now being applied to neuro-oncology have gained general recognition and appreciation

Table 4
Assays

Morphological	Immunological	Molecular	Level
Light microscopy Electron microscopy Histochemistry	Immunocytochemistry Immunofluorescence	In situ hybridization	Tissue, cellular, or subcellular
	Western blots Metabolic labeling & immunoprecipitation	Northern blots Metabolic labeling & nuclear run-off	Molecular

only in the past decade or so.[210] They can be applied at the tissue, cellular, and biochemical levels (Table 4).

Antibody production and the subsequent characterization of virtually all classes of neural antigens has been facilitated by advances in antigen purification and presentation, but especially by the development of the hybridoma technique.[211–212] This approach yields highly specific mAbs to defined antigenic determinants of even complex antigens, regardless of the purity of the immunogen. In vitro immunization permits the generation of mAbs when only small amounts of immunogen are available.[213–215] A number of neural markers were first identified using a "shotgun" immunization of crude cell homogenates of cellular fractions, followed by screening of mAbs against tissue sections or cells in culture.[22,118,120,216–217] or by solid-phase immunoassay.[218,219] A major advantage of this approach is that conformationally sensitive antigens are more likely to be preserved. Furthermore, specialized immunization protocols have been designed to increase the frequency of hybridomas producing antibodies against minor, but potentially interesting, cell surface antigens.[220–225] The use of hybridomas also allows the production of cellularly radiolabeled antibodies[38] and bispecific antibodies made by hybrid hybridomas.[226]

Several options and permutations of techniques are available for immunostaining cells in culture and tissue sections.[208] Indirect immunofluorescence and immunoperoxidase labeling remain the most commonly used procedures for antigen detection and localization. Panels of anti-immunoglobulins recognizing essentially all species of interest, as well as mouse immunoglobin subclasses, are commercially available as pre-tagged conjugates linked to fluorochromes (primarily rhodamine or fluorescein), or to enzymes (e.g., horse radish peroxidase) that catalyze the generation of insoluble products at the antigen-antibody site. Simultaneous labeling of two antigens is therefore possible with the use of heterologous primary antibodies. Improved sensitivity can be attained using a three-step labeling process consisting of primary antibody, followed by biotinylated anti-immunoglobulin, and finally by avidin-conjugated fluorochrome or enzyme. Maximal amplification of signal is provided by the highly sensitive peroxidase-antiperoxidase[208] and avidin-biotin-peroxidase complex labeling methods.[227,228] Dual labeling at the ultrastructural level can be accomplished by using secondary antibodies coupled to colloidal gold particles of two different diameters.[35,47,56]

The examination by immunological techniques can be carried to the molecular level through the use of "Western" immunoblots for proteins, combining polyacrylamide gel electrophoresis and subsequent tranfer of the separated proteins onto nitrocellulose paper.[229] This technique allows the identification of the size of the labeled antigen, and using appropriate standard curves, permits the quantification of antigens. A parallel technique for lipids uses thin layer chromatography (TLC) for separation, followed by immunostaining directly on the TLC plate.[167,230]

Finally, receptor binding sites for neurotransmitters, growth factors, and other ligands can in principle be identified using the elegant anti-idiotypic antibody approach.[66,231]

Some Additional Comments on Neuronal and Glial Markers

Several of the markers listed in Tables 1 and 2 deserve further comment because of their extensive use in cell identification in both developmental neurobiology and neuro-oncology.

Neuron-specific enolase (NSE) has received particular attention as a neuronal marker. This soluble protein is a cell-specific isozyme of the glycolytic enzyme enolase.[107] It is present in CNS neurons and essentially all neuroendocrine, paraneuronal cell types. During development, a switch is made in the gene expression from the α to the γ subunit, providing an index for neural differentiation and neuron maturity; the α subunit predominates in fetal brain, whereas the γ subunit appears at the onset of neurogenesis.

Intermediate Filament Proteins (IF): Intermediate filaments are 8–11 nm diameter elements of the cytoskeleton which are widely distributed among cell types. Five major cell-type-specific classes are recognized, based on immunological and biochemical differences.[154] The expression of IFs is developmentally regulated in CNS neurons and glia. Most, if not all, proliferating neuronal and glial progenitors in the neuroepithelium abundantly express one of these classes, *vimentin.* Subsequently, post-mitotic neuroblasts cease vimentin expression and begin to accumulate *neurofilaments* (comprised of a triplet of proteins), passing through a brief period when both neurofilament and vimentin proteins are present in the same cell.[232] Astrocytes, in contrast, acquire *glial fibrillary acidic protein* (GFAP), the principle subunit of glial intermediate filaments. GFAP expression in vitro can be influenced by a variety of means including cAMP analogues, plating density, serum components, hormones, and growth factors. These and other considerations have led Chiu and Goldman[140] to suggest that "while GFAP is a useful marker, its mere presence is a highly limited definition of an astrocyte or a radial glial cell." GFAP, along with NSE, has been one of the more studied markers in neuro-oncology (below).

S100 protein is a soluble, acidic, calcium-binding protein originally characterized by Moore[104] and co-workers. Though not entirely specific for glial cells, it has found extensive application as a marker in the study of CNS tumors (below).

Cell adhesion molecules. The identification and analysis of molecules that mediate cell-cell interactions is currently in a growth phase. Recently, the field has been somewhat simplified by the conclusion that several of the cell adhesion molecules identified in various laboratories are in fact the same molecules carrying different names (e.g., N-CAM = D2 = BSP-2; 1987 Gordon Conference on "Cell Contact and Cell Adhesion"). Nevertheless, the field is still embryonic and care must be taken in the application of these markers. For example, L1 is found only on post-mitotic neurons and mediates strictly neuron-neuron interactions. N-CAM, on the other hand, is found on both pre- and post-mitotic neurons, as well as on immature astrocytes and oligodendrocytes.[73] In addition to the markers listed in the tables, several other cell adhesion molecules that have mixed cell specificity are under investigation. For example, N-cadherin and NcalCAM are found on neurons, glia, and muscle, and are involved in neuronal cell adhesion and neurite extension.[233,234] Tenascin, cytotactin, and myotendonous antigen, found on glia and fibroblasts, are involved in neuron-glia adhesion and cerebellar neuron migration.[235–237] Finally markers L2/HNK-1 are carbohydrate epitopes present on N-CAM, L1, MAG, and J1, while J3 is present on L1, MAG, and AMOG.[133]

Lipid Antigens. Several lipid membrane antigens have achieved prominence as CNS cell markers. In addition to gangliosides GD_{1b}/GT_{1b}, GQ_{1c}, and GD_3 discussed earlier, ganglioside GM_4 has been described as a CNS myelin and oligodendrocyte specific marker by several laboratories;[179,185,186] however, in cultures of human brain cells, Kim[187] found staining of GFAP positive cells as well. GM_1 is a fairly general marker for neuronal and glial elements of neuroectodermal origin.[238,239] The current extensive studies of cell surface gangliosides as receptor/ligands suggests that additional markers will be found within this class.[240]

Markers for Other Cell Types (Table 3)

Markers for non-neuronal and non-glial cells have also been identified. For example, microvascular endothelial cells are characterized by γ-glutamyltranspeptidase,[198,241] factor VIII antigen[197] or the MESA-l surface antigen.[199] Pericytes, fibroblasts, and leptomeningial cells express fibronectin,[242] and Thy-l can be used as an additional fibroblast marker.[126] Microglia have been identified as phagocytic cells containing nonspecific esterase, acetylated low density lipoprotein receptors, and the Mac-1 and Mac-3 antigens.[4,200]

Molecular Markers

Cloned Genetic Probes

The advent of recombinant DNA technology has opened up a major new approach to the identification of cells of the central nervous system.[243] The investigator is no longer limited to assay terminal cell products, such as lipids and proteins. Using appropriate genetic probes, one can study the expression of specific messenger RNAs (mRNA), the first step in the overall series of reactions of gene expression. Insofar as translational control is an important regulatory phenomenon, cells that are undergoing cell-type specific transcription but not translation can still be identified. This is an especially im-

---

Table 5

Some cDNA Probes for CNS Markers

Acetylcholine receptor (250–251A)
2′,3′-cyclic nucleotide 3′-phosphohydrolase (252)
GABA/benzodiazepine receptor (253)
Glial fibrillary acidic protein (GFAP) (254, 255)
Glycine receptor, strychnine-binding subunit (91)
Myelin associated glycoprotein (MAG) (256–258)
Myelin basic protein (MBP) (259–265)
Nerve growth factor (NGF) (266, 267)
Neurofilament, L (268–270)
Neurofilament protein, mid-size (271)
Neuron-specific enolase (NSE) (272–275)
Neuropeptides (see ref. 248, 276)
Neurotransmitter enzymes (see ref. 245, 248)
Proteolipid protein (PLP) (261, 276–279)
S100 protein (280)

Numbers in parentheses are reference numbers.

portant issue when dealing with tumor cells, for which there is evidence of transformation-induced translational blocks precluding the identification of certain cell-type specific proteins.[244]

The application of these probes parallels immunological analyses (Table 4). At the cellular level in situ hybridization replaces immunocytochemistry.[245,246] At the biochemical level, "Northern" blots replace "Western" immunoblots to detect specific mRNAs and determine their sizes.[247] Metabolic labeling and pulse-chase experiments can also be carried out to study transcription rates and message stability. Thus the concepts, goals, and techniques are basically unaltered; only the molecular target has changed. The extension of these probes and techniques to neuro-oncology is underway.[248,249]

A considerable number of cloned genes and cDNA probes of nervous system specific proteins is already available and is increasing steadily. Some examples are presented in Table 5.

Growth Factors and Oncogenes

The recognition and analysis of human oncogenes, genes coding for growth regulating factors and the associated receptors,[281–283] are having important impacts on the study of human neurotumors.[284] Alteration in the structure, regulation, or number of these genes can lead to abnormal growth. Cytogenetic abnormalities, including translocations, aneuploidy, and at a more detailed level altered banding patterns, are commonly found in tumor cells including glial malignancies[285,286] and may be related to changes in proto-oncogenes.[284] The molecular correlates of these phenomena can be studied by in situ hybridization and restriction fragment polymorphism.

Altered expression of growth factors and their receptors is associated with many human glial and neuronal malignancies.[284,287–289] If a particular alteration is sufficiently common, it may constitute a cell-type marker and become part of the diagnostic panel for specific tumor types. Three oncogenes in particular have relevance for the study of human neurotumors: *erb*-B codes for three of four domains of the EGF receptor (EGF-R),[290] located on chromosome 7;[291] *sis* codes for one of the polypeptides of platelet-derived growth factor (PDGF),[292,293] located on chromosome 22;[294] N-*myc*, a nuclear protein that seems to have multiple activities including transcriptional regulation, located on chromosome 2.[295]

Glial cells express both PDGF and EGF-R. About one-third of primary human gliomas show gene amplification and over-expression of the epidermal growth factor receptor (EGF-R);[296–298] *sis* gene expression is amplified in some gliomas,[299] and the majority of human glioma cell lines tested express PDGF[300,301] or endothelial cell growth factor.[302] The possibility of autocrine growth stimulation[303] has been discussed.[304]

The N-*myc* oncogene is expressed in nearly all neuroblastoma cell lines and in many neuroblastoma tumors.[306,307] High levels of N-*myc* have also been detected in neuroectodermal tumors such as retinoblastoma[308] and small cell lung cancer[309] and glioblastoma.[310] Using in situ hybridization, evidence has been presented that N-*myc* expression is highest in the least differentiated cells in a tumor.[311–314a] The development of antisera to c-*myc* protein epitopes has promise for clinical analysis.[294]

This is still a fledging field that promises to provide diagnostic markers and has considerable impact on our understanding of brain development and pathology.

Some Confounding Factors in Marker Expression

Marker Expression Plasticity

Developmentally or pathologically induced deviations in marker expression can be confounding variables in cell type identification.

An example of plasticity in the expression of markers is found in a comparison of the distribution of GFAP and NSE in normal, reactive, and neoplastic brain cells types.[315] In normal conditions, NSE is found with few exceptions only in neurons and cells of the amine precursor uptake and decarboxylation system. However, it also appears in several neoplasms including glioblastoma, astrocytoma, ependymoma, and medulloblastoma; in these cases, both proteins can be expressed in the same cell.

Progenitor cells can also co-express markers associated with different adult cell types. For example, a bipotential progenitor cell for oligodendrocytes and a type of astrocytes can, under certain conditions, express both galactocerebroside (GC) and GFAP (along with A_2B_5 and tetanus-specific gangliosides).[180,201,316] Upon further maturation, determined in part by environmental signals, these progenitors differentiate into either GFAP-positive, GC-negative astrocytes or GC-positive, GFAP-negative oligodendrocytes, with the concomitant loss of A_2B_5 reactivity and tetanus toxic receptors. Similarly, switches in the expression of subunit proteins such as the developmental switch of α to γ NSE (above) may also occur. Thus the degree of differentiation of the cells in a tumor can be reflected in the pattern of marker expression.

Experimental Modulation of Gene Expression

The expression of markers, in particular by semi-differentiated tumor cells, can be modulated in culture either by the simple isolation from normal in vivo regulatory mechanisms or by design.[175] One recurring method used to accomplish this has been the use of dibutyryl cAMP to elevate intracellular cAMP levels.[140,184,187,317,318] An example from our own recent experience is perhaps instructive. We have examined numerous clonal lines of rodent origin for nervous system specific markers, seeking in particular to identify a cell line that would provide a model for the regulation of myelin gene expression. Most of these cell lines were originally derived from chemically induced rat tumors, in which the transformation event occurred during the last third of gestation.[1,319] As a general rule, these lines express cell-type specific markers that appear relatively early developmentally, but not those that appear later. For example, schwannoma cell line D6P2T expresses cell surface sulfatide, accumulates galactocerebroside internally, and synthesizes the major peripheral myelin glycoprotein P_o, but does not have measurable levels of the mRNA for myelin basic protein. These cells therefore resemble semi-differentiated Schwann cells. Growth of the cells in dibutyryl cAMP leads to the onset of galactocerebroside transport to the surface and the accumulation of mRNA for myelin basic protein.[167,244] Interestingly, MBP itself is not synthesized even when there are substantial levels of MBP-message. It appears that a further translational regulation is present.

Application of Markers to the Analysis of CNS Tumors

The diagnosis and analysis of both experimental and human neural tumors and derived cell lines is increasingly being based on a combination of morphological, biochemical, and immunocytochemical studies.[205,320–325] While many of the markers described above are potentially useful tools in neuro-oncology, a smaller subset of GFAP, NSE, S100 protein, and NF has received particular attention.[326–330a] Among these, GFAP is highly restricted to normal astrocytes and astrocyte-derived tumors, while NF, S100 protein, and NSE may be more broadly found among cell types in neurotumors[210,321,331,332] (see ref. 333 for additional references).

GFAP is found in non-neoplastic normal and reactive astrocytes, Bergmann glia, reactive ependymal cells, and in developing fetal glia, including radial glia, ependymocytes, and immature spinal oligodendrocytes. In neoplastic material, GFAP has been found in astrocytomas, astroblastomas, some ependymomas, astrocytic cells of mixed gliomas, gangliogliomas, mixed gliomas-sarcomas, glioblastomas, medulloblastomas, and certain pinecytomas[204,334–341] (see ref. 323 for additional references). Among more malignant tumors, it is common to find that only a small proportion of the cells are positive for GFAP.[342]

NSE is present at high levels in neuroendocrine tumors, and has found extensive use as a diagnostic tool, particularly for the analysis of the clinical course of small cell lung cancer and pediatric neuroblastoma.[343–345] The better differentiated tumors often have higher levels of the marker under study. For example, a correlation has been found between the degree of differentiation and the levels of neuropeptides such as somatostatin, substance P, vasoactive intestinal peptide, and cholecystokinin.[65,346]

These four markers are often used as a panel, sometimes in conjunction with additional markers.[204,347–349] For example, GFAP is often paired with vimentin, which is found in fibroblasts and many other mesenchymally derived cell types, and in fibrosarcomas, but absent in oligodendroglioma.[350] Meningiomas have been identified as tumors that are positive for vimentin and variably positive for ketatin, but negative for GFAP and S100 protein.[351,352] Finally, malignant astrocytomas and gliomas contain an increased amount of GD_3 ganglioside.[353] Kim[187] has studied human gliomas in culture, finding that 100% of the GC-positive cells were also GD_3-positive, but only 5–10% of GFAP-positive cells stained for GD_3. He concluded that GD_3 is therefore a marker for human oligodendroglioma cells in culture. In this study, neuronal and fibroblast elements were GD_3-negative. Many of these markers are stable in post-mortem brain, though precautions must be taken.[354]

Cell-type specific markers are particularly useful for poorly differentiated neoplasms which have often been difficult to diagnose by other means.[327,354a] The determination of the cellular origin of human acoustic neurinomas, controversial from their first description in the early 1900's until the early 1970's, is an early example in which biochemical and immunological markers were used to determine the predominant cell type of a human tumor. The "neuroectodermal school" held that these tumors arise from and are composed of Schwann cells. The "mesodermal school," in contrast, contended that since this tumor produces collagenous elements and reticulin fibers, it must arise from mesodermal fibroblastic elements, and should therefore be called a peripheral fibroblastoma. Both groups used electron microscopy and tissue culture to support their view. A glial origin was subsequently indicated when it was demonstrated, using biochemical and immunological techniques, that these tumors expressed the markers S100 protein, 2′,3′-cyclic nucleotide 3′-phosphohydrolase, galactocerebroside, and sulfatide.[355,356]

The recent applications of currently less-utilized markers such as the calmodulin-binding protein calcineurin,[108,109] synaptophysin,[357] and apolipoprotein E[358] suggest the potential rapid expansion of the field.

Prospectus

The future of CNS cell-type specific markers for neuro-oncological analysis is promising. The number and variety of markers will continue to increase, particularly in the area of molecular probes of transcriptional activity. Techniques will continue to be modified with resultant improvements in specificity and sensitivity. In particular, further advances can be expected in multiple antigen labeling and ultralocalization techniques. The application of these markers to the diagnosis and management of human neural tumors is currently at a data-gathering stage in which panels of marker expression are being compared to existing criteria of diagnosis. As experience develops, the biochemical, immunological, and molecular parameters will increasingly become the nucleus of the criteria for identifying neurotumor subclasses and predicting clinical prognosis.

REFERENCES

1. Pfeiffer SE. Oligodendrocyte development in culture systems. Adv Neurochem 1984; 5:233–279.
2. Windle WF. Biology of Neuroglia. Springfield, Illinois, Charles C. Thomas, 1958.
3. Bornstein MB, Murray MR. Serial observations on patterns of growth, myelin formation, maintenance and degeneration in cultures of newborn rat and kitten cerebellum. J Biophys Biochem Cytol 1958; 4:499–505.
4. Raff MC, Fields K, Hakamori S, Mirsky R, Pruss R, Winter J. Cell type-specific markers for distinguishing and studying neurons and the major classes of glial cells in culture. Brain Res 1979; 174:283–308.
5. Siegel GJ, Albers RW, Agranoff BW, Katzman R, eds. Basic Neurochemistry. Boston, Little, Brown & Co., 1981.
6. Fonnum FJ. A rapid radiochemical method for the determination of choline acetyltransferase. J Neurochem 1975; 24:407–409.
7. Miki A. Acetylcholinesterase activity in the neural tube of the early chick embryo. Acta Histochem Cytochem 1981; 14:143–152.
8. van Straaten HWM, Hekking JWM, Drukker J. The demonstration of acetylcholinesterase in plastic sections. Its application as a marker of early neuronal development. Acta Histochem 1986; S32:185–190.
9. Wong-Riley M. Changes in the visual system of monocularly sutured or enucleated cats demonstrable with cytochrome oxidase histochemistry. Brain Res 1979; 171:11–28.
10. Ashwell KWS, Webster WS. Vascularity and cytochrome oxidase distribution in the occipital cortex in MAM Ac-induced microencephaly. Develop Brain Res 1987; 33:301–304.
11. DeLaTorre JC. An improved approach to histofluorescence using the SPG method for tissue monoamines. J Neurosci Meth 1980; 3:1–15.
12. Currie DN, Dutton GR. [^{3}H]GABA uptake as a marker for cell type in primary cultures of cerebellum and olfactory bulb. Brain Res 1980; 192:473–481.

13. Schousboe A. Transport and metabolism of glutamate and GABA in neurons and glial cells. Int Rev Neurobiol 1981; 22:1–45.
14. Kanazawa I, Kwak S, Sasaki M, Mizusawa H, Muramoto O, Yoshizawa K, Nukina N, Kitamura K, Kurisaki H, Subita K. Studies on neurotransmitter markers and neuronal cell density in the cerebellar system in oligopontocerebellar atrophy and cortical cerebellar atrophy. J Neurol Sci 1985; 71:193–208.
15. Reynolds R, Herschkowitz N. Selective uptake of neuroactive amino acids by both oligodendrocytes and astrocytes in primary dissociated culture: a possible role for oligodendrocytes in neurotransmitter metabolism. Brain Res 1986; 371:253–266.
16. Cash R, Raisman R, Ploaka A, Aqid V. High and low affinity [^{3}H] imipramine binding sites in control and parkinsonian brains. Eur J Pharmacol 1985; 117:71–80.
17. Tehrani MH, Barnes EM, Jr. Ontogeny of the GABA receptor complex in chick brain: studies in vivo and in vitro. Brain Res 1986; 340:91–98.
18. Brockes J, ed. Neuroimmunology. New York: Plenum Press, 1982.
19. Valentino KL, Winter J, Reichardt LF. Applications of monoclonal antibodies to neuroscience research. Ann Rev Neurosci 1985; 8:199–232.
20. Winter J, Valentino KL, Reichardt LF. Neurobiology. In Weir DM, ed, Applications of Immunological Methods in Biomedical Sciences. Handbook Exptl Immunol, vol. 4, Oxford, Blackwell Scientific, 1986; pp 112.1–112.34.
21. Bock E. Nervous system specific proteins. J Neurochem 1978; 30:7–14.
22. Barnstable CJ, Akagawa K, Hofstein R, Horn JP. Monoclonal antibodies that label discrete cell types in the mammalian nervous system. Cold Spring Harbor Symp Quant Biol 1983; 48:863–876.
23. McKay R, Raff MC, Reichardt LF. Monoclonal antibodies to neural antigens. Cold Spring Harbor, Cold Spring Harbor Laboratory, 1981.
24. Yen S-H, Fields KL. Antibodies to neurofilament, glial filament and fibroblast intermediate filament proteins bind to different cell types in the nervous system. J Cell Biol 1981; 88:115–126.
25. Shaw G, Osborne M, Weber K. An immunofluorescence microscopical study of the neurofilament triplet proteins, vimentin and glial fibrillary acidic protein within the adult rat brain. Eur J Cell Biol 1981; 26:68–82.
26. Osborn M, Giesler N, Shaw G, Weber K. Intermediate filaments. Cold Spring Harbor Symp Quant Biol 1982; 46:413–429.
27. Lee V, Wu HL, Schlaepfer WW. Monoclonal antibodies recognize individual neurofilament triplet proteins. Proc Natl Acad Sci USA 1982; 79:6089–6092.
28. Goldstein ME, Sternberger LA, Sternberger NH. Microheterogeneity ('Neurotypy") of neurofilament proteins. Proc Natl Acad Sci USA 1983; 80:3101–3105.
29. Schlaepfer WW. Neurofilaments: Structure, metabolism, and implications in disease. J Neuropathol Exp Neurol 1987;117–129.
30. Caceres A, Binder LI, Payne MR, Bender P, Rebhun L, Steward O. Differential subcellular localization of tubulin and the microtubule asso-

ciated protein MAP-2 in brain tissue as revealed by immunocytochemistry. J Neurosci 1984; 4:394–410.

31. Huber G, Matus A. Differences in the cellular distributions of two microtubule associated proteins, MAP-1 and MAP-2, in rat brain. J Neurosci 1984; 4:151–160.

32. Shiomura Y, Hirokawa N. Colocalization of microtubule-associated protein 1A and microtubule-associated protein-2 on neuronal microtubules in situ revealed with double-label immunoelectron microscopy. J Cell Biol 1987; 104:1575–1578.

33. Storm-Mathisen J, Leknes AK, Bore AT, Vaaland JL, Edminson P, Huag FMS, Ottersen OP. First visualization of glutamate and GABA in neurons by immunocytochemistry. Nature (London) 1983; 301:917–920.

34. Seguela P, Gefford M, Buijs RM, Lemoal MG. Antibodies against gamma-aminobutyric acid. Specificity studies and immunocytochemical results. Proc Natl Acad Sci USA 1984; 81:3888–3892.

35. van den Pol AN. Dual ultrastructural localization of two neurotransmitter-related antigens: colloidal gold-labeled neurophysin-immunoreactive supraoptic neurons receive peroxidase-labeled glutamate decarboxylase or gold-labeled GABA-immunoreactive synapses. J Neurosci 1986; 5:2940–2954.

36. Consolazione A, Milstein C, Wright B, Cuello AC. Immunocytochemical detection of serotonin with monoclonal antibodies. J Histochem Cytochem 1981; 29:1425–1430.

37. Steinbusch HWM. Distribution of serotonin immunoreactivity in the central nervous system of the rat. Cell bodies and terminals. Neuroscience 1981; 6:557–618.

38. Cuello AC, Priestley JV, Milstein C. Immunocytochemistry with internally labeled monoclonal antibodies. Proc Natl Acad Sci USA 1982; 79:665–669.

39. Senba E, Daddona PE, Watanabe T, Wun JY, Naov JI. Coexistence of adenosine deaminase histidine decarboxylase and glutamate decarboxylase in hypothalamic neurons of the rat. J Neurosci 1985; 5:3393–3402.

40. Crawford GD, Correa L, Salvaterra PM. Interaction of monoclonal antibodies with mammalian choline acetyltransferase. Proc Natl Acad Sci USA 1982; 79:7031–7035.

41. Echenstein F, Thoenen HT. Production of specific antisera and monoclonal antibodies to choline acetyltransferase: Characterization and use for identification of cholinergic neurons. EMBO J 1982; 1:363–68.

42. Levey AI, Armstrong DM, Atweh SF, Terry RD, Wainer BH. Monoclonal antibodies to choline acetyltransferase: Production, specificity, and immunohistochemistry. J Neurosci 1983; 3:1–9.

43. Chan-Palay V, Lin C-T, Palay S, Yamamoto M, Wu J-Y. Taurine in the mammalian cerebellum: Demonstration by autoradiography with [³H] taurine and immunocytochemistry with antibodies against the taurine-synthesizing enzyme, cystein-sulfinic acid decarboxylase. Proc Natl Acad Sci USA 1982; 79:2695–2699.

44. Ross ME, Baetze EE, Rees DJ, Joh TJ. Monoclonal antibodies to catecholamine-neurotransmitter-synthesizing enzymes can be used for immunocytochemistry and immunohistochemistry. In McKay R, Raff MC,

Reichardt LF, eds, Monoclonal Antibodies to Neural Antigens. Cold Spring Harbor, Cold Spring Harbor Laboratory, 1981; pp 101–108.

45. Oertel WH, Schmechel DE, Mugnaini E, Tappaz ML, Kopin IJ. Immunocytochemical localization of glutamate decarboxylase in rat cerebellum with a new antiserum. Neuroscience 1981; 6:2715–2735.

46. Perez de la Mora M, Possani LD, Tapia R, Teran L, Palacios R, Fuxe K, Hökfelt T, Ljungdahl A. Demonstration of central gamma-aminobutyrate-containing nerve terminals by means of antibodies against glutamate decarboxylase. Neuroscience 1981; 6:875–895.

47. van den Pol AN. Tyrosine hydroxylase immunoreactive neurons throughout the hypothalamus receive glutamate decarboxylase immunoreactive synapses: A double pre-embedding immunocytochemical study with particulate silver and HRP. J Neurosci 1986; 6:877–891.

48. Kaneko T, Urade Y, Watanabe Y, Mizuno N. Production, characterization, and immunohistochemical application of monoclonal antibodies to glutaminase purified from rat brain. J Neurosci 1987; 7:302–309.

49. van Orden LS, Burke JP, Redick JA, Rybarczyk KE, van Orden DE, Baker HA, Hartman BK. Immunocytochemical evidence for particulate localization of phenylethanolamine-N-methyl transferase in adrenal medulla. Neuropharmacol 1976; 16:129–133.

50. Armstrong DM, Pickel VM, Joh TH, Reis DJ, Miller RJ. Immunocytochemical localization of catecholamine synthesizing enzymes and neuropeptides in area postrema and medial nucleus tractus solitarius of rat brain. J Comp Neurol 1981; 196:505–517.

51. Swanson LW, Sawchenko PE, Berod A, Hartman BK, Helle KB, van Orden DI. An immunohistochemical study of the organization of catecholaminergic cells and terminal fields in the paraventricular and supraoptic nuclei of the hypothalamus. J Comp Neurol 1981; 196:271–285.

52. Ross ME, Reis DJ, Joh TH. Monoclonal antibodies to tyrosine hydroxylase: Production and characterization. Brain Res 1981; 208:493–498.

52A. Pearson J. Goldstein M, Markey K, Brandeis L. Human brainstem catecholamine neuroanatomy as indicated by immunocytochemistry with antibodies to tyrosine hydroxylase. Neuroscience 1983; 8:3–32.

52B. Iacovitti L, Lee J, Joh TH, Reis DJ. Expression of tyrosine hydroxylase in neurons of cultured cerebral cortex: evidence for phenotypic plasticity in neurons of the CBS. J Neurosci 1987; 7:1264–1270.

53. Hökfelt T, Johansson O, Ljungdahl A, Lundberg JM, Schultzberg M. Peptidergic neurons. Nature 1980; 284:515–521.

54. Vaughn JE, Barber RP, Ribak CE, Houser CR. Methods for the immunocytochemical localization of proteins and peptides involved in neurotransmission. Curr Trends Morphol Tech 1981; 3:33–36.

55. Iversen LL. Neuropeptides: What next? Trends Neurosci 1983; 6:293–294.

56. Joseph SA, Piekut DT. Dual immunostaining procedure demonstrating neurotransmitter and neuropeptide codistribution in the same brain section. Am J Anat 1986; 175:331–342.

57. Davis BJ, Burd GD, Macrides F. Localization of methionine-enkephalin

substance P and somatostatin immunoreactivities in the rat olfactory bulb. J Comp Neurol 1982; 204:377–383.

58. McLean S, Skirboll LR, Pert CVB. Comparison of substance P and enkephalin distribution in rat brain: an overview using radioimmunocytochemistry. Neuroscience 1985; 14:837–852.

59. Pickel VM, Chan J, Milner TA. Autoradiographic detection of [I-125] secondary antiserum: A sensitive light and electron microscopic labeling method compatible with peroxidase immunocytochemistry for dual localization of neural antigens. J Histochem Cytol 1986; 34:707–718.

60. Ljungdahl A, Hokfelt T, Nilsson G. Distribution of substance P-like immunoreactivity in the central nervous system of the rat. I. Cell bodies and nerve terminals. Neuroscience 1978; 3:861–943.

61. Cuello AC, Galfre G, Milstein C. Detection of substance P activity in the central nervous system by a monoclonal antibody. Proc Natl Acad Sci USA 1979; 76:3532–3536.

62. Chan-Palay V. Immunocytochemical detection of substance P neurons, their processes and connections by in vivo microinjections of monoclonal antibodies. Anat Embryol 1979; 156:225–240.

63. Karten HJ, Brecha N. Localization of substance P immunoreactivity in amacrine cells of the retina. Nature 1980; 281:87–88.

64. Boorsma DM, Cuello AC, Von Leeuwen FW. Direct immunocytochemistry with a horse radish peroxidase-conjugated monoclonal antibody against substance P. J Histochem Cytochem 1982; 30:1211–1216.

65. Tam FK. An immunochemical study with neuron-specific-enolase and substance P of human enteric innervation: the normal developmental pattern and abnormal deviations in Hirschsprung's disease and pyloric stenosis. J Pediatric Surg 1986; 21:227–232.

66. Knigge KM, Piekut DT, Berlove DJ, Junig JT, Melrose PA. Staining of magnocellular neurons of the supraoptic and paraventricular nuclei with vasopressin anti-idiotype antibody: a potential method for receptor immunocytochemistry. Mol Brain Res 1987; 2:69–78.

67. Hirn M, Pierres M, Deagostini-Bazin H, Hirsch M, Goridis C. Monoclonal antibody against cell surface glycoproteins of neurons. Brain Res 1981; 214:433–439.

68. Rutishauser U, Hoffman S, Edelman GM. Binding properties of a cell adhesion molecule from neutral tissue. Proc Natl Acad Sci USA 1982; 79:685–689.

69. Edelman GM. Cell adhesion molecules. Science 1983; 219:450–457.

70. Edelman G. Specific cell adhesion in histogenesis and morphogenesis. In Edelman GM, Thiery J-P, eds. The Cell in Contact. New York, John Wiley & Sons, 1985; pp. 139–148.

71. Rutishauser U. Developmental biology of a neural cell adhesion molecule. Nature (London) 1984; 310:549–554.

72. Schachner M, Faissner A, Fisher G, Keilhauer G, Kruse J, Künemund Lindner J, Wernecke H. Functional and structural aspects of the cell surface in mammalian nervous system development. In Edelman GM, Theiry J-P, eds, The Cell in Contact. New York, John Wiley & Sons, 1985; pp. 257–275.

73. Martini R, Schachner M. Immunoelectron microscopic localization of

neural cell adhesion molecules (L1, N-CAM, and MAG) and their shared carbohydrate epitope and myelin basic protein in developing sciatic nerve. J Cell Biol 1986; 103:2439–2448.

74. Murray BA, Hemperly JJ, Prediger EA, Edelman GM, Cunningham BA. Alternatively spliced mRNAs code for different polypeptide chains of the chicken neural cell adhesion molecule (N-CAM). J Cell Biol 1986; 102:189–193.

74A. Cole GJ, Loewy A, Glaser L. Neuronal cell-cell adhesion depends on interactions of N-CAM with heparin-like molecules. Nature (London) 1986; 320:445–447.

75. Lindner J, Rathjen F, Schachner M. L1 mono- and polyclonal antibodies modify cell migration in early postnatal mouse cerebellum. Nature (London) 1983; 305:427–430.

76. Salton SRJ, Richter-Landsberg C, Green LA, Shelanski MJ. Nerve growth factor-inducible large external (NILE) glycoprotein: Studies of a central and peripheral neuronal marker. J Neurosci 1983; 3:441–454.

77. Grumet M, Hoffman S, Chuong C-M, Edelman GM. Polypeptide components and binding functions of neuron-glia adhesion molecules. Proc Natl Acad Sci USA 1984; 81:7989–7993.

78. Rathjen FG, Schachner M. Monoclonal antibody L1 recognizes neuronal cell surface glycoproteins mediating cellular adhesion. In Behan PO, Spreafico F, eds, Neuroimmunology. New York; Raven Press, 1984; pp. 79–88.

79. Stallcup WB, Beasley L. Involvement of the nerve growth factor-inducible large external glycoprotein (NILE) in neurite fasculation in primary cultures of rat brain. Proc Natl Acad Sci 1985; 82:1276–1280.

80. Chuong C-M, Crossin KL, Edelman GM. Sequential expression and differential function of multiple adhesion molecules during the formation of cerebellar cortical layers. 1987; 104:331–342.

81. Chang S, Rathjen FG, Raper JA. Extension of neurites on axons is impaired by antibodies against specific neural cell surface glycoproteins. J Cell Biol 1987; 104:355–362.

82. Rathjen FG, Wolff JM, Frank R, Bonhoeffer F, Rutishauser U. Membrane glycoproteins involved in neurite fasciculation. J Cell Biol 1987; 104:343–353.

82A. Wood JG, Jean DH, Whitaken JN, McLaughlin BJ, Albers RW. Immunocytochemical localization of the sodium, potassium activated ATPase in knife-fish brain. J Neurocytol 1977; 6:571–581.

83. Fambrough DM, Bayne EK. Multiple forms of $(Na^+ + K^+)$-ATPase in chicken. Selective detection of the major nerve, skeletal muscle, and kidney form by a monoclonal antibody. J Biol Chem 1983; 258:1926–1935.

84. Goldin SM, Moczydlowski EG, Papzian DM. Isolation and reconstitution of neuronal ion transport channels. Ann Rev Neurosci 1983; 6:419–446.

85. Chan SY, Hess EJ, Rahaminoff H, Goldin SM. Purification and immunological characterization of a calcium pump from bovine brain synaptosomal vehicles. J Neurosci 1984; 4:1468–1478.

86. Ventner JC, Eddy B, Hall LM, Fraser CM. Monoclonal antibodies detect

the conservation of muscarinic cholinergic receptor structure from *Drosophilia* to human brain and detect possible structural homology with alpha-adrenergic receptors. Proc Natl Acad Sci USA 1984; 81:272–276.

87. Strader CD, Pickel VM, Joh TH, Strohsacker MW, Shorr RGL, Lefkowitz RJ, Caron MG. Antibodies to the β-adrenergic receptor: Attenuation of catecholamine-sensitive adenylate cyclase and demonstration of post-synaptic receptor localization in brain. Proc Natl Acad Sci USA 1983; 80:1840–1844.

88. Schoch P, Richard JG, Haring P, Takacs B, Stahli C, Staehelin T, Haefely W, Mohler H. Colocalization of GABA$_A$ receptor and benzodiazepine receptors in the brain shown by monoclonal antibodies. Nature (London) 1985; 314:168–171.

89. Mamalaki C, Stephenson FA, Barnard EA. The GABA$_A$/benzodiazepine receptor is a heterotetramer of homologous α and β subunits. EMBO J 1987; 6;561–565.

90. Richards JG, Schoch P, Haring P, Takacs B, Mohler H. Resolving GABA$_A$/benzodiazepine receptors: cellular and subcellular localization in the CNS with monoclonal antibodies. J Neurosci 1987; 7:1866–1886.

91. Grenningloh G, Rienitz A, Schmitt B, Methfessel C, Zensen M, Beyreuther K, Gundelfinger ED, Betz H. The strychnine-binding subunit of the glycine receptor shows homology with nicotinic acetylcholine receptors. Nature (London) 1987; 328:215–220.

92. Gomez CM, Richman DP, Berman PW, Burres SA, Arnason BGA, Fitch FW. Monoclonal antibodies against purified nicotinic acetylcholine receptor. Biochem Biophys Res Commun 1979; 88:575–582.

93. Conti-Troncini B, Tzartos S, Lindstrom J. Monoclonal antibodies as probes of acetylcholine receptor structure. 2. Binding to native receptor. Biochemistry 1981; 20:2181–2191.

94. Chandler CE, Parsons LM, Hosang M, Shooter EM. A monoclonal antibody modulates the interaction of nerve growth factor with PC12 cells. J Biol Chem 1984; 259:6882–6889.

95. Eisenbarth GS, Walsh FS, Nirenberg M. Monoclonal antibody to a plasma membrane antigen of neurons. Proc Natl Acad Sci USA 1979; 76:4913–4917.

96. Berg GJ, Schachner M. Electron microscopic localization of A$_2$B$_5$ cell surface antigen in monolayer cultures of murine cerebellum and retina. Cell Tissue Res 1982; 224:637–645.

97. Schnitzer J, Schachner M. Cell type specificity of a neural cell surface antigen recognized by the monoclonal antibody A$_2$B$_5$. Cell Tissue Res 1982; 224:625–636.

98. Kasai N, Yu R. Monoclonal antibody A$_2$B$_5$ is specific to ganglioside GQ$_{1c}$. Brain Res 1983; 277:155–158.

99. Kundu S, Pleatman M, Redwine W, Boyd A, Marcus D. Binding of monoclonal antibody A$_2$B$_5$ to gangliosides. Biochem Biophys Res Commun 1983; 116:836–842.

100. Richardson PJ, Walker JH, Jones RT, Whittaker VP. Identification of a cholinergic-specific antigen Chol-1 is a ganglioside. J Neurochem 1982; 38:1605–1614.

101. Dimpfel W, Huang RTC, Habermann E. Gangliosides in nervous tissue

and binding of ^{125}I-labeled tetanus toxin, a neuronal marker. J Neurochem 1977; 29:329–334.

102. Mirsky R, Wendon LMB, Black P, Stolkin C, Bray D. Tetanus toxin: A cell surface marker for neurones in culture. Brain Res 1978; 148:151–159.

103. Schnitzer J, Schachner M. Expression of Thy-1, H-2, and NS-4 cell surface antigens and tetanus toxic receptors in early postnatal and adult mouse cerebellum. J Neuroimmunol 1981; 1:429–456.

104. Moore BW. Brain specific proteins. In Schnieder D, ed, Proteins of the Nervous System, New York, Raven Press, 1973; pp 1–12.

105. Haan EA, Boss BD, Cowan WM. Production and characterization of monoclonal antibodies against the "brain-specific" proteins 14-3-2 and S-100. Proc Natl Acad Sci USA 1982; 79:7585–7589.

106. Marangos PJ, Polak JM, Pearse AGE. Neuron-specific enolase. A probe for neurons and neuroendocrine cells. Trends Neurosci 1982; 5:193–196.

107. Marangos PJ. Neuron specific enolase, a clinically useful marker for neurons and neuronendocrine cells. Ann Rev Neurosci 1987; 10:269–295.

108. Wood JG, Wallace RW, Whitaker JN, Cheung WY. Immunocytochemical localization of calmodulin and a heat-labile calmodulin-binding protein (CaM-BP80) in basal ganglia of mouse brain. J Cell Biol 1980; 84:66–76.

109. Goto S, Matsukado Y, Mihara Y, Inoue N, Miyamoto E. Calcineurin as a neuronal marker of human brain tumors. Brain Res 1986; 371:237–243.

110. Kelly PT, McGuiness TL, Greengard P. Evidence that the major postsynaptic density protein is a component of a CA^{2+}-calmodulin-dependent protein kinase. Proc Natl Acad Sci USA 1984; 81:945–949.

111. Hendry SHC, Hockfield S, Jones EG, McKay R. Monoclonal antibody that identifies subsets of neurones in the central visual system of monkey and cat. Nature (London) 1984; 307:267–269.

112. Cohen J, Selvendran SY. A neuronal surface antigen is found in the CNS but not in peripheral neurons. Nature 1981; 291:421–423.

113. Miller CA, Benzer S. Monoclonal antibody cross-reactions between *Drosophila* and human brain. Proc Natl Acad Sci USA 1983; 80:7641–7645.

114. Carlin RC, Bartelt DC, Siekevitz P. Identification of fodrin as a major calmodulin binding protein in post synaptic density preparations. J Cell Biol 1983; 96:443–481.

115. Lazarides E, Nelson WJ. Erythrocyte and brain forms of spectrin in cerebellum. Distinct membrane-cytoskeletal domains in neurons. Science 1983; 220:1295–1296.

116. Lazarides E, Nelson WJ. Erythrocyte form of spectrin in cerebellum: Appearance at a specific stage in the terminal differentiation of neurons. Science 1983; 222:931–933.

117. Lazarides E, Nelson WJ, Kasamatsu T. Segregation of two spectrin forms in the chicken optic system: A mechanism for establishing restricted membrane-cytoskeletal domains in neurons. Cell 1984; 36:269–278.

118. Hawkes R, Niday E, Matus A. Monoclonal antibodies identify novel neural antigens. Proc Natl Acad Sci USA 1982; 79:2410–2414.
119. Kitano T, Hashimoto T, Kikkawa U, Ase K, Saito N, Tanaka C, Ichimori Y, Tsukamoto K, Nishizuka Y. Monoclonal antibodies against rat brain protein kinase C and their application to immunocytochemistry in nervous tissues. J Neurosci 1987; 7:1520–1525.
120. Barnstable CJ. Monoclonal antibodies which recognize different cell types in the rat retina. Nature (London) 1980; 286:231–235.
121. Trisler D, Grunwald GB, Moskal J, Darveniza P, Nirenberg M. Molecules that identify cell type or position in the retina. In Behan P, Spreafico F, eds, Neuroimmunology and Neural Diseases. New York, Raven Press, 1984; pp. 89–97.
122. Hockfield S, McKay R. A surface antigen expressed by a subset of neurons in the vertebrate central nervous system. Proc Natl Acad Sci USA 1983; 80:5758–5761.
123. Goelz SE, Nestler EJ, Chehrazi B, Greengard P. Distribution of protein I in mammalian brain as determined by a detergent-based radioimmune assay. Proc Natl Acad Sci USA 1981; 78:2130–2134.
124. Matthew WD, Tsavaler L, Reichardt LF. Identification of a synaptic vesicle-specific membrane protein with a wide distribution in neuronal and neurosecretory tissue. J Cell Biol 1981; 91:257–269.
125. Williams AF, Barclay AN, Letarte-Muirhead M, Morris RJ. Rat Thy-1 antigens from thymus and brain: their tissue distribution, purification, and chemical composition. Cold Spring Harbor Symp Quant Biol. 1977; 41:51–61.
126. Mirsky R. The use of antibodies to define and study major cell types in the central and peripheral nervous system. In Brockes J, ed, Neuroimmunology. New York, Plenum Press, 1982; pp. 141–182.
127. Kemshead JT, Ritter MA, Colmore SF, Greaves MF. Human Thy-1: Expression on the cell surface of neuronal and glial cells. Brain Res 1982; 236:451–461.
128. Morris RJ. The surface antigens of nerve cells. In Pfeiffer SE ed, Neuroscience Approached Through Cell Culture. Boca Raton, CRC Press, 1982; pp. 1–49.
129. Morris R. Thy-1 in developing nervous tissue. Dev Neurosci 1985; 7:133–160.
130. Arimatsu Y, Naegele JR, Barnstable CJ. Molecular markers of neuronal subpopulations in layers 4, 5, and 6 of cat primary visual cortex. J Neurosci 1987; 7:1250–1263.
131. Langley OK, Ghandour MS. An immunocytochemical investigation of non-neuronal enolase in cerebellum: A new astrocyte marker. Histochem J 1981; 13:137–148.
132. Langley OK, Ghandour MS, Vincendon G, Gombos G, Warecka K. Immunoelectron microscopy of α_2-glycoprotein: An astrocyte-specific antigen. J Neuroimmunol 1982; 2:131–143.
133. Antonicek H, Persohn E, Schachner M. Biochemical and functional characterization of a novel neuron-glia adhesion molecule that is involved in neuronal migration. J Cell Biol 1987; 194:1587–1595.
134. Boyles JK, Pitas RE, Wilson EM, Mahley RW, Taylor JM. Apolipopro-

tein E associated with astrocytic glia of the central nervous system and with non-myelinating glia of the peripheral nervous system. J Clin Invest 1985; 1501–1513.

135. Pitas RE, Boyles JK, Lee SH, Foss D, Mahley RW. Astrocytes synthesize apolipoprotein E and metabolize apolipoprotein E-containing lipoproteins. Biochim Biophys Acta 1987; 917:148–161.

136. Eng LF, Vanderhaeghen JJ, Bignami A, Gerstl B. An acidic protein isolated from fibrous astrocytes. Brain Res 1971; 28:351–354.

137. Ludwin SK, Kosek JC, Eng LF. The topographical distribution of S-100 and GFA protein in the adult rat brain: An immunohistochemical study using horseradish peroxidase-labeled antibodies. J Comp Neurol 1976; 165:197–208.

138. Bignami A, Dahl D. Specificity of the glial fibrillary acidic protein for astroglia. J Histochem Cytochem 1977; 25:466–499.

139. Pegram CN, Eng LF, Wikstrand CJ, McComb RD, Lee YL, and Bigner DD. Monoclonal antibodies reactive with epitopes restricted to glial fibrillary acidic proteins of several species. Neurochem Pathol 1985; 3:119–138.

140. Chiu FC, Goldman JE, Regulation of glial fibrillary acidic protein (GFAP) expression in CNS development and in pathological states. J Neuroimmunol 1985; 8:283–292.

141. Norenberg MD, Martinez-Herandez A. Fine structural localization of glutamine synthetase in astrocytes of rat brain. Brain Res 1979; 161:303–310.

142. McGeer PL, McGeer EG. Amino acid neurotransmitters. In Siegel G, Albers RW, Agranoff BW, Katzman R, eds, Basic Neurochemistry. Boston, Little Brown & Co, 1981; pp. 233–253.

143. Lagenaur C, Sommer I, Schachner M. Subclass of astroglia recognized in mouse cerebellum by monoclonal antibody. Develop Biol 1980; 79:367–378.

144. Sommer I, Lagenaur C, Schachner M. Recognition of Bergmann glial and ependymal cells in the mouse nervous system by monoclonal antibody. J Cell Biol 1981; 90:448–458.

145. Bartlett PF, Nobel MD, Pruss RM, Raff MC, Rattray S, Williams CA. Rat neural antigen-2 (RAN-2): A cell surface antigen on astrocytes, ependymal cells, Müller cells and leptomeninges defined by a monoclonal antibody. Brain Res 1981; 204:339–351.

146. Wechsler W, Pfeiffer SE, Swenberg JA, Koestner A. S-100 protein in methyl- and ethylnitrosourea induced tumors of the rat nervous system. Acta Neuropath (Berl). 1973; 24:287–303.

147. Wechsler W, Ramadan MA, Pfeiffer SE. Morphologic and biochemical characteristics of transplantable neurogenic tumors induced by N-ethyl-N-nitrosourea in inbred BD IX rats. J Natl Cancer Inst 1979; 62:811–817.

148. Ghandour MS, Langley OK, Labourdette G, Vincedon B, Gombos G. Specific and artifactual cellular localizations of S100 protein: An astrocyte marker in rat cerebellum. Dev Neurosci 1981; 4:68–78.

149. Solter D, Knowles BB. Monoclonal antibody defines a stage-specific

mouse embryonic antigen (SSEA-I). Proc Natl Acad Sci USA 1978; 75:5565–5569.

150. Lagenaur C, Schachner M, Solter D, Knowles B. Monoclonal antibody SSEA-1 is specific for a subpopulation of astrocytes in mouse cerebellum. Neurosci Lett 1982; 31:181–184.

151. Pruss R. Thy-1 antigen on astrocytes in long-term cultures of rat central nervous system. Nature (London) 1979; 280:688–690.

152. Chiu FC, Norton WT, Fields KL. The cytoskeleton of primary astrocytes in culture contains actin, glial fibrillary acid protein, and the fibroblast-type filament protein, vimentin. Neurochem 1981; 37:147–155.

153. Dahl D, Rueger DC, Bignami A, Weber K, Osborn M. Vimentin, the 57,000 molecular weight protein of fibroblast filaments, is the major cytoskeletal component in immature glia. Eur J Cell Biol 1981; 24:191–196.

154. Osborn M, Ludwig-Festl M, Weber K, Bignami A, Dahl L, Bayrenther K. Expression of glial and vimentin type intermediate filaments in cultures derived from human glial material. Differentiation 1981; 19:262–267.

155. Schnitzer J, Francke WW, Schachner M. Immunocytochemical demonstration of vimentin in astrocytes and ependymal cells of the developing and adult mouse nervous system. J Cell Biol 1981; 90:435–447.

156. Mirsky R, Winter J, Abney ER, Pruss RM, Gavrilovic J, Raff MC. Myelin-specific proteins and glycolipids in rat Schwann cells and oligodendrocytes in culture. J Cell Biol 1980; 84:483–494.

157. Norton WT, ed. Oligodendroglia: Advanced Neurochemistry, vol 5. New York, Plenum Press, 1986; pp. 351.

158. Raff MC, Mirsky R, Fields K, Lisak R, Dorfman Silberberg D, Gregson N, Leibowitz S, Kennedy M. Galactocerebroside is a specific cell surface antigenic marker for oligodendrocytes in culture. Nature (London) 1978; 274:813–816.

159. Ranscht B, Clapshaw PA, Price J, Noble M, Seifert W. 1982. Development of oligodendrocytes and Schwann cells studied with a monoclonal antibody against galactocerebroside. Proc Natl Acad Sci USA 1982; 79:2709–2713.

160. Dawson G, Sundarraj N, Pfeiffer SE. Synthesis of myelin glycosphingolipids (galactosylceramide and galactosyl (3-O-sulfate) ceramide (sulfatide) by cloned cell lines derived from mouse neurotumors. J Biol Chem 1977; 252:2777–2779.

161. Sommer I, Schachner M. Monoclonal antibodies (01 to 04) to oligodendrocyte cell surfaces: An immunocytological study in the central nervous system. Dev Biol 1981; 83:311–327.

162. Singh H, Pfeiffer SE. Myelin-associated galactolipids in primary cultures from dissociated fetal rat brain: biosynthesis, accumulation, and cell surface expression. J Neurochem 1985; 45:1371–1381.

163. Lisak R, Pleasure D, Silberberg D, Manning M, Saida T. Investigation of glial cells in semithin sections. Brain Res 1981; 223:107–122.

164. Kim SU, Sato D, Silberberg DH, Pleasure DE, Rorke LB. Long-term culture of human oligodendrocytes. J Neurol Sci 1983; 62:295–301.

165. Pleasure D, Kim SU, Silberberg DH. In vitro studies of oligodendroglial lipid metabolism. Adv Neurochemistry 1984; 5:175–189.
166. Morell P, Toews AD. In vivo metabolism of oligodendroglial lipids. Adv Neurochem 1984; 5:47–75.
167. Bansal R, Pfeiffer SE. Regulated galactolipid synthesis and cell surface expression in Schwann cell line D6P2T. J Neurochem 1987; 1902–1911.
168. Kumpulainen T, Nystrom SHM. Immunohistochemical localization of carbonic anhydrase isoenzyme C in human brain. Brain Res 1981; 220:220–225.
169. Cammer W, Zimmerman TR, Jr. Glycerolphosphate dehydrogenase, glucose-6-phosphate dehydrogenase, lactate dehydrogenase and carbonic anhydrase activities in oligodendrocytes and myelin: comparisons between species and CNS regions. Dev Brain Res 1983; 6:21–26.
170. Cammer W. Oligodendrocyte-associated enzymes. Adv Neurochem 1984; 5:199–225.
171. Langley OK, Ghandour MS, Vincedon G, Gombos G. Carbonic anhydrase: An ultrastructural study in rat cerebellum. Histochem J 1980; 12:473–483.
172. Poduslo SE, Norton WT. Isolation and some chemical properties of oligodendroglia from calf brain. J Neurochem 1972; 19:727–736.
173. Pfeiffer SE, Wechsler W. Biochemically differentiated neoplastic clone of Schwann cells. Proc Natl Acad Sci USA 1972; 69:2885–2889.
174. Carnegie PR, Sims NR. Proteins and enzymes of myelin. In Field EJ, ed. Multiple Sclerosis. A Critical Conspectus. Baltimore, University Park Press, 1977; pp. 182–188.
175. Sundarraj N, Schachner M, Pfeiffer SE. Biochemically differentiated mouse glial lines carrying a nervous system specific cell surface antigen (NS-I). Proc Natl Acad Sci USA 1975; 72:1927–1931.
176. Sprinkel TJ, Sheedlo HJ, Buxton TB, Rissing JP. Immunochemical identification of 2′,3′-cyclic nucleotide 3′-phosphodiesterase in central and peripheral nervous system myelin, the Wolfgram protein fraction, and bovine oligodendrocytes. J Neurochem 1983; 41:1664–1671.
177. Sternberger NH. Patterns of oligodendrocyte function seen by immunocytochemistry. Adv Neurochem 1984; 5:125–165.
177A. Kim SU, McMorris FA, Sprinkle TJ. Immunofluorescence demonstration of 2′-3′-cyclic nucleotide 3′-phosphodiesterase in cultures of oligodendrocytes of mouse, rat, and human. Brain Res 1984; 300:195–199.
178. Bansal R, Pfeiffer SE. Developmental expression of 2′-3′-cyclic nucleotide 3′-phosphohydrolase in dissociated fetal rat brain cultures and rat brain. J Neurosci Res 1985; 14:21–34.
179. Yu R, Iqbal K. Sialoslygalactosyl ceramide as a specific marker for human myelin and oligodendroglial perikarya: Gangliosides of human myelin, oligodendroglia and neurons. J Neurochem 1979; 32:293–300.
180. Goldman JE, Geier SS, Hirona M. Differentiation of astrocytes and oligodendrocytes from germinal matrix cells in primary cultures. J Neurosci 1986; 6:52–60.
181. Goldman JE, Hirano M, Yu RK, Seyfried TN. GD3 ganglioside is a glycolipid characteristic of immature neuroectodermal cells. J Immunol 1984; 7:179–192.

182. Leveille PJ, McGinnis JF, Maxwell DS, DeVellis J. Immunocytochemical localization of glycerol-3-phosphate dehydrogenase in rat oligodendrocytes. Brain Res 1980; 196:287–305.
183. Fisher M, Gapp DA, Kozak LP. Immunohistochemical localization of sn-glycerol-3-phosphate dehydrogenase in Bergmann glia and oligodendroglia in the mouse cerebellum. Dev Brain Res 1981; 1:341–354.
184. Weingarten DP, Kumar S, Bressler J, deVellis J. Regulation of differentiated properties of oligodendrocytes. Adv Neurochem 1984; 5:299–326.
185. Ledeen RW, Yu R, Eng L. Gangliosides of human myelin. Sialosylgalactosyl ceramide as a major component. J Neurochem 1973; 21:829–839.
186. Seifried T, Glaser G, Yu R. Cerebral, cerebellar and brain stem gangliosides in mice susceptible to audiogenic seizures. J Neurochem 1978; 31:21–27.
187. Kim SU. Antigen expression by glial cells grown in culture. J Neuroimmunol 1985; 8:255–282.
188. Quarles RH. Myelin-associated glycoprotein in development and disease. Dev Neurosci 1983/84; 6:285–303.
189. Barbarese E, Braun PE, Carson JH. Identification of prelarge and presmall basic proteins in mouse myelin and their structural relationship to large and small basic proteins. Proc Natl Acad Sci USA 1977; 74:3360–3364.
190. Barbarese E, Pfeiffer SE. Developmental regulation of myelin basic protein in dispersed cultures. Proc Natl Acad Sci USA 1981; 78:1953–1957.
191. Hartman BK, Agrawal HC, Agrawal D, Kalmbach S. Development and maturation of central nervous system myelin: Comparison of immunohistochemical localization of proteolipid protein and basic protein in myelin and oligodendrocytes. Proc Natl Acad Sci USA 1982; 79:4217–4220.
192. Benjamins JA. Protein metabolism of oligodendroglial cells in vivo. Adv Neurochem 1984; 5:87–116.
193. Schwob VS, Clark HB, Agrawal D, Agrawal HC. Electron microscopic immunocytochemical localization of myelin proteolipid protein and myelin basic protein to oligodendrocytes in rat brain during myelination. J Neurochem 1985; 45:559–571.
194. Lees MB, Sakura JD, Sapirstein VS, Curatolo W. Structure and function of proteolipids in myelin and non-myelin membranes. Biochem Biophys Acta 1979; 559:209–230.
195. Agrawal HC, Hartman BK. Proteolipid protein and other proteins of myelin. In Bradshaw RA, Schneider DM eds, Proteins of the Nervous System. New York. Raven Press, 1980, pp. 145–169.
196. Connor JR, Fine RD. The distribution of transferrin immunoreactivity in the rat central nervous system. Brain Res 1986; 368:319–328.
197. Bowman PD, Betz AL, Ar D, Wolinsky JS, Penney JB, Shivers RR, Goldstein GW. Primary culture of capillary endothelium from rat brain. In Vitro 1981; 17:353–362.
198. Ghandour MS, Langley OK, Varga V. Immunohistological localization

of γ-glutamyltranspeptidase in cerebellum at light and electron microscope levels. Neurosci Lett 1980; 20:125–129.

199. Ghandour S, Langley K, Gombos G, Hirn M, Hirsch MR, Goridis C. A surface marker for murine vascular endothelial cells defined by monoclonal antibody. J Histochem Cytochem 1982; 30:165–170.

200. Giulian D, Baker TJ. Characterization of ameboid microglia isolated from developing mammalian brain. J Neurosci 1986; 6:2163–2178.

201. Raff MC, Miller RH, Nobel M. A glial progenitor cell that develops in vitro into an astrocyte or an oligodendrocyte depending on culture medium. Nature (London) 1983; 303:390–396.

202. Loffner F, Lohmann SM, Walckhoff B, Walter U, Hamorecht B. Immunocytochemical characterization of neuron-rich primary cultures of embryonic rat brain cells by established neuronal and glial markers and by monospecific antisera against cyclic nucleotide-dependent protein kinases and the synaptic vesicle protein synapsin. Brain Res 1986; 363:2005–2021.

203. Hockfield S, McKay R. Identification of major cell classes in the developing mammalian nervous system. J Neurosci 1985; 5:3310–3328.

204. Reifenberger G, Mai J, Krajewski Wechsler W. Distribution of anti-LEU-7, anti-LEU-11a and anti-LEU-M1 immunoreactivity in the brain of the adult rat. Cell Tiss Res 1987; 248:305–313.

205. Reifenberger G, Szymas J, Wechsler W. Differential expression of glial- and neuronal-associated antigens in human tumors of the central and peripheral nervous system. Acta Neuropathol (Berl) (in press).

206. Szymas J, Reifenberger G, Wechsler W. Leu-1 immunoreactivity in the human brain: discrimination between differentiated tumors and between neoplastic and brain tissue. Naturwissenschaften 1987; 74:188–190.

207. Cuello AC. Immunohistochemistry. IBRO Handbook Series: Methods in the Neuroscience. New York, John Wiley & Sons, 1983.

208. Sternberger LA. Immunocytochemistry. New York, John Wiley & Sons, 1986.

209. Weir DM, Herzenberg LA, Blackwell C, Herzenberg LA, eds. Applications of Immunological Methods in Biomedical Sciences, Vol 4. Oxford, Blackwell Scientific Publications, 1986.

210. DeArmond SJ, Eng LF. Immunohistochemistry: Techniques and application to neuro-oncology. Prog Exp Tumor Res 1984; 27:92–117.

211. Köhler G, Milstein C. Continuous cultures of fused cells secreting antibody of predefined specificity. Nature (London) 1975; 256:495–497.

212. Yelton DE, Scharff M. Monoclonal antibodies. A powerful tool in biology and medicine. Ann Rev Biochem 1981; 50:657–680.

213. Luben RA, Mohler MA. In vitro immunization as an adjunct to the production of hybridomas producing antibodies against the lymphocyte osteoclast activating factor. Mol Immunol 1980; 17:635–639.

214. Luben RA, Brazeau P, Böhlen P, Guillemin R. Monoclonal antibodies to hypothalmic growth hormone-releasing factor with picomoles of antigen. Science 1982; 218:887–889.

215. Boss BD. An improved in vitro immunization procedure for the pro-

duction of monoclonal antibodies against neural and other antigens. Brain Res 1984; 291:193–196.

216. Sternberger LA, Harwell LW, Sternberger NH. Neurotypy: Regional individuality in rat brain detected by immunocytochemistry with monoclonal antibodies. Proc Natl Acad Sci USA 1982; 79:1326–1330.

217. Gard AL, Dutton GR. Myelin-specific domain on the plasmalemma of oligodendroglia: differential expression in the rat and hypomyelinating mouse mutants jumpy and quaking. J Neurosci Res 1987; 17:329–343.

218. Hirn M, Demierre M, Goridis C. A solid-phase radioimmunoassay for detecting antibodies to brain cell surface antigens. Brain Res Bull 1981; 7:441–444.

219. Gard AL, Pigott R, Dutton GR. A solid-phase β-galactosidase ELISA for detecting and quantifying monoclonal antibody binding to dissociated cell cultures of postnatal rodent cerebellum. J Neurosci Meth 1983; 8:51–60.

220. Kennet RH, Gilbert F. Hybrid myelomas producing antibodies against a human neuroblastoma antigen present on fetal brain. Science 1979; 203:1120–1121.

221. Milstein C, Lennox E. The use of monoclonal antibody techniques in the study of developing cell surfaces. Curr Top Dev Biol 1980; 14:1–31.

222. Fox PC, Berenstein EH, Siraganian RP. Enhancing the frequency of antigen-specific hybridomas. Eur J Immunol 1981; 11:431–434.

223. Springer TA. Monoclonal antibody analysis of complex biological systems: Combination of cell hybridization and immunoadsorbents in a novel cascade procedure and its application to the macrophage cell surface. J Biol Chem 1981; 256:3833–3839.

224. Matthew WD, Patterson PH. The production of a monoclonal antibody which blocks the action of a neurite outgrowth promoting factor. Cold Spring Harbor Symp Quant Biol 1983; 48:625–631.

225. Thalhamer J, Frend J. Passive immunization: A method of enhancing the immune response against antigen mixtures. J Immunol Meth 1985; 80:7–13.

226. Milstein C. Cuello AC. Hybrid hybridomas and their use in immunohistochemistry. Nature (London) 1983; 305:537–540.

227. Hsu SM, Raine L, Fanger H. A comparative study of the PAP method and avidin-biotin-complex method for studying polypeptide hormones with radioimmunoassay antibodies. Am J Clin Pathol 1981; 75:734–738.

228. Hsu S-M, Raine L, Fanger H. Use of avidin biotin peroxidase complex (ABC) in immunoperoxidase techniques. A comparison between ABC and unlabeled antibody (PAP) procedures. J Histochem Cytochem 1981; 29:577–580.

229. Towbin H, Staehelin T, Gordon J. Electrophoretic transfer of proteins from polyacrylamide gels to nitrocellulose sheets: Procedure and some applications. Proc Natl Acad Sci USA 1979; 76:4350–4354.

230. Saito M, Kasai N, Yu RK. In situ immunological determination of basic carbohydrate structures of gangliosides on thin-layer plates. Anal Biochem 1985; 148:54–58.

231. Gaulton GN, Co MS, Royer H-D, Greene MI. Anti-idiotypic antibodies as probes of cell surface receptors. Mol. Cell Biochem 1985; 65:5–21.

232. Schwob JE, Farber NB, Gottlieb DI. Neurons of the olfactory epithelium in adult rats contain vimentin. J Neurosci 1986; 6:208–217.
233. Hatta K, Takagi S, Futjisawa H, Takeichi M. Spatial and temporal expression pattern of N-cadhedrin cell adhesion molecules correlated with morphogenetic processes of chicken embryos. Dev Biol 1987; 120:215–227.
234. Bixby JL, Pratt RS, Lilien J, Reichardt LF. Neurite outgrowth on muscle cell surfaces involved extracellular matrix receptors as well as Ca^{2+}-dependent and -independent cell adhesion molecules. Proc Natl Acad Sci USA 84:2555–2559.
235. Chiquet M, Fambrough DM. Chick myotendinous antigen. II A novel extracellular glycoprotein complex consisting of large disulfide-linked subunits. J Cell Biol 1984; 98:1937–1946.
236. Chiquet-Ehrismann R, Mackie EJ, Pearson CA, Shakura T. Tenascin: an extracellular matrix protein involved in tissue interactions during fetal development and oncogenesis. Cell 1986; 47:131–139.
237. Grumet M, Hoffman S, Crossin KL, Edelmann GM. Cytotactin, an extracelular matrix protein of neural and non-neural tissue that mediates glia-neuron interaction. Proc Natl Acad Sci USA 1985; 82:8075–8079.
238. Willinger M, Schachner M. GM_1 ganglioside as a marker for neuronal differentiation in mouse cerebellum. Dev Biol 1980; 74:101–117.
239. Asou H, Brunngraber EG. Absence of ganglioside GM_1 in astroglial cells from 21-day-old rat brain. Immunohistochemical, histochemical, and biochemical studies. Neurochem Res 1983; 8:1045–1047.
240. Althaus HH, Seifert W, eds. Glial-Neuronal Communication in Development and Regeneration. Berlin, Springer-Verlag, 1987.
241. Shine HD, Haber B. Immunocytochemical localization of γ-glutamyl transpeptidase in the rat CNS. Brain Res 1981; 217:339–349.
242. Schachner M, Schoonmaker G, Hynes RO. Cellular and subcellular localization of LETS protein in the nervous system. Brain Res 1978; 158:149–158.
243. Suttcliffe JG, Milner RJ, Shinnick TM, Bloom FE. Identifying the protein products of brain-specific genes using antibodies to chemically synthesized peptides. Cell 1983; 33:671–682.
244. Yang IK, Pfeiffer SE, Carson JH. Reciprocal regulation of myelin P_o glycoprotein and myelin basic protein gene expression by cAMP. (Submitted.)
245. Han VKM, Snouweart J, Towle AC, Lund PK, Lauder JM. Cellular localization of tyrosine hydroxylase mRNA and its regulation in the rat adrenal medulla and brain by in situ hybridization with an oligodeoxyribonucleotide probe. J Neurosci Res 1987; 17:11–18.
246. Liesi P, Julian JP, Vilia P, Grosvald F, Reichardt L. Specific detection of neuronal cell bodies: in situ hybridization with biotin-labeled neurofilament cDNA probe. J Histochem Cytochem 1986; 34:923–926.
247. Maniatis T, Fritsch EF, Sambrook J. Molecular Cloning. Cold Spring Harbor: Cold Spring Harbor Laboratory, 1982.
248. Hayden MR, Nichols JL. Molecular genetic approaches to the study of the nervous system. Dev Neurosci 1983/84; 6:189–214.

249. Breakefield XO, Cambi F. Molecular genetic insights into neurologic diseases. Ann Rev Neurosci 1987; 10:535–594.
250. Merle JP, Sebbane R, Gardner S, Lindstrom J. cDNA clone for the subunit of the acetylcholine receptor from the mouse muscle cell line BC3H-1. Proc Natl Acad Sci USA 1983; 80:3845–3849.
251. McCarthy MP, Earnest JP, Young EF, Choe S, Stroud RM. The molecular neurobiology of the acetylcholine receptor. Ann Rev Neurosci 1986; 9:383–413.
251A. Boulter J, Evans K, Goldman D, Martin G, Treco D, Heinemann S, Patrick J. Isolation of a cDNA clone coding for a possible neural nicotinic acetylcholine receptor α-subunit. Nature (London) 1986; 319:368–374.
252. Bernier L, Alvarez F, Norgard M, Sabatini DD, Colman DR. Cloning and characterization of myelin CNP cDNAs. Trans Am Soc Neurochem 1986; 17:106.
253. Schofield PR, Darlison MG, Fujita N, Burt DR, Stephenson FA, Rodriguez H, Rhee LM, Ramachandran J, Reale V, Glencorse TA, Seeburg PH, Barnard EA. Sequence and functional expression of the GABA$_A$ receptor shows a ligand-gated receptor super-family. Nature (London) 1987; 328:221–227.
254. Lewis SA, Balcarek JM, Krek V, Shelanski M, Cowan NJ. Sequence of a cDNA clone encoding mouse glial fibrillary acidic protein: Structural conservation of intermediate filaments. Proc Natl Acad Sci USA 1984; 81:2743–2746.
255. Dewhurst S, Stevenson M, McComb RD, Volsky DJ. Expression of glial fibrillary acidic protein in human glioma cell lines as detected by molecular hybridization. Acta Neuropathol (Berl) 1987; 74:383–386.
256. Salzer J, Bernier L, Colman DR. Isolation of rat MAG clones. Trans Am Soc Neurochem 1986; 17:106.
257. Salzer JL, Holmes WP, Colman DR. Complete amino acid sequence of the MAG proteins: homology to the immunoglobulin gene superfamily. J Neurochem (Suppl) 1987; S33A.
258. Lai C, Nave K-A, Brow M, Noronha AB, Quarles RH, Bloom FE, Sutcliffe JG, Milner RJ. The two forms of 1B236/MAG arise by alternate splicing and are developmentally regulated. J Neurochem (Suppl) 1987; S145B.
259. Roach A, Boylan K, Horvath S, Prusiner SB, Hood LE. Characterization of cloned cDNA representing rat myelin basic protein: Absence of expression in brain of shiverer mutant mice. Cell 1983; 34:799–806.
260. Zeller NK, Hunkeler MJ, Campagnoni AT, Sprague J, Lazzarini RA. Characterization of mouse myelin basic protein messenger RNAs with a myelin basic protein cDNA clone. Proc Natl Acad Sci USA 1984; 81:18–22.
261. Lemke G. Molecular biology of the major myelin genes. Trends Neurosci 1986; 9:266–270.
262. Kimura M, Inoko H, Katsuki M, Ando A, Sato T, Hirose T, Takashima H, Inayama S, Okano H, Takamatsu K, Mikoshiba K, Tsukada Y, Wanatabe I. Molecular genetic analysis of myelin-deficient mice: Shiverer mutant show deletion in gene(s) coding for myelin basic protein. J Neurochem 1985; 44:692–696.
263. Takahashi N, Roach A, Teplow DB, Pruisner SB, Hood L. Cloning and

characterization of the myelin basic protein gene from mouse: One gene can encode both 14 Kd and 18.5 Kd MBPs by alternate use of exons. Cell 1985; 42:139–148.

264. Saxe DF, Takahashi N, Hood L, Simon I. Localization of the human basic protein gene (MBP) to region 18q → 22qter by in situ hybridization. Cytogenet Cell Genet 1986; 39:246–249.

265. Akowitz AA, Barbarese E, Scheld K, Carson JH. Structure and expression of myelin basic protein gene sequences in the *mld* mutant mouse: reiteration and rearrangement of the MBP gene. Genetics 1987; 116:447–464.

266. Scott J, Selby M, Urdea M, Quiroga M, Bell GI, Rutter WJ. Isolation and nucleotide sequence of a cDNA encoding the precursor of mouse nerve growth factor. Nature (London) 1983; 302:538–540.

267. Ullrich A, Gray A, Wood WI, Hayflick J, Seeburg PH. Isolation of a cDNA clone coding for the gamma-subunit of mouse nerve growth factor using a high-stringency selection procedure. DNA 1984; 3:387–392.

268. Lewis SA, Cowan NJ. Genetics, evolution and expression of the 68,000-mol-wt neurofilament protein: Isolation of a cloned cDNA probe. J Cell Biol 1985; 100:843–850.

269. Julien J-P, Ramachandran K, Grosveld F. Cloning a cDNA encoding the smallest neurofilament protein from the rat. Biochim Biophys Acta 1985; 825:398–404.

270. Julien J-P, Meyer D, Flavell D, Hurst J, Grosveld F. Cloning and developmental expression of the murine neurofilament gene family. Mol Brain Res 1986; 1:243–250.

271. Myers MM, Lazzarini RA, Lee VM-Y, Schlaepfer WW, Nelson DL. The human mid-size neurofilament subunit: a repeated protein sequence and the relationship of its gene to the intermediate filament gene family. EMBO J 1987; 6:1617–1626.

272. Sakimura K, Kushiya E, Obinata M, Odani S, Takahashi Y. Molecular cloning and the nucleotide sequence of cDNA for neuron-specific enolase messenger RNA of rat brain. Proc Natl Acad Sci USA 1985; 82:7453–7457.

273. Sakimura K, Kushiya E, Obinata M, Takahashi Y. Molecular cloning and the nucleotide sequence of cDNA to mRNA for non-neuronal enolase (αα enolase) of rat brain and liver. Nucl Acids Res 1985; 13:4365–4378.

274. Ginns EI, Miller N, Martin BM, Fong K, Abrahamson L, Winfield S, Marangos PJ. Isolation and sequence analysis of cDNA clones for human non-neuronal and neuron specific enolase. Fed Proc 1986; Vol. 45.

275. Martin BM, Marangos PJ, Merkle-Lehman D, Gins EI. Structural studies of human neuron-specific enolase. Fed Proc 1986; 45:1848.

276. McKay RDG. Molecular approaches to the nervous system. Ann Rev Neurosci 1983; 6:527–546.

277. Milner RJ, Lai C, Nave K-A, Lenoir D, Ogata J, Sutcliffe JG. Nucleotide sequences of two mRNAs for rat brain myelin proteolipid protein. Cell 1985; 42:931–939.

277A. Naismith AL, Hoffman-Chudzik E, Tsui LC, Riordan JR. Study of the expression of myelin proteolipid protein (lipophilin) using a cloned complementary DNA. Nucl Acids Res 1985; 13:7413–7425.

278. Willard HF, Riordan JR. Assignment of the gene for myelin proteolipid protein to the X chromosome: Implications for X-linked myelin disorders. Science 1985; 230:940–942.
279. Gardinier MV, Macklin WB, Diniak AJ, Deininger PL. Cloning and expression of rat myelin proteolipid mRNA. Mol Cell Biol 1986; 6:3755–3762.
280. Kuwano R, Usui H, Maeda T, Araki K, Yamakuni T, Kurihara T, Takahashi Y. Tissue distribution of rat S-100 α and β subunit mRNAs. Mol Brain Res 1987; 2:79–82.
281. Bishop JM. Cellular oncognes and retroviruses. Ann Rev Biochem 1983; 52:301–354.
282. Bishop JM. Viral oncogenes. Cell 1985; 42:23–38.
283. Varmus H. The molecular genetics of cellular oncogenes. Ann Rev Genet 1984; 18:553–612.
284. Shapiro JR. Biology of gliomas: Heterogeneity, oncogenes, growth factors. Semin Oncol 1986; 13:4–15.
285. Biedler JL, Ross RA, Shanske S, et al. Human neuroblastoma cytogenetics: Search for significance of homogeneously staining regions and double minute chromosomes. Adv Neuroblastoma Res 1980; 4:81–96.
286. Rosen N, Israel MA. Genetic abnormalities as biological tumor markers. Semin Oncol 1987; 14:213–231.
287. Hopkins CR, Hughes RC, eds. Growth Factors: Structure and Function. Cambridge, The Company of Biologists, Ltd., 1985.
288. Westermark B, Nister M, Heldin CH. Growth factors and oncogenes in human malignant glioma. Neurol Clin 1985; 3:785–799.
289. Breakefield XO, Stern DF. Oncogenes in neural tumors. Trends Neurosci 1986; 9:150–155.
290. Downward J, Yarden Y, Mayer E, Scrace G, Totty N, Stockwell P, Ulrich A, Schlessinger J, Waterfield MD. Close similarity of epidermal growth factor receptor of v-*erb*-B oncogene protein sequences. Nature (London) 1984; 307:521–527.
291. Shimizu N, Kondo I, Gamou S, Behzadin MA, Shimizy Y. Genetic analysis of hyperproduction of epidermal growth factor receptors in human epidermoid carcinoma A431 cells. Somatic Cell Mol Genet 1984; 10:45–53.
292. Doolittle RF, Hunkapiller MW, Hood LE, Devare SG, Robbins KC, Aaronson SA, Antoniades HN. Simian sarcoma virus *onc* gene, v-*sis*, is derived from the gene (or genes) encoding a platelet-derived growth factor. Science 1983; 221:275–277.
293. Waterfield MD, Scrace GT, Whittle N, Stroobant P, Johnsson A, Wateson A, Wastermark B, Heldin C-H, Huang JS, Deul TF. Platelet-derived growth factor is structurally related to the putative transforming protein p28^{sis} of simian sarcoma virus. Nature (London) 1983; 304:35–39.
294. Swan DC, McBride OW, Robbins KC, Keithley DA, Reddy EP, Aaronson SA. Chromosomal mapping of the simian sarcoma virus *onc* gene analogue in human cells. Proc Natl Acad Sci USA 1982; 79:4691–4695.
295. Slamon DJ, Boone TC, Seeger RC, Keith DE, Chazin V, Lee HC, Souza LM. Identification and characterization of the protein encoded by the human N-*myc* oncogene. Science 1986; 232:768–772.

296. Libermann TA, Razon N, Bartal AD, Yarden Y, Schlessinger J, Soreq H. Expression of epidermal growth factor receptors in human brain tumors. Cancer Res 1984; 44:753–760.
297. Libermann TA, Nusbaum HR, Razon N, Kris R, Lax I, Soreq H, Whittle N, Waterfield M, Ullrich A, Schlessinger J. Amplification, enhanced expression and possible rearrangement of the EGF receptor gene in primary human brain tumors of glial origin. Nature (London) 1985; 313:144–147.
298. Libermann TA, Nusbaum HR, Razon N, Kris R, Lax I, Soreq H, Whittle N, Waterfield MD, Ullrich A, Schlessinger J. Amplification and over-expression of the EGF receptor gene in primary human glioblastomas. J Cell Sci 1985; 3:161–172.
299. Eva A, Robbins KC, Andersen PR, Srinivasan A, Tronick SR, Reddy EP, Ellmore NW, Galen AT, Lautenberger JA, Papas TS, Westlin EH, Wong-Stahl R, Gallo RC, Aaronson SA. Cellular gene analogous to retroviral *onc* genes are transcribed in human tumour cells. Nature (London) 1982; 295:116–119.
300. Betsholtz C, Johnson A, Heldin C-H, Westermark B, Lind P, Urdea MS, Eddy R, Shows TB, Philpott K, Mellor AL, Knott TJ, Scott J. cDNA sequence and chromosomal localization of human platelet-derived growth factor A-chain and its expression in tumor-cell lines. Nature (London) 1986; 320:695–699.
301. Nister M, Heldin C-H, Westermark B. Clonal variation in the production of a platelet-derived growth factor-like protein and expression of cor-responding receptors in a human malignant glioma. Cancer Res 1986; 46:332–340.
302. Libermann TA, Friesel R, Jaye M, Lyall RM, Westermark R, Drohan W, Schmidt A, Maciac T, Schlessinger J. An angiogenic growth factor is expressed in human glioma cells. EMBO J 1987; 6:1627–1632.
303. Sporn MB, Todaro GJ. Autocrine secretion and malignant transfor-mation of cells. N Engl J Med 1980; 303:878–880.
304. Mohamed AN, Pu P-Y, Shipiro WR, Shapiro JR. Correlation of BCNU resistance in human glioma cells with over-representation of chromo-some 22 and production of a factor resembling platelet-derived growth factor (PDGF). Proc Am Assoc Cancer Res 1985; 26:32.
305. Nister M, Heldin C-H, Wasteson A, Westermark B. A glioma-derived analog to platelet-derived growth factor: Demonstration of receptor competing activity and immunological cross-reactivity. Proc Natl Acad Sci USA 1984; 81:926–930.
306. Schwab M, Alitalo K, Klempnauer KH, Varmus HE, Bishop JM, Gilbert F, Brodeur G, Goldstein M, Trent J. Amplified DNA with limited ho-mology to *myc* cellular oncogene is shared by human neuroblastoma cell lines and a neuroblastoma tumor. Nature (London) 1983; 305:245–248.
307. Brodeur GM, Seeger RC. Gene amplification in human neuroblastomas: Basic mechanisms and clinical implications. Cancer Genet Cytogenet 1986; 19:101–111.
308. Lee W, Murphree AL, Benedict WF. Expression and amplification of the N-*myc* gene in primary retinoblastoma. Nature 1984; 309:458–460.

309. Nau MM, Brooks BJ Jr, Carney DN, Gazdar AF, Batty JF, Sausville EA, Minna JD. Human small cell lung cancers show amplification and expression of the N-*myc* gene. Proc Natl Acad Sci USA 1986; 83:1092–1096.

310. Trent J, Meltzer P, Rosenblum M, Harsh G, Kinzler K, Mashal R, Feinberg A, Vogelstein B. Evidence for rearrangement, amplification, and expression of c-*myc* in a human glioblastoma. Proc Natl Acad Sci USA. 1986; 83:470–473.

311. Schwab M, Ellison J, Busch M, et al. Enhanced expression of the human N-*myc* gene consequent to amplification of DNA may contribute to malignant progression of neuroblastoma. Proc Natl Acad Sci USA 1984; 81:4940–4944.

312. Brodeur GM, Seeger RC, Schwab M. Amplification of N-*myc* in untreated human neuroblastomas correlates with advanced disease stage. Science 1984; 224:1121–1124.

313. Seeger RC, Brodeur GM, Gather H, Dalton A, Siegel SE, Wong KY, Hammond D. Association of multiple copies of the N-*myc* oncogene with rapid progression of neuroblastomas. N Engl J Med. 1985; 31:1111–1116.

314. Grady-Leopardi EF, Schwab M, Ablin AR, Rosenau W. Detection of N-*myc* oncogene expression of human neuroblastoma by in situ hybridication and blot analysis: relationship to clinical outcome. Cancer Res 1986; 46:3196–3199.

314A. Rosen N, Reynolds CP, Thiele CJ, Biedler JL, Israel MA. Increased N-*myc* expression following progressive growth of neuroblastoma. Cancer Res 1986; 46:4139–4142.

315. Vinores SA, Rubinstein LJ. Simultaneous expression of glial fibrillary acidic (GFA) protein and neuron-specific enolase (NSE) by the same reactive or neoplastic astrocytes. Neuropathol Appl Neurobiol 1985; 11:349–359.

316. Choi Kim. Expression of glial fibrillary acid protein in immature oligodendroglia. Science 1984; 223:407–409.

317. Haynes LW, Weller RO. Induction of some features of glial differentiation in primary cultures of human gliomas by treatment with dibutyryl cyclic AMP. Br J Exp Pathol 1978; 59:259–276.

318. Morris RJ, Gower S, Pfeiffer SE. Thy-1 cell surface antigen on cloned cell lines of the rat and mouse: stimulation by cAMP and by butyrate. Brain Res 1980; 183:145–149.

319. Pfeiffer SE, Betschart B, Cook J, Mancini P, Morris R. Glial cell lines. In Federoff S, Hertz L, eds, Cell, Tissue and Organ Cultures in Neurobiology. New York, Academic Press, 1978; pp. 287–346.

320. Kennedy PGE. Neural cell markers and their applications to neurology. J Neuroimmunol 1982; 2:35–53.

321. Bonnin JM, Rubinstein LJ. Immunohistochemistry of central nervous system tumors; its contributions to neurosurgical diagnosis. J Neurosurg 1984; 60:1121–1133.

322. McComb RD, Bigner DD. The biology of malignant gliomas: a comprehensive survey. Clin Neuropathol 1984; 3:93–106.

323. Bullard DE, Gillespie GY, Mahaley MS, Bigner DD. Immunobiology of human gliomas. Semin Oncol 1986; 13:994–1009.
324. Longo DL, ed. Tumor Markers. Sem Oncology 1987; 14:1–234.
325. Wechsler W. Experimental malignant gliomas: pathology and transplantation biology of ENU-induced rat tumors. In Grundman E, Bock WJ, Wechsler W, eds. GBK Symp 17, in press. Stuttgart, Gustav Fisher, 1987.
326. Benda P. Proteine S-100 et tumeurs cerebrates humaines. Rev Neurol 1968; 118:368–372.
327. Haglid K, Carlsson C-A, Stavrou D. An immunological study of human brain tumors concerning the brain specific proteins S-100 and 14.3.2. Acta Neuropathol 1973; 24:187–196.
328. Dohan FC, Kornblith PL, Wellum GR, Pfeiffer SE, Levine L. S-100 protein and 2′,3′-cyclic nucleotide 3′-phosphohydrolase in human brain tumors. Acta Neuropathol (Berl) 1977; 40:123–128.
329. Nakajima T, Kameya T, Tsumuraya M, Shimosato Y, Kato K. Enolase distribution in human brain tumors, retinoblastoma and pituitary adenomas. Brain Res 1984; 308:215–222.
330. Laerum OD, Mork SJ, Haugen A, Bock E, Rosengren L, Haglid K. Differentiation markers (S-100, GFAP, NSE and D2) in fetal rat brain cells during malignant transformation in cell culture. J Neuro-Oncol 1985; 3:137–146.
330A. Nakamura Y, Becker LE, Marks A. Distribution of immunoreactive S-100 protein in pediatric brain tumors. J Neuropathol Exp Neurol 1983; 42:136–145.
331. Velasco ME, Dahl D, Roessmann V, Gambetti P. Immunohistochemical localization of glial fibrillary acidic protein in human glial neoplasms. Cancer 1980; 45:484–494.
332. Eng LF, DeArmond SJ. Immunochemistry of the glial fibrillary acidic (GFA) protein. Progr Neuropathol 1983; 5:19–38.
333. Britt RH, Lyons BE, Eng LF, Bigner SH, Bigner DD. Immunohistochemical study of glial fibrillary acidic protein in avian sarcoma virus-induced gliomas in dogs. J Neuro-Oncol 1985; 3:53–59.
334. Jacque CM, Vinner C, Kujas M, Raoul M, Racadot J, Baumann NA. Determination of glial fibrillary acidic protein (GFAP) in human brain tumors. J Neurol Sci 1978; 35:147–155.
335. van der Meulen JDM, Houthoff HJ, Ebels EJ. Glial fibrillary acidic protein in human gliomas. Neuropathol Appl Neurobiol 1978; 4:177–190.
336. Duffy PE, Huang Y-Y, Rapport MM, Graf L. Glial fibrillary acidic protein in giant cell tumors of brain and other gliomas. A possible relationship to malignancy, differentiation and pleomorphism of glia. Acta Neuropathol (Berl) 1980; 52:51–57.
337. Bignami A, Schoene WC. Glial fibrillary acidic protein in human brain tumors. In DeLellis RA, ed. Diagnostic Immunohistochemistry. Mason Monographs in Diagnostic Pathology, New York, Masson Publishing, 1981; 2:213–224.
338. Marsden HB, Kumar S, Kahn J, Anderson BJ. A study of glial fibrillary acidic protein (GFAP) in childhood tumors. Int J Cancer 1983; 31:439–445.

339. Pasquier B, Lachard A, Pasquier D, Coudere P, Delpech B, Courel M-N. Glial fibrillary acidic protein (GFA) in central nervous system tumors. An immunohistochemical study of 207 cases. 1st Part: Astrocytomas, glioblastomas, ependymomas, papillomas of the choroid plexus. Ann Pathol 1983; 3:127–136.
340. Herpers MJHM, Budka H. Glial fibrillary acidic protein (GFAP) of oligodendroglial tumors: gliofibrillary oligodendroglioma and transitional oligoastrocytoma as subtypes of oligodendroglioma. Acta Neuropathol (Berl) 1984; 64:265–272.
341. Paetau A, Virtanen I. Cytoskeletal properties and endogenous degradation of glial fibrillary acidic protein and vimentin in cultured human glioma cells. Acta Neuropathol (Berl) 1986; 69:73–80.
342. Bigner DD. Biology of gliomas: potential clinical implications of glioma cellular heterogeneity. Neurosurgery 1981; 9:320–326.
343. Kivela T. Neuron-specific enolase in retinoblastoma. An immunohistochemical study. Acta Ophthalmol 1986; 64:19–25.
344. Cooper EH. Neuron specific enolase: a marker of (small cell) cancers of neuronal and neuroendocrine origin. Biomed Pharmacother 1985; 39:165–166.
345. Bates SE, Longo DL. Use of serum tumor markers in cancer diagnosis and management. Semin Oncol 1987; 14:102–138.
346. Allen JM, Hoyle NR, Yeats JC, Ghatei MA, Thomas DGT, Bloom SR. Neuropeptides in neurological tumours. J Neuro-Oncol 1985; 3:197–202.
347. Garson JA, Coakham HB, Kemshead JT, Brownell B, Harper EI, Allan P, Bourne S. The role of monoclonal antibodies in brain tumour diagnosis and cerebrospinal fluid (CSF) cytology. J Neuro-Oncol 1985; 3:165–171.
348. Wada C, Kurata A, Hirose R, Tazaki Y, Kan S Ishihara Y, Kameya T. Primary leptomeningeal ependymoblastoma. J Neurosurg 1986; 64:968–973.
349. Blobel GA, Gould VE, Moll R, Lee I, Huszar M, Geiger B, Franke WW. Coexpression of neuroendocrine markers and epithelial cytoskeletal proteins in bronchopulmonary neuroendocrine neoplasms. Lab Invest 1985; 52:39–51.
350. Yung WA, Luna M, Borit A. Vimentin and glial fibrillary acidic protein in human brain tumors. J Neuro-Oncol 1985; 3:35–38.
351. Holden J, Dolman CL, Chung A. Immunohistochemistry of meningiomas including the angioblastic type. J Neuropathol Exp Neurol 1987; 46:50–56.
352. Nakamura M, Inoue HK, Ono N, Kunimine H, Tamada J. Analysis of hemangiopericytic meningiomas by immunohistochemistry, electron microscopy and cell culture. J Neuropathol Exp Neurol 1987; 46:57–71.
353. Eto Y, Shinoda S. Gangliosides and neutral glycosphingolipids in human brain tumors. Specificity and their significance. Adv Exp Med 1982; 152:279–290.
354. Ritchie T, Scully SA, DeVellis J, Noble EP. Stability of neuronal and

glial marker enzymes in post-mortem rat brain. Neurochem Res 1985; 11:383–392.

354A. DeLellis RA, Dayal Y. The role of immunohistochemistry in the diagnosis of poorly differentiated malignant neoplasms. Semin Oncol 1987; 14:173–192.

355. Pfeiffer SE, Kornblith PL, Cares HL, Seals J, Levine L. S-100 protein in human acoustic neurinomas. Brain Res 1972; 41:187–193.

356. Pfeiffer SE, Sundarraj N, Dawson G, Kornblith PL. Human acoustic neurinomas: nervous system specific biochemical parameters. Acta Neuropathol (Berl) 1979; 47:27–31.

357. Wiedenmann B, Franke WW, Kuhn C, Moll R, Gould VE. Synaptophysin: a marker protein for neuroendocrine cells and neoplasms. Proc Natl Acad Sci USA 1986; 83:3500–3504.

358. Gibicke-Haerter PJ, Darby JK, Shooter EM, Riccardi VM, Weisgraber KH, Boyles JK, Mahley RW. Apolipoprotein E synthesis in neurofibrosarcomas and schwannoma cell cultures from two individuals with neurofibromatosis. Exp Neurol 1987; 95:323–335.

2

Parameters of Glial Differentiation: Modulation by Neoplastic Transformation and Tumor Promoters

Deborah Benzil, Alan Hirschfeld,
and Joseph Bressler

To understand cancer is to gain access to the logic of the system
which imposes on cells the constraints of the organism.
—*The Logic of Life: A History of Heredity,* Francois Jacob, 1976,
Vintage Books

Introduction

We believe the constraints alluded to in this quote by the Nobel Laureate, Francois Jacob, are those which control cellular differentiation. In numerous studies, researchers have found that neoplastic cells very often express properties of fetal cells.[1] In addition, there are examples of neoplastic cell lines which differentiate in culture and lose the ability to express various neoplastic-related properties. There are yet other examples in which cells lose the ability to express differentiated properties while acquiring the expression of neoplastic properties after stimulation with tumor promoters.[2]

Our laboratory is particularly interested in differentiation and

From: Kornblith PL, Walker MD (editors). Advances in Neuro-Oncology. Futura Publishing Company, Inc., Mount Kisco, NY, © 1988.

transformation in glial cells. We have studied several properties of differentiation in primary astroglial cultures, as well as in transformed human and rat glial cultures. Understanding how differentiation is altered during transformation of cells may lead to new approaches in the chemotherapy of glial tumors.

Factors that control glial differentiation may also be important in the ontogeny of glial tumors; these are likely to differ from factors that play a role in the differentiation of other cell types. Little is known about the initial transforming signal and the ensuing pattern of progression of glial tumors. Recent epidemiological studies indicate an increased relative risk of brain tumors in rubber plant workers,[3] chemists,[4] and workers in the petrochemical industry.[5] No single carcinogen has been uncovered in any of these exposure groups. To date, the only carcinogen directly linked to an increased risk of central nervous system (CNS) tumors is vinyl chloride. The evidence for this exists in both epidemiological studies[6] as well as animal exposure models.[7] Many other compounds have been shown to induce CNS tumors in various animal models[8]; so far, none have been linked to human tumors. Studies on differentiation may lead to insight into which subpopulation of glial cells are most susceptible to transformation, as well as which factors are probable causes of this transformation. In addition, studies on differentiation, specifically the effects of various substances on the progress or arrest of differentiation, may lead to the discovery of some common mode of action which is specific to the CNS.

The specific questions addressed in this chapter are: (1) What markers of glial differentiation are altered in transformed glial cell lines? (2) Do chemicals known to affect glial cells quantitatively or qualitatively alter expression of differentiation properties? (3) What common mechanisms are there by which properties of differentiation are altered? (4) What can we learn about the ontogeny of central nervous system tumors through the study of differentiation properties? and (5) What new approaches to chemotherapy are possible given a greater understanding of glial differentiation?

Experimental Evidence

To determine which glial-specific properties are altered during the transformation process, we first measured various properties before and after transformation of glial cells. In one series of studies, enriched oligodendroglial-derived cells were isolated from pregnant rats which were treated with either ethynitrosourea (ENU) or solvent.[9] Cell lines were established which were positive or negative for tumorigenicity as tested in sublethally irradiated syngeneic hosts (Table 1). We found two oligodendroglial-specific markers, 2'3'cyclic nucleotide phosphohydrolase (CNPase) and lactate dehydrogenase inducibility,[10] fully expressed in the tumorigenic cell lines. Another oligodendroglial marker, glycerol phosphate dehydrogenase (GPDH) inducibility,[11] was not expressed in any of the tumorigenic cell lines.

Similar types of studies were conducted using an enriched astroglial-derived population, though the results were not as clear.[12] First, the astroglial-derived cell lines were found to spontaneously transform in culture. In other words, cells from both ENU-treated as well as solvent-treated pregnant rats underwent neoplastic transformation at similar passage numbers. In characterizing the pretransformed cells we found that they were negative for glial fibrous acidic protein (GFAP) and GPDH inducibility but positive for glutamine synthetase (GS) inducibility, an astroglial marker.[13] The transformed cells were no longer inducible for GS but were now, surprisingly, inducible for GPDH. We have been unable to clone the pretransformed cells and, as such, these cell lines represent a heterogenous cell population. We are, therefore, unsure whether the transformation event selected for a GPDH-positive cell or if the transformation induced GPDH-negative cells to become GPDH-positive. Overall, these studies demonstrated to us that only a select number of differentiated

Table 1
Loss of Differentiated Function in Transformed Glial Cells

Cell Line	Tumorigenic	CNPase[1]	GPDH[2]	GS[2]	LDH[2]
Oligodendroglial	yes	265 ± 15	N.D.	N.D.	1.8
Astroglial derived	no	N.E.	N.D.	7.2	N.D.
Astroglial derived	yes	N.E.	4.8	N.D.	1.6

[1] Units of enzyme (nmol of substrate used per minute at 30°C) divided by protein concentration. Primary oligodendroglial cultures exhibit 441 ± 11 units of activity, (see McCarthy and de Vellis, 1980). N.E. = not examined.
[2] Fold increase in specific activity of enzyme after cells are stimulated with dexamethasone (GPDH annd GS) or Bt$_2$cAMP (LDH). N.D. = none detected.

properties of glial cells are lost during transformation. We also felt that GPDH inducibility might be an important key in deciphering the relationship between differentiation and neoplasia.

In order to further test this relationship, we have conducted studies in GPDH regulation, using the C6 rat glioma cell line. We use these cells because they also express other glial specific properties.[14] We have found that phorbol ester (PE) tumor promoters inhibit the expression of GPDH induction in the C6 rat glioma cell lines.[15] The inhibition of GPDH inducibility by phorbol ester tumor promoters was due either to a decrease in the transcription or to translation of GPDH-specific mRNA. A strong correlation was found between the ability of various PEs to inhibit GPDH induction with their ability to promote mouse skin tumors as well as their ability to bind to the phorbol ester receptor (Table 2). In addition, the ED_{50} found for phorbol 12 myristate 13 acetate (PMA) to inhibit GPDH induction was comparable to the Ki needed in competition receptor studies. It was therefore suggested that the PE receptor was involved in the inhibition of GPDH inducibility.

In vivo, tumor promotion can be divided into two events, termed stage I and stage II.[16] Though PMA is active during both stages, mezerin[17] and phorbol retinoic acid (PRA)[18] are weak stage I promoters but potent stage II promoters. We found mezerin and PRA to

Table 2
Relative Potency of Tumor Promoters[1,2]

Compound	Promotion	GPDH	PE-Receptor
PMA	1	1	1.0
4B-phorbol 12, 13 dibutyrate	72–180	2	112
4B-phorbol 12, 13 dibenzoate	20–100	3	98
4B-phorbol 12, 13 diacetate	200	N.D.	8,500
Mezerin	49	0.08	10.0
PRA	50	0.08	1.0

[1] Tumor promoters were compared to PMA in regards to their relative ability to affect tumor promotion in mouse skin, inhibit GPDH induction after dexamethasone stimulation in C6 cells, and inhibit [³H]PDBu binding to the PE receptor in mouse brain.
[2] Data from promotion and receptor studies were taken from Blumberg P, 1980, see references.

be five to ten times more active than PMA in inhibiting GPDH induction (Table 2).[19] In order to explain why mezerin and PRA are more active than PMA, we hypothesized that they may be acting through an alternate PE receptor.

One known receptor for the PE tumor promoters is the protein kinase C (PKC),[20] a calcium activated phospholipid-dependent protein kinase which is endogenously activated by diacylglycerols (DG).[21] DG are generated during the phosphatydylinositol cycle.[22] We reasoned that the alternate PE receptor might not be PKC and thus not activated by DG. We therefore asked whether GPDH inducibility was also inhibited by elevating intracellular DG levels.

Two approaches can be used to raise DG levels in whole cells. One is to use a semi-permeable DG such as 1-oleoy-2-acetyl-rac-glycerol (OAG). In this case, OAG enters the cells and directly elevates DG levels and thus activates the enzyme; OAG was ineffective in inhibiting GPDH induction. The other approach is to stimulate the cells to elevate endogenous DG levels. We found two methods in which DG levels could be raised in C6 glioma cells (Table 2). Treating cells with 2-bromo-octanoate[23] blocks the conversion of DG to triacylglycerols resulting in a buildup of DG. Alternatively, cells treated with phospholipase C (C. perfringens) hydrolyze phosphatidylcholine to 1,2-diglyceride and phosphorylcholine and thereby raise DG levels.[24] Under both conditions, the DG generated competitively inhibited (^{3}H)PDBU in binding to the PE receptor. We also found that the treated cells exhibited less GPDH induction than the untreated cells. Other types of phospholipases were ineffective, indicating that we were not observing an effect of nonspecific membrane pertubation. It is unclear why OAG was ineffective. This may be related to the relatively long incubation time needed to observe activity; OAG may be quickly degraded in the cell and fail to effect long-term PKC-related characteristics. Regardless, we conclude from these studies that the PKC was involved in the PMA-mediated inhibition of GPDH induction though this does not exclude the possibility that there is an alternative receptor which is also effective.

PE tumor promoters may affect GPDH induction by attenuating cAMP levels. cAMP has been shown to be a competence factor during GPDH induction,[25] and PE inhibit the β-adrenergic response in C6 rat glioma cells[26,27] (Table 3). Since we were aware that PKC was important in the inhibition of GPDH induction, we asked if this enzyme was also important in inhibiting the β-adrenergic response. Another reason why this was important was that other investigators

Table 3
Elevated Diglyceride Levels Inhibit GPDH Induction in C6 Rat
Glioma Cells

Reagent	Diglycerides[1]	GPDH Induction[2]	Percent Inhibition of [³H]PDBu Binding
OAG	N.E.[3]	N.D.[4]	N.D.
2-bromo-octanoate (1 mM)	1.7	66 ± 5	45 ± 6
Phospholipase C (0.1 μ/ml)	2.7	68 ± 7	53 ± 5

[1] Fold increase compared to untreated cells.
[2] Percent inhibition of stimulated GPDH activity when compared to stimulated cells which were not treated with the reagents.
[3] Not examined.
[4] No inhibition detected.

using lymphoma cells[28] and pinealocytes[29] found that activated PKC augmented the β-adrenergic response. It seemed paradoxical that in some cell types, PKC activation inhibited the β-adrenergic response, while in other cells it led to an augmentation of this response. We found that with DG activation of PKC in phospholipase C and 2-bromo-octanoate treated cells, there were lower levels of cAMP after isoproterenol stimulation than in untreated cells. We also found that the forskolin response was diminished in PMA, phospholipase C, or 2-bromo-octanoate treated cells, indicating that the inhibition was nonreceptor-mediated.[30] The inhibition was also not related to changes in phosphodiesterase activity indicating that the lower cAMP levels were not due to an increased rate of cAMP degradation. In contrast to our results, other investigators found that the PMA-mediated inhibition of the β-adrenergic response in C6 glioma cells occurred at the level of the receptor.[31] Broken preparations of PMA-treated cells did not exhibit a change in the activity of the catalytic or regulatory subunit of adenylate cyclase. In sucrose gradient analysis of membrane β-receptors, they found that PMA-treated cells exhibited more receptors in a light membrane fraction than nontreated cells. These results suggested that PMA induced the internalization of the β-receptor, so less receptor was available for stimulation at the cell surface. Our results do not disagree with these investigators with respect to changes in receptor mobility but they do conflict with respect to the possibility that the regulatory or catalytic subunit is impaired after PMA treatment. We found that the forskolin response, which is distal to the receptor, was attenuated in whole, PMA-treated cells. Kasis et al., in reconstitution experiments using membrane preparations, found that there was no change in the activity of the regulatory subunits, nor was there change in sodium fluoride stimulated adenylate cyclase activity. These differences may he attributed to the methods of exploring the β-adrenergic system. These other investigators treated whole cells, but assayed individual proteins in a broken cell preparation; in our work, however, we have studied whole cells. Forskolin is believed to only activate the catalytic subunit of adenylate cyclase in broken cell preparations, but activates the catalytic subunit and the regulatory subunit in whole cells.[30] Why these differences exist is not established. We therefore conclude that PMA effects the β-adrenergic systeln at least at two sites, the receptor site, and the regulatory subunit site.

Another approach this laboratory has taken to gain a better understanding of the interrelationship between cAMP and PE, is to study their respective protein kinases and their phosphorylation substrates. There are many biological effects attributed to stimulation of the PKC and protein kinases A (PKA). Our laboratory has studied phosphorylation profiles in C6 cells following stimulation with either PMA or forskolin (Table 4). We have found similarities and differences

Table 4

PKC Activators Affect cAMP Production in C6 Rat Glioma Cells[1]

PKC Activator	Isoproterenol (10 μM0	Forskolin (50 μM)	Phosphodiesterase Activity
PMA (50 nM)	48 ± 5	34 ± 4	N.D.[2]
Phospholipase C (0.1 units/ml)	95 ± 6	95 ± 8	N.D.
2-bromo-octanoate (1 mM)	N.E.[3]	49 ± 5	N.E.

[1] Percent inhibition of stimulated cAMP levels when compared to levels in stimulated cells which were not treated with a PKC activator.
[2] No change in activity detected.
[3] Not examined.

in the molecular weight classes of proteins phosphorylated after PMA and forskolin stimulation. For example, proteins of a molecular weight class of 80,000 and 25,000 are phosphorylated under both conditions. Unlike PMA, forskolin stimulates the phosphoylation of proteins with a molecular weight class of 35,000, while PMA stimulates the phosphorylation of proteins with a molecular weight class 90,000, 45,000, and 30,000. Since cAMP is important for GPDH induction, and PMA inhibits this event, those proteins which are uniquely phosphorylated by PMA may play a role in the inhibition of this response.

Another parameter of differentiation studied in our laboratory is S-100 protein expression. S-100 protein(s) is actually a group of dimeric proteins, with a molecular weight of 21,000, composed of the combination of at least three immunologically distinct subunits.[32] The highest concentration of S-100 protein is found in neural tissue, where it is particularly enriched in astrocytes.[33] The specific function of S-100 is still largely unknown. It may play a role in microtubule assembly,[34] act as a calcium-dependent modulator of protein phosphorylation,[35] and or regulate GABA transport across cell membranes.[36] In tissue culture, as C6 cells become confluent, their S-100 content increases.[37]

In one series of studies we asked whether sodium butyrate (NaBu) would inhibit the cAMP-dependent induction of S-100 protein levels. We chose to look at NaBu because previous work by Weingarten et al., demonstrated that in C6 cells, NaBu will inhibit the glucocorticoid-mediated induction of GPDH,[38] yet increase GS levels.[39] Since GPDH inducibility in the rat is an oligodendroglial specific property and GS is localized to the astrocyte, we felt that NaBu may stimulate C6 cells to undergo astrocytic differentiation. Using this reasoning, we explored the possibility that another marker of astrocytic differentiation, S-100 protein, would be elevated by NaBu treatment. This was not the case. In fact, NaBu had no effect on basal S-100 levels, though it inhibited by 82% the induction of S-100 protein after stimulation with isoproterenol and theophylline. In a human glioma cell line, NaBu inhibited the basal S-100 protein levels. Other short-chain fatty acids such as sodium proprionate and sodium isobutyrate were less efficient inhibitors than NaBu, a finding consistent with results reported in other systems.[40,41]

Several different effects induced by NaBu on cells in culture have been described.[40,41] All or some of these effects may be important for NaBu to affect the changes we observed. We were particularly puzzled, however, by the reports describing the ability of NaBu to potentiate the β-adrenergic response in HeLA cells.[42] How could a drug that augments cAMP response inhibit the expression of two properties that are dependent on high cAMP levels, i.e., S-100 expression and GPDH inducibility. We consequently investigated the effects of NaBu at 1 mM on the β-adrenergic response in C6 cells. An overnight incubation with NaBu inhibited the β-adrenergic response by 61%. The inhibition was not effected through the β-receptor since the forskolin response was also inhibited by 65%. At present, we do not know whether NaBu has altered the transcriptional activity of genes whose products are important for increasing cAMP levels or uncoupled the adenylate cyclase catalytic subunit from its regulatory subunit. These possibilities are currently under investigation.

Conclusions and General Discussion

Neoplastic cells differ from their normal counterparts in their phenotypic expression; endogenous genes may be repressed while there is inappropriate expression of genes related to tumor growth and spread. One observable result is the loss of the ability of the cells to express differentiated properties. Histopathologists have used immunohistochemical techniques to identify the expression of differentiated properties, such as the expression of GFAP, in astroglial-derived tumors as one determinant of staging. In general, a greater degree of differentiation translates into lower staging and thus a more promising prognosis.[43,44]

The work of our laboratory, along with that of other laboratories, sheds some new insights into the transformation process in glial cells and suggests some specific areas for future research. First, there are several markers of glial differentiation which are predictably altered in transformed glial cell lines; namely, GS and GPDH inducibility are altered while CNPase activity and LDH inducibility remain intact. In addition, alteration of the expression of these differentiated properties by chemicals is variable and seems to be highly cell lineage specific. For example, NaBu seems to induce differentiation in some cell lines,[45] but our studies suggest an opposite effect in cell lines of glial origin. Caution needs to be exercised in labeling chemicals as "differentiating agents" since the global ability to promote differentiation is not likely.

In contrast to this great variability, our studies in glial cells seem to indicate that there may be a common mechanism by which expression of differentiated properties are controlled; namely, that they are controlled through modulating cAMP levels. Though the importance of cAMP in differentiating glioma cells has been suggested, the evidence for such an effect was poor.[46] Our studies with S-100 levels and GPDH inducibility show a common link of alteration of cAMP levels. This is likely to be somewhat glial-specific since, as noted above, other nonglial cell lines show exactly opposite responses. cAMP may regulate expression of differentiated properties and transformation through control of intercellular communication. Evidence for this is suggested by studies which demonstrate that cAMP modulates de novo synthesis of gap junctional proteins.[47] Studies also demonstrate that pMA inhibits intercellular communication though the mechanism of this action is not yet known.[48]

Some conclusions regarding the ontonogy of brain tumors can also be made. It is generally accepted that neoplastic transformation involves the loss of differentiated properties along with the acquisition of phenotypic expression of several tumor related factors. Whether this transformation targets multipotential stem cells or causes reversion of already mature cells is still unknown; our studies indicate that the latter is at least possible. Tumor promoters are capable of causing this kind of reversion in cell cultures. We believe that available epidemiology studies suggest that certain industrial chemicals might act as in vivo tumor promoters in much the same way as PMA affects cells in vitro.

Relating to future chemotherapeutic modalities, our studies indicate that manipulation of cAMP levels may be more fruitful than the use of "differentiating agents" in treating gliomas. In some cell types, differentiating agents have shown more promise. Retinoic acid, a differentiating agent for leukemic cell lines,[49] has been used with success in several case reports of myeloplastic disorders and acute promyelocytic leukemia.[50,51] Synergism has been demonstrated in leukemic cell cultures between retinoic acid and cAMP elevating agents.[52] Polar solvents such as DMSO are currently in phase-two clinical trials for their use as differentiating agents but success has been very limited.[53] Recent studies with tamoxifen and clomiphene, effective chemotherapeutic agents in mammary tumors, show them both to be inhibitors of PKC.[54] PKC control of cellular differentiation and/or cAMP levels may be the mechanism through which these two drugs inhibit the growth and spread of mammary tumors.

Future studies, such as those using mutant cell lines unresponsive to stimulation with PMA, cAMP, and NaBu will hopefully shed even more light on the intricate process of cellular differentiation and neoplastic transformation and aid in developing more directed chemotherapeutic modalities.

REFERENCES

1. Potter VR. Phenotypic diversity in experimental hepatomas, the content of partially blocked ontogeny. Br J Cancer 1978; 38:1.
2. Blumberg P. In vitro studies on the mode of action of the phorbol esters, potent tumor promoters. Part 1. CRC Crit Rev Toxicol 1980; 153–197.
3. Mancuso TF. Epidemiological investigation of occupational cancers in the rubber industry. In: Levinson C, ed. New Multinational Health Hazards, 80–136.
4. Olin GR, Ahlbom A. Cancer mortality among three Swedish male academic cohorts: Chemists, architects and mining engineers/metallurgists. Ann NY Acad Sci 1982; 381:197–201.
5. Maltoni C, Cilbertie A, Carreti D. Experimental contributions in identifying brain potential carcinogens in the petrochemical industry. Ann NY Acad Sci 1982; 381:216–249.
6. Maltoni C. Predictive value of carcinogenesis bioassays. Ann NY Acad Sci 1976; 271:431–443.
7. Waxweiler RJ, Stringer W, Wagoner JK, Jones J, Falk H, Carter C. Neoplastic risk among workers exposed to vinyl chloride. Ann NY Acad Sci 1976; 271:40–48.
8. Ward JM, Rice JM. Naturally and chemically induced brain tumors of rat and mice in carcinogenesis assays. Ann NY Acad Sci 1982; 381:304–319.
9. Bressler JP, Cole R, de Vellis J. Neoplastic transformation of oligodendrocytes from the newborn rat in vitro. Cancer Res 1983; 49:709–715.
10. McCarthy KD, de Vellis J. Preparation of separate astroglial and oligodendroglial cell cultures from rat cerebral tissue. J Cell Biol 1980; 85:890–902.
11. Leveille PJ, McGinnis JF, Maxwell DS, de Vellis J. Immunocytochemical localization of glycerol-3–phosphate dehydrogenase in rat oligodendrocytes. Brain Res 1980; 196:287–305.
12. Bressler JP, de Vellis J. Neoplastic transformation of rat astrocytes in culture. Brain Res 1984; 348:21–27.
13. Bell KP, Norenberg MD. Glutamine synthethase: slial localization in brain. Science 1977; 195:1356–1358.
14. Benda P, Lightbody L, Sato G, Levine L, Sweet W. Differentiated rat glial cell strain in tissue culture. Science 1968; 161:370.
15. Bressler JP, Weingarten D, Kornblith PL. Glucocorticoid-mediated increases in glycerol phosphate dehydrogenase activity is inhibited by the phorbol ester tumor promoters. J Neurochem 1985; 45:1268–1272.
16. Boutwell RC. Some biological aspects of skin carcinogenesis. Prog Exp Tumor Res 1964; 4:207–250.

17. Slaga TJ, Fischer SM, Nelson K, Gleason GL. Studies on the mechanism of skin tumor promotion: Evidence for several stages in promotion. Proc Natl Acad Sci, USA 1980; 77:3659–3663.
18. Furstenberger G, Berry DL, Sorg B, Marks F. Skin tumor promotion by phorbol esters is a two-stage process. Proc Natl Acad Sci, USA 1981; 78:7722–7726.
19. Leach KL, Frost MM, Blumberg PM, Bressler JP. Second stage tumor promoters: Effect of 3H phorbol 12,13-dibutyrate binding and glycerol phosphate dehydrogenase activity in C6 rat glioma cells. (submitted for publication).
20. Castagna M, Takai Y, Kaibuchi K, Sano K, Kikkawa U, Nishizuka Y. Direct activation of calcium and phospholipid-dependent protein kinase by tumor promoting phorbol esters. J Biol Chem 1982; 257:7847–7851.
21. Kishmimoto A, Takai Y, Mori T, Kikkawa U, Nishizuka Y. Direct activation of calcium-activated, phospholipid-dependent protein kinase by diacylglycerol, its possible relation to phosphatidylinositol turnover. J Biol Chem 1980; 255:2273–2276.
22. Hokin LE. Receptors and phosphoinositide-generated second messengers. Ann Rev Biochem 1985; 54:205–235.
23. Mayorek N, Bar-Tana J. Inhibition of diacylglycerol acyltransferase by 2-bromo-octanoate in cultured rat hepatocytes. J Biol Chem 1981; 260:6528–6532.
24. Stahl WL. Phospholipase C purification and specificity with respect to individual phospholipids and brain microsomal membrane phospholipids. Arch Biochem Biophys 1973; 154:47–55.
25. Breen GAM, McGinnis JF, de Vellis J. Modulation of HC induction of GPDH by N(6), 0(2)-dibutyryl cAMP, norepinephrine and isobutylmethylxanthine in rat brain cell cultures. J Biol Chem 1978; 253:2554–2562.
26. Mallorga P, Tallman JF, Henneberry RF, Hiate F, Strittmatter WT, Axelrod J. Mecaprine blocks B-adrenergic agonist-induced desensitization in astrocytoma cells. Proc Natl Acad Sci 1980; 77:1341–1345.
27. Brostrom MA, Brostrom CO, Brotman LA, Lee CS, Wolff DJ, Geller HM. Alterations of glial tumor cell Ca^{2+} metabolism and Ca^{2+}-dependent cAMP accumulation by phorbol myristate acetate. J Biol Chem 1982:257:675S-6765.
28. Bell JD, Buston IL, Brunton LL. Enhancement of adenylate cyclase activity in S49 lymphoma cells by phorbol esters. J Biol Chem 1985; 260:2625–2628.
29. Sugden D, Vanecek J, Klein DC, Thomas TP, Anderson WB. Activation of protein kinase C potentiates isoprenaline-induced cyclic AMP accumulation in rat pinealocytes. Nature 1985; 213:259–61.
30. Seamen KB, Wetzel B. Interaction of forskolin with dually regulated adenylate cyclase. Adv Cyclic Nucleotide Protein Phosphoryl 1984; 17:91–99.
31. Kassis S, Zaremba T, Patel J, Fishman PH. Phorbol esters and β-adrenergic agonists mediate desensitization of adenylate cyclase in rat glioma C6 cells by distinct mechanisms. J Biol Chem 1985; 260:8911–8917.
32. Mahdik SP, Korenovsky, Rapport MM. Heterogeneity of S-100 proteins: Subunit compositions. J Neurochem 1979; 33:751–762.

33. Ludwin SK, Kosek JC, Eng LF. The topographical distributions of S-100 and GFA proteins in the adult rat brain; An immunohistochemical study using horseradish peroxidase-labeled antibodies. J Comp Neurol 1976; 165:197–208.
34. Baudier J, Briving C, Denium J, Haglid K, Sorskog K, Wallin M. Effect of S-100 proteins and calmodulin on Ca2+-induced disassembly of brain microtubules in vitro. FEBS Lett 1982; 147:165–167.
35. Qi D-F, Kuo JR. S-100 modulates Ca(2+)-independent phosphorylation of an endogenous protein (Mr
9K) in brain. J Neurochem 1984; 43:256–260.
36. Hyden H, Lange PW, Larsson S. S-100 in the regulation of GABA transport across the nerve cell membrane. J Neurol Sci 1980; 45:303–316.
37. Labourdette G, Mandel P. S-100 protein in monolayer cultures of glial cells: Basal level in primary and secondary cultures. Biochem Biophys Res Comm 1978; 85:1307–1313.
38. Weingarten D, de Vellis J. Selective inhibition by sodium butyrate of the glucocorticoid induction of glycerol phosphate dehydrogenase in glial cultures. Biochem Biophys Res Comm 1980; 93:1297–1304.
39. Weingarten D, Kumar S, de Vellis J. Paradoxical effects of sodium butyrate on the glucocorticoid inductions of glutamine synthetase and glycerol phosphate dehydrogenase in C6 cells. FEBS Lett 1981; 126:289–291.
40. Prasad KN, Sirha PK. Effect of sodium butyrate on mammalian cells in culture: A review. In vitro 1976; 12:125–132.
41. Sealy L, Chalkley R. The effect of sodium butyrate on histone modification. Cell 1978; 14:115–121.
42. Tallman JF, Smith CC, Henneberry RC. Induction of functional adrenergic receptors in HeLa cells. Proc Natl Acad Sci 1977; 74:873–877.
43. Ramaekers FCS, Puts JJG, Moesker O, Kant A, Huysmans A, Haag D, Jap PHK, Herman CJ, Vooijs GP. Antibodies to intermediate filament proteins in the immunohistochemical identification of human tumours: An overview. Histochem J 1983; 15:691–713.
44. Frame MC, Freshney RI, Vaughan PFT, Graham DI, Shaw R. Interrelationship between differentiation and malignancy-associated properties in glioma. Int J Physiol 1984; 49:269–280.
45. McCue PA, Gobler ML, Sherman MI, Cohen BN. Sodium butyrate induces histone hyperacetylation and differentiation of murine embryonal carcinoma cells. J Cell Biol 1980; 98:602–608.
46. Gumerlock MK, Smith BH, Pollock LA, Kornblith PL: Chemical differentiation of cultured human glioma cells: Morphologic and immunologic effects. Surg Forum 1981: Vol. XXXII.
47. Kanno Y. Modulation of cell communication and carcinogenesis. Jpn J Physiol 1985; 35:693–707.
48. Yamasaki H, Aguelon-Pegouries A, Enomoto T, Martel N, Furstenberger G, Marks F. Comparative effects of a complete tumor promoter, TPA, and a second-stage tumor promoter, PRA, on intercellular communication, cell differentiation and cell transformation. Carcinogenesis 1985; 6:1173–1179.
49. Nilsson B. Probable in vivo induction of differentiation by retinoic acid

of promyelocytes in acute promyelocytic leukemia. Br J Haematol 1984; 57:365–371.

50. Daenen S, Vellenga E, van Dobbenburgh OA, Halls MR. Retinoic acid as antileukemic therapy in a patient with acute promyelocytic leukemia and aspergillus pneumonia. Blood 1986; 67:559–561.

51. Fontana JA, Rogers JS, Durham JP. The role of 13 cis-retinoic acid in the remission induction of a patient with acute promyelocytic leukemia. Cancer 1986; 57:209–217.

52. Fontana J, Munoz M, Durham J. Potentiation between intracellular cyclic-AMP-elevating agents and inducers of leukemic cell differentiation. Leukemia Res 1985; 9:1127–1132.

53. Spremulli EN, Dexter DL. Polar solvents: A novel class of antineoplastic agents. J of Clin Oncol 1984; 2:227–240.

54. O'Brian CA, Liskamp RM, Solomon DH, Weinstein IB. Triphenylethylenes: A new class of protein kinase C inhibitors. JNCI 1986; 76:1243–1246.

3
Deciphering Human Brain Tumor Antigenicity

Duncan K. Fischer, Raj K. Narayan,
and Terence L. Chen

Introduction

Over the past 15 years various polyclonal and monoclonal antibodies have been raised against malignant human brain tumors. These research efforts have often been confounded by broad antigenic cross-reactivity and by the heterogeneity of these tumors. Nevertheless, these approaches have become increasingly sophisticated, paralleling advances in available technology. While some doubt still exists over the existence of a truly tumor-specific protein, efforts aimed at the identification of tumor-associated markers may yet be worthwhile. This chapter summarizes the progress made in these areas, tabulates currently reported antibodies, and explores additional methods for deciphering the underlying composition of human brain tumor antigenicity.

An Overview

Primarily because of their considerable potential for diagnostic and therapeutic applications, the search for brain tumor markers that

From: Kornblith PL, Walker MD (editors). Advances in Neuro-Oncology. Futura Publishing Company, Inc., Mount Kisco, NY, © 1988.
Acknowledgments: The material covered in this chapter was recently reviewed by these authors for the *Journal of Neurosurgery*. While the data presented here are substantially similar, we have expanded and updated the text and added appropriate references. The overlapping material, figures, and tables are being reproduced with permission.

are specific for central nervous system (CNS) malignancy has received considerable attention over the past 15 years. A tumor marker may be defined as a cellular or viral product which is either unique to, or present in higher concentrations in transformed cells as compared to normal cells of the same lineage. Truly specific tumor markers that are present only on neoplastic cells are neoantigens, of which the T-antigens encoded by DNA tumor viruses serve as some of the best examples. Such a marker may be a polypeptide, a carbohydrate, a glycolipid, or a glycoprotein. Certain tumor markers have been found to be related to fetal or differentiation antigens. Such antigens are expressed in greater abundance in cells of common embryologic ancestry, yet can vary depending upon the stage of differentiation.[38]

Primary CNS tumors occur with an incidence approaching 15,000 cases each year in the United States.[121] Despite advances in radiotherapy and the development of chemotherapeutic agents, the survival rate for most malignant brain tumors remains poor. The 2-year survival for glioblastoma multiforme is less than 15–20%.[131] Thus, there is still an urgent need to develop alternative approaches for the treatment of these malignancies. One avenue of great promise is to (1) identify markers or a panel of markers reliably associated with the neoplasm, and (2) employ conjugated polyclonal or monoclonal antibodies directed against these antigens to deliver radioisotopes, drugs, or cytotoxic agents selectively to the tumor cells. This approach may yield both a more specific delivery system for drugs, as well as immunological marker assays permitting the earlier diagnosis of suspected primary or recurrent neoplasms at which time existing conventional treatments would have a greater likelihood of success because of a smaller tumor burden. Moreover, the specific immunological reagents developed against tumor-associated markers could lead to a more detailed biochemical and molecular characterization of tumor antigens, and possibly provide further insight into their relationship to CNS oncogenesis, growth, and progression. The study of membrane surface antigens may provide clues regarding the influence of these antigens upon cell-cell recognition, interaction, and immunosurveillance. Similarly, the characterization of nuclear antigens may help elucidate the underlying processes of genetic regulation and organization.

This chapter addresses the advances achieved in identifying and characterizing brain tumor-associated antigens. In the interests of brevity, the polyclonal and monoclonal reagents generated so far by various laboratories working in the field have been concisely presented in tabular form, and some of their distinctive and potentially useful reactivites have been summarized graphically. The strategies and limitations of immunological as well as direct biochemical identification are discussed, and additional novel genetic approaches are proposed.

Polyclonal Reagents

The earliest attempts to identify glioblastoma antigens were those of Siris and Hass who prepared antisera against an alcohol extract of glioblastoma tissue and a solubilized glioblastoma homogenate, respectively.[50,122] In each case, however, substantial reactivity was present against normal brain antigens. The use of autogenous glioma implants to stimulate patients' immunological response against their own tumors was also unsuccessful in generating reactive sera.[13,47] However, the pioneering clinical studies of Mahaley and colleagues demonstrated that radioiodinated rabbit antihuman glioma antibodies infused in the internal carotid artery could localize preferentially to recurrent glioma cells as measured in tissue fractions, autoradiography, and external brain scans.[35,79,80] This provided considerable impetus to develop other polyclonal reagents which could potentially identify brain tumor markers and thus aid in diagnosis, screening for recurrence, and hopefully immunotherapy, particularly at a time when other laboratories were reporting altered cell-mediated immunity in CNS tumor patients and the possible existence of blocking factors.[19,70]

An early and novel approach involved autoimmunization of patients with saline extracts of their own gliomas to produce human antiglioblastoma sera which detected an alpha-lipoproteinous carcino-fetal glial antigen (CFGA) which, however, was subsequently found to be also present in fetal brain (Table 1).[127,128] The preparation of rabbit heteroantisera against lyophilized glioblastoma tissue and an astrocytoma line #301, which after extensive absorptions possessed little or no cross-reactivities against normal cells, yet reacted with a very high percentage of glioma or astrocytoma lines, lent support to the possibility of tumor-specific markers.[29,130] The existence of glioma-specific membrane antigens and a human astrocytoma-associated antigen (HAAA) was thus proposed (Table 1).[29,32,130]

However, rabbit antisera made in other laboratories against glioma extracts or homogenates cross-reacted with normal fetal brain

Table 1
Brain Tumor-Associated Antigens

Antigen or Polyclonal Antibody	Immunogen	Type of Polyclonal Reagent	Assays
CFGA (carcino-fetal glial antigen)	Autoimmunization of patients with saline extracts of own tumor	Human antisera	DID, absorptions
HAAA (human astrocytoma-associated antigen)	Cells of astrocytoma line 301	Rabbit heteroantiserum (absorbed × 4 with AB)	Dye exclusion cytotoxicity, absorptions
Glioma-specific membrane antigens	Lyophilized glioblastoma tissue (one tumor)	Rabbit heteroantisera	IIF, DID, absorptions
Glioblastoma-associated antigen	Saline extracts of glioblastoma	Rabbit heteroantisera	DID, IEP, absorptions
Meningioma-associated embryonic antigen	Saline extract of 8–10 wk. embryonic brain	Rabbit heteroantisera	DID, IEP, absorptions
Glioblastoma/reactive glia-associated antigen "G" Astrocytoma-associated antigen "A"	NA	Sera from patients	IIF, absorptions
Malignant glial tumor-associated antigen(s)	NA	Sera from glioma patients	IIF, absorptions
Human brain tumor cell surface antigens	Glioma tissue homogenate & sediment	Rabbit heteroantisera	MHA, Ouchterlony, absorptions
Lack of glioblastoma- or meningioma-associated antigens	Triton X-100/sodium barbital extracts of glioblastoma & meningioma tissue	Rabbit heteroantisera	Absorptions, quantitative IEP
HB (human brain) antigen	Homogenate of fetal brain (14 wk. gestation)	Rabbit heteroantiserum	IIF, indirect RIA, absorptions
CGSA (complex glia specific antigen)	Adult rat brain homogenate	Rabbit heteroantisera	IIF, absorptions
Brain tumor surface antigens	NA	Autologous patients' sera	IIF
Medulloblastoma TSA (tumor-associated surface antigens)	Medulloblastoma (BC) tissue cells	Rabbit heteroantisera	Immunocytoadhesion (rosette formation), absorptions
A.C. & B.C. (class I) astrocytoma antigens	NA	Autologous human sera	MHA, IA, anti-C3-MHA, protein A assay, absorptions

Detected by Polyclonal Reagents

Molecular Identification	Neoplastic Cells Present in	Normal Cells Cross-Reactive With	Laboratory
Lipoprotein (alpha-1-mobility)	7/7 G, 4/4 A, 0/2 MN, 0/2 E tumor extracts	Fetal brain	Trouillas, 1971; Trouillas, 1972
ND	7/7 A, 0/3 MN lines; 2/2 A tissue homogenates	None detected after absorptions	Coakham, 1974; Coakham & Lakshmi, 1975
ND	15/15 G lines (3 IIF patterns)	None detected after absorptions	Wahlstrom et al., 1974
Beta-mobility	13/16 G, 2/2 A, 0/3 MN, 0/2 neurinoma saline tissue extracts	Embryonic brain (8–10 wk.)	Kehayov, 1976
ND	5/6 MN, 0/16 G, 0/2 A, 0/2 neurinoma saline tissue extracts	Embryonic brain (8–10 wk.)	Kehayov et al., 1976
ND	7/7 sera on G (3 lines), 6/7 sera on A (1 line) cultures for "G" antigen	6/7 sera on a reactive glial line; 3/3 healthy donor sera also reactive with G cultures	Solheid et al., 1976
ND	2/17 sera for autologous surface antigens, 5/21 sera for autologous cytoplasmic antigens, & 10/21 sera for allogeneic cytoplasmic antigens of G cells	None with normal brain tissue	Sheikh et al., 1977
ND	5/5 G, 3/3 MN, 2/2 A, 2/2 E, 2/2 neurinomas, 1/1 OL cultures	Fetal brain, HeLa cells	Miyake et al., 1977
ND	Glioblastoma & meningioma tissue extracts	Adult liver (yet not in AB or FB)	Dittmann et al., 1977
ND	2/2 N lines, 6/6 N tissues, 0/22 leukemic blasts, one embryonal rhabdomyosarcoma line	5–10% of normal PBL, 0/7 thymocytes	Casper et al., 1977
ND	10/10 G, 5/5 A, 8/8 OL, 2/2 anaplastic G, 1/1 Sch, 0/6 MN tissues	AB (esp. astrocytes)	Lach & Weinrauder, 1978
ND	9/14 G, 2/9 A, 1/1 E, 2/2 SR, 0/6 MN tissues or cultures	ND	Boker, 1978
ND	3/3 MB, 1/1 OL, 1/1 E, 1/3 G, 0/3 A, 0/2 MN fresh tissue cells	None detected after absorptions (FB & fetal tissues not tested)	Sato et al., 1978
ND	Autologous A.C. & B.C. astrocytoma cells only	None detected (including in FB & a normal glial line TF), except autologous fibroblasts (A.C. only)	Pfreundschuh et al., 1978

Table 1

Antigen or Polyclonal Antibody	Immunogen	Type of Polyclonal Reagent	Assays
AJ-aut (class II) astrocytoma antigen	NA	Autologous human sera	MHA, IA, anti-C3-MHA, protein A assay, absorptions
CGA (common glioma antigen), GEA (glioembryonic antigen)	NA	Patients' peripheral blood lymphocytes	Lymphocyte-mediated microcytotoxicity, monolayer absorptions
Glioma-associated specificities M5-30, M5-2	Glioma line U-251 MG	Primate (Macaca fascicularis) antisera	^{14}C-nicotinamide release microcytotoxicity, absorptions
ONA (onconeural antigen)	Cells from neuroblastoma line LA-N-1	Rabbit heteroantisera	^{131}I-SPA, absorptions
Native glioma antigens	NA	Patients' sera & peripheral blood leucocytes	IIF, leucocyte adherence inhibition (LAI) assay
FONA-1, FONA-2 (fetal onconeural antigens)	First trimester fetal brain tissue	Rabbit heteroantiserum	^{131}I-SPA, absorptions
Glioma-associated membrane antigens	Triton X100 extract of plasma membranes from glioma tissue (for rabbit immunizations)	Rabbit heteroantisera, Ig fraction of glioma patients' sera	EM, SDS-PAGE, DID, counter current electrophoresis, absorptions
Glioma-associated antigen N.A.	NA	Autologous patients' sera	Microcytotoxicity, IA, absorptions
Restricted glioma-associated antigen	Membrane-enriched fractions of glioma line LN-18	Rabbit heteroantiserum	^{51}Cr-release cytotoxicity, absorptions
AJ-nat astrocytoma-related antigen	NA	Serum from healthy, nontransfused male donor 537	IA, anti-C3-MHA, protein A assay, absorptions
Tumor-associated antigen(s)	NA	Autologous patients' sera	Microcytotoxicity

The reported polyclonal and monoclonal reagents are summarized in chronological order, including their reactivities in neoplastic as well as normal cells. All lines and tissues are of human origin unless indicated otherwise. The designation x/y indicates x lines or tissues positive out of y tested.

G = glioma/glioblastoma; A = astrocytoma; N = neuroblastoma; R = retinoblastoma; E = ependymoma; MB = medulloblastoma; MN = meningioma; M = melanoma; Sch = schwannoma; SR = sarcoma; OL = oligodendroglioma; PNET = primitive neuroectodermal tumor; PBL = peripheral blood lymphocytes; RBC = red blood cells; AB = adult brain; FB = fetal brain; Kd = kilodaltons; MHA = mixed

(*continued*)

Molecular Identification	Neoplastic Cells Present in	Normal Cells Cross-Reactive With	Laboratory
ND, yet serologically related to AH, a GD2 ganglioside	14/14 A, 6/9 M, 2/2 N, 3/3 SR lines	None detected (including in FB & a normal glial line TF)	Pfreundschuh et al., 1978; Watanabe et al., 1982
ND	All cultures of glial tumors (CGA); anaplastic glioma & melanoma cultures (GEA)	Fetal glial cells (GEA)	Levy, 1978
ND	7/12 G (M5-30), 3/11 G (M5-2), 0/2 MN, 0/2 M, 0/2 N lines	None detected after absorptions with AB & FB	Wikstrand & Bigner, 1979
ND	Homogenates of 10/10 N, 7/7 Wilms' tumor, 5/8 SR, 2/3 oat cell carcinoma, 1/6 M tissues	Adult brain & adrenal	Seeger et al., 1979
ND	3 M KCl extracts of G, MN, pituitary adenoma by LAI	Adult brain	Sheikh et al., 1979; Apuzzo et al., 1981
ND	FONA-1: Homogenates of 10/12 N, 1/1 leiomyosarcoma tissues & many other tumor tissues to a lesser extent	First trimester fetal brain	Danon et al., 1980
70 Kd, 55 Kd, 30 Kd, 10 Kd	Extracts of 20/20 G tissues	None detected (including in AB & FB) after absorptions	Birkmayer & Stass, 1980
ND	10/13 G, 3/6 MN, M, N cultures	Fetal brain & fibroblasts (22 wk. gestation)	Coakham et al., 1980
ND	7/16 G lines (after absorption with M lines), 4/7 G lines (after absorption with AB)	None detected after absorptions (including one with FB cells)	Schnegg et al., 1981
ND	7/7 A, 4/6 M, 2/2 N, 1/1 SR, 1/2 renal cancer, 1/1 cervical cancer lines	Fetal brain	Pfreundschuh et al., 1982
ND	Cultured glioma lines	None detected (autologous fibroblast cultures tested)	Kornblith et al., 1983

hemadsorption assay; SPA = Staphylococcal protein A assay; RIA = radioimmunoassay; IA = immune adherence assay; IIF = indirect immunofluorescence; IEP = immunoelectrophoresis; wk. = week; sup. = supernatant; PEG = polyethylene glycol; PAP = peroxidase anti-peroxidase immunohistochemical technique; NA = not applicable; ND = not determined; C3 = 3rd component of complement; DID = double immunodiffusion; SDS-PAGE = sodium dodecyl sulfate polyacrylamide gel electrophoresis; Ig = immunoglobulin; EM = electron microscopy; ENU = ethylnitrosourea. This table is based on reference 42.

or adult liver.[40,60,87] Rabbit heteroantisera specific for medulloblastoma tumor-associated surface antigens (TSA) were also reported, but these sera were not adequately tested against fetal brain as well as other fetal tissues.[105] Nevertheless, later preparations of rabbit antisera generated against membranes of glioma tissue and a glioma line still reacted with glioma cells after absorptions with normal tissues including brain,[11,109] and identified strong candidates for glioma-related polypeptides at 70, 55, 30, and 10 kilodaltons.[11] Moreover, two nonhuman primate antisera made against a glioma line still reacted with 7/12 and 3/11 glioma cell lines respectively, following adult and fetal brain absorptions, thereby suggesting the possible existence of glioma-associated specificities distinct from normal brain determinants.[134]

The study of the reactivities of patients' sera and peripheral blood lymphocytes against their own tumor cells and tumor lines revealed immunological responses against glioma and/or astrocytoma cells by a wide variety of assays including indirect immunofluorescence,[15,115,123] mixed hemadsorption, immune adherence, and protein A assays,[97] lymphocyte-mediated cytotoxicity,[74] leukocyte adherence inhibition,[5,116] and microcytotoxicity.[31,67] Some of these assays also demonstrated cross-reactivities with autologous fibroblasts, adult brain, or fetal brain and tissues (Table 1). Part of the difficulty lay in the considerable number and quantity of antigens that normal and malignant brain tissue share in common. Thus, for example, when fetal brain was used as the immunogen, the rabbit antisera readily detected antigens in a high percentage of neuroblastoma cells (Table 1).[28,33]

Nevertheless, the analysis of autologous reactivities permitted an elegant classification of cultured astrocytoma cell surface antigens into at least three classes using the sera of 30 astrocytoma patients.[97] Class I antigens, such as those identified by the sera of patients A.C. and B.C., could be detected only on autologous astrocytoma cells, whereas the far more common class III antigens were found to be broadly distributed on normal and neoplastic cells by astrocytoma patients' sera. Class II astrocytoma cell surface antigens such as AJ-aut were present on astrocytomas as well as shared by some neuroblastoma and melanoma cells. AJ-aut (for AJ-autologous antibody) was subsequently shown to be closely related serologically to the human melanoma antigen AH, a probable GD2 ganglioside,[133] and has a counterpart antigen AJ-nat (for AJ-natural antibody) detected by certain healthy donor sera.[98] These cell-surface determinants shared by cells of neuroectodermal origin, first detected with polyclonal reagents, would soon be confirmed with monoclonal antibodies (Table 2) on a broad variety of neural crest-derived tumors.

In part due to complex cross-reactivities, possible heterogeneity in antigenic expression, and the large number of related antigens identified by xenogeneic immunization, polyclonal serologic methodologies have not been able to clearly define a single glioma-specific antigen to date. However, the difference between an "absolute" specificity and a "therapeutically functional" specificity which can be exploited clinically in a particular patient may be most pertinent to the above serologic analysis. Perhaps one can disregard an immunological reagent's cross-reactivities with fetal brain and with other tumor cells, if in the clinical setting it is functionally specific for a patient with a single tumor type and does not bind to adult brain or to other normal tissues.

Monoclonal Reagents

With the development of hybridoma technology[65] yielding potentially unlimited quantities of monoclonal antibodies secreted by indefinitely proliferating hybrid lines, a new era was envisioned in the investigation of tumor antigens. It was hoped that carefully screened monoclonal antibodies, synthesized by a clonal population originating from one antibody-producing cell (and thus directed against a single antigenic determinant), would be able to overcome the complexities of antigenic cross-reactivities previously detected by polyclonal serologic analysis. Furthermore, it was hoped that monoclonal reagents would aid in deciphering interspecies brain antigens such as INMA (interspecies neural membrane antigens)[1] and MBA–2 (mouse brain antigen-2),[83] and would shed light on the possible transformation-associated changes in the expression of various nervous system-specific proteins such as S–100[54,88,89] neuron-specific enolase 14-3-2,[14,81,90] the astroglial-marker glial fibrillary acidic protein GFAP,[8,36,41] alpha-2 glycoprotein (NSA3 or hyaluronectin),[37,46,132] and the neuron-marker neurofilament polypeptides.[72,106] Moreover, it was hoped that analysis with monoclonal antibodies would help unravel the potential immunological role of lymphocyte subpopulations that infiltrate gliomas in effecting an immunosuppression from within an environment of partial immunological privilege.[4] Using OKT and Leu monoclonal antibodies as reagents in flow cy-

Table 2
Brain Tumor-Associated Antigens

Antigen or Monoclonal Antibody	Immunogen	Type of Monoclonal Reagent	Assays
PI 153/3	Cells of neuroblastoma line IMR6	Murine hybridoma sup. & ascites	Microcytotoxicity, indirect RIA, absorptions
PI 125/10	Cells of neuroblastoma line IMR6	Murine hybridoma sup. & ascites	Microcytotoxicity, indirect RIA, absorptions
R_{24}	Cells of melanoma line SK-MEL-28	Murine hybridoma sup. & sera from tumor-bearing nu/nu mice	MHA, absorptions
19-19	Cells of melanoma line SW 691	Murine hybridoma sup.	Indirect RIA, MHA, absorptions
Nu4B	Cells from SW 691 x mouse fibroblast IT 22 somatic cell hybrid (691-I-5-Nu)	Murine hybridoma sup.	Indirect RIA, MHA, absorptions
7.51 and 7.60	Cells of melanoma line CaCL 78-1	Murine hybridoma sup.	MHA, absorptions
BF7 and GE2	Cells of glioma line LN-18	Murine hybridoma sup.	Indirect RIA, absorptions, immunoprecipitation
CG12	Cells of glioma line LN-18	Murine hybridoma sup.	Indirect RIA, absorptions
165	Cultured melanoma cells	Murine hybridoma sup.	Indirect ^{131}I-labeled SPA, absorptions
376	Cultured melanoma cells	Murine hybridoma sup.	Indirect ^{131}I-labeled SPA, absorptions
4D2cl 6	Homogenate of 20 wk. gestation fetal brain	Murine hybridoma sup. & ascites	Cell surface indirect RIA, ^{14}C-nicotinamide release cytotoxicity, PAP, IIF, absorptions
7H10cl 4	Homogenate of 20 wk. gestation fetal brain	Murine hybridoma sup. & ascites	Cell surface indirect RIA, ^{14}C-nicotinamide release cytotoxicity, PAP, IIF, absorptions
1H8cl 2	20 wk. gestation fetal brain homogenate	Murine hybridoma sup. & ascites	Cell surface indirect RIA, ^{14}C-nicotinamide release cytotoxicity, PAP, IIF, absorptions
1H8cl 3	20 wk. gestation fetal brain homogenate	Murine hybridoma sup. & ascites	Cell surface indirect RIA, ^{14}C-nicotinamide release cytotoxicity, PAP, IIF, absorptions

Detected by Monoclonal Antibodies

Molecular Identification	Neoplastic Cells Present In	Normal Cells Cross-Reactive With	Laboratory
ND	6/6 N, 1/2 R, 1/1 G cell lines	Large amounts in FB; small amounts in AB, fetal spleen, null ALL, some B-ALL & normal B cells	Kennett & Gilbert, 1979; Kennett et al., 1980
ND	6/6 N, 1/2 R, 1/1 G cell lines; hepatoma SKHep-1, fibrosarcoma HT1080, lymphoblastoid SCBM cell lines	Fetal fibroblast line IMR90	Kennett & Gilbert, 1979
Glycolipid determinants	16/16 M, 2/5 A lines	Weak reactivity with adult brain and melanocytes	Dippold et al., 1980
ND	31/44 M cell lines & early cultures; 4/7 A (RIA), 1/2 A (MHA) lines	None detected	Herlyn et al., 1980
ND	45/46 M cell lines & early cultures; 6/7 A (RIA), 1/2 A (MHA) lines	1/4 normal fibroblast lines by RIA & MHA	Herlyn et al., 1980
ND	8/8 M, 3/3 N, 4-5/5 G, 4-5/5 R lines; 3/3 M & 2/2 R tissues	Fetal brain	Liao et al., 1981
48 Kd	49-55/62 G, 3-4/10 MN, 2/2 Sch, 1-2/11 M, 0-1/2 MB lines	Normal reactive astrocytes, colon carcinoma line Lovo	Schnegg et al., 1981b; de Tribolet et al., 1984
ND	28/62 G, 10/11 M, 2/3 N, 1/2 MB, 1/2 Sch, 2/10 MN lines	Adult and fetal brain (FB > AB)	Schnegg et al., 1981b; de Tribolet et al., 1984
ND	3/4 M, 2/3 G, 1/4 SR, 0/10 N cell lines	Fetal lung, kidney, colon, muscle	Seeger et al., 1981
ND	2/4 M, 3/3 G, 3/4 SR, 4/10 N cell lines	Adult lung; fetal liver, lung, kidney, colon, muscle	Seeger et al., 1981
ND	5/14 G, 1/2 M, 1/3 N, 0/1 MB lines by RIA; 13/13 G, 1/1 N tissues by PAP	1/5 fetal fibroblast lines by RIA; adult spleen & fetal brain, liver, spleen by PAP	Wikstrand & Bigner, 1982
ND	13/14 G, 0/2 M, 1/3 N, 1/1 MB lines by RIA; 13/13 G, 1/1 N tissues by PAP	Adult spleen & fetal brain, liver, spleen, thymus by PAP	Wikstrand & Bigner, 1982
ND	7/14 G, 2/3 N, 0/2 M, 1/1 MB lines by RIA; 9/15 G tissues by PAP	2/3 fetal fibroblast lines by RIA; fetal brain & spleen by PAP	Wikstrand et al., 1982
ND	9/14 G, 2/3 N, 1/2 M, 1/1 MB lines by RIA; 12/15 G tissues by PAP	Adult spleen & fetal brain, liver, spleen by PAP	Wikstrand et al., 1982

Table 2

Antigen or Monoclonal Antibody	Immunogen	Type of Monoclonal Reagent	Assays
AJ225	Cells from astrocytoma line SK-MG-1	Murine hybridoma sup. & sera from tumor-bearing nu/nu mice	MHA, absorptions, immunoprecipitation
AO10	Cells from astrocytoma line SK-AO2	Murine hybridoma sup. & tumor-bearing nu/nu mice sera	MHA, absorptions
AJ8	Cells from astrocytoma line SK-MG-1	Murine hybridoma sup. & tumor-bearing nu/nu mice sera	MHA, absorptions
AO122	Cells from astrocytoma line SK-AO2	Murine hybridoma sup. & sera from tumor-bearing nu/nu mice	MHA, absorptions, immunoprecipitation
OFA-I-2 (oncofetal antigen-immunogenic) L72	EBV transformation of PBLs of a melanoma patient	Human B-lymphoblastoid cell line sup. & partially purified IgM fractions	IA, absorptions
Me1-5, Me1-14, Me3-TB7, Me4-F8, Me5-D5	Membrane-enriched fractions from melanoma lines Me-43 or IGR-3	Murine hybridoma sup. & ascites	Indirect RIA, absorptions
G13-C6	Whole cells from glioma line LN-18	Murine hybridoma sup. & ascites	Indirect RIA, absorptions
P-64 peptide, 217c	Rat C6 glioma cells	Murine hybridoma sup.	Direct ^{131}I- & ^{125}I-labeled SPA; immunoprecipitation
LGL1-1C3, LGL1-1C6, LGL1-1D6, LGL7-1A2, LGL10-3B5	PEG fusion of intratumoral (glioma) lymphocytes from patients with human myeloma line LICR-LON-HMy2	Human hybridoma sup.	Indirect RIA
UJ127:11	16 wk. gestation fetal brain homogenate	Murine hybridoma sup. & ascites	IIF, indirect RIA, immunoprecipitation, absorptions
UJ13A	16 wk. gestation fetal brain homogenate	Murine hybridoma ascites	Indirect RIA, IIF, absorptions

(*continued*)

Molecular Identification	Neoplastic Cells Present In	Normal Cells Cross-Reactive With	Laboratory
145 Kd	16/16 A, 1/10 M, 2/4 renal carcinoma, 1/17 epithelial cancer, T-cell leukemia MOLT-4 cell lines	Melanocytes	Cairncross et al., 1982
ND	7/16 A, 3/10 M, 2/2 N, 2/17 epithelial cancer, T-cell leukemia MOLT-4 cell lines	Adult & fetal brain	Cairncross et al., 1982
ND	9/16 A, 4/10 M, 0/2 N, 4/17 epithelial cancer cell lines	Melanocytes; adult & fetal skin fibroblasts	Cairncross et al., 1982
265 Kd	9/16 A, 8/10 M, 0/2 N cell lines	Adult & fetal brain; melanocytes; adult & fetal skin fibroblasts	Cairncross et al., 1982
Cell surface glycolipid ganglioside GD2	16/26 M, 6/8 G, 5/8 N cell lines	Fetal brain	Irie et al., 1982; Cahan et al., 1982
Protein determinants abolished by trypsin, unaffected by tunicamycin or neuraminidase	Ranging from 10/12–12/12 (11/11) M, 12/30–23/36 (18/28) A, & 1/3–3/3 N cell lines	None detected (Me5-D5 not tested with FB)	Carrel et al., 1982; de Tribolet et al., 1984
Trypsin-sensitive protein determinant as above	8/9 M, 9/13 G, 1/3 N cell lines	Fetal brain	Carrel et al., 1982
64 Kd	1/1 human glial tumor line; C6 rat glioma cells; ENU-induced transformed rat oligodendrocytes; spontaneously transformed rat astrocytes; two rodent hepatoma lines (weak binding)	Weak binding to a primary rat hepatocyte line & rat liver tissue	Peng et al., 1982; Luner & de Vellis, 1986
ND	1/1 G, 1/1 colon carcinoma, & 1-2/2 lung carcinoma lines; positive radiolocalization with 1D6 of recurrent G in patient	None detected in PBL, RBC, or fibroblasts, except weak binding of 1D6 & 1A2 to PBL and fibroblasts/RBC, respectively (AB & FB not tested)	Sikora et al., 1982, 1983, 1985; Phillips et al., 1982, 1983; Sikora, 1984
220–240 Kd glycoprotein	10/10 Sch, 8/10 MB, 8/8 N, 1/40 G, 0/18 A, 0/8 M, 0/14 E, 0/6 OL, 0/16 MN, 0/3 PNET tissues	AB, FB, kidney tubules, adrenal medulla, esophagus & colon nerve fiber plexi	Kemshead et al., 1983; Garson et al., 1985; Coakham et al., 1985
ND	40/40 G, 18/18 A, 14/14 E, 6/6 OL, 10/10 Sch, 14/16 MN, 10/10 MB, 8/8 N, 3/3 PNET, 0/8 M tissues; positive radiolocalization of tumors in 3/5 patients	AB, FB, adrenal medulla, nerve fiber plexi, optic & peripheral nerves, adult thyroid epithelium, fetal kidney tubules, primary cultures of fetal myoblasts, cerebellum of many mammals	Allan et al., 1983; Garson et al., 1985; Coakham et al., 1985; Davies et al., 1985

Table 2

Antigen or Monoclonal Antibody	Immunogen	Type of Monoclonal Reagent	Assays
GMEM (glioma-mesenchymal extracellular matrix antigen), 81C6	Cell suspensions of glioma line U-251 MG	Murine hybridoma sup. & ascites	Cell surface indirect RIA, IIF, PAP, absorptions, immunoprecipitation
M148	Homogenate of medulloblastoma tissue	Murine hybridoma ascites	IIF, immunoprecipitation
GMEM-related antigen 2A6	Medulloblastoma-derived line TE-671	Murine hybridoma sup. & ascites	Avidin-biotin-peroxidase

The reported polyclonal and monoclonal reagents are summarized in chronological order, including their reactivities in neoplastic as well as normal cells. All lines and tissues are of human origin unless indicated otherwise. The designation x/y indicates x lines or tissues positive out of y tested.

G = glioma/glioblastoma; A = astrocytoma; N = neuroblastoma; R = retinoblastoma; E = ependymoma; MB = medulloblastoma; MN = meningioma; M = melanoma; Sch = schwannoma; SR = sarcoma; OL = oligodendroglioma; PNET = primitive neuroectodermal tumor; PBL = peripheral blood lymphocytes; RBC = red blood cells; AB = adult brain; FB = fetal brain;

tometric immunofluorescence and immunoperoxidase methods has already revealed a relative suppressor-cytotoxic T lymphocyte predominance in peripheral blood as well as in tumor parenchyma of glioma patients.[68,129] This may help explain, in part, the depression of cell-mediated immunity and the possible presence of blocking factors reported earlier in patients with intracranial tumors.[19,70]

However, the results of numerous monoclonal antibody studies (Table 2) have largely supported the earlier findings with polyclonal antibodies of antigens common to cells of neuroectodermal origin. Many of the antiglioma or anti-astrocytoma monoclonal antibodies such as CG12, AO10, and G13-C6 possessed broad reactivities against glioma, melanoma, and neuroblastoma cells, as well as fetal brain (Table 2).[24,27,38,110] For example, the reactivity profiles of two out of four different anti-astrocytoma murine monoclonals (AO10 and AJ8) are very similar in their binding to astrocytoma, melanoma, and epithelial cancer lines (Fig. 1).[24] AO10 and AO122 also cross-reacted

(continued)

Molecular Identification	Neoplastic Cells Present In	Normal Cells Cross-Reactive With	Laboratory
230 Kd (210 Kd minor band) glycoprotein	14/16 G, 1/7 M, 1/3 N, 2/6 SR lines by RIA; 10/11 G, 1/6 A, 4/4 M, 2/2 fibrosarcoma, 1/1 Wilms' tumor, 1/1 ovarian carcinoma tissues by PAP; positive radiolocalization of G line in athymic mice & rats	8/9 fetal & adult fibroblast lines; adult kidney, spleen, liver; fetal spleen & liver; mesenchymal cells	Bourdon et al., 1983, 1984; McComb & Bigner, 1985; Bullard et al., 1986
130 Kd & 110 Kd glycoproteins IIb/IIIa in platelet membranes	2/3 N lines; 4/6 MB, 1/2 N, 4/4 Ewing SR, 3/3 rhabdomyosarcoma, 1/1 hepatoblastoma, 1/1 teratocarcinoma tissues	Platelets & megakaryocytes (brain not tested)	Jones et al., 1984
ND	9/10 G, 1/4 MB tissues	Mesenchymal cells	McComb & Bigner, 1985

Kd = kilodaltons; MHA = mixed hemadsorption assay; SPA = Staphylococcal protein A assay; RIA = radioimmunoassay; IA = immune adherence assay; IIF = indirect immunofluorescence; IEP = immunoelectrophoresis; wk. = week; sup. = supernatant; PEG = polyethylene glycol; PAP = peroxidase antiperoxidase immunohistochemical technique; NA = not applicable; ND = not determined; C3 = 3rd component of complement; DID = double immunodiffusion; SDS-PAGE = sodium dodecyl sulfate polyacrylamide gel electrophoresis; Ig = immunoglobulin; EM = electron microscopy; ENU = ethylnitrosourea; nu/nu = nude. This table is based on reference 42.

with fetal and adult brain (Table 2). Nevertheless, astrocytoma determinants were clearly present since several of the murine monoclonals were capable of immunoprecipitating proteins from labeled astrocytoma cell extracts; AJ225 and AO122 precipitated 145 and 265 Kd polypeptides, respectively.[24]

The nature of the immunogen appeared immaterial to the outcome of the reactivity profile. When 20-week gestation fetal brain (for 4D2cl 6 and 1H8cl 3) or membranes from melanoma lines (for Me1-5, Me1-14, Me3-TB7, Me4-F8, and Me5-D5) served as the sensitizing immunogen in murine hybridoma production, the resulting monoclonals also recognized a broad range of neural crest-derived cells, including glioma, melanoma, and neuroblastoma lines (Table 2).[25,27,38,135,137] Shared antigens were also detected in hematopoietic and lymphoid cells (Table 2),[24,63,135] including CALLA,[26,48] HLA-DR,[26] and platelet glycoprotein IIb-IIIa.[56] In retrospect, this brain-hematopoietic cross-reactivity was somewhat more understandable

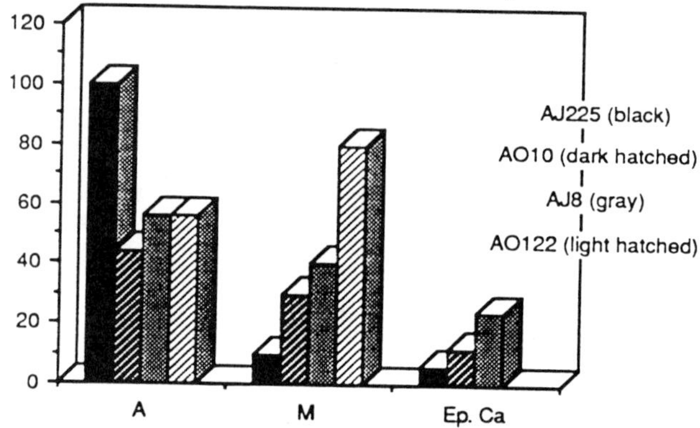

Figure 1. The reactivity profiles of anti-astrocytoma (AJ225, AO10, AJ8, AO122) murine monoclonal antibodies (MAbs) reacting with astrocytoma, melanoma, and epithelial cancer (Ep. Ca) cell lines.[42] The ordinate of the graph is in percentages. A mean of 14.3 cell lines were examined by mixed hemadsorption assay per tumor type. These data were derived from the primary literature referenced in Table 2.

since the Thy-1 antigen had previously been shown to be shared by thymocytes, certain leukemias, and brain.[6,101] The extensive sharing of antigenic determinants by CNS tumor tissue and hematopoietic cells has recently been once again confirmed by indirect immuno-fluorescence using a panel of monoclonal antibodies raised against human hemopoietic cells.[22]

Nevertheless, the anti-astrocytoma monoclonal antibody analysis did yield particularly rewarding dividends concerning astrocyte differentiation. At least nine distinct astrocytoma cell surface antigenic systems were defined, of which two, the determinants AO10 and AJ8, were expressed in a mutually exclusive fashion on the astrocytoma lines examined.[24] Nine out of nine AJ8-positive astrocytoma cell lines were GFAP-negative, whereas over half (57%) of AO10-positive lines also expressed GFAP. Since prior evidence suggested that the expression of GFAP correlated with an increasingly more differentiated state of cells in the astrocyte lineage,[57] it was proposed that AJ8, AO10, and GFAP typing may help to determine whether astrocytic elements were precursor, immature, or mature astrocytes.[24] AJ8$^+$ AO10$^-$ GFAP$^-$ expression would characterize undifferentiated precursors, while an AJ8$^-$ AO10$^+$ GFAP$^+$ antigen typing would identify differentiated mature astrocytes. Intermediate stages would represent in part the approximately 40% of AJ8$^-$ AO10$^+$ lines which were GFAP$^-$. Thus monoclonal antibodies against astrocytoma cell surface antigens have helped not only to classify the antigen systems of these tumor lines, but have also suggested their state of differentiation. A typing scheme such as this to determine differentiation status, if found reliable, could play an important role in neuropathology for the diagnosis and assessment of patient prognosis.

It was also readily apparent that certain monoclonal antibodies possessed distinctive "discordant" reactivities which could offer potential diagnostic benefits as part of an antibody panel. For example, AJ225 was far more "astrocytoma-specific" because of its lower reactivities with melanoma and epithelial cancer lines than the other three anti-astrocytoma monoclonal antibodies (Fig. 1). Conversely, AO122 reacted with 80% of melanoma lines and 0/17 of epithelial cancer lines (Fig. 1). These data immediately suggested that monoclonal reagents, particularly as part of an immunological panel, could specifically differentiate between tumor types as well as between tumor lines and thus provide an initial basis for comparison and subsequent characterization.

Examples of such discordance, which could serve both diagnostic and neuropathological investigations, were searched out among the other reported monoclonal reagents (Table 2, Fig. 2). As in Figure 1 above, the data reported in the primary literature has been summarized in bar graph format by these authors.[42] Murine monoclonals UJ127:11 and UJ13A against fetal brain homogenate were quite disparate in their reactivity profiles to glioma, ependymoma, and meningioma tissues (Fig. 2A). Whereas UJ13A was pan-neuroectodermal (pan-NE) in its reactivity, UJ127:11 was far more restricted and reacted principally with neural tumors, such as medulloblastoma and neuroblastoma, and very infrequently with glioma, ependymoma, or meningioma tissues.[2,30,45,61] UJ13A will most probably have limited clinical application because of its lack of specificity.

Discordance in melanoma reactivity was noted in the antiglioma line monoclonals G13-C6 and 81C6 (Fig. 2B). G13-C6 reacted with a very high percentage (89%) of melanoma lines by RIA, while glial-associated 81C6, which identifies the glioma-mesenchymal extracellular matrix antigen GMEM, reacted with a low percentage (14%) of such melanoma lines by RIA.[17,27] Both monoclonal reagents identified shared neuroectodermal antigens common to glioma and neuroblastoma lines (Fig. 2B). Yet, the cross-reactivity of 81C6 with he-

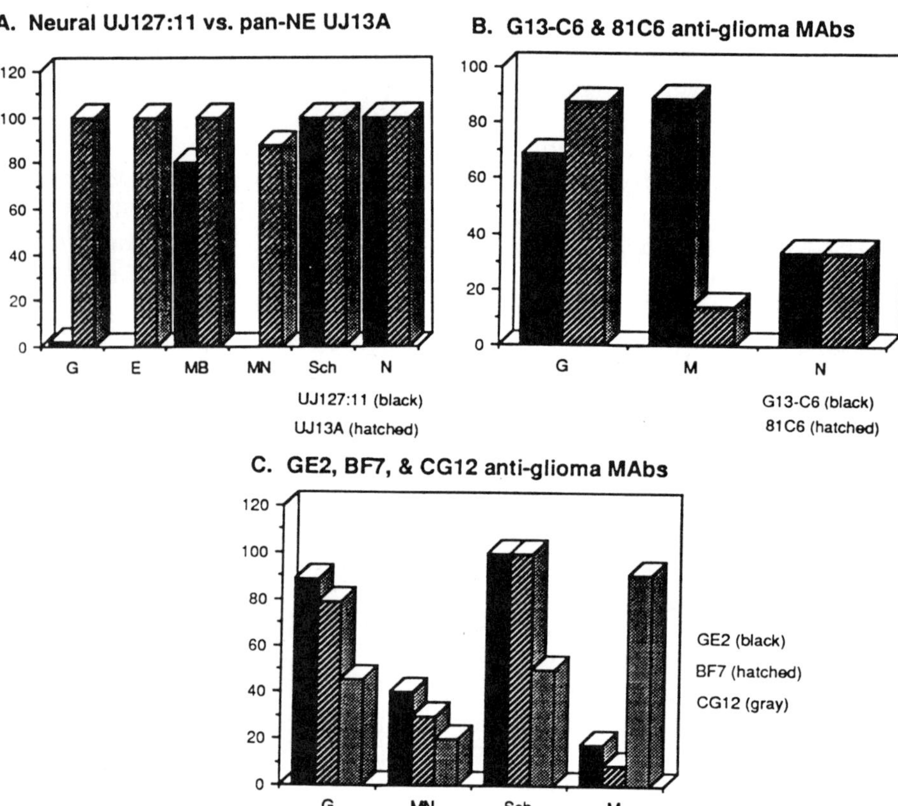

Figure 2. The reactivity profiles of antifetal brain (UJ127:11, UJ13A) and antiglioma (G13-C6, 81C6, GE2, BF7, CG12) murine monoclonal antibodies (MAbs) reacting with different percentages (bar graph ordinate) of a variety of tumor lines or tissues.[42] (A) A mean of 16.3 tissues were examined by indirect RIA, indirect immunofluorescence, or immunoperoxidase techniques per tumor type. (B) A mean of 8.5 lines were tested by indirect RIA per tumor type. (C) A mean of 21.25 lines were examined by indirect RIA per tumor type. The data were derived from the primary literature on these monoclonals referenced in Table 2. The same cell line and tissue abbreviations are employed as in Tables 1 and 2.

patic tissues (Table 2) suggests that liver localization may restrict its clinical usefulness.

Discordance in glial versus melanoma reactivity was also apparent in the antiglioma line monoclonals BF7, GE2, and CG12 (Fig. 2C). Only CG12 identified antigens in a large fraction of melanoma lines; the reactivity profiles of GE2 and BF7 were more "glial-specific" and revealed reactivities with higher percentages of glioma and schwannoma lines.[38,110] Clearly panels of monoclonal antibodies are needed, since "discordant" reactivities may represent the limit of monoclonals' specificity when it comes to highly conserved and shared neuroectodermal and differentiation antigens.

The difference between "absolute" and "therapeutically functional" specificities, as mentioned before, is also very pertinent to the use of monoclonal reagents in the clinical setting. Monoclonal antibodies that are "cross-reactive" with fetal brain and various tumor cells may nevertheless be therapeutically efficacious in a particular patient with a single tumor type, provided that they do not react extensively with normal adult tissues.

Probably the strongest evidence to date for possible glioma-specific tumor markers has come not from human but rather from animal model systems. Monoclonal antibodies have detected antigens apparently specific for chemically induced rat glioma cells.[73,124] Recently, the putatively tumor-specific murine monoclonal 217c raised against C6 rat glioma cells[96] has been shown to immunoprecipitate a 64 Kd polypeptide only from the immunizing C6 rat glioma line and chemically induced oligodendrocyte or spontaneously transformed astrocyte rat lines, yet not from control cell lines.[78] However, the applicability and relevance of data derived from animal cell lines to the clinical setting still needs to be clearly demonstrated.

Cytogenetic Heterogeneity

For decades, investigators have long noted and described the recurrent theme of cytogenetic heterogeneity in tumors of all organ systems, including those of the CNS. A variety of karyotypic abnormalities are found among individual tumors of the same phenotype.[104] Furthermore, individual tumors are often amalgamations of diploid and aneuploid cells with multiple subpopulations of cytogenetically aberrant clones.[114] Cytogenetic heterogeneity is certain to contribute to antigenic differences and thus complicate the quest for reliable tumor markers.

This intratumor heterogeneity is the result of multiple generations of cell division acting in tandem with a variety of other factors in a complex and dynamic fashion. Some of these factors may be the inherently unstable genetic character of neoplastic cells[138] coupled with natural (e.g., nutritional, vascular perfusion, immunosurveillance, etc.) or externally imposed (e.g., chemotherapy, radiation) selective conditions, which even in themselves, may vary from one location to another within the same tumor. A well-known example is that tumor cells in areas of relative hypoxia are more resistant to X-irradiation than cells in areas of adequate oxygenation. This heterogeneity, not surprisingly, often results in tumor progression as the more malignant clones are selected through this dynamic process.[9] This is frequently observed by the coupling of biologically aggressive behavior such as chemotherapy resistance and increased metastatic potential, with the appearence of ever increasing chromosomal abnormalities and histological pleomorphism.

A number of specific chromosomal abnormalities are frequently seen in primary tumors of the central nervous system.[114] Karyotypic studies of tumors of glial origin often display the presence of "double minute" chromosomes,[69] an overrepresentation of chromosome #7, an underrepresentation of chromosome #10 or #22, and breaks in the short arm of chromosome #9.[10,77] Similarly, studies of meningiomas[82,112] and acoustic neuromas[113] often demonstrate loss of genetic material from chromosome #22. The frequent abnormality seen with chromosome #22 suggests the existence of a common underlying mechanism of oncogenesis among these primary CNS tumor types, perhaps with a deregulative or a permissive role being served by this chromosomal anomaly. New, or previously repressed antigens may be thus expressed.

The presence of "double minute" chromosomes or multiple copies of chromosome #7 suggests that gene dosage or gene amplification plays an important role, possibly in conjunction with oncogenes.[12,51,108] These not only may have a causative relationship in the oncogenesis of gliomas, but may also confer a selective advantage as well. Indeed, investigators have demonstrated amplification of the cellular oncogene *c-myc* in the "double minute" chromosomes of a human glioblastoma-derived cell line.[126] Moreover, a novel cellular gene, termed *gli* and located on chromosome #12, has recently been found to be highly amplified and transcribed in a malignant glioma and its derived cell line, each of which contained numerous double minute chromosomes.[64] The locus of the epidermal growth factor receptor has also been mapped to chromosome #7[66] and aberrant receptor kinase activity[76] has been shown to occur.

As more information becomes available about the human genome[58] and as the tools of molecular biology become increasingly more powerful,[7] understanding CNS neoplastic processes will be based on ever more fundamental principles. Biochemical and genetic dissection of CNS tumors will serve as a basis for understanding and advancing the therapy for this devastating disease.

The Immunological Approach and its Limitations

There are several underlying premises basic to the immunological approach which must be met in order for it to succeed. First, the tumor marker must be consistently associated with the brain neoplasm, either because the marker is unique to the transformed cells or is present in greater abundance in them as compared to normal brain. Second, the marker must be sufficiently antigenic for the current methods of developing polyclonal and monoclonal antibodies to be successful. This may be a problem when dealing with low abundance, sequestered, cell-cycle specific, or lipid-associated antigens. These factors, coupled with the likely immunocompromised state of patients with a malignancy and the potential difficulty in antigen presentation both due to the blood-brain barrier and the absence of a CNS lymphatic system, may account for only a small minority of glioma patients developing a measurable humoral response against their neoplasm.[84] Immunosurveillance and effector arm function may also be less efficient in "immunologically privileged sites" such as the brain.[86] Third, there are technical difficulties such as the separation of blood elements and endothelium from the tumor tissue preparation. This problem can be circumvented in part by the use of tumor cell tissue culture lines which are composed of relatively homogeneous cell populations. The advantage of using a tumor cell line must be weighed against the observation that cells in culture may express antigens differently, both qualitatively and quantitatively, than cells in vivo. This is especially problematic with tissue culture lines of high passage number. Fourth, the developed immunological reagents must be monospecific, high-titered, and possess high affinity association constants. Monoclonality does not rule out cross-reactivity.[18] A monoclonal antibody, which for example exquisitely binds to an epitope within a domain common to many cellular proteins, would be extensively cross-reactive and thus not useful because of its lack of specificity. Moreover, a particular antibody species may bind to several dissimilar antigenic determinants, a property termed "linked specificities."[102] Fifth, the above approach, although promising, depends upon a reliable and clinically convenient delivery system.[21] Although the blood-brain barrier (BBB) appears to be somewhat permeable in the vicinity of the tumor as evidenced by contrast enhancement on CT scans, it may nevertheless prove to be a formidable deterrent to the delivery of antibodies. The data from many clinical studies may be obscured by limitations in the delivery system. Modification of the blood-brain barrier, intra-arterial therapy, and use of conjugated Fab immunoglobulin fragments may help overcome this obstacle.[94] Difficulty in interpretation of clinical results may be compounded by the host's generation of anti-antibodies as well as the interaction of immunoglobulins with immune modifiers such as the endogenous interleukins. Finally, it should be pointed out that many normal brain proteins are highly antigenic since they are relatively isolated from the immune system by the blood-brain barrier. Consequently, any efforts to raise a high-titered antibody against a CNS-associated tumor is liable to lead to cross-reaction with normal brain tissue resulting in an autoimmune allergic encephalitis.[95]

A number of factors may have contributed to the lack of tumor type specificity exhibited by the reported monoclonal reagents (Table 2). First, a large number and amount of cellular constituents, particularly structural ones, are commonly shared. Murine hybridoma production against human antigens involves xenogeneic immunization which can emphasize antibody manufacture against certain common cell surface components. In part, this problem, as well as that of patients producing antibodies against murine immunoglobulins, can be solved by developing human hybridomas.[117-120] Secondly, some of the complexities detected in monoclonal as well as polyclonal serologic analysis may have arisen from the marked phenotypic heterogeneity of human glioma lines and their cell subpopulations.[125,136] The development of a stem cell assay system is one potential way to help minimize the effect of cell line heterogeneity in the testing of chemotherapeutic agents.[103] Finally, monoclonality does not rule out cross-reactivity,[18] and the exquisite binding of monoclonal antibodies to a particular epitope is irrelevant if that epitope is part of a common domain shared by many molecules.

Direct Biochemical and Genetic Identification

Due to the complexity and number of proteins present in tumors, and the limitations of protein separation techniques, most workers have chosen to raise antibodies to glioma tissues without attempting to identify and isolate the specific proteins against which these antibodies are directed. Other more direct approaches to identifying tumor-associated antigens are now within the realm of possibility. The introduction and refinement of two-dimensional gel electrophoresis (2DE) and silver staining has resulted in renewed interest in the fingerprinting of proteins in various biological materials.[3] These two-dimensional protein patterns provide not only the molecular weights and isoelectric points of the constituent polypeptides, but also semi-quantitative information on their relative amounts. Using these techniques, normal CNS proteins in rat brain were only recently described.[53] Subsequently, these techniques were applied to normal human brain and demonstrated a fairly constant protein pattern associated with different samples of normal human cerebral cortex.[91] These particular gels displayed proteins with molecular weights ranging from 14 to 100 Kd and isoelectric points of 4.7 to 7.0. Initially, almost none of the over 150 "spots" seen on the gels were known, but using immunoblotting and co-migration techniques several of the major spots have been identified (Fig. 3A).[92] A wide variety of human brain tumors have recently been studied using 2DE, and this investigation has revealed that the different tumor types have fairly characteristic protein patterns which differ substantially from that seen in normal brain.[93] Moreover, application of these techniques has demonstrated large amounts of GFAP in astrocytomas, a prominent vimentin complex in meningiomas, and neuron-specific enolase in medulloblastomas.[93] Of particular significance, characteristic protein profiles were found for high- and low-grade astrocytomas, juvenile astrocytomas, ependymomas, and medulloblastomas, and each tumor profile contained certain polypeptide spots that were not detected or were clearly reduced in normal human cortex (Fig. 3B).[93] Efforts are now underway in our laboratory to isolate these tumor-associated proteins from the malignant astrocytoma gels. The production of polyclonal and monoclonal antibodies against the proteins eluted from these singly excised spots may yield reagents capable of specifically binding certain CNS tumors.

There are several potential limitations associated with the above approach. First, several polypeptides lie outside the molecular weight

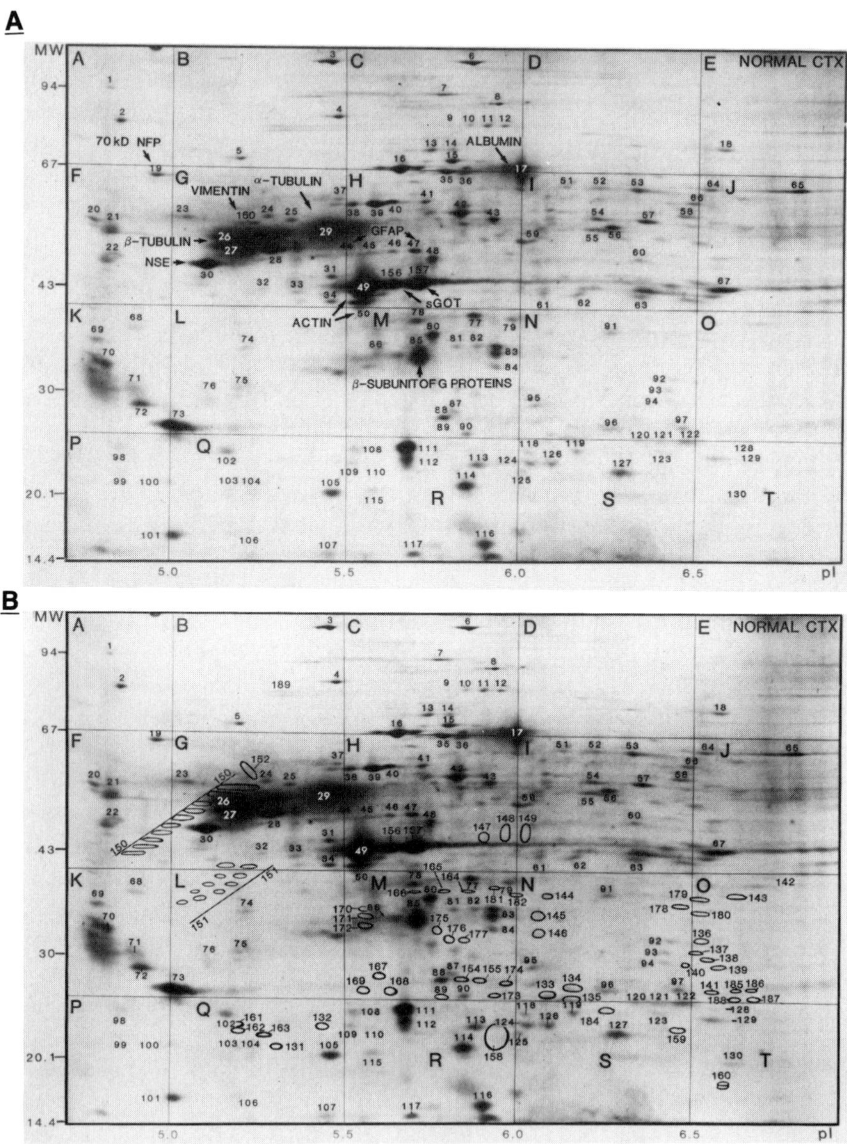

Figure 3. Silver-stained two-dimensional gel of normal human cerebral cortex (A), including polypeptide spots whose identities have been established.[42,92,93] The positions of potential tumor-associated polypeptides (B), identified on gels of astrocytomas, ependymomas, and medulloblastomas, have been superscribed onto the normal gel pattern.[42,92,93]

and pI range that must arbitrarily be chosen for such studies, and thus may escape detection. Second, not all proteins lend themselves to separation by 2DE because of their solubility, charge, or staining characteristics. Third, polypeptides initially identified as possibly tumor-associated may later be found to be present in body organs other than the brain. Finally, several of the tumor-associated proteins may be cytosolic or nuclear in location rather than on the tumor cell surface membrane. While this would obviously limit their usefulness as "target" proteins, they could nevertheless yield important data relating to the metabolism and composition of the tumor.

Another direct approach which could complement the above study would be the cDNA cloning[49] of ribonucleic acid from fresh brain tumor tissue into an efficient expression vector such as lambda-gt 11.[139,140] Using subtraction hybridization or labeled RNA from normal human brain, as well as both seronegative and extensively absorbed antitumor sera, can serve as controls in the screening process to identify potentially unique genetic inserts and their products. Monospecific sera, in turn, can be generated against these genetically dissected products, before returning the investigation to tumor tissue. The genetic dissection of complex antigenic systems by employing recombinant cloning coupled with gene transfer techniques has already proven successful in the unequivocal identification of a transformation-associated nuclear antigen of Epstein-Barr virus.[43,44] Thus, genetic dissection can contribute significantly to the specificity attained by immunological means alone.

Conclusions

The advances made in identifying and characterizing human brain tumor-associated antigens using both polyclonal sera and monoclonal antibodies have been reviewed. In neither case were truly brain tumor-specific antigens documented. Rather, broadly shared neuroectodermal and common differentiation antigens were detected in glioma, astrocytoma, neuroblastoma, melanoma, and hematopoietic cells. Yet, discordant reactivity profiles were noted among certain monoclonal antibodies that would make these reagents potentially useful in tumor diagnosis and therapy, possibly as part of an antibody panel. Attempts at the direct identification of tumor markers using two-dimensional electrophoresis and cDNA cloning are new approaches to address this problem of major biological and clinical significance.

REFERENCES

1. Akeson R, Seeger RC. Interspecies neural membrane antigens on cultured human and murine neuroblastoma cells. J Immunol 1977; 118:1995–2003.
2. Allan PM, Garson JA, Harper EI, et al. Biological characterization and clinical applications of a monoclonal antibody recognizing an antigen restricted to neuroectodermal tissues. Int J Cancer 1983; 31:591–598.
3. Anderson L, Anderson N. Some perspectives on two-dimensional protein mapping. Clin Chem 1984; 30:1898–1905.
4. Apuzzo MLJ, Mitchell MS. Immunological aspects of intrinsic glial tumors. J Neurosurg 1981; 55:1–18.
5. Apuzzo MLJ, Sheikh KMA, Weiss MH, et al. The utilization of native glioma antigen in the assessment of cellular and humoral immune responses in malignant glioma patients. Acta Neurochir 1981; 55:181–200.
6. Barclay AN, Letarte-Muirhead M, Williams AF, et al. Chemical characterization of the Thy–1 glycoproteins from the membranes of rat thymocytes and brain. Nature 1976; 263:563–567.
7. Barlow D, Lehrach H. Genetics by gel electrophoresis: the impact of pulsed field gel electrophoresis on mammalian genetics. TIG 1987; 3:167–171.
8. Bignami A, Eng LF, Dahl D, et al. Localization of the glial fibrillary acidic protein in astrocytes by immunofluorescence. Brain Res 1972; 43:429–435.
9. Bigner D. Biology of gliomas: potential clinical implications of glioma cellular heterogeneity. Neurosurgery 1981; 9:320–326.
10. Bigner S, Friedman H, Biegel J, et al. Specific chromosomal abnormalities characterize four established cell lines derived from malignant human glioma. Acta Neuropathol 1986; 72:86–97.
11. Birkmayer GD, Stass HP. Humoral immune response in glioma patients: a solubilized glioma-associated membrane antigen as a tool for detecting circulating antibodies. Int J Cancer 1980; 25:445–452.
12. Bishop JM. The molecular genetics of cancer. Science 1987; 235: 305–311.
13. Bloom WH, Carstairs KC, Crompton MR, et al. Autologous glioma transplantation. Lancet 1960; 2:77–78.
14. Bock E, Dissing J. Demonstration of enolase activity connected to the brain specific protein 14–3–2. Scand J Immunol 1975; 4(suppl2):31–36.
15. Boker D-K. Zur immunofluoreszenz menschlicher hirntumoren. Acta Neurochir 1978; 41:363–371.
16. Bourdon MA, Coleman RE, Blasberg RG, et al. Monoclonal antibody localization in subcutaneous and intracranial human glioma xenografts: paired-label and imaging analysis. Anticancer Res 1984; 4:133–140.

17. Bourdon MA, Wikstrand CJ, Furthmayr H, et al. Human glioma-mesenchymal extracellular matrix antigen defined by monoclonal antibody. Cancer Res 1983; 43:2796–2805.
18. Brown NA. Prospects for human monoclonal antibodies: a critical perspective. Yale J Biol Med 1982; 55:297–303.
19. Brooks WH, Netsky MG, Normansell DE, et al. Depressed cell-mediated immunity in patients with primary intracranial tumors. J Exp Med 1972; 136:1631–1647.
20. Bullard DE, Adams CJ, Coleman RE, et al. In vivo imaging of intracranial human glioma xenografts comparing specific with nonspecific radiolabaeled monoclonal antibodies. J Neurosurg 1986; 64:257–262.
21. Bullard DE, Bourdon M, Bigner DD. Comparison of various methods for delivering radiolabeled monoclonal antibody to the normal rat brain. J Neurosurg 1984; 61:901–911.
22. Budka H, Majdic O, Knapp W. Cross-reactivity between human hemopoietic cells and brain tumors as defined by monoclonal antibodies. J Neuro-Oncol 1985; 3:173–179.
23. Cahan LD, Irie RF, Singh R, et al. Identification of a human neuroectodermal tumor antigen (OFA-I–2) as ganglioside GD2. Proc Natl Acad Sci USA 1982; 79:7629–7633.
24. Cairncross JG, Mattes MJ, Beresford HR, et al. Cell surface antigens of human astrocytoma defined by mouse monoclonal antibodies: identification of astrocytoma subsets. Proc Natl Acad Sci USA 1982; 79:5641–5645.
25. Carrel S, Accolla RS, Carmagnola AL, et al. Common human melanoma-associated antigen(s) detected by monoclonal antibodies. Cancer Res 1980; 40:2523–2528.
26. Carrel S, de Tribolet N, Gross N. Expression of HLA-DR and common acute lymphoblastic leukemia antigens on glioma cells. Eur J Immunol 1982; 12:354–357.
27. Carrel S, de Tribolet N, Mach JP. Expression of neuroectodermal antigens common to melanomas, gliomas, and neuroblastomas. Acta Neuropathol 1982; 57:158–164.
28. Casper JT, Borella L, Sen L. Reactivity of human brain antiserum with neuroblastoma cells and nonreactivity with thymocytes and lymphoblasts. Cancer Res 1977; 37:1750–1756.
29. Coakham H. Surface antigen(s) common to human astrocytoma cells. Nature 1974; 250:328–330.
30. Coakham GB, Garson JA, Brownell B, et al. Diagnosis of cerebral neoplasms using monoclonal antibodies. Prog Exp Tumor Res 1985; 29:57–77.
31. Coakham HB, Kornblith PL, Quindlen EA, et al. Autologous humoral response to human gliomas and analysis of certain cell surface antigens: in vitro study with the use of microcytotoxicity and immune adherence assays. J Natl Cancer Inst 1980; 64:223–233.
32. Coakham GB, Lakshmi MS. Tumour-associated surface antigen(s) in human astrocytomas. Oncology 1975; 31:233–243.
33. Danon YL, Seeger RC, Maidman JE. Fetal neural antigens on human neuroblastoma cells. J Immunol 1980; 124:2925–2929.

34. Davies AG, Richardson RB, Bourne S, et al. The delivery of radiolabelled MAb to human primary cerebral tumours. In: Second workshop on monoclonal antibodies in neuro-oncology. J Neuroimmunol 1985; 10:182.

35. Day ED, Lassiter S, Woodhall B, et al. The localization of radioantibodies in human brain tumors. Cancer Res 1965; 25:773–778.

36. Delpech B, Delpech A, Vidard MN, et al. Glial fibrillary acidic protein in tumours of the nervous system. Br J Cancer 1978; 37:33–40.

37. Delpech B, Halavent C: Characterization and purification from human brain of a hyaluronic acid-binding glycoprotein, hyaluronectin. J Neurochem 1981; 36:855–859.

38. de Tribolet N, Carrel S, Mach JP. Brain tumor-associated antigens. Prog Exp Tumor Res 1984; 27:118–131.

39. Dippold WG, Lloyd KO, Li LTC, et al. Cell surface antigens of human malignant melanoma: definition of six antigenic systems with mouse monoclonal antibodies. Proc Natl Acad Sci USA 1980; 77:6114–6118.

40. Dittmann L, Axelsen NH, Norgaard-Pedersen B, et al. Antigens in human glioblastomas and meningiomas: search for tumour and onco-foetal antigens. Estimation of S-100 and GFA protein. Br J Cancer 1977; 35:135–141.

41. Eng LF, Vanderhaeghen JJ, Bignami A, et al. An acidic protein isolated from fibrous astrocytes. Brain Res 1971; 28:351–354.

42. Fischer DK, Chen TL, Narayan RK. Immunological and biochemical strategies for the identification of brain tumor-associated antigens. J Neurosurg 1988; 68:165–180.

43. Fischer DK, Miller G, Gradoville L, et al. Genome of a mononucleosis Epstein-Barr virus contains DNA fragments previously regarded to be unique to Burkitt's lymphoma isolates. Cell 1981; 24:543–553.

44. Fischer DK, Robert MF, Shedd D, et al. Identification of Epstein-Barr nuclear antigen polypeptide in mouse and monkey cells after gene transfer with a cloned 2.9 kilobase pair subfragment of the genome. Proc Natl Acad Sci USA 1984; 81:43–47.

45. Garson JA, Coakham HB, Kemshead JT, et al. The role of monoclonal antibodies in brain tumour diagnosis and cerebrospinal fluid (CSF) cytology. J Neuro-Oncol 1985; 3:165–171.

46. Girard N, Tayot J, Delpech B, et al. Brain glycoprotein in tumours of the nervous system. J Neuropathol Exp Neurol 1980; 39:88–98.

47. Grace JT, Perese DM, Metzgar RS, et al. Tumor autograft responses in patients with glioblastoma multiforme. J Neurosurg 1961; 18:159–167.

48. Greaves MF, Brown G, Rapson NT, et al. Antisera to acute lymphoblastic leukemia cells. Clin Immunol Immunopathol 1975; 4:67–84.

49. Gubler U, Hoffman BJ. A simple and very efficient method for generating cDNA libraries. Gene 1983; 25:263–269.

50. Hass WK. Soluble tissue antigens in human brain tumor and cerebrospinal fluid. Arch Neurol 1966; 14:443–447.

51. Heim S, Mitelman F. Nineteen of 26 cellular oncogenes precisely localized in the human genome map to one of the 83 bands involved in primary cancer-specific rearrangements. Hum Genet 1987; 75:70–72.

52. Herlyn M, Clark WH, Jr, Mastrangelo MJ, et al. Specific immunoreactivity of hybridoma-secreted monoclonal anti-melanoma antibodies to

cultured cells and freshly derived human cells. Cancer Res 1980; 40:3602–3609.

53. Heydorn WE, Creed GJ, Goldman D, et al. Mapping and quantitation of proteins from discrete nuclei and other areas of the rat brain by two-dimensional gel electrophoresis. J Neurosci 1983; 3:2597–2606.

54. Hyden H, McEwen B. A glial protein specific for the nervous system. Proc Natl Acad Sci USA 1966; 55:354–358.

55. Irie RF, Sze LL, Saxton RE. Human antibody to OFA-I, a tumor antigen, produced in vitro by Epstein-Barr virus-transformed human B-lymphoid cell lines. Proc Natl Acad Sci USA 1982; 79:5666–5670.

56. Jones D, Fritschy J, Garson J, et al. A monoclonal antibody binding to human medulloblastoma cells and to the platelet glycoprotein IIb-IIIa complex. Br J Haematol 1984; 57:621–631.

57. Juurlink BHJ, Fedoroff S, Hall C, et al. Astrocyte cell lineage. I. Astrocyte progenitor cells in mouse neopallium. J Comp Neurol 1981; 200:375–391.

58. Kao F-T. Human genome structure. Int Rev Cytol 1985; 96:51–88.

59. Kehayov IR. Tumour-associated water soluble antigen(s) in human glioblastoma demonstrated by immunodiffusion and immunoelectrophoresis. Ann Immunol (Inst Pasteur) 1976; 127C:703–716.

60. Kehayov I, Botev B, Vulchanov V, et al. Demonstration of a phase (stage)-specific embryonic brain antigen in human meningioma. Int J Cancer 1976; 18:587–592.

61. Kemshead JT, Fritschy J, Garson JA, et al. Monoclonal antibody UJ 127:11 detects a 220,000–240,000 kdal glycoprotein present on a subset of neuroectodermally derived cells. Int J Cancer 1983; 31:187–195.

62. Kennett RH, Gilbert F. Hybrid myelomas producing antibodies against a human neuroblastoma antigen present on fetal brain. Science 1979; 203:1120–1121.

63. Kennett RH, Jonak Z, Bechtol KB. Characterization of antigens with monoclonal antibodies. Prog Cancer Res Ther 1980; 12:209–219.

64. Kinzler KW, Bigner SH, Bigner DD, et al. Identification of an amplified, highly expressed gene in a human glioma. Science 1987; 236:70–73.

65. Kohler G, Milstein C. Continuous cultures of fused cells secreting antibody of predefined specificity. Nature 1975; 256:495–497.

66. Kondo I, Shimizu N. Mapping of the human gene for epidermal growth factor receptor (EGFR) on the p13-q22 region of chromosome 7. Cytogenet Cell Genet 1983; 35:9–14.

67. Kornblith PL, Coakham HB, Pollock LA, et al. Autologous serologic responses in glioma patients. Cancer 1983; 52:2230–2235.

68. Kril MP, Apuzzo MLJ. Observations in the study of T-lymphocyte subsets by monoclonal antibodies and flow cytometric analysis in intracranial neoplastic disorders. Clin Neurosurg 1983; 30:125–136.

69. Kucheria K. Double minute chromatin bodies in a subependymal glioma. Br J Cancer 1968; 22:696–697.

70. Kumar S, Taylor G, Steward JK, et al. Cell-mediated immunity and blocking factors in patients with tumours of the central nervous system. Int J Cancer 1973; 12:194–205.

71. Lach B, Weinrauder H. Glia-specific antigen in the intracranial tumors. Immunofluorescence study. Acta Neuropathol (Berl) 1978; 41:9–15.
72. Lazarides E. Intermediate filaments as mechanical integrators of cellular space. Nature 1980; 283:249–256.
73. Lee FH, Hwang KM. Antibodies as specific carriers for chemotherapeutic agents. Cancer Chemother Pharmacol 1979; 3:17–24.
74. Levy NL. Specificity of lymphocyte-mediated cytotoxicity in patients with primary intracranial tumors. J Immunol 1978; 121:903–915.
75. Liao DK, Clarke BJ, Kwong PC, et al. Common neuroectodermal antigens on human melanoma, neuroblastoma, retinoblastoma, glioblastoma and fetal brain revealed by hybridoma antibodies raised against melanoma cells. Eur J Immunol 1981; 11:450–454.
76. Libermann T, Nusbaum H, Razon N, et al. Amplification, enhanced expression, and possible rearrangement of EGF receptor gene in primary human brain tumors of glial origin. Nature 1985; 313:133–147.
77. Lubs H, Salmon J. The chromosome complement of human solid tumors. II. Karyotypes of glial tumors. J Neurosurg 1965; 22:160–168.
78. Luner SJ, de Vellis J. Immunoprecipitation of a M_r 64,000 glial tumor-associated antigen by monoclonal antibody 217c. Cancer Res 1986; 46:863–865.
79. Mahaley MS, Jr, Mahaley JL, Day ED. The localization of radioantibodies in human brain tumors. II. Radioautography. Cancer Res 1965; 25:779–793.
80. Mahaley MS, Jr. Immunological studies with human gliomas. J Neurosurg 1971; 34:458–459.
81. Marangos PJ. Clinical studies with neuron-specific enolase. In: Advances in Neuroblastoma Research, Evans AE, D'Angio GJ, Seeger RC, eds. Alan R. Liss, Inc., New York, 1985; pp. 285–294.
82. Mark J. Chromosomal abnormalities and their specificity in human neoplasms: an assessment of recent observations by banding techniques. Adv Cancer Res 1977; 24:165–222.
83. Martin SE, Martin WJ. Interspecies brain antigen detected by naturally occurring mouse anti-brain autoantibody. Proc Natl Acad Sci USA 1975; 72:1036–1040.
84. Martin-Achard A, Diserens AC, de Tribolet N, et al. Evaluation of the humoral response of glioma patients to a possible common tumor-associated antigen(s). Int J Cancer 1980; 25:219–224.
85. McComb RD, Bigner DD. Immunolocalization of monoclonal antibody-defined extracellular matrix antigens in human brain tumors. J Neuro-Oncol 1985; 3:181–186.
86. Medawar PB. Immunity to homologous grafted skin, Part 3 (Fate of skin homografts transplanted to brain, to subcutaneous tissues and to anterior chamber of the eye.). Br J Exp Pathol 1948; 29:58–69.
87. Miyake E, Kitamura K, Nomoto K, et al. An attempt to detect cell surface antigens in cultured human brain tumors by mixed hemadsorption test. Acta Neuropathol (Berl) 1977; 37:27–29.
88. Moore BW. A soluble protein characteristic of the nervous system. Biochem Biophys Res Commun 1965; 19:739–744.
89. Moore BW, McGregor D. Chromatographic and electrophoretic frac-

tionation of soluble proteins of brain and liver. J Biol Chem 1965; 240:1647–1653.

90. Moore BW, Perez VJ. Specific acidic proteins of the nervous system. In: Physiological and Biochemical Aspects of Nervous Integration, Carlson FD, ed. Englewood Cliffs, NJ, Prentice-Hall, 1968; pp. 343–359.

91. Narayan RK, Heydorn WE, Creed GJ, et al. Proteins in normal, irradiated, and postmortem human brain quantitatively compared by using two-dimensional gel electrophoresis. Clin Chem 1984; 30:1989–1995.

92. Narayan RK, Heydorn WE, Creed GJ, et al. Identification of major proteins in human cerebral cortex and brain tumors. J Protein Chem 1985; 4:375–389.

93. Narayan RK, Heydorn WE, Creed GJ, et al. Protein patterns in various malignant human brain tumors by two-dimensional gel electrophoresis. Cancer Res 1986; 46:4685–4694.

94. Neuwelt EA, Specht D, Hill SA. Permeability of human brain tumour to ^{99m}Tc-glucoheptonate and ^{99m}Tc-albumin: implications for monoclonal antibody therapy. J Neurosurg 1986; 65:194–198.

95. Paterson PY. Experimental autoimmune (allergic) encephalomyelitis: induction, pathogenesis, and suppression. In: Textbook of Immunopathology, Miescher PA, Muller-Eberhart HJ, eds. New York, Grune and Stratton, 1976; pp. 179–213.

96. Peng WW, Bressler JP, Tiffany-Castiglioni E, et al. Development of a monoclonal antibody against a tumor-associated antigen. Science 1982; 215:1102–1104.

97. Pfreundschuh M, Shiku H, Takahashi T, et al. Serological analysis of cell surface antigens of malignant human brain tumors. Proc Natl Acad Sci USA 1978; 75:5122–5126.

98. Pfreundschuh M, Rohrich M, Piotrowshi W, et al. Natural antibodies to cell-surface antigens of human astrocytoma. Int J Cancer 1982; 29:517–521.

99. Phillips J, Alderson T, Sikora K, et al. Localisation of malignant glioma by a radiolabelled human monoclonal antibody. J Neurol Neurosurg Psych 1983; 46:388–392.

100. Phillips J, Sikora K, Watson JV: Localisation of glioma by human monoclonal antibody. Lancet 1982; 2:1214–1215.

101. Reif AE, Allen JM. The AKR thymic antigen and its distribution in leukemias and nervous tissues. J Exp Med 1964; 120:413–433.

102. Richards FF, Konigsberg WH, Rosenstein RW, et al. On the specificity of antibodies. Science 1975; 187:130–137.

103. Rosenblum ML, Massimo AG, Wilson CB, et al. Stem cell studies of human malignant brain tumors. Part 1: Development of the stem cell assay and its potential. J Neurosurg 1983; 58:170–176.

104. Sakurai M, Sandberg A. Correlation of karyotypes with clinical features of acute myeloblastic leukemia. Cancer 1976; 37:285–299.

105. Sato K, Raimondi AJ, Dray S, et al. Comparison of tumor-associated surface antigens on cells from medulloblastomas and from other neoplasms of the human nervous system. Child's Brain 1978; 4:83–94.

106. Schlaepfer WW, Lee V, Wu HL. Assessment of immunological properties of neurofilament triplet proteins. Brain Res 1981; 226:259–272.

107. Seeger RC, Zeltezer PM, Rayner SA. Onco-neural antigen: a new neural differentiation antigen expressed by neuroblastoma, oat cell carcinoma, Wilms' tumor, and sarcoma cells. J Immunol 1979; 122:1548–1555.
108. Schmidek H. The molecular genetics of nervous system tumors. J Neurosurg 1987; 67:1–16.
109. Schnegg JF, de Tribolet N, Diserens AC, et al. Characterization of a rabbit anti-human malignant glioma antiserum. Int J Cancer 1981; 28:265–269.
110. Schnegg JF, Diserens AC, Carrel S, et al. Human glioma-associated antigens detected by monoclonal antibodies. Cancer Res 1981; 41:1209–1213.
111. Seeger RC, Rosenblatt HM, Imai K, et al. Common antigenic determinants on human melanoma, glioma, neuroblastoma, and sarcoma cells defined with monoclonal antibodies. Cancer Res 1981; 41:2714–2717.
112. Seizinger B, de la Monte S, Atkins L, et al. Molecular genetic approach to human meningioma: loss of genes on chromosome 22. Proc Natl Acad Sci USA 1987; 84:5419–5423.
113. Seizinger B, Martuza L, Gusella J. Loss of genes on chromosome 22 in tumorigenesis of human acoustic neuroma. Nature 1986; 322:644–647.
114. Shapiro J. Biology of gliomas: heterogeneity, oncogenes, growth factors. Semin Oncol 1986; 13:4–15.
115. Sheikh KMA, Apuzzo MLJ, Kochsiek KM, et al. Malignant glial neoplasms: definition of a humoral host response to tumor-associated antigen(s). Yale J Biol Med 1977; 50:387–403.
116. Sheikh KMA, Apuzzo MLJ, Weiss MH. Specific cellular immune responses in patients with malignant gliomas. Cancer Res 1979; 39:1733–1738.
117. Sikora K. The characterisation of gliomas using human monoclonal antibodies. Expl Cell Biol 1984; 52:189–195.
118. Sikora K, Alderson T, Phillips J, et al. Human hybridomas from malignant gliomas. Lancet 1982; 1:11–14.
119. Sikora K, Alderson T, Ellis J, et al. Human hybridomas from patients with malignant disease. Br J Cancer 1983; 47:135–145.
120. Sikora K, Alderson T, Chan S, et al. Monoclonal antibodies and glioma. Prog Exp Tumor Res 1985; 29:45–49.
121. Silverberg E, Lubera J. Cancer statistics. CA-A Cancer J Clin 1987; 37:2–19.
122. Siris JH. Concerning the immunological specificity of glioblastoma multiforme. Bull Neurol Inst NY 1936; 4:597–601.
123. Solheid Cl, Lauro G, Palladini G. Two separate membrane-bound antigens on human glioma cells in tissue culture detected with sera from glioma patients by immunofluorescence. J Neurol Sci 1976; 30:55–64.
124. Stavrou D, Suss C, Bilzer T, et al. Monoclonal antibodies reactive with glioma cell lines derived from experimental brain tumors. Eur J Cancer Clin Oncol 1983; 19:1439–1449.
125. Studer A, de Tribolet N, Diserens AC, et al. Characterization of four human malignant glioma cell lines. Acta Neuropathol (Berl) 1985; 66:208–217.

126. Trent S, Meltzer P, Rosenblum M, et al. Evidence for rearrangement, duplication and expression of c-myc in a human glioblastoma. Proc Natl Acad Sci USA 1986; 83:470–473.

127. Trouillas P. Carcino-fetal antigen in glial tumours. Lancet 1971; 2:552.

128. Trouillas P. Immunologie des tumeurs cerebrales: l'antigene carcino-foetal glial. Ann Inst Pasteur 1972; 122:819–828.

129. von Hanwehr RI, Hofman FM, Taylor CR, et al. Mononuclear lymphoid populations infiltrating the microenvironment of primary CNS tumors. J Neurosurg 1984; 60:1138–1147.

130. Wahlstrom T, Linder E, Saksela E, et al. Tumor-specific membrane antigens in established cell lines from gliomas. Cancer 1974; 34:274–279.

131. Walker MD, Green SB, Byar DP, et al. Randomized comparisons of radiotherapy and nitrosoureas for the treatment of malignant glioma after surgery. N Engl J Med 1980; 303:1323–1329.

132. Warecka K, Bauer H. Studies on "brain-specific" proteins in aqueous extracts of brain tissue. J Neurochem 1967; 14:783–787.

133. Watanabe T, Pukel CS, Takeyama H, et al. Human melanoma antigen AH is an autoantigenic ganglioside related to G_{D2}. J Exp Med 1982; 156:1884–1889.

134. Wikstrand CJ, Bigner DD. Surface antigens of human glioma cells shared with normal adult and fetal brain. Cancer Res 1979; 39:3235–3243.

135. Wikstrand CJ, Bigner DD. Expression of human fetal brain antigens by human tumors of neuroectodermal origin as defined by monoclonal antibodies. Cancer Res 1982; 42:267–275.

136. Wikstrand CJ, Bigner SH, Bigner DD. Demonstration of complex antigenic heterogeneity in a human glioma cell line and eight derived clones by specific monoclonal antibodies. Cancer Res 1983; 43:3327–3334.

137. Wikstrand CJ, Bourdon MA, Pegram CN, et al. Human fetal brain antigen expression common to tumors of neuroectodermal tissue origin. J Neuroimmunol 1982; 3:43–62.

138. Wolman S. Cytogenetic heterogeneity: its role in tumor evolution. Cancer Genet Cytogenet 1986; 19:129–140.

139. Young RA, Davis RW. Efficient isolation of genes by using antibody probes. Proc Natl Acad Sci USA 1983; 80:1194–1198.

140. Young RA, Davis RW. Yeast RNA polymerase II genes: isolation with antibody probes. Science 1983; 222:778–782.

4

Brain Tumor Angiogenesis

*Henry Brem, Rafael J. Tamargo,
Christopher Guerin, Steven S. Brem,
and Harold Brem*

Introduction

Our understanding of the role of brain tumor neovascularization has increased over the past several years. A brain tumor, like other solid tumors, passes through two distinct phases: (1) an avascular phase and (2) a vascular phase.[1,2] The mechanism by which tumors progress from the avascular to the vascular stage theoretically lends itself to major therapeutic applications. For instance, the chemicals that tumors produce to elicit a neovascular response, the angiogenic factors,[3] can be used as clinical markers of the presence of a tumor that has progressed into the vascular phase. Most importantly, tumor growth can be disrupted by inhibiting angiogenesis and depriving the tumor of its blood supply. By understanding the mechanism by which tumors progress from the avascular to the vascular phase, the potential exists for reversing this progression and thereby forcing vascular tumors into the avascular phase.

Tumors deprived of their blood supply cannot exist as a three-dimensional masses larger than 0.5–0.6 mm^3.[4] Furthermore, established tumors can be forced to regress using angiogenesis inhibitors.[5] Several inhibitors of neovascularization have been found. Angio-

From: Kornblith PL, Walker MD (editors). Advances in Neuro-Oncology. Futura Publishing Company, Inc., Mount Kisco, NY, © 1988.
This work has been supported by the Andrew W. Mellon Foundation, the NIH Grant # NS01058-01, The American Cancer Society Grant # IN-llW, and the Association for Brain Tumor Research Fellowship in memory of Steven Lowe.

genesis inhibitors have been isolated from cartilage[6] and vitreous.[7] Cortisone, dexamethasone, and medroxyprogesterone have been shown to block tumor neovascularization and tumor growth in the rabbit cornea.[8] Protamine sulfate has been shown to inhibit angiogenesis.[9] More recently, the combination of heparin or heparin fragments and cortisone has been shown to be a powerful inhibitor of angiogenesis.[5]

We will discuss the potential applications of these findings to brain tumors. This review is divided into three sections. The first will review the background and experimental information on the basic understanding of the avascular/vascular phases and the role of the angiogenic factors. The second will discuss the potential applications of angiogenesis tumor markers. The third will review the findings on the inhibitors of tumor angiogenesis.

Background of Tumor Angiogenesis

Several distinct events must occur for a tumor to develop. A tumor begins as a single cell. The cell can be transformed by a variety of mechanisms, for instance, chemical or viral.[10] Regardless of the mechanism of transformation, the malignant cell replicates rapidly and forms a population of abnormal cells. These cells aggregate as a three-dimensional mass which receives its nutrition by diffusion. The avascular mass continues to proliferate until it reaches approximately 10^6 cells, corresponding to a spheroid 3–4 mm in diameter.[11] At this size, the limitations on the inward diffusion of oxygen and nutrients and the outward diffusion of metabolic by-products prevent further growth of the spheroid; the proliferation of the cells on the periphery is balanced by the death and necrosis of the cells at the core. At this stage the tumor is considered dormant in terms of further growth.

In order to continue to grow, the tumor must induce the proliferation of host capillary endothelial cells by producing angiogenic factors. The capillary endothelial cells migrate toward the tumor and proliferate to form new vessels.[12] When the tumor vessels reach the tumor mass, the tumor is released from its growth restrictions and proliferates at its maximal genetic capability. At this point the rate of growth changes from linear to exponential and the tumor expands rapidly. Only vascular tumors are clinically significant, since tumors only 3–4 mm in diameter would rarely produce symptoms. The point at which the tumor makes a transition between being a dormant nodule and then a vascular mass represents a natural control point at which tumor progression can be stopped. Furthermore, the tumor's angiogenic factors provide markers of a malignancy that has progressed beyond the avascular stage.

The restrictions on growth reponsible for the avascular spheroid has been studied by Folkman and Hochberg.[11] The initial discovery was made by Folkman while studying tumors transplanted to organ perfusion systems.[13,14] Folkman observed that in these systems tumors never grew beyond a few millimeters despite being viable. He also noted that there was endothelial degeneration in the perfused tissues and therefore no vascular response to the tumor angiogenic factors.

The growth of tumor cells in two dimensions is unrestricted, provided an unlimited surface area, and adequate nutrients. By contrast, Folkman and Hochberg showed that cellular spheroids growing in three dimensions in soft agar are self-regulated. In their study,[11] the multicellular spheroids grew to a diameter of 3–4 mm, containing approximately 10^6 cells, and then entered a dormant growth phase. The restrictions imposed by the inward diffusion of oxygen and nutrients and the outward diffusion of metabolic wastes prevented further growth; the proliferation of the cells at the periphery was balanced by the death and necrosis of those in the center.

The experiment by Folkman and Hochberg suggested that tumors without a blood supply cannot progress beyond a certain volume for biological reasons. Greene and Arnold[15] had previously demonstrated that fragments of human glioblastoma, less than 1 mm in diameter, survived for over 9 months in the anterior chamber of the guinea pig eye remote from blood vessels. During this time there was no change in the tumor size, metastatic spread, or detectable damage to the host. Similarly, Gimbrone et al.[4] demonstrated that tumors without a blood supply cannot progress beyond a certain size by implanting the rabbit V2 carcinoma in the anterior chamber of the rabbit eye. The resulting tumor spheroids floated in the aqueous humor of the anterior chamber and grew to reach a volume of 0.5–0.6 mm^3 and then became dormant. If the spheroids, however, were surgically implanted on the vascular bed of the iris, they became vascularized and entered a phase of exponential growth.

The avascular phase can exist for many years and is self-limiting unless the tumor can produce angiogenic factors that will stimulate the host capillary endothelial cells to proliferate. The rapid, exponential growth phase is responsible for clinical symptoms.

Angiogenesis as a Tumor Marker

A transformed cell may develop the ability to produce angiogenic factors and induce a neovascular response before it becomes overtly malignant.[16–19] Therefore, angiogenic factors can be used as preneoplastic markers or as indicators of a tumor that is progressing into the vascular stage. The purification, sequencing, and cloning of several angiogenic factors in the past 3 years,[3] since Shing et al.[20] described a simple technique for isolating tumor-derived endothelial cell growth factors, brings us closer to being able to screen for these factors as tumor markers. As shown in Table 1, different varieties of angiogenic factors are being identified: the heparin-binding factors include acidic and basic fibroblast growth factors (FGFs) and the nonheparin-binding factors include alpha and beta transforming growth factors (TGFs). In addition, there are other factors still poorly characterized that cannot be assigned to either category, such as the

Table 1
Angiogenic Factors

Heparin-Binding Factors
    Endothelial cell growth factor (ECGF)
    Acidic fibroblast growth factor (acidic FGF)
    Basic fibroblast growth factor (basic FGF)
Nonheparin-Binding Factors
    Angiogenin
    Transforming growth factor—Alpha (TGF-α)
    Transforming growth factor—Beta (TGF-β)
    Epidermal growth factor (EGF)
Other Angiogenic Factors
    Low molecular weight endothelial mitogens
    Endothelial cell chemotactic factors
    Lipids (e.g., PGE_1 and PGE_2)
Modulators of Angiogenesis
    Heparin
    Copper

From reference 3.

endothelial cell chemotactic factors, as well as modulators of angiogenesis, such as heparin and copper, whose roles remain unclear.

Brem, Cotran, and Folkman[1] studied the angiogenesis response to malignant brain tumors. An objective grading system was developed which quantitated the vascularity of tumors. The formula took into account three factors: (1) vasoproliferation in the tumor, (2) endothelial cell hyperplasia, and (3) endothelial cytology. They then classified several solid tumors along a spectrum. The glioblastoma multiforme was the most "endothelial-rich" tumor studied. Chondrosarcomas, by contrast, were rated as "endothelial-poor."

The microscopic angiogenesis grading system was then compared to the standard Kernohan grading system for astrocytomas.[21] For each increasing degree of anaplasia as determined by the Kernohan system, there was a corresponding increase in the angiogenesis score. Furthermore, the angiogenesis score correlated well with postoperative survival.

These findings suggested that tumor angiogenesis is critical in determining the malignant potential of the tumor. The next question to be addressed was whether tumor angiogenesis could be used as a marker system. This assertion was tested by Brem, Jensen, and Gullino[16] by implanting in the rabbit iris pieces of tissue obtained during breast biopsies to rule out malignant disease. The degree of neovascularization elicited by the implants was assessed by slit-lamp stereo microscopy and by histological examination. It was found that whereas normal lobules, atypical lobules, fibrocystic masses, and fibroadenomas did not stimulate angiogenesis, the malignant tumors elicited an angiogenic response. Of particular interest were the implants of hyperplastic lobules. It has been shown that clinically 17% of these lesions transform into carcinomas. Brem, Jensen, and Gullino observed that 20% of their implanted hyperplastic lobules were positive for angiogenesis. This finding suggests that angiogenesis is a reflection of the malignant potential of a neoplasm.

A similar technique was used by Brem et al.[22] to evaluate the angiogenic potential of human brain tumors. Biopsy samples were implanted in the rabbit cornea and evaluated for their ability to elicit an angiogenesis response. A variety of tumors such as acoustic neuromas, hemangioblastomas, angioblastic meningiomas, and glioblastomas induced angiogenesis in 95% of the corneas. By contrast, low grade astrocytomas produced angiogenesis in only 13% of the corneas. Of interest was that whereas 14% of pituitary adenomas produced neovascularization similar to that of the low grade astrocytomas, two recurrent chromophobe adenomas produced neovascularization in 78% of the corneas. An extensive study of the recurrent chromophobe adenomas utilizing histological and ultrastructural techniques failed to reveal any differences between these tumors and the more benign pituitary adenomas. These results suggested that the aggressive potential of these lesions was accurately reflected by their angiogenic behavior in the rabbit cornea.

Having shown that the angiogenesis response associated with a tumor could be assessed by studying a sample of the tumor in the rabbit iris and cornea, the question arose whether the fluid surrounding a malignancy possessed angiogenesis activity and could be used to assess this activity without actually removing the tumor. Tapper et al.[23] studied the aqueous humor of patients undergoing anterior chamber taps. The samples were placed in the chick chorioallantoic membrane and evaluated in terms of their angiogenic response. The aqueous humor of 15 patients with nonmalignant disease such as cataracts and glaucoma was evaluated and only one (7%) was positive for angiogenesis. By contrast, the aqueous humor of 23 patients with malignant disease in the eye (retinoblastomas, choroidal melanomas, and a metastatic breast carcinoma to the iris) was similarly evaluated and 18 (78%) of the samples were positive. Therefore, angiogenesis was shown to be an activity which could be isolated from the fluid surrounding the tumor without having the tumor itself available.

Chodak et al.[24] similarly studied the urine of patients with malignancies of the genitourinary system. Since angiogenic factors have been shown to induce migratory behavior of endothelial cells, Chodak et al. evaluated the in vitro migration of endothelial cells as an index of angiogenic activity. Whereas the urine of normal controls elicited little or no migration, the urine of patients with transitional cell carcinomas of the bladder induced a mean increase of 50% in the migratory behavior of the endothelial cells. In two patients who eventually were found to have recurrent tumor, an increase in endothelial cell migration was documented before the tumors became clinically detectable.

Brem, Patz, and Tapper[25] similarly evaluated the migration-stimulating activity of the cerebrospinal fluid (CSF) of patients with brain tumors. The migratory activity of 3T3 cells plated on gold-coated coverslips showed a tenfold increase when bathed by the CSF of patients with gliomas (17 patients) as compared to the response when bathed with CSF from patients with aneurysms, arteriovenous malformations, trauma, metabolic and degenerative disorders, and systemic diseases (79 patients).

In summary, angiogenesis has been shown to be a reflection of the clinical and pathological behavior of malignancies and to be useful not only as a correlative of the histological appearance of these lesions, but also as a tumor marker that may be superior to the present methods used to predict the biological behavior of the tumor.

Inhibition of Tumor Angiogenesis

The remainder of this chapter will focus on the role of neovascularization in the development of brain tumors and on the potential of anti-angiogenesis therapy for the control of tumor growth.

By 1975 there was ample experimental evidence suggesting that a tumor would remain as a small avascular nodule until it elicited an angiogenesis response, became vascularized, and entered a phase of exponential growth. It was thought that the transition from the avascular to the vascular stage represented a natural control point. There were, however, no known inhibitors of angiogenesis.

Brem and Folkman[6] demonstrated that cartilage contains an inhibitor of angiogenesis. Although some cartilage is vascularized in the human embryo, its blood vessels disappear after birth.[26–28] Mature cartilage is a relatively avascular tissue that contains very few cells and consists almost entirely of an extracellular matrix composed of water, collagen, and protein polysaccharide complexes. In mice, carcinomas induced in the ear by chemical carcinogens never infiltrate the cartilage, but grow instead in tissue surrounding the cartilage.[29] Williams[30] made the incidental observation that the V2 carcinoma implanted in the rabbit ear did not seem to induce neovascularization. Eisenstein et al.[31] demonstated that cartilage resists invasion by blood vessels and that it loses this property when extracted with guanidine. These observations suggested the possibility that a factor capable of inhibiting vascular growth might reside in neonatal cartilage.

Brem and Folkman transplanted fresh rabbit neonatal cartilage on the chick chrioallantoic membrane (CAM) and observed that a zone of inhibition lacking new blood vessels developed around the implant. Similarly, when cartilage was placed adjacent to the Walker 256 carcinosarcoma on the CAM, it inhibited tumor angiogenesis. Pre-existing blood vessels were unaffected by the presence of cartilage.

This suggested that cartilage inhibited the proliferation of new blood vessels but did not affect pre-existing, stable blood vessels.

The phenomenon of cartilage inhibition of tumor angiogenesis was studied quantitatively in the rabbit cornea model. Intracorneal pouches were created to a distance of 1 mm from the vascular limbus. A piece of cartilage was placed at the bottom of the pouch and a piece of V2 carcinoma placed above it. The cartilage implant decreased the rate of tumor-elicited capillary growth by an average of 75% and prevented tumor vascularization completely in 28% of the samples. Control samples consisting of V2 carcinoma and boiled cartilage always showed a brisk angiogenesis response. It was demonstrated that in the zone around the cartilage, a chemical was present that prevented the proliferation of new blood vessels without apparent toxicity to the sensitive tissues of the rabbit cornea and the chick CAM.

Subsequently, Langer et al.[32] isolated a factor from cartilage that inhibited tumor-induced angiogenesis and restricted tumor growth. The factor was isolated in a fraction containing several protein species with a major component having a molecular weight of about 16,000. Langer et al.[33] infused this factor in the carotid artery of rabbits with an intracorneal tumor implant. The infusion of the cartilage inhibitor disrupted tumor growth in the ipsilateral cornea without any apparent toxicity to the tissues. Further applications of this promising angiogenesis inhibitor, however, have been hampered by the large quantities of cartilage required to extract adequate quantities of the inhibitor and by the laborious isolation procedure.

Another biological inhibitor of angiogenesis was isolated from vitreous, also an avascular tissue. Brem et al.[7] incorporated a vitreous extract in a sustained release polymer matrix and implanted the matrix in the rabbit cornea together with the V2 carcinoma. The vitreous extract released from the polymer inhibited tumor-induced neovascularization. It has been postulated that the vitreous inhibitor may be responsible for suppressing the proliferation of blood vessels in the retina. Furthermore, diabetic retinopathy, which is characterized by the proliferation of retinal vessels, may result from an imbalance between a neovascularization factor produced by the hypoxic retina and the angiogenesis inhibitor present in vitreous.

The difficulties associated with the extraction of angiogenesis inhibitors from cartilage and vitreous prompted the search for a clinically available inhibitor. Gross et al.[8] showed that cortisone, dexamethasone, and medroxyprogesterone inhibit tumor neovascularization and growth when administered in high doses in a sustained release polymer matrix implanted in the rabbit cornea. By contrast, estradiol and testosterone had no effect.

Subsequently, Taylor and Folkman[9] found that protamine is a specific inhibitor of angiogenesis. The observation that mast cells accumulated at the site of a tumor implant in the CAM prior to the ingrowth of the capillary sprouts[34] suggested that a product of mast cells may be involved in the facilitation of angiogenesis. This product was eventually shown to be heparin, which facilitates angiogenesis but cannot initiate it, and the known antagonist of heparin, protamine, became a candidate as an inhibitor of angiogenesis. The significant toxicities associated with this compound, however, precluded its systemic use against primary tumors.

A fortuitous finding led to the discovery that the combination of heparin and cortisone was a powerful inhibitor of angiogenesis.[5] The local administration of these drugs resulted in angiogenesis inhibition in the CAM and the rabbit cornea. Their systemic administration resulted in regressions and cures of several lethal tumors implanted in mice.

Surprisingly, neither the glucocorticoid and mineralocorticoid properties of cortisone, nor the anticoagulant properties of heparin are relevant to antiangiogenesis. When heparin is substituted by heparin-derived oligosaccharides and these are administered with cortisone, the antiangiogenesis effect is maintained. The oral administration of heparin, which destroys its anticoagulant activity, results in the release of heparin fragments into plasma[35] which, in the presence of cortisone, are antiangiogenic. Conversely, Crum, Szabo, and Folkman[36] showed that cortisone can be substituted with several "angiostatic steroids" that lack any glucocorticoid and mineralocorticoid properties and which have been shown to be anti-angiogenic in the presence of heparin or heparin-derived oligosaccharides.

Recently, a number of investigators have attempted to induce the regression of tumors with the systemic administration of the combination of heparin and cortisone. These studies, however, have yielded conflicting results. Folkman et al.[5] obtained tumor regression and increased survival in mice given heparin and cortisone systemically. Sakamoto et al.[37] documented tumor growth inhibition in mice, but failed to obtain tumor regression or increased survival. Ziche et al.[38] reported tumor growth inhibition in mice treated with systemic cortisone acetate alone.

The addition of heparin enhanced this effect only slightly. No regressions were observed. Penhaglion and Camplejohn[39] reported the transient inhibition of tumor growth in mice treated with systemic cortisone acetate alone and did not observe potentiation of this effect when heparin was added. No tumor regressions were obtained either.

The different results of these four studies may be due to the variability in the antiangiogenic properties of heparins obtained from different sources. Commercial heparin is a heterogeneous mixture of glycosaminoglycans.[40] Heparins from different sources vary in their anticoagulant properties. Similarly, different heparins have been shown to have different antiangiogenic activities. Whereas different heparins can be rendered equally antiangiogenic when administered locally by increasing the dose of the weakest species, only certain heparins are antiangiogenic when administered systemically in the drinking water.[5,36]

Although Ingber, Madri, and Folkman[41] have demonstrated that the administration of angiostatic steroids and heparin results in the dissolution of the capillary basement membrane, the mechanism by which these compounds induce angiogenesis inhibition remains largely unknown.

The current concepts in antiangiogenesis therapy are being successfully applied in animal brain tumor models. Brem and Zagzag[42] have shown that growth of the V2 carcinoma implanted in the brain of hypocupremic rabbits is markedly inhibited. These animals have been depleted of copper by the administration of penicillamine, a copper chelator, and by a low copper diet. Copper has been previously shown to be an important modulator of angiogenesis.[3] Tamargo, Leong, and Brem[43] have demonstrated that the growth of the rat 9L gliosarcoma can be significantly inhibited by the localized, sustained administration of heparin and cortisone incorporated in a biodegradable polymer matrix implanted at the site of tumor growth. This study demonstrates that the growth of a malignant glioma can be disrupted using angiogenesis inhibitors.

Future Perspectives in Tumor Angiogenesis

The fields of angiogenesis in general and of tumor angiogenesis in particular have evolved dramatically in the past 15 years since Folkman published his first article on tumor angiogenesis.[2] Current research efforts are defining angiogenesis as a highly complex and tightly regulated system. In the past few years, several angiogenesis factors have been isolated, purified, and in some instances even cloned. In addition to the capillary endothelial cell, other cells such as mast cells and pericytes seem to be involved in the control of angiogenesis. The complex relationships within this array of cellular and humoral elements are currently under intense investigation. The complexity of the angiogenesis system may very well rival that of the clotting system. Angiogenesis may be the final result of a complex angiogenesis cascade. The process may be disrupted by interfering with several steps of the cascade.

As the structure of the angiogenesis system becomes clearer, we may come to understand how cartilage, vitreous, protamine, corticosteroids, and the combination of angiostatic steroids and heparin fragments inhibit tumor angiogenesis and may learn how to use these agents more effectively. As our current therapeutic thinking shifts away from directly challenging the tumor cell and focuses on modulating host responses that either support or inhibit tumor growth, angiogenesis inhibitors may emerge as a mainstay in the armamentarium of biological response modifiers.

Summary

Through our understanding of the role of neovascularization in the progression of brain tumors, we have learned that tumors pass through two distinct phases, an avascular followed by a vascular phase. The investigation of this progression has led to important applications. The avascular and vascular phases serve as markers for the biological activity of the tumor. This has been assessed morphologically by grading tumors according to the degree of angiogenesis and experimentally by assaying the angiogenesis response of different tumors and evaluating the angiogenesis properties of fluid in contact with tumors. This has been applied to a variety of human malignant brain tumors. By increasing our understanding of angiogenesis, we will be able to better control brain tumor growth.

REFERENCES

1. Brem S, Cotran R, Folkman J. Tumor angiogenesis: A quantitative method for histologic grading. JNCI 1972; 48:347–356.
2. Folkman J. Anti-angiogenesis: New concept for therapy of solid tumors. Ann Surg 1972 ; 175:409–416.

3. Folkman J, Klagsbrun M. Angiogenic factors. Science 1987; 235:442–447.
4. Gimbrone MA, Leapman SB, Cotran RS, Folkman J. Tumor dormancy in vivo by prevention of neovascularization. J Exp Med 1972; 136:261–276.
5. Folkman J, Langer R, Linhardt RJ, Haudenschild C, Taylor S. Angiogenesis inhibitionand tumor regression caused by heparin or a heparin fragment in the presence of cortisone. Science 1983; 221:719–725.
6. Brem H, Folkman J. Inhibition of tumor angiogenesis mediated by cartilage. J Exp Med 1975; 141:427–439.
7. Brem S, Preis I, Langer R, Brem H, Folkman J. Inhibition of neovascularization by an extract derived from vitreous. Am J Ophthalmol 1977; 84:323–328.
8. Gross J, Azizkhan RG, Biswas C, Bruns RR, Hsieh DST, Folkman J. Inhibition of tumor growth, vascularization, and collagenolysis in the rabbit cornea by medroxyprogesterone. Proc Natl Acad Sci USA 1981; 78:1176–1180.
9. Taylor S, Folkman J. Protamine is an inhibitor of angiogenesis. Nature 1982; 297:307–312.
10. Laerum OD, Mork SJ, De Ridder L. The transformation process. Prog Exp Tumor Res 1984; 27:17–31.
11. Folkman J, Hochberg M. Self-regulation of growth in three dimensions. J Exp Med 1973; 138:745–753.
12. Ausprunk DHy Folkman J. Migration and proliferation of endothelial cells in preformed and newly formed blood vessels during tumor angiogenesis. Microvasc Res 1977; 14:53–65.
13. Folkman J, Long DM, Becker FF. Growth and metastasis of tumor in organ culture. Cancer 1963; 16:453–467.
14. Folkman J, Cole P, Zimmerman S. Tumor behavior in isolated perfusion organs: In vitro growth and metastases of biopsy material in rabbit thyroid and canine intestinal segment. Ann Surg 1966; 164:491–502.
15. Greene HSN, Arnold H. The homologous and heterologous transplantation of brain and brain tumor. J Neurosurg 1945; 2:315–331.
16. Brem S, Jensen HM, Gullino PM. Angiogenesis as a marker of preneoplastic lesions of the human breast. Cancer 1978; 41:239-244.
17. Gimbrone MA, Gullino PM. Neovascularization induced by intraocular xenografts of normal, preneoplastic, and neoplastic mouse mammary tissues. JNCI 1976; 56:305–318.
18. Maiorana A, Gullino PM. Acquisition of angiogenic capacity and neoplastic transformation in the rat mammary gland. Cancer Res 1978; 38:4409–4414.
19. Ziche M, Gullino PM. Angiogenesis and neoplastic progression in vitro. JNCI 1982; 69:483–487.
20. Shing Y, Folkman J, Sullivan R, Butterfield C, Murray J, Klagsbrun M. Heparin affinity: Purification of a tumor derived capillary endothelial cell growth factor. Science 1984; 223:1296–1298.
21. Brem S. The role of vascular proliferation in the growth of brain tumors. Clin Neurosurg 1976; 23:440–453.
22. Brem H, Thompson D, Long DM, Patz A. Human brain tumors: Differences in ability to stimulate angiogenesis. Surg Forum 1980; 31:471–473.

23. Tapper D, Langer R, Bellows AR, Folkman J. Angiogenesis capacity as a diagnostic marker for human eye tumors. Surgery 1979; 86:36–40.
24. Chodak GW, Haudenschild C, Gittes RF, Folkman J. Angiogenic activity as a marker of of neoplastic and preneoplastic lesions of the human bladder. Ann Surg 1980; 192:762–771.
25. Brem H, Patz J, Tapper D. Detection of human central nervous system tumors: Use of migration-stimulating activity of the cerebrospinal fluid. Surg Forum 1983; 34:532–534.
26. Blackwood HJJ. Vascularization of the condylar cartilage of the human mandible. J Anat 1965; 99:551–563.
27. Coventry MB, Ghormley RK, Kernohan JW. The intervertebral disc. Its microscopic anatomy and pathology. Part I. Anatomy, development, and physiology. J Bone Joint Surg 1945; 27:105-112.
28. Haraldsson S. The vascular pattern of a growing and full-grown human epiphysis. Acta Anat 1962; 48:156–167.
29. Dontenwill W, Chevalier HJ, Reckzeh G. Growth of carcinomas in the region of the cartilage. JNCI 1973; 50:291–293.
30. Williams RG. The vascularity of normal and neoplastic grafts in vivo. Cancer Res 1951; 11:139–144.
31. Eisenstein R, Sorgente N, Soble LW, Miller A, Kuettner KE. The resistance of certain tissues to invasion: Penetrability of explanted tissues by vascularized mesenchyme. Am J Pathol 1973; 73:765–774.
32. Langer R, Brem H, Falterman K, Klein M, Folkman J. Isolation of a cartilage factor that inhibits tumor neovascularization. Science 1976; 193:70–72.
33. Langer R, Conn H, Vacanti J, Haudenschild C, Folkman J. Control of tumor growth in animals by infusion of an angiogenesis inhibitor. Proc Natl Acad Sci USA 1980; 77:4331–4335.
34. Kessler DA, Langer RS, Pless NA, Folkman J. Mast cells and tumor angiogenesis. Int J Cancer 1976; 18:703–709.
35. Kragh-Larsen A, Lund DP, Langer R, Folkman J. Oral heparin results in the appearance of heparin fragments in the plasma of rats. Proc Natl Acad Sci USA 1986; 83:2964–2968.
36. Crum R, Szabo S, Folkman J. A new class of steroids inhibits angiogenesis in the presence of heparin or a heparin fragment. Science 1985; 230:1375–1378.
37. Sakamoto N, Tanaka NG, Tohgo A, Osada Y, Ogawa H. Inhibitory effects of heparin plus cortisone acetate on endothelial cell growth both in cultures and in tumor masses. JNCI 1987; 78:581–585.
38. Ziche M, Ruggiero M, Pasquali F, Chiarugi VP. Effects of cortisone with and without heparin on angiogenesis induced by prostaglandin El and by S180 cells, and on growth of murine transplantable tumours. Int J Cancer 1985; 35:549–552.
39. Penhaglion M, Camplejohn RS. Combination heparin plus cortisone treatment of two transplanted tumors in C3H/He mice. JNCI 1985; 74:869–873.
40. Jaques LB. Determination of heparin and related sulfated mucopolysaccharides. Methods Biochem Anal 1977; 24:203–312.
41. Ingber DE, Madri JA, Folkman J. A possible mechanism for inhibition

of angiogenesis by angiostatic steroids: Induction of capillary basement membrane dissolution. Endocrinology 1986; 119:1768–1775.
42. Brem S, Zagzag D. The control of neoplasia in the brain by angiosuppression: Copper depletion prevents neovascularization and inhibits tumor growth. Presented at The Annual Meeting of the American Association of Neurological Surgeons, May 3–7, 1987, Dallas, Texas.
43. Tamargo RJ, Leong KW, Brem H. Inhibition of growth of the 9L glioma by the local sustained release of angiogenesis inhibitors. Presented at The Annual Meeting of the American Association of Neurological Surgeons, May 3–7, 1987, Dallas, Texas.

5

Brain Tumors and the Fibrinolytic Enzyme System

Raymond Sawaya and
Robert Highsmith

Introduction

Brain tumors constitute a group of heterogeneous neoplasms with complex and poorly understood biology. Research efforts directed at improving our understanding of these tumors and ultimately our therapeutic results have focused on the development of improved animal and tissue culture models and more recently on the recognition of tumor associated antigens.[30,48] The study of the biochemical phenomena associated with brain tumors has been restricted to the analysis of the metabolic pathways of glycolysis and has therefore been limited in scope. In this chapter, we summarize our efforts, supported by a pertinent but scattered literature, of studying the role played by the fibrinolytic enzyme system in brain tumor biology.

Numerous pathophysiological mechanisms are undoubtedly involved in the neoplastic process, and claims that any single enzymatic

From: Kornblith PL, Walker MD (editors). Advances in Neuro-Oncology. Futura Publishing Company, Inc., Mount Kisco, NY, © 1988.

This work was made possible in part by a grant from the Veterans Administration and by research grant HL 31543 from the NIH. The authors wish to recognize the following individuals who have either participated in or have influenced this research: Craig Cummins, Marcia Gallagher, Sue Green, Paul Kornblith, Ilona Ormsby, and Mario Zuccarello. Our thanks are also extended to Ms. Anita Tolle and Ms. Betty Guttridge for their excellent secretarial assistance.

system is responsible for the biological changes associated with the transformation of a cell cannot be supported by a careful and comprehensive review of the literature. However, to understand the various intricate and complex mechanisms characteristic of the neoplastic cell, it is essential to analyze each individual biological system while at the same time recognizing the role played by related systems.

The selection of the fibrinolytic enzyme system for our studies is based on its recognized role in cancer biology, its ubiquitous nature, and the potency of its constituents enzymes. In addition, direct ties are known to exist between this enzyme system and the other enzyme systems also associated with the neoplastic transformation. It is not surprising therefore that the biological functions affected by changes in the fibrinolytic enzyme system have covered a wide spectrum ranging from tumor growth to tumor invasiveness, tumor hemorrhage, and tumor host interactions leading to serious coagulopathies and thromboembolic complications.

In this chapter we will review some aspects of our current understanding of the fibrinolytic enzyme system, review the literature dealing with brain tumors, and consider the pathophysiological and therapeutic implications that may derive from this analysis.

The Fibrinolytic Enzyme System

Introduction

The traditional view of the fibrinolytic pathway has focused on those events resulting in the dissolution of intravascular deposits of fibrin, the end product of the coagulation system. As a necessary prerequisite to this process, the inactive zymogen (plasminogen) must first be converted by limited proteolysis (plasminogen activator) to an active serine protease (plasmin) (Fig. 1). Once evolved in plasma, plasmin may hydrolyze a variety of protein substrates, including coagulation factors V and VIII as well as fibrinogen and fibrin and several constituents of the extracellular matrix. However, the half-life of free plasmin in plasma is extremely brief due to its very rapid inhibition by α_2-antiplasmin, accompanied by an additional large array of protease inhibitors in plasma. The elucidation of the mechanisms by which in vivo fibrinolysis occurs, despite the molar excess

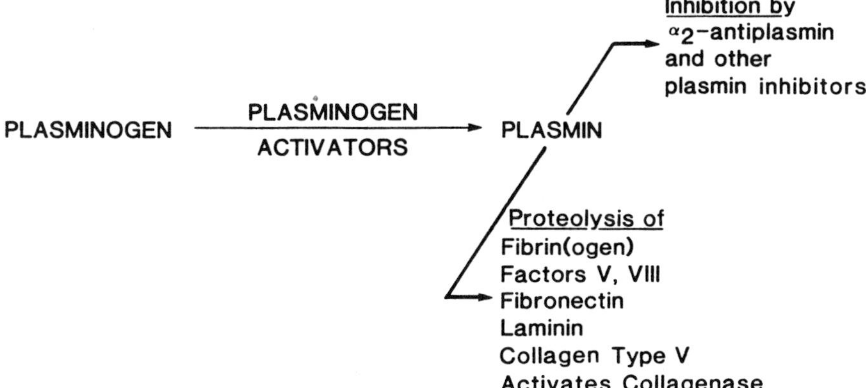

Figure 1. Summary of some of the physiological effects of plasminogen-dependent fibrinolysis.

of inhibitors, has been the subject of numerous intense and fruitful investigations in the past few years and will be reviewed later in this section.

Although most attention in the past has focused on the fibrinolytic properties of plasmin, it now appears that this endopeptidase may have an important role in other extracellular processes that require proteolysis. In favor of this concept is the fact that many other enzyme systems such as the inflammatory response, kinin generation, and complement activation are frequently tandem to the clotting and fibrinolytic sequences. In addition, the rather ubiquitous nature of plasminogen activators (PA) throughout the body tissues and the relative abundance of plasminogen which is delivered to the tissues via the blood stream, support a potential regulatory role that this enzyme system may play in extracellular proteolytic events. Thus, it is not surprising that the synthesis and release of plasminogen activator, the trigger of the fibrinolytic sequence, has been implicated in a variety of physiological and pathological events such as follicular rupture during ovulation,[18] macrophage, and granulocyte migration,[238] trophoblast invasion,[222] mammary gland involution[159] and the expression of the malignant phenotype.[54,61,63,170,239] The latter role will be discussed later in this chapter in regard to the interaction of fibrinolytic factors with neoplasia of the central nervous system.

Plasminogen

Plasminogen, formerly referred to as profibrinolysin, is the inactive zymogen of the fibrinolytic system and circulates in plasma at a concentration of approximately 2.0 μM or 175 μg/ml. Human plasminogen is a single chain glycoprotein with a molecular weight of approximately 90,000 and has about 2% carbohydrate. The zymogen exists in plasma in two major molecular forms which differ primarily in their carbohydrate content and in the presence or absence of sialic acid. The complete primary amino acid sequence of plasminogen has now been completed mostly by Magnusson's laboratory[218] and by Wallen and Wiman.[264] The molecule is stabilized by 24 disulfide bridges and contains 790 amino acid residues, of which about 60% are folded into a repeating series of five triple loop structures called "kringles."[218] This region of the molecule possesses considerable sequence homology with the human clotting zymogen, prothrombin; its integrity is very important for it is the locus for binding of plasminogen to the fibrin molecule during clot lysis[271] as well as being the primary site of interaction with α_2-antiplasmin.[268] The amino acid lysine also binds to this region of the plasminogen molecule, a fact which forms the basis for the affinity purification of the zymogen on columns of insolubilized lysine.[66] Native human plasminogen has an NH_2-terminus glutamic acid residue and is therefore commonly referred to as Glu-plasminogen.[253] However, limited proteolysis in this portion of the molecule results in the formation of Lys-plasminogen with lysine at the NH_2-terminal.[253] The COOH-terminal amino acid is asparagine.[192]

Turnover studies[53] in normal humans using radioiodinated zymogen preparations indicate a plasma half-life of about 2 days for native plasminogen. Interestingly, the disappearance rate for Lys-plasminogen is much faster at 0.8 days. On the average, approximately 55% of the plasma pool of plasminogen is catabolized per day. The primary site of synthesis of plasminogen in the human is most likely the parenchymal cell of the liver.[25] However, several studies[15,95,96,175,176] have provided indirect evidence which suggests considerable species variation as well as possible multiple sites of synthesis and/or storage. For instance, the eosinophilic granules of bone marrow cells[15,175] and other granulocytes[176] and the kidney[95] have been implicated as possible alternative sites of synthesis.

Plasminogen can be rapidly synthesized as evidenced by complete restoration within 12–24 hours following depletion during thrombolytic therapy.[95] Furthermore, circulating levels of the zymogen appear to be tightly regulated as evidenced by the precise re-establishment of plasma levels following depletion.[96] Animal studies by Highsmith and Kline,[96] using cross-injection techniques, suggest that restoration of plasma plasminogen levels following depletion may be mediated by the release of a blood-borne humoral-like substance. Plasminogen levels can be quantitated indirectly by caseinolytic, esterolytic, or fibrinolytic assays[250] following its conversion to plasmin with either urokinase or streptokinase. Direct measurements of immunoreactive plasminogen levels by radioimmunoassay[179] or immunodiffusion[135] are more frequently utilized than enzymatic assays, due largely to the presence in plasma of inhibitors directed against plasmin and plasminogen activators.

Plasminogen Activators and the Activation of Plasminogen

Plasminogen activation can occur by any one of several different mechanisms (Fig. 2). Endogenous or "intrinsic" activation occurs concomitant with the contact activation of factor XII (Hageman factor) during coagulation.[183] Factor XIIa or its active biological fragments do not directly convert plasminogen to plasmin but rather indirectly via their action on the kallikrein system. Kallikrein, formed by limited proteolysis of prekallikrein (Fletcher factor) by factor XIIa, can directly activate plasminogen to plasmin. High molecular weight kininogen (Fitzgerald factor) serves as an additional cofactor to these reactions by greatly enhancing the rate of kallikrein formation. Also, these reactions are most likely accountable for the activation of the complement system and the inflammatory response which accompany blood vessel injury. It should be noted, however, that these reactions have been confirmed almost entirely with purified proteins or with clotting assays using plasmas deficient in one of the factors. More importantly, the physiological significance of this pathway to the overall fibrinolytic mechanism is not clearly understood.

The second and biologically most important pathway of plasminogen activation is that achieved by the blood-borne or tissue and vessel wall-derived plasminogen activators. The precise origin(s) of the blood-borne plasminogen activators has been long debated and has led to a somewhat bewildering terminology. For example, the elevated levels of PA in plasma following exercise, venous occlusion, stress, or in postmortem blood have been variously termed blood PA,

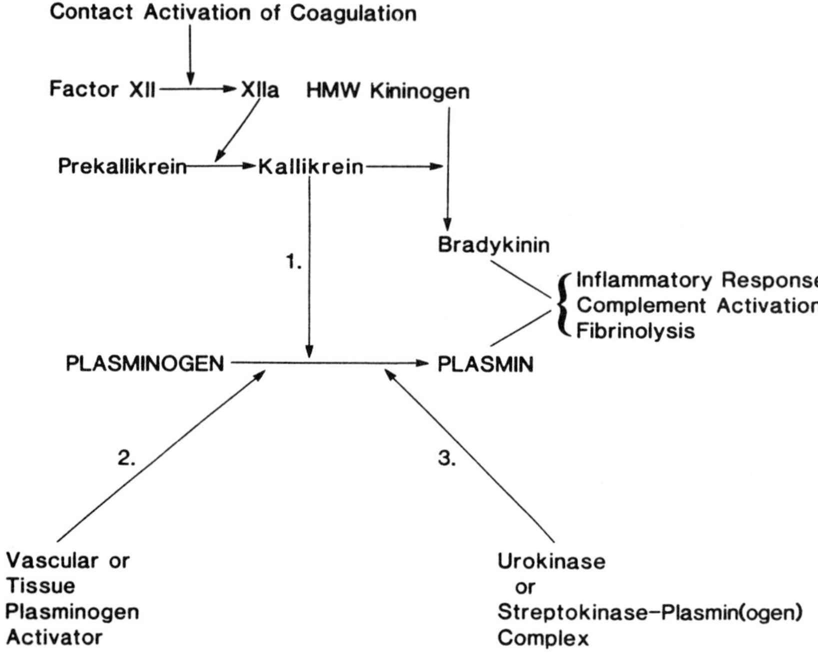

Figure 2. Common mechanisms of activation of the fibrinolytic enzyme system.

vascular PA, endothelious-derived PA.[51] In addition, plasminogen activators are present tightly bound in many organs, tissues, and secretions so that their extraction usually requires the use of chaotropic agents and extensive homogenization procedures.[49] Although precise biochemical comparisons of purified forms of the various vascular PA have not been completed, it appears very likely that the endothelial cell-derived blood-borne PA are in fact immunologically identical to the tissue type PA.[49,181,187,251] Tissue plasminogen activator (t-PA) is a serine protease of molecular weight approximately 70,000 and in its native state, is composed of two disulfide-linked polypeptide chains.[49,187,251] In addition, t-PA is uniquely suited for playing a key role as a fibrinolytic activator because of its high affinity for the fibrin molecule.[227] The plasma t-PA antigen concentration has been reported to be about 6–7 ng/ml in resting normal individuals when measured by an immunoradiometric assay.[189] However, considerably more t-PA probably exists in plasma as a complex with a fast-acting anti-activator.[219] The physiological importance of t-PA can be inferred from the association of depressed plasma fibrinolytic activity with thrombotic or atherosclerotic disease.[164–166] Following venous occlusion, the level of t-PA in plasma increases markedly. It is generally agreed that the source of the t-PA is most likely the venous endothelial cell. The ability of endothelial cells to release plasminogen activator in response to a standardized venous occlusion forms the basis of a test of "fibrinolytic capacity."[153] Utilizing this procedure, several investigators have found that patients with chronic thrombotic episodes display an impaired ability to release PA.[104] Futhermore, the high risk of recurrent thrombosis in these patients appears to be lessened by compounds which stimulate the release of t-PA.[154] Thus, a growing body of evidence strongly suggests that the t-PA of vascular tissue is intimately involved in the maintenance of vessel patency.

A third pathway of plasminogen activation can be accomplished by the exogenous PA, urokinase (UK) and streptokinase (SK). Although these two activators have been extensively studied and used therapeutically as thrombolytic agents, they clearly play no role in the normal vasculature since SK is a bacterial by-product and urokinase, while produced by the human kidney, does not gain access to the peripheral circulation. Numerous excellent reviews of these two PA have been published; only a few salient properties will be discussed here. Urokinase is a serine protease with trypsin-like specificity.[126,212] It is produced by the renal tubular epithelium and is therefore present in human urine. Human embryonic kidney cells also produce UK when cultured in vitro.[14,20] Two molecular weight forms of UK have been reported[216] corresponding to approximately 32,000 and 54,000 daltons. The smaller form is most likely a result of limited proteolysis of the larger form.[25] The mechanism by which UK activates plasminogen is essentially the same as that discussed below for t-PA. However, UK is clearly different from t-PA both antigenically[188] and in terms of its interaction with the fibrin molecule.[33] It should also be noted that while UK is usually considered an exogenous activator, there is recent convincing evidence[127] that there exists in cultured endothelial cells a molecule which is immunochemically identical to urinary UK. This endothelium-derived activator is generally referred to as UK-type PA as distinct from the tissue-type activator (t-PA). Whether the UK-type plasminogen activator is released in vivo or if it has any role in intravascular fibrinolysis remains unclear.

Streptokinase (SK) is a single-chain protein of molecular weight 47,000[58,65] which is produced by the Hancefield group C strain of B-hemolytic streptococci.[229] Early studies[44,144] on the properties of this protein led to the discovery of the plasminogen-plasmin system as the potential proteolytic pathway of plasma responsible for directing fibrinolysis. The term "streptokinase" is a misnomer in that the protein is not a kinase in a biochemical sense, nor is it an enzyme. Yet, when added to human plasma or to purified human plasminogen, SK results in the rapid quantitative conversion of plasminogen to plasmin, a process known to require enzymatic proteolysis. This apparent paradox has been the subject of intense studies for many years and has now been largely resolved.[184] We now know that SK, in a highly species specific manner, rapidly forms a complex with plasminogen in an equimolar 1:1 ratio. The complex then acquires the properties of an enzyme by formation of an active center in the plasminogen (free and complexed with SK) to either free plasmin or to an SK-plasmin complex which itself is an excellent activator of plasminogen. Thus, SK is classified as an indirect activator of plasminogen and is considerably different than UK or t-PA in that it requires preformation of a complex with plasmin(ogen). SK has been widely used as a thrombolytic agent and, at relatively high doses, has resulted in considerable success when administered by coronary catheterization immediately following coronary thrombosis.[68] However, SK is antigenic in humans and often elicits undesirable side effects.[68] In addition, SK resembles UK in that neither possess the high affinity for fibrin(ogen) that typifies the t-PA molecule.

Independent of the activator molecule (t-PA, UK or SK-plasmin complex), the critical event occurring during the transition of native Glu-plasminogen to plasmin is the hydrolysis of a single arginyl-valyl peptide bond (Arg_{560}–Val_{561}) in the COOH-terminal portion of plasminogen.[51] While there is universal agreement on the requirement for cleavage of this bond, other studies using purified proteins indicate that additional proteolysis may occur so that the precise temporal sequence of plasminogen activation, particularly in vivo, is not yet totally resolved.

Plasminogen activators can be quantified by a variety of techniques using esters, synthetic polypeptide chains coupled to chromogenic cleaving groups as well as whole proteins as substrates. Most assays are two-stage in nature in that they require a preincubation for the activation of added plasminogen in the first stage followed by the quantification of plasmin formed in the second stage. Unfortunately, the relative activities of different plasminogen activators are highly variable in different assay systems depending on: (1) the presence of fibrin(ogen); (2) the plasminogen concentration and the form of plasminogen (Glu- or Lys-) used; (3) the presence or absence of detergents such as SDS or Triton X-100 which may potentiate the activity of t-PA; and (4) the pH and ionic strength of the assay buffers. Hopefully, the impending establishment of an international standard will alleviate these problems. Be that as it may, perhaps the most useful and direct measurements are the various immunological assays using commercially available antibodies to the specific PA. Several approaches can thus be utilized including direct immunoradiometric determination of PA antigen levels[189] or enzymatic assay following immunodepletion of a specific PA molecule. Another interesting approach which is gaining wide usage is a zymographic method[87] or modifications thereof. These techniques involve SDS-PAGE of plasminogen activator-containing samples in gels containing plasminogen or other substrates either copolymerized or applied as an overlay. The method is useful because it allows simultaneous correlation of PA activity with molecular weight heterogeneity.

Inhibitors of Fibrinolysis

Human plasma is richly endowed with an abundance of naturally occurring protease inhibitors. The biological importance of these inhibitors in opposing intravascular proteolysis is quickly appreciated when one considers the pathological consequences of their deficiency states. For example, antithrombin deficiency is clearly associated with thromboembolic disease[71] and conversely, an α_2-antiplasmin deficit is manifested as a severe hemorrhagic tendency.[68] The major well-characterized proteinase inhibitors, their molecular weights and plasma concentrations are listed in Table 1. Nearly all of the inhibitors have broad specificities in that they will inhibit, to varying degrees, almost all plasma proteases. However, their specific names are primarily derived from that protease which is most rapidly inhibited or the protease which was being investigated at the time of discovery of the inhibitor.

The fibrinolytic system has two major protease components which are subject to regulation by protease inhibitors: PA molecule has been hampered by the inability of clot lysis assays to differentiate plasminogen activator inhibition from plasmin inhibition. Thus,

Table 1
Plasma Proteinase Inhibitors

Inhibitor	Molecular Weight (daltons)	Plasma Concentration (μM)
α_2-antiplasmin	67,000	1.0
Cl-inhibitor	107,000	1.6
inter-α-trypsin inhibitor	165,000	3.0
α_2-macroglobulin	725,000	3.4
antithrombin	62,000	4.7
α_1-antichymotrypsin	70,000	7.1
α_1-antitrypsin	55,000	23.6

until recently, unequivocal identification of the specific targets at which inhibitors act has been difficult. With the advent of better assay systems, the chemistry and relevance of specific plasmin inhibitors has been well established. The certainty of the existence and role of specific PA inhibitors, while not as strong, appears to be growing despite being the subject of considerable debate. A review of antiplasmins will be given first, followed by a discussion of putative inhibitors directed against plasminogen activators.

Inhibitors of Plasmin

During the past 10 years, an extensive literature has developed in regard to the role played by the various plasma protease inhibitors in opposing the action of plasmin.[3] In purified systems, nearly all of the inhibitors listed in Table 1 demonstrate antiplasmin activity with varying rates of inhibition. However, convincing evidence has been recently reviewed[4] and has established that in vivo, the physiologically most important and most recently discovered antiplasmin is α_2-antiplasmin. Although earlier studies[5,8,52] hinted at the existence of this inhibitor, its definitive role as the major plasma antiplasmin was reported nearly simultaneously by three independent groups of investigators in 1976.[50,147,149] For some time, this inhibitor was variously termed α_2-plasmin inhibitor, the immediate or fast acting plasmin inhibitor or α_2-antiplasmin. The latter term has now gained wide acceptance and immunochemical evidence has confirmed the identity of these inhibitor prepartions.[50,93] α_2-Antiplasmin is a single chain glycoprotein that co-migrates with α_2-globulins upon electrophoresis.[45] The inhibitor has a molecular weight of approximately 70,000 and contains about 13% carbohydrate.[45] Structural studies suggest that the molecule is very hydrated and highly asymetric[269]; the NH_2-terminal amino acid sequence is Asn-Gln-Glu-Gln-Val while that for the COOH-terminus is Phe-Leu.[269] The concentration of α_2-antiplasmin in pooled normal plasma is approximately 1 μM with significantly depressed levels occurring with severe liver disease, intravascular coagulation or following thrombolytic therapy.[36]

During the reaction between plasmin and α_2-antiplasmin, a very stable 1:1 stoichiometric complex of molecular weight 150,000 is formed.[45] The active site of the enzyme is tightly blocked as evidenced by its lack of both esterolytic as well as proteolytic activity.[45] The reaction between enzyme and inhibitor proceeds in two sequential steps.[7,268] In the first step, a reversible complex is formed by noncovalent binding between the inhibitor and the lysine binding sites on the B-chain of plasmin. Next, an irreversible and probably covalent bond is formed between the active site of plasmin and the reactive center on the inhibitor. The rate of interaction of plasmin and α_2-antiplasmin is extremely rapid and is one of the fastest protein-protein interactions ever described.[266] The precise molecular mechanism of interaction of plasmin and its primary inhibitor have been detailed elsewhere.[4,50] In addition to the direct inhibition of plasmin by complex formation, α_2-antiplasmin has two other properties of importance in the regulation of fibrinolysis. α_2-Antiplasmin interferes with the adsorption of plasminogen to fibrin[7] and the inhibitor is cross-linked to the fibrin molecule by factor XIIIa during coagulation.[197] The net effect of these properties is to bestow specificity to the interaction between the inhibitor, plasminogen, PA, and fibrin. These properties also account for the great effectiveness of α_2-antiplasmin as an inhibitor of fibrinolysis in vivo as compared to the other known antiproteases.

In normal plasma, the concentration of plasminogen is approximately 1.5- to 2.0-fold greater than α_2-antiplasmin. Therefore, upon extensive activation of plasminogen to plasmin during thrombolytic therapy, one can effectively exhaust the available pool of α_2-antiplasmin. Under these conditions, it is generally felt that the excessive plasmin formed is effectively inhibited by α_2-macroglobulin.[4] However, this general assumption has been challenged by a recent report using newer methodology,[92] which indicated that significant amounts of α_2-macroglobulin-plasmin complexes were formed before α_2-antiplasmin was fully saturated. It was also noted that significant quantitative differences in the amount of plasmin bound by α_2-antiplasmin vs. α_2-macroglobulin could be obtained depending on whether preformed plasmin was added to plasma versus in vivo activation of plasminogen to plasmin. Thus, some degree of uncertainty remains as to the precise quantitative role that α_2-macroglobulin plays in the inhibition of plasmin in plasma.

Inhibitors of Plasminogen Activators

As alluded to earlier, methodological problems have prevented the unequivocal differentiation of antiplasmin from antiactivators, largely because the measurement of the latter can be greatly influenced by the presence of antiplasmins. Endogenous or "intrinsic" activators of plasminogen (factor XIIa-induced fibrinolysis) can be inhibited in vitro by Cl-esterase inhibitor,[112] antithrombin-heparin mixtures[220] and α_2-macroglobulin.[142] However, since the physiological significance of this activation pathway to the overall fibrinolytic mechanism remains speculative, so does the potential role of its inhibitors.

The exogenous activators, SK and UK, are inhibited to varying degrees and by different mechanisms when added to human plasma. The reported half-life of UK in vivo is 9 to 17 min and 27 to 60 min in vitro[75]; thus, plasma clearance of UK seems to play a key role. In purified systems, nearly all of the well-characterized protease inhibitors (α_2-macroglobuin, α_1-antitrypsin, α_2-antiplasmin and antithrombin) have weak, but significant, inhibitory activity towards UK.[51] However, convincing evidence for a fast-acting inhibitor specifically directed toward UK in plasma is not available. Since SK alone does not possess biological activity, it cannot be inhibited per se. Interestingly, even when complexed with plasmin(ogen), the activator complex is unreactive toward α_2-antiplasmin[36] which may help to explain the therapeutic usefulness of this activator complex. Perhaps the major route of neutralization of SK in vivo is by endogenous antibodies directed against SK, particularly in subjects with recent streptococcal infections.[51] The anti-SK antibody titers are quite variable in individuals and sufficient SK must be administered to neutralize the antibody before affecting significant plasminogen activation.

A great deal of experimentation has been completed, with some-what conflicting results, on inhibitors of vascular- or tissue-type PA. As early as the 1950s, it was proposed that the vascular PA circulated as a reversible activator-inhibitor complex which dissociated in the presence of fibrin.[148] This model was attractive for it helped to explain the rapid dissolution of fibrin in plasma and the enhancing effect of fibrin on plasminogen activation. However, convincing evidence of the existence of such a system has been lacking and we now know that the latter effect is most likely due to the enhanced binding affinity of t-PA and plasminogen to the fibrin molecule.[267] Nevertheless, recent evidence in the last few years has produced a strong argument for the existence of a fast-acting specific inhibitor of t-PA in plasma. For example, when t-PA was added to human plasma at concentrations equivalent to that occurring during venous occlusion, the t-PA was rapidly inactivated with a half-life of about 1 min.[118] The rapid inhibition of t-PA in human plasma has been confirmed by other investigators.[39,40,244] Studies on the inactivation of t-PA in plasma have been greatly assisted by the development of an accurate and sensitive method for quantifying t-PA in plasma.[40,270] Using this method, the inhibitor has now been partially characterized.[266] The molecular weight of the plasma inhibitor is about 50,000 and it appears to form a 1:1 stoichiometric complex with t-PA. Relatively low concentrations of the newly described t-PA inhibitor were found in healthy individuals. Interestingly, however, in many patients with ongoing thrombosis, coronary artery disease or during normal pregnancy, the t-PA inhibitor values were significantly elevated,[265] suggesting a potential important role of this inhibitor in the etiology of thrombosis. The precise physiological role of the circulating t-PA inhibitor and its relationship to yet another recently described inhibitor synthesized by endothelial cells in culture[131] remains to be established.

Summary: Regulation of Fibrinolysis In Vivo

Regulation of the fibrinolytic enzyme system involves numerous protein-protein interactions which historically have been somewhat bewildering. However, during the past few years our basic knowledge from experimentation on these interactions at the molecular level now permits the construction of a model for the regulation of fibrinolysis in vivo.[51] The data listed below represent key findings which are instrumental in formulating this regulatory model: (1) Plasminogen specifically binds with high affinity to fibrin via the lysine binding sites (Kringle structures) on the zymogen. (2) The physiologically most important plasminogen activator (t-PA) also binds strongly to fibrin and the rate of plasminogen activation by t-PA is enhanced by fibrin. (3) α_2-Antiplasmin rapidly and irreversibly inhibits free plasmin and interacts with both the enzyme and zymogen via the lysine binding sites on plasmin(ogen). (4) A newly described inhibitor of t-PA rapidly and irreversibly inhibits free t-PA. (5) Fibrinogen can inhibit the plasmin-α_2-antiplasmin interaction by competing for binding to the lysine binding sites of plasmin(ogen). Utilizing this information, the following model can be formulated which is reasonably consistent with the literature. Activation of plasminogen in normal plasma by the exogenous activators UK or SK results in the generation of plasmin which, unless in excess, will be irreversibly inhibited by α_2-antiplasmin. Thus, under normal conditions, α_2-antiplasmin protects fibrinogen from proteolysis by plasmin. However, when fibrin is formed in vivo, t-PA, plasminogen and plasmin molecules are bound to the fibrin surface and thereby protected from inhibition. More efficient fibrinolysis is obtained with t-PA as the triggering mechanism due mainly to its high binding affinity for fibrin. Following the infusion of t-PA (or presumably after appropriate triggering and release of t-PA-like molecules from the endothelial cell), the activator binds rapidly at the site of fibrin deposition and activates the surface bound plasminogen to plasmin. Circulating free t-PA is achieved without significant systemic fibrinogenolysis by the in situ generation of plasmin protected from circulating α_2-antiplasmin. Although not completely tested, this model is supported by numerous in vivo studies which have been recently reviewed.[51] Futhermore, recent clinical studies [19] using recombinant t-PA [167] in the successful treatment of coronary thrombosis lends credence to this model being operative in vivo.

Plasminogen Activators in Brain Tumors

At the beginning of this century, investigators noted that explants of cancer tissue consistently caused proteolytic degradation and dissolution of plasma clots.[35,74] It was not until the mid-1970s, however, that the extracellular proteolytic activity of cancer cells was conclusively linked to the release of PA by the transformed cells. Normal cells transformed by oncogenic viruses were shown to produce abundant amounts of PA prior to the histological recognition of the malignant phenotype.[42,161,239] The methodology used in the assessment of the fibrinolytic activity of the neoplastic tissue has varied. Early reports have demonstrated the fibrinolytic capacity of normal and neoplastic tissues placed on fibrin plates, and have consistently shown that the neoplastic tissue's content of PA exceeded that found in the corresponding normal tissue.[185] Differences in PA production between malignant and benign neoplastic tissues have not been as consistent;[260] however, recent studies have been more sophisticated in identifying the MW and the immunological types of PA contained in various neoplastic tissues and are more likely to provide a better understanding of the characteristics and of the role played by PA in neoplasia.[81,138,177,252,263]

Studies on PA in brain tumors have been restricted, with few exceptions, to tissue culture models of rat and human glioma cell lines (Table 2). The earliest reports demonstrating an association between brain tumors and fibrinolysis originated from Dr. Kraus' laboratories and involved the measurement of lysis zones produced by fresh human brain tumor samples placed on fibrin plates.[24,114,117] Lysis zones were prominent with medulloblastoma, meningioma, and metastasis, variable with glioblastoma, and small with ependymoma. Necrotic tissue associated with glioblastoma lacked the ability to produce lysis on fibrin plates.[114]

Tovi et al.[232] compared the fibrinolytic and thromboplastic activities of meningiomas and gliomas and found higher fibrinolytic activity in meningioma tissue. Since plasmin inhibitors could be present to a variable degree in some of the tumors studied, fibrin plate assays have a limited value in accurately assessing the content of PA in brain tumor tissue.

In two consecutive studies, Wilson and Dowdle studied the PA production of a large variety of cultured human brain tumors.[259,260] The results emphasized the fact that PA synthesis is not the exclusive property of malignant cells; however, the rate of PA secretion by normal cerebral tissue was considerably lower than that found with malignant brain tumors. On the other hand, cell cultures of benign neoplasms secreted PA at rates comparable to those derived from malignant cells.

Hince and Roscoe detected high levels of plasminogen-dependent fibrinolytic activity in cell lines derived from an ethylnitrosourea-induced glioma of the rat brain and confirmed the low fibrinolytic activity detected in normal brain.[98] A positive correlation was found between the level of fibrinolytic activity, growth in agar and tumor-

Table 2
Brain Tumors and Plasminogen Activators

Author/Year	Tissue Source	Tissue Type	MW Determination	Immunological Determination	P.A. Activity Measurement	Assay System
Bock et al. 1970	Fresh Human Tumors	Brain Glioblastoma Astrocytoma Ependynoma	NO	NO	YES	Fibrin Plate
Koos et al. 1971	Fresh Human Tumors	Glioblastoma Astrocytoma Metastatic Meningioma Others	NO	NO	YES	• Fibrin Plate • Todd's Fibrin Slide
Tovi et al. 1975	Fresh Human Tumors	Meningioma Glioblastoma	NO	NO	YES	Todd's Fibrin Slide
Wilson et al. 1977	Human Tissue Culture	Nrain Glioblastoma Astrocytoma Meningioma Pituitary Adenoma Others	NO	NO	YES	^{125}I-Fibrin Plates
Hince, Roscoe. 1978	Rat Tissue Culture	Enu-induced Glioma	NO	NO	YES	Fibrin overlay method
Zanker et al. 1978	Rat Tissue Culture	C_6 Glioma $SDIG_1$ Glioma	NO	NO	YES	^{125}I-Fibrin Plate

Tucker et al. 1978	Human Tissue Culture	Glioblastoma Meningioma	NO	YES	YES	^{125}I-Fibrin Plate
Wilson et al. 1978	Human Tissue Culture	Brain Glioblastoma Astrocytoma Melanoma Meningioma Others	NO	NO	YES	^{125}I-Fibrin Plate
Higuchi. 1979	Fresh Human Tumors	Meningioma Glioblastoma Metastatic Craniopharyngioma Others	NO	NO	YES	Fibrin Plate
Hince, Roscoe. 1980	Rat Tissue	Normal Brain Enu-induced Glioma	NO	NO	YES	H^3-Fibrinogen Plate
Zankeret al. 1980	Rat and Rabbit Tissue Culture	Glioma	NO	NO	YES	^{125}I-Fibrin Plate
Wilson et al. 1980	Human Tissue Culture	Glioblastoma Meningioma Melanoma Other	YES	YES	NO	• ^{125}I-Fibrin Plate • Electrophoresis
Soreq, Miskin. 1981	Fresh Rodent Tissue	• Brain • Rat Glioma	YES	NO	YES	• ^{125}I-Fibrin Plate • Overlay Method • Electrophoresis
Bykowska et al. 1981	Rat Tissue Culture	Glioma	YES	YES	YES	• Electrophoresis • Fibrin Plates

Table 2   (*continued*)
Brain Tumors and Plasminogen Activators

Author/Year	Tissue Source	Tissue Type	MW Determination	Immunological Determination	P.A. Activity Measurement	Assay System
Nielsen et al. 1982	Human Tissue Culture	Glioblastoma	YES	YES	YES	• ^{125}I-Fibrin Plate • Electrophoresis
Dano et al. 1982	Human Tissue Culture	Glioblastoma Melanoma	YES	YES	YES	• Immunofluorescence • ^{125}I-Fibrin Plate • Electrophoresis
Liepkalns et al. 1982	Human Tissue Culture	• Glioblastoma • Fetal Brain	NO	NO	YES	^{125}I-Fibrin Plate
Gilbert, Wachsman. 1982	Human Tissue Culture	Neuroblastoma	YES	YES	YES	• ^{125}I-Fibrin Plate • Fluorogenic Assay • Electrophoresis
Sawaya, Highsmith	Fresh Human Tissue	Brain Glioblastoma Astrocytoma Metastatic Meningioma Acoustic Neuroma	YES	NO	YES	Zymography

igenicity of the cell line. Of interest is the fact that the enhanced fibrinolytic activity was detected in the latent period before the histological appearance of tumors or the ability of cells to form colonies in agar. In a subsequent study, these authors have shown that despite higher cell-associated PA in the glioma cell line than in the normal brain line, PA secretion in the harvest fluid was similar for both cell lines.[99]

Zanker et al. have demonstrated that the most intense fibrinolytic activity of rat glioma cells coincided with mitotic waves,[274] and that fibrin degradation products are engulfed in the cytoplasma of glioma cells raised on a fibrin layer.[275] Migration inhibition of glioma cells growing on fibrin-coated filters was accomplished with tranexamic acid, a fibrinolytic inhibitor. These authors have also shown that cultures reaching a high passage level exhibit a tendency for low PA activity.

The first attempt at immunologically identifying brain tumor PA was made by Tucker et al., who used human glioblastoma, ependymoblastoma, meningioma, and normal brain cell lines.[233] Cells cultured from normal adult brain showed no detectable fibrinolytic activity. Anti-urokinase immunoglobulin G failed to inhibit the PA activity of the human brain tumor preparations, leading the authors to conclude that brain tumor PA is antigenically different from urokinase.

Higuchi studied the fibrinolytic activity of 11 cystic brain tumors as compared to 18 solid brain tumors and four normal brains and concluded that cystic brain tumor tissues contained much higher fibrinolytic activity than solid brain tumors or normal brain.[97] The significance of these results remains uncertain.

The MW identification of PA present in normal brain and in brain tumors was first reported by Wilson et al., who indicated that normal brain tissue contained a predominant form of PA with a MW of 60 K similar to u-PA, while normal brain tumors in culture produced additional MW forms of 70 K, >95 K, and 38 K.[261] Because of the small number of samples, no particular trend could be detected for each brain tumor type. PA produced by normal brain tissue and by tumors of ectodermal or mesenchymal origin were inhibited by anti-urokinase antibody, a finding conflicting with that described by Tucker et al.[233]

In a study of PA in rodent brain, Soreq and Miskin were able to correlate PA activity with cell bodies in neuronal-enriched regions and in endothelial, meningeal, and ependymal layers. Homogenates of mature mouse brain contained a major MW band of about 80 K and a minor band of 50 K.[217] The 80 K band co-migrated with the PA from a differentiated mouse neuroblastoma tumor. There was a two-fold increase in PA activity observed in homogenates of cerebellar tissue few days following x-irradiation of the brain, while no effect was demonstrated on the PA activity of meningeal cells. In an important study, Bykowska et al. have purified the PA produced by cultured rat glioma cell line and showed that the amino acid composition of the brain tumor PA and its affinity to bind to fibrin were similar to those of the tissue-type PA.[32] The MW of the brain tumor PA were 60 K and 30 K, similar to u-PA even though the immunological identity of the PA was related to t-PA and not to urokinase, a finding supporting the results reported by Tucker et al.[233] and at variance with the results of Wilson et al.[261]

In 1982, two groups of investigators studied PA production by established human glioblastoma cell lines. Liepkalns et al. demonstrated a three-fold increase in the glioma cell-associated PA as compared to fetal neural cells, and over 20-fold increase in cell released PA.[128] This latter finding is in disagreement with the results of Hince and Roscoe reported previously.[99]

Nielsen et al. have identified a 52 K MW form of PA derived from a human glioblastoma cell line and have shown that the enzyme is released in an inactive form, therefore, suggesting that methodological differences may account for the variations in brain tumor PA MW reported from various centers.[152] In a follow-up study, this group of investigators used an antibody raised against the 52 K MW form of PA to evaluate the immunofluorescence staining of cultured glioblastoma cells.[62] The fluorescence was located in the cytoplasm of the cells, and marked variations in the staining intensity were observed between the individual cells. The main advantage of the immunohistochemical method is the ability to distinguish the histological affinity of different types of PA.

Our studies of brain tumor PA were done on fresh human samples collected in the operating room. A total of 58 samples were analyzed using a zymographic technique developed in our laboratory.[204] The histological types of tumors selected included metastatic, glioblastoma, acoustic neuroma, meningioma, low grade glioma, and normal brain. The PA activity was highest in metastatic tissue and acoustic neuroma, followed by glioblastoma, meningioma, and low grade glioma. All tumor samples had a mean PA activity greater than that of normal brain, although statistical significance could be demonstrated only for the first two tumor types. The MW pattern for each type of brain tumor was uniquely different with few exceptions. All samples contained a 60 K MW form. All primary brain tumors contained PA forms with MW of 68 K or 74 K or both, while none of the metastatic tumors contained PA with similar MW. The 84 K MW form was most characteristic of the meningioma group while the 94 K and 36 K MW forms were characteristic of the malignant brain tumors and of the acoustic neuroma. The finding of multiple MW forms of PA in non-CNS neoplastic tissue has been previously described with values ranging from 28 K to 165 K,[2,21,41,70,246] raising several unanswered questions. For instance, are the larger PA forms the product of different genes, or are they aggregates of the smaller forms? The precise cellular origin of the various forms of brain tumors PA is not known. Undoubtedly, some cells uniformly present in all of our tumor samples account for some of the PA detected. For example, the 60 K form, present in all tumor extracts might be produced in part by endothelial cells which are certainly present in each of the tumor extracts. However, the finding of consistent differences among the groups is more in favor of tumor cell-specific forms of PA. This theory is also supported by the variablity in MW patterns seen within the glioblastoma group, a tumor known for its heterogeneous cell population.

Our studies demonstrate a lack of association between a specific MW form of PA and the malignant phenotype since extracts of acoustic neuroma, a benign tumor, consistently contained lytic bands at 36 K and 94 K similar to those seen in metastatic tumors and in glioblastoma. On the other hand, differences were evident within the glioma group where low grade glioma can in most circumstances be differentiated from the highly malignant glioma since the former contains fewer PA forms and has a lower fibrinolytic capacity.

Tumor-associated PA can also be differentiated immunologically. The urokinase type of PA (u-PA) is generally associated with PA forms of MW 30 K and 60 K while the tissue-type of PA (t-PA) is associated with PA MW of 70 K. Other MW forms are of uncertain type and may be associated with either u-PA or with other unspecified forms of PA. Preliminary data from our laboratory indicate that both PA forms are present in fresh human brain tumors and that some MW forms do not immunoreact with antibodies directed against either type of PA (Fig. 3). Our findings are also supported by those of Colombi et al. who studied human breast tumors and reported PA forms different from the urokinase and the melanoma tissue type PA.[55]

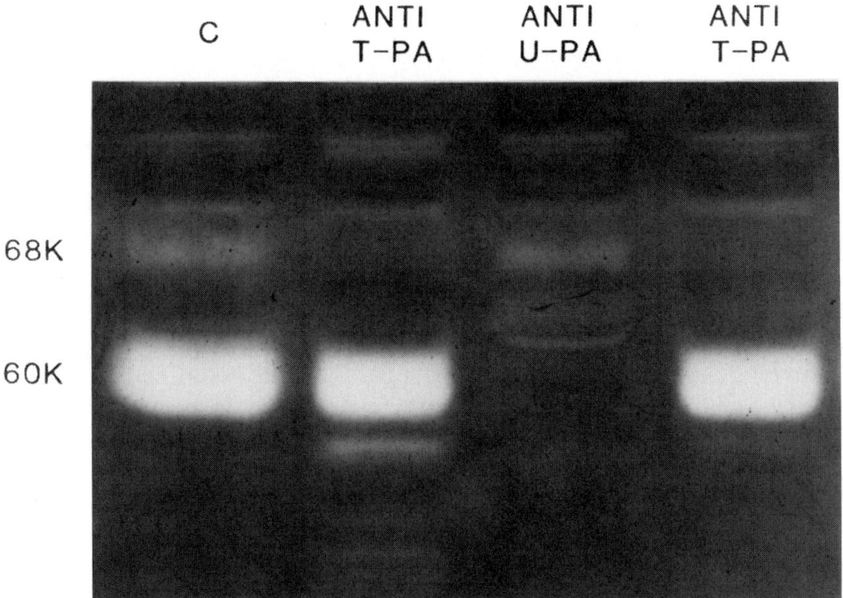

Figure 3. Antigenic specificity of various molecular weight PA in a meningioma demonstrated on an SDS-Page. C = Tumor homogenate alone. Anti t-PA = tumor homogenate preincubated with antimelanoma (right) or antiuterine (left) t-PA antibodies. Anti u-PA = tumor homogenate preincubated with anti-u-PA antibodies. Note the lack of immunoreactivity of the higher molecular weight PA forms.

Plasmin Inhibitors in Brain Tumors

Inhibitors of various elements of the fibrinolytic system have been detected in primary carcinoma of the liver, bladder, ovary, and lung.[120] Proteolytic inhibitory activity in leukemic cells and malignant breast tissue was also related to the presence of specific factors, most of which inhibit fibrinolysis.[236] Those factors include α_1-antitrypsin (AAT), α_1-antichymotrypsin, α_2-macroglobulin, α_2-antiplasmin, and antithrombin III. Additionally, the fibrin-stabilizing factor (factor XIII) was also found to possess fibrinolytic inhibitory activity.[237] Such a factor was produced by a spontaneously developed plasma cell tumor.[201]

Reports dealing with brain tumors have generally focused on the fibrinolytic activity of such tumors placed on fibrin plates. The degree of lysis produced is dependent on the presence of fibrinolytic inhibitors within the tumors, although cross-incubation experiments reported by few investigators failed to reveal the presence of fibrinolytic inhibitors in cultured glioma cells or in samples of fresh human brain tumors.[97,114]

Our first observation of the presence of plasmin inhibitors in brain tumors was made using a spectrophotometric assay to quantitate the hydrolytic effect of plasmin on the synthetic substrate CBZ-lysine. The addition of homogenized brain tumor samples produced a marked inhibition of the hydrolysis caused by a standard amount of plasmin. This inhibition was noted with meningioma and glioblastoma and was negligible with metastatic, acoustic neuroma, and normal brain.[201]

In order to identify the specific type of plasmin inhibitor present in brain tumor tissue, we have used immunodiffusion assays with various antibodies to the common plasmin inhibitors and found positive precipitation with AAT antibody in 68% of a total of 77 tumors, while none of the samples precipitated with α_2-macroglobulin antibody.[205] Marked differences in AAT positivity among the various histological groups of brain tumors were noted. For instance, all acoustic neuromas were positive for AAT, while only 50% of meningiomas were positive for AAT. The results for metastatic, glioblastoma, and low grade glioma were 91%, 78%, and 71%, respectively. There were no statistically significant differences noted between the group of patients with tumors positive for AAT and the patients with tumors negative for AAT in regard to age, sex, Karnofsky index, duration of symptoms, size of tumor, prothrombin time, partial thromboplastin time, platelet count, or erythrocyte sedimentation rate. Statistically significant differences were, however, found in the PA activity of the tumor (p = 0.001), the degree of peritumoral brain edema as detected on CT scan (p = 0.05), and the preoperative serum fibrinogen level (p = 0.02), all three parameters being more prominent in the group of patients with AAT-positive tumors.

The source and the significance of the presence of AAT in brain tumors are unknown. AAT is the major serine protease inhibitor of human plasma and has a broad range of enzyme inhibitory activity.[27] It has been described in normal tissues including the liver, histiocytes, mast cells, nerves, and gastrointestinal cells.[13,205,215] In neoplastic tissues, it is described mainly in hepatocellular carcinoma, liver sarcoma, ovarian malignancies, gastric carcinoid, hemangioblastoma, and osteoblastoma. In addition, CSF and serum AAT levels have been elevated in some patients with brain tumors.[77,140,256] It is our hypotheses that AAT is actively produced by the tumor cells. In support of this hypothesis is the fact that none of the tumors studied had detectable amounts of α_2-macroglobulin, therefore precluding the possibility of a passive transfer of AAT from the serum due to a breakdown in the blood brain barrier. The lack of differences in the blood parameters of patients with AAT-positive tumors compared to those with negative AAT is against the possibility of a nonspecific acute-phase reaction being responsible for the AAT positivity. Finally, recent work in our laboratory has demonstrated positive AAT cyto-plasmic immunostaining of brain tumor cells using peroxidase antiperoxidase technique. The lack of extracellular staining in several tumors studied is against the possibility of an exogenous source for AAT.[277]

The detection of plasmin inhibitors in brain tumors depends largely on the methodology used. In many instances, tumors positive for AAT have shown little or no plasmin inhibitory activity in our biological assay (i.e., acoustic neuromas) and, similarly, tumors showing marked plasmin inhibitory activity have not immuno-reacted with any of the antibodies against the common natural plas-min inhibitors. In view of the important role played by protease in-hibitors and their relationship to the proteolytic activities detected in brain tumors, there is a great need for further investigation in this field with particular attention paid to the various components of the fibrinolytic enzyme system present within each tumor sample (Fig. 4).

Pathophysiologic Significance

The fibrinolytic enzyme system is intricately related to several other enzyme systems including the coagulation, kininogen, prosta-glandin, and complement systems (Fig. 2).[22,27,85,109,254] In addition, several proteolytic enzymes have functions mimicking fibrinolysis or acting in concert with the fibrinolytic enzyme system.[86,156,198] In this section, we will describe some of the pathophysiological mechanisms associated with brain tumors and highlight the possible role played by the fibrinolytic enzymes in their genesis.

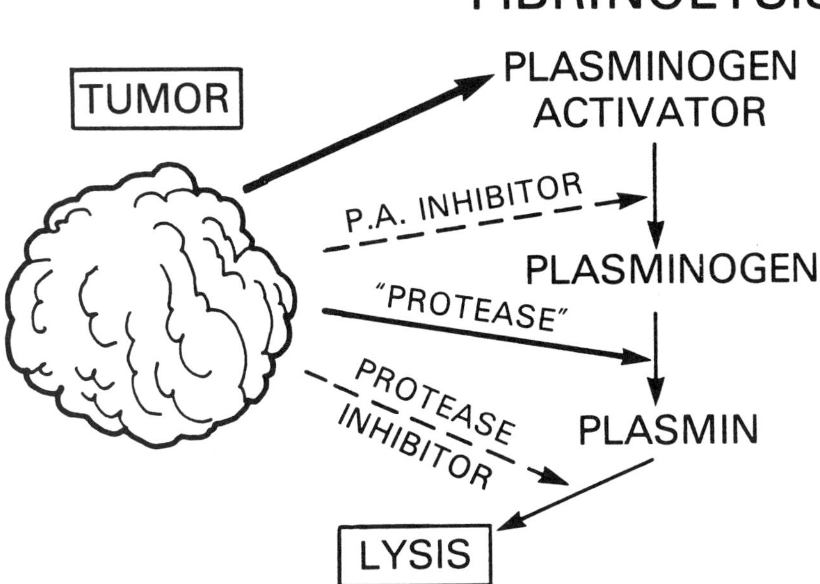

Figure 4. Fibrinolytic activators and inhibitors secreted by or contained within the neoplastic tissue.

Coagulation Disorders

Alterations of hemostasis in cancer patients have been described extensively,[22,101,186,245,254] and in systematic studies, hemostatic abnormalities have been detected in as many as 95% of patients.[182] The underlying mechanisms are complex and frequently unexplained; however, in some instances, procoagulant and fibrinolytic factors released by the neoplastic cells are assumed to be partially responsible for the altered hemostatic system.[201]

Hemostatic disorders in brain tumor patients have rarely been described. In fact, in a recent review Weick stated that "there have been no reports of primary brain tumors being associated with intravascular coagulation."[254] Our own review of the literature indicates that hemostatic abnormalities have been reported in patients with both primary and secondary brain tumors[199] and in neuroblastoma.[141]

The earliest report of coagulation abnormality was described in

1952 by Nathanson and Savitsky who showed an increased platelet adhesive index in six out of eight patients with brain tumors.[151] This finding was subsequently confirmed by Millac, who demonstrated a higher percentage of adhesive platelets in patients with malignant brain tumors than in those with benign brain tumors.[143] Morozov published the first detailed coagulation study of 45 patients with benign and malignant brain tumors and concluded that in patients with benign brain tumors there was a tendency toward a reduction in the coagulant properties of the blood without change in the fibrinolytic activity, while in patients with malignant tumors there was a moderate increase in the fibrinolytic activity of the blood.[145,146] Kraus recognized the occurrence of hyperfibrinolytic states during neurosurgical procedures and recommended the use of a wide-spectrum protease inhibitor to treat this condition.[116,117]

In a guinea pig model of an intracerebral transplantable glioblastoma, Hurt et al. have demonstrated various coagulation changes consistent with disseminated intravascular coagulation and secondary hyperfibrinolysis and concluded that a clot-promoting substance was probably released either from the tumor or the adjacent neural tissue causing the clotting abnormalities seen in the animals.[102]

Scharrer and Hubner have specifically studied the plasma fibrinolytic activity of 45 patients with brain tumors and found a mild elevation in the fibrinolytic activity of patients with primary brain tumors and a moderate reduction of this activity in patients with metastatic disease.[206] Burgman et al. studied the blood coagulation properties of 53 patients harboring a glial tumor and found an increase in the coagulation and in the viscosity of the blood both parameters being accentuated in the postoperative period.[31] Van Der Sande et al. have most recently shown a postoperative increase in the coagulation abnormalities in 18 patients with intracranial pathology.[242] The main abnormality was that of an elevated FDP level which tended to be higher with more extensive intracranial procedures. Finally, several individual reports have described various coagulopathies in patients with either primary or metastatic brain tumors (Table 3). The presumed hemostatic disorders included acute and chronic DIC, acute fibrinolysis, and hypercoagulable states, and the outcome has generally been fatal.[37,73,132,139,173,196,199,213,243]

Thromboembolic Complications

Since the early report of Trousseau in 1865, a direct association between malignancies and thromboembolic complications (TEC) has

Table 3
Summary of Cases with Coagulopathy

Author Year	Age/Sex	Diagnosis	Brain Tumor Site	Presumed Hemostatic Disorder	Treatment
Fountain 1960	36 M	Metastatic Carcinoma of Bronchus	Posterior Fossa-Meninges	Acute DIC	Fibrinogen
MacGee 1970	49 F	Metastatic Carcinoma of Breast	Cerebellum	Acute Fibrinolysis	Fibrinogen, EACA
	NS	Metastatic Tumor	Posterior Fossa	Acute DIC	NS
Chacornac 1973	NS	Glioma	NS	Acute Fibrinolysis	NS
Vardi 1974	19 F	Oligodendroglioma	Left parieto-temporal	Acute DIC	Heparin
Finelli 1976	45 F	Primary reticulum cell sarcoma	Left parieto-occipital	Hypercoagulable state	—
Matjasko 1977	23 F	Oligodendroglioma	Third ventricle	Acute DIC	Heparin, FFP
Sack 1977	50 M	Metastatic Carcinoma of Bronchus	Right parietal	Chronic DIC	Heparin, Warfarin
Sawaya 1983	39 M	Metastatic Carcinoma of Lung	Left cerebellar	Chronic DIC	Heparin, Platelets
Siddiqui 1983	36 F	Malignant Astrocytoma	Right frontal	Acute DIC	Heparin
Portugal 1984	52 F	Melanotic meningioma	posterior fossa	Acute DIC	Heparin Cryoprecipitate Fibrinogen

M = male; F = female; NS = not stated; DIC = disseminated intravascular coagulation; EACA = aminocaproic acid; FFP = fresh frozen plasma.

been well established and, next to bacterial infections, constitutes the main cause of death in patients with solid tumors.[196] Thromboembolic complications in patients with brain tumors have not received sufficient attention. In 1960 Wetzel et al. reviewed a series of 6,065 neurosurgical autopsies and found a 3% incidence of fatal postoperative pulmonary emboli.[257] Patients with brain tumors were not specifically identified. In another autopsy study involving 334 patients with primary intracranial neoplasms, the incidence of venous thrombosis was 27.5%—statistically different from the 17% incidence for a control neurosurgical group.[110] Of particular importance is the fact that of the group of patients with thrombosis, 38% were not postsurgical patients. There have been several clinical studies confirming the high incidence of postoperative thrombophlebitis in neurosurgical patients and in patients with brain tumors, particularly the malignant astrocytoma type.[38,108,195,235,241] We have retrospectively analyzed a series of 36 patients with malignant brain tumors and TEC and found a high percentage of thrombi occurring in fully ambulatory patients or in the nonparalytic leg and frequently in situations unrelated to any surgical intervention (manuscript in preparation).

The location of the intracranial neoplasm is of particular significance. Brisman et al., reviewing 1,000 cases of brain tumors, found that patients with a suprasellar tumor had a higher incidence of TEC than those with a tumor in other locations.[28] Similarly the report by Blabey et al. of four children with ileofemoral thrombophlebitis and central nervous system pathology revealed two patients with a suprasellar neoplasm[23] and the report of Sjoberg et al. described seven patients with Cushing syndrome suffering from thromboembolic complications.[214] We have recently reported such an occurrence in a patient with a craniopharyngioma who died suddenly from a massive pulmonary embolism prior to his planned operation.[200]

The types of brain tumors more commonly associated with TEC have not been previously identified. In an ongoing clinical project involving 46 patients harboring a malignant glioma, a metastatic brain tumor or a meningioma postoperative deep venous thrombosis is being detected using I^{125} fibrinogen leg scanning. Preliminary results have so far shown that while over 70% of patients with meningioma and over 60% of patients with malignant glioma had a positive fibrinogen scan, only 20% of the patients with metastatic disease to the brain had a positive fibrinogen leg scan. These findings are of great significance since our results described earlier have shown that metastatic tumors to the brain have a higher fibrinolytic activator activity and a lower fibrinolytic inhibitory activity than malignant glioma or meningioma tissue.

The mechanisms by which an intracranial tumor influences the hemostatic balance in the blood of the host are multiple and the role that each one plays in any individual case has yet to be determined.[155,201] Perhaps the most convincing mechanism involves the production by the tumor of factors that activate the coagulation system or that inhibit the fibrinolytic system. Procoagulants have been found in brain tumors[97,232] and tissue culture studies have demonstrated that procoagulant material and platelet aggregating material are shed by the cells into the culture medium.[69,106] The production by brain tumors of factors that inhibit the fibrinolytic system has also been demonstrated as detailed earlier.[201,205]

The ability of the central nervous system to influence the hemostatic balance was recognized by Cannon as early as 1914,[200] Kudrjashov described in a series of animal experiments the presence of a physiological antiplasmin reflex humoral mechanism responsible for the defense of the organisms against thrombogenic substances.[119] The exact location of the center for the control of the blood coagulation is not fully established. However, the hypothalamic-basal ganglia region may constitute a major component of this system. Indeed, the stimulation of this region led to an increase in plasma factor VIII,[89] and electrical stimulation of the basal ganglia-diencephalic region resulted in shortening of the venom clotting time.[57]

More recently, a hypothalamic-pituitary system that stimulates the release of PA in the rat has been described.[88,174] The pathways involved in the regulation of blood coagulation by the central nervous system seem to include additionally the brain stem, the spinal cord, and the autonomic nervous system.[57,89,119]

In summary, TECs occur commonly in patients with primary brain tumors and are the result of tumor-host interactions either as a direct response to the production by the tumors of factors capable of altering the hemostatic balance or indirectly through interference with the hypothalamic-diencephalic center for the control of blood coagulation and fibrinolysis.

Finally, our findings of elevated plasma fibronectin levels in patients with brain tumors are interesting since fibronectin, through its opsonic capabilities, can enhance the clearance by the reticulum endothelial system of cell debris, immune complexes, and degradation products of fibrinogen and fibrin that result from the local interactions between the tumor and the host.[202] Elevated plasma fibronectin levels in patients with brain tumors may, therefore, represent an early indicator of a disturbed hemostatic balance.

Brain Tumor Hemorrhage

Spontaneous intracranial hemorrhage in patients with brain tumors has been widely reported. The incidence has varied between 1.3 and 15% and hemorrhages have been associated with most histological types.[60,79,83,84,91,113,125,136,157,225,249,255,272] In many instances, the hemorrhage was the presenting event responsible for the demise of the patient.[100,208,276] In order of relative frequency, choroid plexus papilloma and metastatic tumors, especially choriocarcinoma and melanoma, are most frequently associated with spontaneous hemorrhages.[136] Pituitary adenomas are also considered to be prone to spontaneous hemorrhages.[225] Intraventricular neoplasms are responsible for almost 50% of the hemorrhagic tumors, followed by base of the skull tumors.[79]

The mechanisms responsible for the hemorrhage have included various promoting factors such as rate of growth, vascularization, infarction and necrosis, vascular invasion and mechanical stretching.[79,249] Although it is unquestionable that such mechanistic factors have been described histologically in a variety of brain tumors, it seems more logical that a local disturbance of the hemostatic balance in favor of a hyperfibrinolytic state is at least partly responsible for the spontaneous hemorrhagic event.[6,26,130]

Plasminogen activators have been directly incriminated at the source of hemorrhagic disorders[130] and our own studies detailed earlier have demonstrated an increased production of PA by metastatic as well as primary brain tumors.[204] Involvement of the fibrinolytic system has rarely been considered as an initiating factor in brain tumor hemorrhage and further studies will be required to demonstrate the specific mechanisms involved.

Tumor Growth Invasiveness and Metastasis

Factors important to tumor growth invasiveness and metastasis include host immunological response, host hormonal environment and the intrinsic biological potential of the tumor. The role played by the fibrinolytic enzyme system is applicable to the latter factor as demonstrated by a growing body of experiments.[34,150,158]

Secretion of PA by tumor cells provides an attractive mechanism for initiating the breakdown of barriers to tumor growth and spread.[46,156,198] This enzyme is a serine protease whose pH optimum (pH 7.5) is close to that of extracellular fluid. Its substrate, plasminogen, exists in the body fluids, and the product of its action, plasmin, is a proteolytic enzyme of broad specificity. Plasmin degrades several types of structural constituents including basement membrane glycoproteins (Fig. 1).[129,156,198]

The observation that fibrin is found in the extracellular spaces of tumor tissue has suggested that fibrin deposition may represent an additional barrier to the spread of the neoplastic tissue and that enhanced tumor fibrinolytic activity may provide the neoplastic tissue with the capability to overcome this barrier.[169] In addition, the finding of phagocytized fibrin degradation products within brain tumor cells indicates that the enhanced fibrinolytic activity associated with neoplasia may promote tumor growth and spread via the provision of nutritional elements.[275]

The importance of fibrinolysis in the growth of a glioblastoma cell line implanted subcutaneously in nude mice was indirectly demonstrated following the oral administration of a competitive inhibitor of plasminogen activation.[203] The growth rate of the tumors in the control animals was significantly higher than that in the treated animals (Table 4).

In view of the increasingly recognized role of PA in malignancy

Table 4
Antifibrinolytic Therapy of an Experimental Glioblastoma

Animal Group	Number of Mice	Drug	Rate of Tumor Growth (cumm/day)	Mean Survival (days)
A	9	5% EACA	0.47 ⎫ NS	60.0 ⎫ NS
B	10	2.5% EACA	0.55 ⎰ ⎱ $p < 0.05$	61.3 ⎰ ⎱ $p < 0.05$
C	10	0.9% Benzyl alcohol	0.81 ⎭	50.7 ⎭

EACA = aminocaproic acid; NS = not significant.

and metastasis, it seemed paradoxical to find high PA production in benign primary brain tumors such as acoustic schwannoma and meningioma. In addition, primary malignant brain tumors which are also rich in fibrinolytic activity are recognized for their low potential to metastasize.[1] This seemingly paradoxical finding can be best explained by the fact that the process of tumor metastasis involves a sequence of events which may require the production by the tumor cells of various proteolytic enzymes including PA.[34] In addition, the type of PA produced by brain tumors may influence its ability to spread since t-PA, for instance, was found to have greater transformation enhancing activity than u-PA.[64] The presence of fibrinolytic inhibitors may also influence the metastatic potential of the neoplasm as shown by Malone et al., who found that tumor spread correlated directly with tumor activation of fibrinolysis and inversely with inhibition of fibrinolysis.[134]

Finally, although primary brain tumors rarely metastasize secondary brain tumors present an increasingly challenging problem, the treatment of which could benefit from an improved understanding of the mechanisms involved in metastasis.

Immunosuppression

Cellular and humoral immune responses in patients harboring malignant glial tumors have been the subject of numerous studies.[9] Although previous studies have indicated the presence of circulating antibodies, in vitro microcytotoxicity assay of the immune responses in individuals with astrocytoma demonstrated evidence of significant cytotoxicity in 65% of sera tested.[115] Positive results were more frequently obtained in lower-grade astrocytoma, suggesting the presence of an altered immune response secondary to immunosuppressive agents. Studies by Brooks et al. also indicated a significant degree of anergy during the preoperative period in patients with anaplastic gliomas.[29] The concept of immunoblocking factors was reviewed recently by Apuzzo and Mitchell, who have described blocking factors which may activate suppressor T-cells and suppressor macrophages which elaborate prostaglandins capable of impairing the proliferation of T-cell precursors.[9]

Kikuchi and Neuwelt described the presence of immunosuppressive factors in brain-tumor cyst fluid suggesting that brain tumor cells produce lymphocyte-suppressive factors which may be released into the blood.[111]

Several indirect observations suggest that the fibrinolytic enzyme system may be responsible at least in part for the altered immune response detected in patients with brain tumors. Fibrin(ogen) degradation products (FDP) were found to be immunosuppressant via the inhibition of lymphocyte protein synthesis.[82,172] FDP are found in brain tumor cyst fluids.[97] Moreover, PA were found to have an immune-modulating function since the presence of PA was inhibitory to the natural killer-mediated lysis of target tissue and to the specific cell-mediated cytotoxicity reactions.[284] This inhibitory role is thought to provide the means for a tumor self-defense in the face of what might otherwise be a successful anti-tumor immune reaction mounted by the host.[172,226,248]

A similar concept of tumor self-defense was proposed in our study of AAT in brain tumors as suggested by the results of Weiss et al.[256] and the extensive review of Breit et al.[27] AAT is capable, for instance, of inhibiting the cytotoxic reactions of lymphocytes including antibody-dependent cell-mediated cytotoxicity, T-cell-mediated cytotoxicity and natural killer activity.[27] The role of AAT in regulating the complement system by inhibiting its activation is of great significance since the complement system is thought to be the major initiator and amplifier of both immune- and nonimmune-mediated tissue injury.

Peritumoral Brain Edema

Peritumoral brain edema occurs commonly in humans as documented by computerized tomography scanning and is a potential cause of morbidity and mortality.[80] Despite the important clinical significance of this phenomenon, little attention has been given to elucidate its specific pathogenic mechanism.

Peritumoral brain edema is considered to be a secondary event developing as the consequence of an altered blood-brain barrier permeability by the tumor.[16] The leakage of serum proteins across tumor vessels is thought to depend upon the vascularization of the tumor and the permeability of the vessel wall.[103] It is very likely that specific factors produced by the tumor are responsible for the brain edema. A vascular permeability factor that promotes the accumulation of ascites fluid was described by Senger et al.[210] These same authors have more recently reviewed the close interactions between microvascular permeability and extravascular fibrin deposition, coagulation and fibrinolysis.[56,69] Secretory-excretory phenomenon was described in a study on meningioma associated with brain edema; however, the nature of the excreted material was not identified.[171] The microvascular permeability enhancing activity of fibrin(ogen) degradation products is well demonstrated and is similar to the enhancing activity described with bradykinin, an enzyme closely linked to the fibrinolytic system.[78,133,233,240]

In a recent limited study, Quindlen et al. found a positive correlation between brain edema and the fibrinolytic activity as detected on a fibrin plate.[178] In our own study of 39 patients, we were able to demonstrate a definite but weak correlation between the occurrence and degree of peritumoral brain edema, and the degree of fibrinolytic activity of the tumoral tissue, suggesting that PA-induced fibrinolysis is only partially responsible for the edema associated with brain tumors.[204] Other factors, possibly including the bradykinin system or even PA-independent fibrinolysis by elastase-like neutral proteases may be involved in the production of peritumoral brain edema.[86,133,240]

Radiation Effect

Radiation therapy to the brain is a common form of treatment for most unresectable brain tumors. The side effects of early edema and delayed radiation necrosis are clinically important but pathophysiologically obscure.[121] It has recently been demonstrated that neural tissue subjected to radiation therapy shows an enhanced PA activity in the short term following irradation. On the other hand, both Astedt et al. and Svanberg et al. have shown that large irradiated vessels have a prolonged decrease in PA-dependent fibrinolytic activity.[10,224] In a study of the radiation effect on the fibrinolytic activity of dog's liver, Henderson et al. were able to demonstrate a dramatic loss of fibrinolytic activity from all hepatic vessels with the exception of the major portal branches.[94]

The intriguing observation of Rizzoli and Pagnanelli of a dramatic response of delayed radiation necrosis of the brain to heparin may suggest that the loss of PA production by the brain is responsible for this frequently fatal disease.[191] In our study of PA activity in 13 malignant brain tumor tissue samples, we looked specifically at the subset of tumors previously irradiated and found that four of the six samples with lytic activity below the mean level for this group were derived from tumors which had been irradiated within 6 months of the surgery, while only one of the seven samples with lytic activity above the mean level for this group was derived from a tumor which was irradiated 3 years previously.[204]

More studies will be required to elucidate further the direct effect of brain radiation therapy on the local fibrinolytic system especially as it relates to radiation-induced edema and necrosis.

Clinical Applications

Diagnostic and Prognostic Applications

The potential use of PA production as a marker for human neoplasia was the subject of several studies. In a detailed analysis, Roblin stated that "for PA expression to be clinically useful in cancer detection, either PA levels generated by malignant tissues in vivo must be significantly higher than PA levels of normal tissues, or malignancy must produce detectable concentrations of a particular type of PA in locations where it is not normally present."[193] In a previous section, we have reported the findings of Hince and Roscoe[98] of higher PA production by rat glioblastoma than by rat brain, and our own findings of higher PA activity in malignant glioma than in low grade glioma or in normal brain. However, as our study demonstrated, PA activity alone failed to differentiate between acoustic neuroma, a benign tumor, and metastatic brain tumors. With further refinements in our assays, we were able to demonstrate convincing zymographic differences between several major types of brain tumors. Other authors have studied the relationship between multiple forms of PA in human breast tumors and the presence of metastasis in lymph nodes, suggesting that PA molecular weight patterns when correlated with PA activity may provide important prognostic information.[55] Similarly, the type of PA detected in the neoplastic tissue may also have prognostic significance since t-PA was found to exert transformation-enhancing activity which was lacking with u-PA.[64] We have also demonstrated that additional types of PA are present in some brain tumors (Fig. 3) which provide an exciting potential for the immunological detection of PA in body fluids as well as in histological sections.[122,231]

The use of monoclonal antibodies in the diagnosis of brain tumors has become a reality.[30,48] A radioimmunoassay detecting antigen CA 125 has also been used to monitor the course of epithelial ovarian cancer,[17] and a similar assay was applied to the detection of PA released by ovarian tumor in culture medium, in the blood of nude mice with ovarian tumor grafts and in the blood of patients with ovarian carcinoma.[11] More sophisticated immunoradiometric assays have also been applied to measure human t-PA as well as t-PA-inhibitors complexes in human plasma.[189,190]

Finally, immunohistochemical localization of t-PA and u-PA has been demonstrated for the first time in tissue sections using a peroxidase method and monospecific antibodies to PA.[122] Such studies have not yet been applied to brain tumors.

Therapeutic Applications

Hemorrhagic Disorders

Intraoperative bleeding during neurosurgical procedures has been associated with neoplastic disorders and has presented a frustrating and frequently challenging problem to the neurosurgeon.[37,117] Although a direct link between the hemorrhagic tendency of the tumors and the hyperfibrinolytic state has not yet been convincingly demonstrated, several indirect observations, detailed in the previous sections, make this hypothesis quite plausible.

Previous authors have suggested that the excessive intraoperative hemorrhage was due to the activation of the fibrinolytic system leading at times to overt coagulopathies, and have therefore proposed the use of a wide spectrum protease inhibitor to treat this hemorrhagic disorder.[37,117,232] A heightened awareness of the pathophysiologic mechanisms of the underlying hemorrhagic disorders in neurosurgery is essential if a rapid and effective treatment is to be applied. The demonstration of the type of coagulopathy responsible for the excessive hemorrhage requires a detailed coagulation profile which cannot be practically accomplished within the time frame of the surgical procedure; however, such an analysis could provide us with significant data to be used in future studies and possibly in the empiric treatment of the presumed hemorrhagic disorder.[230]

Thromboembolic Complications

Thromboembolic complications occur frequently in patients with brain tumors either in the postoperative period (meningioma, glioblastoma) or at the time of tumor recurrence and progression (glioblastoma). The treatment of the TEC is similar to the standards outlined for patients with other disorders and should rely primarily on prophylactic measures. Among such measures, intermittent calf compression has demonstrated its effectiveness without the added hemorrhagic risks associated with the administration of low dose heparin.[235] This form of prophylaxis is best suited for the perioperative period because of the obligatory period of bed rest and the limited period of risk. In patients with progressive brain tumors, especially those with preserved neural function, other forms of prophylaxis are required. From a theoretical standpoint, a wide spectrum protease inhibitor with antifibrinolytic and anticoagulant properties may be used for this purpose.[67] Studies documenting the effectiveness of such therapy are still needed.

Brain Edema

Systemic steroids are routinely administered to treat the peritumoral brain edema. The mechanism by which the edema is reduced is unknown; however, recent data have shown that links do exist between steroid receptors and PA,[228] and that dexamethasone, a steroid most commonly used to treat brain edema, has an inhibitory effect on PA.[105] Myeloid leukemic cells treated with dexamethasone had a reduction in their PA activity to less than 25% of control.[262] Laug found that the same drug at a concentration of 10^{-8} molar completely inhibited u-PA production and secretion by endothelial cells whereas t-PA production remained unaffected.[124] In a glioma tissue culture model, Freshney demonstrated marked reductions (4–22%) in PA production following the administration of dexamethasone.[76] Dano et al. have also shown that dexamethasone reduced the PA content of a glioblastoma cell line along with a reduction in its immunofluorescence while progesterone affected neither parameter.[62] The mechanism of action of dexamethasone on the peritumoral brain edema may be through the induction of an inhibitor of PA similar to that seen in rat hepatoma cells.[59,209]

The clinical implications of these findings may be of great importance if we consider the potential side-effects of dexamethasone therapy especially during long-term administration.[72] If the beneficial effect of dexamethasone on the peritumoral brain edema is via its inhibition of PA, then a more direct and specific inhibitor of PA may obviate the risks associated with glucocorticoid therapy.

Antineoplastic Therapy

The notion that the ability of malignant tumors to invade and destroy normal tissues may be due to the production of specific proteolytic enzymes have led numerous investigators to study the effect of various protease inhibitors on the growth, spread, and metastasis of several tumors implanted in animals.[234] Antifibrinolytic drugs have generally significantly reduced the tumor growth rate and have decreased the number of spontaneous metastasis derived from experimental tumors.[123,168,169,194,203,207,221,258,274] However, in studies on the lodgement of tumor cells in lung after an intravenous tumor cell injection, antifibrinolytic drugs were found to enhance metastasis formation, presumably because of the microthrombus formation around intravascularly trapped tumor cells.[47,169,234] We have reported the results of our study on the effect of a synthetic fibrinolytic inhibitor, epsilon amino caproic acid (EACA) on the growth of a malignant brain tumor transplanted subcutaneously in nude mice.[203] The tumor produced PA and showed histologic characteristics similar to those of the original tumor. There was no statistical difference between the treated and the control groups as regards to the age of the animals at the time of tumor transplantation, the interval implant-treatment time, or the tumor volume at the time of treatment. Statistically significant differences between the groups, however, indicated that the treated animals had longer mean survival time and had a lower rate of tumor growth (Table 4). These findings support the hypothesis that the fibrinolytic system plays a role in the growth and development of malignant gliomas and that interference with the fibrinolytic system may have a therapeutic role.

The results of malignant brain tumor therapy remain deceptive and our understanding of the biology of brain tumors is far from comprehensive.[211] Therefore, the clinical implications of our study may be of great significance. The effective treatment of patients with advanced carcinoma using fibrinolytic inhibitors as adjuvent therapy has been reported,[12,90] and in a recent study, antibodies to PA inhibited the metastasis in an animal model of a human carcinoma.[160] It is likely, therefore, that with current technology, specific monoclonal antibodies against brain tumor PA could be produced and tested for therapeutic use.[180]

Summary

This review has clearly demonstrated the intricate involvement of the fibrinolytic enzyme system in brain tumor biology. The specific mechanisms by which this enzyme system affects the various biological events described in this chapter remain unelucidated. From a basic descriptive standpoint, PA forms should be identified and correlated with their histological distribution, the nature of the tumor, and its biological behavior. Plasmin inhibitors undoubtedly present in brain tumors should also be characterized. Plasmin inhibitory activity should be quantitated and taken into consideration whenever PA activity is measured in tumor tissue. In view of the seriousness and frequency of the hemorrhagic and thromboembolic events associated with brain tumors, a greater understanding of the role played by all the constituents of the hemostatic balance should be considered (Fig. 5). Such studies will have to include not only

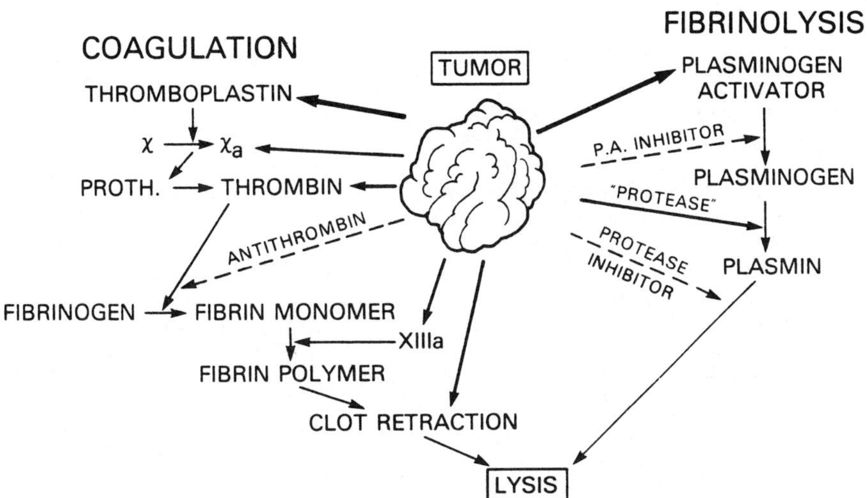

Figure 5. Complex balance of fibrinolytic and coagulation enzymes intimately involved in the pathophysiological mechanisms associated with the neoplastic process.

elements of the coagulation cascade but also the kininogen and prostaglandin systems. However, regardless of the influence exerted by these related enzyme systems, the fibrinolytic enzymes are potent and ubiquitous enzymes and have been shown to be intimately related to the neoplastic process. A better understanding of their role in brain tumor growth and spread is likely to lead to specific therapeutic measures.

REFERENCES

1. Alvord EC Jr. Why do gliomas not metastasize? Arch Neurol 1976; 33:73–75.
2. Angles-Cano E, Boyer B, Gisselbrecht S, Debre P. Heterogeneity of plasminogen activator expression in various Moloney virus-induced tumor cell lines. Lack of correlation with tumor growth and cell phenotype. Int J Cancer 1984; 33:277–280.
3. Aoki N. Natural inhibitors of fibrinolysis. Prog Cardiovasc Dis 1979; 21:267–286.
4. Aoki N, Harpel PC. Inhibitors of the fibrinolytic enzyme system. Semin Thromb Haemost 1984; 10:24–41.
5. Aoki N, Moroi M. Distinction of serum inhibitor of activator-induced clot lysis from α_1-anti-trypsin. Proc Soc Exp Biol Med 1974; 146:567–570.
6. Aoki N, Saito H, Kamiya T, Koie K, Sakata Y, Kobakura M. Congenital deficiency of α_2 plasmin inhibitor associated with severe hemorrhagic tendency. J Clin Invest 1979; 63:877–884.
7. Aoki N, Sakata Y. Influence of α_2-plasmin inhibitor on adsorption of plasminogen to fibrin. Thromb Res 1980; 19:149–155.
8. Aoki N, von Kaulla KN. Human serum plasminogen antiactivator: Its distinction from antiplasmin. Am J Physiol 1971; 220:1137–1145.
9. Apuzzo MLJ, Mitchell SM. Immunological aspects of intrinsic glial tumors. J Neurosurg 1981; 55:1–18.
10. Astedt B. Bergentz SE, Svanberg L. Effect of irradiation on the plasminogen activator content in rat vessels. Experientia 1974; 30:1466–1467.
11. Astedt B. Immunological detection of tumor plasminogen activator in biological markers of neoplasia: Basic and applied aspects. Ruddon, ed. Amsterdam, Elsevier North Holland Inc., 1978; p.481–489.
12. Astedt B, Mattsson W, Trope C. Treatment of advanced breast cancer with chemotherapeutics and inhibition of coagulation and fibrinolysis. Acta Med Scand 1977; 201:491–493.
13. Bagdasarian A, Wheeler J, Stewart GJ, Ahmed SS, Colman RW. Isolation of α_1-protease inhibitor from human normal and malignant ovarian tissue. J Clin Invest 1981; 67:281–291.
14. Barlow GH, Lazer L. Characterization of the plasminogen activator isolated from human embryo kidney cells: comparison with urokinase. Thromb Res 1972; 1:201–208.

15. Barnhart MI, Riddle JM. Cellular localization of profibrinolysin (plasminogen). Blood 1963; 21:306–321.
16. Bartkowski HM. Peritumoral edema. Prog Exp Tumor Res 1984; 27:179–190.
17. Bast RC Jr, Klug TL, St. John E, Jenison E, Niloff JM, Lazarus H, Berkowit RS, Leavitt T, Griffiths T, Parker L, Zurawski VR, Knapp RC. A radioimmunoassay using a monoclonal antibody to monitor the course of epithelial ovarian cancer. N Engl J Med 1983; 309:883–887.
18. Beers WH, Strickland S, Reich E. Ovarian plasminogen activator: Relationship to ovulation and hormonal regulation. Cell 1975; 6:387–394.
19. Bergmann SR, Fox KAA, Ter-Pogossian MM, Sobel BE, Collen D. Clot-selective coronary thrombolysis with tissue-type plasminogen activator. Science 1983; 220:1181–1183.
20. Bernik MB, Kwaan HC. Origin of fibrinolytic activity in cultures of human kidney. J Lab Clin Med 1967; 70:650–655.
21. Bernik MB, Wijngaards G, Rijken D. Production by human tissues in culture of immunologically distinct multiple molecular weight forms of plasminogen activators. Ann NY Acad Sci 1981; 370:592–596.
22. Bick RL. Alterations of hemostatasis associated with malignancy. Semin Thromb Haemost 1978; 5:1–26.
23. Blabey RG, Weil R III, Santulli TV. Iliofemoral thrombophlebitis associated with central nervous system pathology. Am J Surg 1975; 130:315–316.
24. Bock F, Kraus H, Blumel G, Koos W. L'activite fibrinolytique des tumours cerebrales. Neuro Chirurgie 1970; 16:542–547.
25. Bohmfalk JR, Fuller GM. Plasminogen is synthesized by primary cultures of rat hepatocytes. Science 1980; 209:408–410.
26. Booth NA, Bennett B, Wijngaards G, Grieve JHK. A new life-long hemorrhagic disorder due to excess plasminogen activator. Blood 1983; 61:267–275.
27. Breit SN, Wakefield D, Robinson JP, Luckhurst E, Clark P, Penny R. The role of α_1-antitrypsin deficiency in the pathogenesis of immune disorders. Clin Immunol Immunopathol 1985; 35:363–380.
28. Brisman R, Mendell J. Thromboembolism and brain tumors. J Neurosurg 1973; 38:337–338.
29. Brooks WH, Netsky MG, Normasuell DE, et al. Depressed cell-mediated immunity in patients with primary intracranial tumors. Characterization of a humoral immunosuppressive factor. J Exp Med 1972; 136:1631–1647.
30. Bullard DE, Bigner DD. Applications of monoclonal antibodies in the diagnosis and treatment of primary brain tumors. J Neurosurg 1985; 63:2–16.
31. Burgman GP, Kachkov IA, Vial'tseva Shcherbakova GG. The state of blood coagulation in patients with glial tumors of the brain. Zh Vopr Neirokhir 1979; 3:34–39.
32. Bykowska K, Rijken DC, Collen D. Purification and characterization of the plasminogen activator secreted by a rat brain tumor cell line in culture. Thromb Haemost 1981; 46:642–644.
33. Camiolo SM, Thorsen, Astrup T. Fibrinogenolysis and fibrinolysis with

tissue plasminogen activator, urokinase, streptokinase-activated human globulin and plasmin. Proc Soc Exp Biol Med 1971; 138:277–280.

34. Carlsen SA, Ramshaw IA, Warrington RC. Involvement of plasminogen activator production with tumor metastasis in a rat model. Cancer Res 1984; 44:3012–3016.

35. Carrel A, Burrows MT. Cultivation in vitro of malignant tumors. J Exp Med 1911; 13:571–575.

36. Cederholm-Williams SA, DeCook F, Lijnen HR, Collen D. Kinetics of the reactions between streptokinase plasmin and α_2-antiplasmin. Eur J Biochem 1979; 100:125–132.

37. Chacornac R. Fibrinolyse et coagulopathie de consommation en Neurochirurgie. Neurochirurgie 1973; 19:265–269.

38. Chaika VT, Raevskii VP, Kant II, Polenov AL. Thromboembolic complications in patients with cerebral tumors and cerebral cranial traumas. Vopr Neirokhir 1970; 34:35–39.

39. Chmielewska J, Ranby M, Wiman B. Determination of tissue plasminogen activator in plasma. Evidence for a rapid inhibitor. Thromb Haemostat 1983; 50:193.

40. Chmielewska J, Ranby M, Wiman B. Evidence for a rapid inhibitor to tissue plasminogen activator in plasma. Thromb Res 1983; 31:427–436.

41. Christman JK. Multiple forms of plasminogen activator. In: Biological markers of neoplasia: basic and applied aspects. Ruddon, ed. Amsterdam, Elsevier North Holland. 1978; pp. 433–449.

42. Christman JK, Acs G. Purification and characterization of a cellular fibrinolytic factor associated with oncogenic transformation: the plasminogen activator from SV-40-transformed hamster cells. Biochim Biophys Acta 1974; 340:339–347.

43. Christman JK, Acs G, Silagi S, Silverstein SC. Plasminogen activator: biochemical characterization and correlation with tumorigenicity. In: Proteases and Biological Control. E. Reich R Shaw (Eds). Cold Spring Harbor Laboratory. 1975; pp. 827–839.

44. Christensen LR, Macleod CM. A proteolytic enzyme of serum: characterization activation and reaction with inhibitors. J Gen Physiol 1945; 28:559–566.

45. Christensen U, Clemmensen I. Kinetic properties of the primary inhibitor of plasmin from human plasma. Biochem J 1977; 163:389–391.

46. Cliffton ER. Effect of fibrinolysin on spread of cancer. Fed Proc 1966; 25:89–93.

47. Cliffton EE, Agostino DA. Effect of inhibitors of fibrinolytic enzymes on development of pulmonary metastases. J Natl Cancer Inst 1964; 33:753–763.

48. Coakham HR, Garson JA, Brownell B, Kemshead JT. Monoclonal antibodies as reagents for brain tumor diagnosis: a review. J Roy Soc Med 1984; 77:780–787.

49. Cole ER, Bachmann FW. Purification and properties of a plasminogen activator from pig heart. J Biol Chem 1977; 252:3729–3737.

50. Collen D. Identification and some properties of a new fast-reacting plasmin inhibitor in human plasma. Eur J Biochem 1976; 69:209–216.

51. Collen D. On the regulation and control of fibrinolysis. Thrombos Haemost 1980; 43:77–89.
52. Collen D, DeCock F, Verstraete M. Immunochemical distinction between antiplasmin and α_1-antitrypsin. Thromb Res 1975; 7:245–249.
53. Collen D, Verstraete M. Molecular biology of human plasminogen. II. Metabolism in physiological and some pathological conditions in man. Thromb Diath Haemorrh 1975; 34:403–408.
54. Colombi M, Dano K, Reich E. Serine enzymes released by cultured neoplastic cells. J Exp Med 1978; 147:745–757.
55. Colombi M, Barlanti S, Magdelenat H, Fiszer-Szafarz B. Relationship between multiple forms of plasminogen activator in human breast tumors and plasma and the presence of metastases in lymph nodes. Cancer Res 1984; 44:2971–2975.
56. Colvin RB, Dvorak HF. Role of the clotting in cell-mediated hypersensitivity. J Immunol 1975; 114:377–387.
57. Correll JW. Central neural structures and pathways important for control of blood clotting: evidence for release of antiheparin factor. Bibl Anat 1969; 10:433–441.
58. Crum R, DeRenzo EC, Siiteri PK, Hutchings BI, Bell PH. Preparation and certain properties of highly purified streptokinase. J Biol Chem 1967; 242:533–539.
59. Cwikel BJ, Barouski-Miller B, Coleman PL, Gelehrter TD. Dexamethasone induction of an inhibitor of plasminogen activator in HTC hepatoma cells. J Biol Chem 1984; 259:6847–6851.
60. Dagi TF, Maccabe JJ. Metastatic trophoblastic disease presenting as a subarachnoid hemorrhage: report of two cases and review of the literature. Surg Neurol 1980; 14:175–184.
61. Dano K, Reich E. Serine enzymes released by cultured neoplastic cells. J Exp Med 1978; 147:745–757.
62. Dano K, Dabelsteen E, Nielsen LS, Kaltoft K, Wilson EL, Zeuthen J. Plasminogen activating enzyme in cultured glioblastoma cells. J Histochem Cytochem 1982; 30:1165–1170.
63. Dano K, Andreason PA, Grondahl-Hansen J, Kristensen P, Nielson LS, Skriver L. Plasminogen activators, tissue degradation and cancer. Adv Cancer Res 1985; 44:139–266.
64. De Petro G, Vartio T, Salonen EM, Vaheri A, Barlati S. Tissue type plasminogen activator but not urokinase exerts transformation-enhancing activity. Int J Cancer 1984; 33:563–567.
65. DeRenzo EC, Siiteri PK, Hutchings BI, Bell PH. Preparation and certain properties of highly purified streptokinase. J Biol Chem 1967; 242:533–539.
66. Deutsch DG, Mertz ET. Plasminogen purification from human plasma by affinity chromatography. Science 1970; 170:1095–1096.
67. Dubber HC, McNicol GP, Douglas AS. In vitro and in vivo studies of Trasylol. Thromb Diath Haemorrh 1966; 20:173.
68. Duckert F. Thrombolytic therapy. Semin Thromb Haemost 1984; 10:87–103.
69. Dvorak HF, Senger DR, Dvorak AM, Harvey VS, McDonagh J. Regu-

lation of extravascular coagulation by microvasular permeability. Science 1985; 227:1059–1061.

70. Evers JL, Patel J, Madeja JM, Schneider SL, Hobika GH, Camiolo SM, Markus C. Plasminogen activator activity and composition in human breast cancer. Cancer Res 1982; 42:219–226.

71. Egeberg 0. Inherited anti-thrombin deficiency causing thrombophilia. Thromb Diath Haemorrh 1965; 13:516–530.

72. Fast A, Alon M, Weiss S, Zer-Aviv FR. Avascular necrosis of bone following short-term dexamethasome therapy for brain edema. J Neurosurg 1984; 61:983–985.

73. Finelli PF. Remote cerebral infarction as a presenting manifestation of brain tumor (primary reticulum cell sarcoma): case report. Military Med 1976; 141:548–550.

74. Fisher A. The cultivation of malignant tumor cells indefinitely outside the body. Cancer Res 1925; 9:62–70.

75. Fletcher AP, Alkjaersig N, Sherry S, Genton E, Hirsh J, Bachmann F. The development of urokinase as a thrombolytic agent: Maintenance of a sustained thrombolytic state in man by its intravenous infusion. J Lab Clin Med 1965; 65:713–731.

76. Freshney RI. Effects of glucocorticoids on glioma cells in culture. ExpCell Biol 1984; 52:286–292.

77. Galvez S. Farcas A, Monari M. The concentration of alpha–1–antitrypsin in cerebrospinal fluid and serum in a series of 40 intracranial tumors. Clin Chim Acta 1979; 91:191–196.

78. Gerdin B, Saldeen T. Effect of fibrin degradation products on microvascular permeability. Thromb Res 1978; 13:995–1006.

79. Gil R, Le Fevre J-P. Les hemorragies meningees au cours des tumeurs intracraniennes. interet des formes (pseudo-aneurysmales). Semin Hop Paris 1970; 46:3505–3512.

80. Gilbert JJ, Paulseth JE, Coates RK, Malott D. Cerebral edema associated with meningiomas. Neurosurgery 1983; 12:599–605.

81. Gilbert LC, Washsman JT. Characterization and partial purification of the plasminogen activator. Biochim Biophys Acta 1982; 704:450–460.

82. Girmann G, et al. Immunosuppression by micromolecular fibrinogen degradation products in cancer. Nature 1976; 259:399–401.

83. Glass B, Abbott KH. Subarachnoid hemorrhage consequent to intracranial tumors. Arch Neurol Psychiatry 1955; 73:369–379.

84. Globus JH, Sapirstein M. Massive hemorrhage into brain tumor. JAMA 1942; 120:348–352.

85. Goodwin JS. Prostaglandins and host defense in cancer. Med Clin North Am 1981; 65:829–844.

86. Gramse M, Bingenheimer C, Schmidt W, Egbring R, Havemann K. Degradation products of fibrinogen by elastase-like neutral protease from human granulocytes. J Clin Invest 1978; 61:1027–1033.

87. Granelli-Piperno A, Reich E. A study of proteases and protease-inhibitor complexes in biological fluids. J Exp Med 1978; 148:223–234.

88. Granelli-Piperno A, Reich E. Plasminogen activators of the pituitary gland: enzyme characterization and hormonal modulation. J Cell Biol 1983; 97:1029–1037.

89. Gunn CG, Hampton JW. CNS influence on plasma levels of factor VIII activity. Am J Physiol 1967; 212:124–130.
90. Guthrie D, Ross WM, Latner AL, Turner GA, Way S. Effective treatment of a patient with an advanced carcinoma of the cervix with a combination of bromocriptine and aprotinin. Br J Clin Prac 1981; 35:330–332.
91. Harada K, Kiya K, Matsumura S, Mori S, Vozumi T. Spontaneous intracranial hemorrhage caused by oligodendroglioma: a case report and review of the literature. Neurol Med Chir (Tokyo) 1982; 22:81–84.
92. Harpel PC. α_2-Plasmin inhibitor and α_2-macroglobulin-plasmin complexes in plasma. Quantitation by an enzyme-linked differential antibody immunosorbent assay. J Clin Invest 1981; 68:46–55.
93. Hedner U, Gallimore M. Two human immunochemically distinct fibrinolytic inhibitors. Thromb Haemost 1977; 38:145.
94. Henderson BW, Bicher, Johnson RJ. Loss of vascular fibrinolytic activity following irradiation of the liver—an aspect of late radiation damage. Radiat Res 1983; 95:646–652.
95. Highsmith RF, Kline DL. Kidney: Primary source of plasminogen after acute depletion in the cat. Science 1971; 174:141–142.
96. Highsmith RF, Kline DL. Plasminogen restoration by the kidney mediated by a plasma factor. Am J Physiol 1973; 225:1032–1037.
97. Higuchi H. Tissue coagulation system and fibrinolytic activity of brain tumors. Neurol Med Chir 1979; 19:509–516.
98. Hince TA, Roscoe JP. Fibrinolytic activity of cultured cells derived during ethylnitrosourea-induced carcinogenesis of rat brain. Br J Cancer 1978; 37:424–433.
99. Hince TA, Roscoe JP. Differences in pattern and level of plasminogen activator production between a cloned cell line from an ethylnitrosourea-induced glioma and one from normal adult rat brain. J Cell Physiol 1980; 104:199–207.
100. Hinton DR, Dolan E, Sima AF. The value of histopathological examination of surgically removed blood clot in determining the etiology of spontaneous intracerebral hemorrhage. Stroke 1984; 15:517–520.
101. Hirsh J. Hypercoagulability. Semin Hematol 1977; 14:409–425.
102. Hurt JP, Odom MH, Perlmutt L, Krigman MK. Blood clotting changes in guinea pigs with a heterologous intracranial neoplasm. Lab Invest 1970; 23:179–183.
103. Hurter T. Experimental brain tumors and edema in rats. Exp Pathol 1984; 26:41–48.
104. Isacson S, Nilsson IM. Defective fibrinolysis in blood and vein walls in recurrent "idiopathic" venous thrombosis. Acta Chir Scand 1972; 138:313–319.
105. Isotalo H, Tryggvason K, Vierikko A, Vihko R. Plasminogen activators and steroid receptor concentrations in normal, benign, and malignant breast and ovarian tissues. Anticancer Res 1983; 3:331–336.
106. Jamieson GA, Bastida E, Ordinas A. Mechanisms of platelet aggregation by human tumor cell lines. In: Interaction of platelets and tumor cells. Jamieson G. ed. New York, Alan R Liss, 1982; pp. 405–413.
107. Jensen RH, Bigbee WL, Zimmerman AL, King EB. Plasminogen acti-

vator as a diagnostic marker for preneoplastic cells in human gynecologic specimens. Acta Cytol 1979; 23:105–113.

108. Joffe SN. Incidence of postoperative deep vein thrombosis in neurosurgical patients. J Neurosurg 1975; 42:201–203.

109. Karmali RA. Prostaglandins and cancer. CA 1983; 33:322–332.

110. Kayser-Gatchalian MC, Kayser K. Thrombosis and intracranial tumors. J Neurol 1975; 209:217–224.

111. Kikuchi K, Neuwelt EA. Presence of immunosuppressive factors in brain-tumor cyst fluid. J Neurosurg 1983; 59:790–799.

112. Kluft C. Elimination of inhibition in euglobulin fibrinolysis by use of flufenamate. Involvement of C1-activator. Haemostasis 1977; 6:351–369.

113. Kohli CM, Crouch RL. Meningioma with intracerebral hematoma. Neurosurgery 1984; 15:237–240.

114. Koos W, Valencak E, Kraus H, Blumel G, Bock F. L'activite'fibrinolytique relevee dans les tumeurs intra-craniennes. Neurochirurgie 1971; 17:549–558.

115. Kornblith PL, Dohan FC, Wood WC, et al. Human astrocytoma: serum-mediated immunologic response. Cancer 1974; 33:1512–1519.

116. Kraus H. The problem of blood coagulation disturbances with neurosurgery. Acta Neurochir 1969; 20:123–130.

117. Kraus H. Fibrinolytic activity of cerebral tumors and the treatment of a tendency to hemorrhage. Arch Neurol Neurochir Psychiatr 1971; 108:27–31.

118. Kruithof EKO, Ransijn A, Bachmann F. Inhibition of tissue plasminogen activator by human plasma. In: Progress in fibrinolysis. Davidson JF, Bachman F, Bouvier CA, Kruithof EKO, eds. Edinburgh, Churchill Livingstone 1983; 6:362–366.

119. Kudrjashov BA, Kalishevska TM. Existence and significance of a reflex-humoral antiplasmin system in the organism. Nature 1963; 198:763–764.

120. Kwaan HC, McFadzean R, McFadzean, AJS. Antifibrinolytic activity in primary carcinoma of the liver. Clin Sci 1959; 18:251–261.

121. Lampert, PW, Davis RL. Delayed effects of radiation on the human central nervous system. Neurology 1964; 14:912–917.

122. Larsson A, Astedt B. Immunohistochemical localization of tissue plasminogen activator and urokinase in the vessel wall. J Clin Pathol 1985; 38:140–145.

123. Latner AL, Longstaff E, Pradhan K. Inhibition of malignant cell invasion in vitro by a proteinase inhibitor. Br J Cancer 1973; 27:460–464.

124. Laug WE. Glucocorticoids inhibit plasminogen activator production by endothelial cells. Thromb Haemost 1983; 50:888–892.

125. Lazaro RP, Messer HD, Brinker RA. Intracranial hemorrhage associated with meningioma. Neurosurgery 1981; 8:96–101.

126. Lesuk A, Terminiello L, Traver JH, Geoff JL. Biochemical and biophysical studies of human urokinase. Thromb Diath Hemorrh 1967; 18:293–297.

127. Levin EG, Loskutoff DJ. Cultured bovine endothelial cells produce both

urokinase and tissue-type plasminogen activators. J Cell Biol 1982; 94:631–636.
128. Liepkalns VS, Liepkalns-Icard, Sommer AM, Quigley JP. Properties of cloned human glioblastoma cells. J Neurol Sci 1982; 57:257–264.
129. Liotta LA, Goldfarb RH, Brundage R, Siegal GP, Terranova V, Garbisa S. Effect of plasminogen activator (urokinase), plasmin, and thrombin on glycoprotein and collagenous components of basement membrane. Cancer Res 1981; 41:4629–4636.
130. Lisiewicz J. Mechanisms of hemorrhage in leukemias. Semin Thromb Hemostas 1978; 4:241–267.
131. Loskutoff DJ, van Mourik JA, Erickson LA, Lawrence D. Detection of an unusually stable fibrinolytic inhibitor produced by bovine endothelial cells. Proc Natl Acad Sci USA 1983; 80:2956–2960.
132. MacGee EE, Bernell WR. Acute fibrinolysis following craniotomy and removal of metastatic tumor of the cerebellum. J Neurosurg 1970; 32:578–580.
133. Maier-Hauff, Baethmann K, Lange AJ, Schurer L, Unterberg A. The kallikrein-kinin system as mediator in vasogenic brain edema. J Neurosurg 1984; 61:97–106.
134. Malone JM, Gervin AS, Moore WS, Keown K. Tumor interaction with the fibrinolytic system. J Surg Res 1979; 26:581–589.
135. Mancini G, Carbonara AO, Herermans JF. Immunological quantitation of antigens by single radial immunodiffusion. Immunochemistry 1965; 2:235–246.
136. Mandybur TI. Intracranial hemorrhage caused by metastatic tumors. Neurology 1977; 27:650–655.
137. Mann BS, Geddes JF. The nature of cytoplasmic inclusions in cerebellar haemangioblastomas. Acta Neuropathol 1985; 67:174–176.
138. Markus G, Kohga S, Camiolo SM, Madega JM, Ambrus JL, et al. Plasminogen activators in human malignant melanoma. J Natl Cancer Inst 1984; 72:1213–1222.
139. Matjasko MJ, Ducker TB. Disseminated intravascular coagulation associated with removal of a primary brain tumor. J Neurosurg 1977; 47:476–480.
140. Matsuura H, Nakazawa S. Prognostic significance of serum α_1-acid glycoprotein in patients with glioblastoma multiforme. A preliminary communication. J Neurol Neurosurg Psychiatry 1985; 48:835–837.
141. McMillian, CW, Gaudry CL, Holemans R. Coagulation defects and metastatic neuroblastoma. J Pediatr 1968; 72:347–350.
142. McConnel DJ. Inhibitors of kallikrein in human plasma. J Clin Invest 1972; 51:1611–1623.
143. Millac P. Platelet stickiness in patients with intracranial tumors. Br Med J 1967; 4:25–26.
144. Milstone JH. A factor in normal human blood which participates in streptococcal fibrinolysis. J Immunol 1941; 42:109–120.
145. Morozov VV. The coagulative and anti-coagulative blood systems in cerebral tumors of a supratentorial localization. Zh Nevropatol Psikhiatr im S.S.K. 1968; 68:505–509.
146. Morozov VV. Blood coagulation properties in patients with supraten-

torial tumors during pre- and post-operative periods. Vopr Neirokhir 1970; 34:56–60.

147. Moroi M, Aoki N. Isolation and characterization of alpha-plasmin inhibitor from human plasma. A novel proteinase inhibitor which inhibits activator-induced clot lysis. J Biol Chem 1976; 251:5956–5965.

148. Mullertz S. Mechanism of activation and effect of plasmin in blood. Ph.D. thesis, Copenhagen. Eijnar Munxsgaard, 1956.

149. Mullertz S, Clemmensen I. The primary inhibitor of plasmin in human plasma. Biochem J 1976; 159:545–553.

150. Nagy B, Ban J, Brdar B. Fibrinolysis associated with human neoplasia. Production of plasminogen activator by human tumors. Int J Cancer 1977; 19:614–620.

151. Nathanson M, Savitsky JP. Platelet adhesive index studies in multiple sclerosis and other neurologic disorders. Bull NY Acad Med 1952; 28:462–468.

152. Nielsen LS, Hansen JG, Skriver L, Wilson EL, Kaltoft K, Zeuthen J, Dano K. Purification of zymogen to plasminogen activator from human glioblastoma cells by affinity chromatography with monoclonal antibody. Biochemistry 1982; 21:6410–6415.

153. Nilsson IM, Pandolfi M. Assay of fibrinolytic activity of the vessel wall. In: Progress in chemical fibrinolysis and thrombolysis. Davidson JF, Samama M, Desnoyers PC, eds. New York, Raven Press, 1976; 2:1–13.

154. Nilsson IM. Phenformin and ethylestrenol in recurrent venous thrombosis. In: Progress in Chemical Fibrinolysis and Thrombolysis. Davidson JF, Samama M, Desnoyers PC, eds. New York, Raven Press, 1975; pp. 1:1–12.

155. Odom MH, Hurt JP, Krigman MR. The induction of thrombosis in guinea pigs by a brain tumor. Lab Invest 1972; 27:550–554.

156. O'Grady LO, Upfold LI, Stephens RW. Rat mammary carcinoma carinoma cells secrete active collagenase and activate latent enzyme in the stroma via plasminogen activator. J Cancer 1981; 28:509–515.

157. Oldberg E. Hemorrhage into gliomas. Arch Neurol Psychiatr 1933; 30:1061–1073.

158. Orenstein NS, Buczynski A, Dvorak HF. Cryptic and active plasminogen activators secreted by line 10 tumor cells in culture. Cancer Res 1983; 43:1783–1789.

159. Ossowski L, Biegel D, Reich E. Mammary plasminogen activator. Correlation with involution, hormonal modulation and comparison between normal and neoplastic tissue. Cell 1979; 16:929–940.

160. Ossowski L, Reich E. Antibodies to plasminogen activator inhibit tumor metastasis. Cell 1983; 35:611–619.

161. Ossowski L, Unkeless JC, Tobia A, Quigley JP, Rifkin DB, Reich E. An enzymatic function associated with transformation of fibroblasts by oncogenic viruses. J Exp Med 1973; 137:112–126.

162. Ossowski L, Vassalli JD. Plasminogen activator in normal and malignant cells. A comparison of enzyme levels and of hormonal responses. In: Biological Markers of Neoplasia: Basic and Applied Aspects. Ruddon, ed., Elsevier North Holland, Amsterdam, 1978; pp. 473–479.

163. Palmer PE, Ucci AA, Wolfe HJ. Expression of protein markers in malignant hepatoma. Cancer 1980; 45:1424–1431.
164. Pandolfi M, Isacson S, Nilsson IM. Low fibrinolytic activity in the walls of veins of patients with thrombosis. Acta Med Scand 1969; 186:1–5.
165. Paramo JA, Alfaro MJ, Rocha E. Postoperative changes in the plasmatic levels of tissue-type plasminogen activator and its fast-acting inhibitor-relationship to deep vein thrombosis and influence of prophylaxis. Thromb Haemost 1985; 54:713–716.
166. Peabody RA, Tsapogas MJ, Wu KT. Altered endogenous fibrinolysis and biochemical factors in atherosclerosis. Arch Surg 1974; 109:309–313.
167. Pennica D, Holmes WE, Kohr WJ, Harkins RN, Vehar GA, Ward CA, Bennett WF, Yelverton E, Seeburg PH, Heyneker HL, Goeddel DV, Collen D. Cloning and expression of human tissue-type plasminogen activator DNA in E. coli. Nature 1983; 301:214–221.
168. Peterson HI. Experimental studies on fibrinolysis in growth and spread of tumour. Acta Chir Scand 1968; 394:3–42.
169. Peterson HI. Fibrinolysis and antifibrinolytic drugs in the growth and spread of tumors. Cancer Treat Rev 1977; 4:213–217.
170. Peterson HI, Kjartansson I, Korsan-Bengtsen K, Rudenstam CM, Zettergren L. Fibrinolysis in human malignant tumors. Acta Chir Scand 1973; 139:219–223.
171. Philippon J, Foncin JF, Grobb R, Srour A, Poisson M, Pertuiset BF. Cerebral edema associated with meningiomas. Possible role of a secretory-excretory phenomenon. Neurosurgery 1984; 14:295–301.
172. Plow EF, Freaney D, Edgington TS. Inhibition of lymphocyte protein synthesis by fibrinogen-derived peptides. J Immunol 1982; 128:1595–1599.
173. Portugal JR, Alencar A, Brito LC, Carvalho P. Melanotic meningioma complicated by disseminated intravascular coagulation. Surg Neurol 1984; 21:275–281.
174. Prowse CV, Dow RC, Fink G. A hypothalamic-pituitary system that stimulates the release of plasminogen activator in the rat. Brain Res 1984; 299:133–138.
175. Prokopowicz LJ, Stormorken H. Fibrinolytic activity of leukocytes in smears of bone marrow and peripheral blood. Scand J Haematol 1968; 5:129–137.
176. Prokopowicz LJ, Rejniak L, Niewiarowski S. Influence of cytostatic agents on fibrinolytic and proteolytic enzymes and on phagocytosis of guinea pig leucocytes. Experientia 1967; 23:813–814.
177. Quigley JP. Phorbol ester-induced morphological changes in transformed chick fibroblasts. Evidence of direct catalytic involvement of plasminogen activator. Cell 1979; 17:131–141.
178. Quindlen EA, Bucher A. Correlation of tumor plasminogen activator with peritumoral cerebral edema. J Neurosurg 1987; 66:729–733.
179. Rabiner SF, Goldfine ID, Hart A, Summaria L, Robbins KC. Radiommunoassay of human plasminogen and plasmin. J Lab Clin Med 1969; 74:265–271.
180. Rajput B, Degen SF, Reich E, Waller EK, Axelrod J, Eddy RL, Shows

TB. Chromosome locations of human tissue plasminogen activator and urokinase genes. Science 1985; 230:672–674.

181. Ranby M, Bergsdorf N, Pohl G, Wallen P. Isolation of two variants of native one-chain tissue plasminogen activator. FEBS Lett 1982; 146:289–292.

182. Rasche H, Dietrich M. Hemostatic abnormalities associated with malignant diseases. Eur J Cancer 1977; 13:1053–1064.

183. Ratnoff OD. The surface-mediated initiation of blood coagulation and related phenomena. In: Haemostasis: Biochemistry, Physiology and Pathology. Ogston D, Bennett B, eds. London, John Wiley, 1977; pp. 25–55.

184. Reddy KNN. Mechanism of activation of human plasminogen by streptokinase. In: Fibrinolysis. Kline DL, Reddy KNN, eds. Boca Raton, FL, CRC Press, 1980; pp. 71–94.

185. Reich E. Activation of plasminogen. A widespread mechanism for generating localized extracellular proteolysis. In: Biological Markers of Neoplasia: Basic and Aplied Aspects. Ruddon, ed. Elsevier North Holland, Amsterdam, 1978; pp. 491–500.

186. Rickles FR, Edwards RL. Activation of blood coagulation in cancer. Trousseau's syndrome revisited. Blood 1983; 62:14–31.

187. Rickli EE, Zaugg G. Isolation and purification of highly enriched tissue plasminogen activator from pig heart. Thromb Diath Haemorrh 1970; 23:64–76.

188. Rijken DC, Wijngaards G, Zaal-de Jong M, Welbergen J. Purification and partial characterization of plasminogen activator from human uterine tissue. BiochimBiophys Acta 1979; 580:140–153.

189. Rijken DC, Juhan-Vague I, DeCock F, Collen D. Measurements of human tissue-type plasminogen activator by a two-site immunoradiometric assay. J Lab Clin Med 1983; 101:274–284.

190. Rijken C, Juhan-Vague I, Collen D. Complexes between tissue-type plasminogen activator and proteinase inhibitors in human plasma, identified with an immunoradiometric assay. J Lab Clin Med 1983; 101:285–294.

191. Rizzoli HV, Pagnanelli DM. Treatment of delayed radiation necrosis of the brain. J Neurosurg 1984; 60:589–594.

192. Robbins KC, Summaria L, Hsieh B, et al. The peptide chains of human plasmin. Mechanism of activation of human plasminogen to plasmin. J Biol Chem 1967; 242:2333–2342.

193. Roblin R. Plasminogen activator production as a possible biological marker for human neoplasia. Some fundamental questions. In: Biological Markers of Neoplasia: Basic and Applied Aspects. Ruddon, ed, Elsevier North Holland, Amsterdam, 1978; pp. 421–432.

194. Rudenstam CM, Goteborg. Effect of fibrinolytic and antifibrinolytic therapy on the dissemination of experimental tumours. Bibl Anat 1967; 9:418–424.

195. Ruff RL, Posner JB. The incidence of systemic venous thrombosis and the risk of anticoagulation in patients with malignant gliomas. Ann Neurol 1981; 10:92.

196. Sack GH, Levin J, Bell WR. Trousseau's syndrome and other manifes-

tations of chronic dissemiated coagulopathy in patients with neoplasms. Clinical, pathophysiologic, and therapeutic features. Medicine 1977; 56:1–37.

197. Sakata Y, Aoki N. Cross-linking of α_2-plasmin inhibitor to fibrin by fibrin stabilizing factor. J Clin Invest 1980; 65:290–297.

198. Salo T, Liotta LA, Keski-Oja J, Turpeenniemi-Hujanen T, Tryggvason K. Secretion of basement membrane collagen degrading enzyme and plasminogen activator by transformed cells-role in metastasis. Int J Cancer 1982; 30:669–673.

199. Sawaya R, Donlon JA. Chronic disseminated intravascular coagulation and metastatic brain tumor. A case report and review of the literature. Neurosurgery 1983; 12:580–584.

200. Sawaya R, Decourteen-Meyers G, Copeland B. Massive preoperative pulmonary embolism and suprasellar brain tumor. Case report and review of the literature. Neurosurgery 1984; 15:566–571.

201. Sawaya R, Cummins CJ, Kornblith PL. Brain tumors and plasmin inhibitors. Neurosurgery 1984; 15:795–800.

202. Sawaya R, Cummins CJ, Smith BH, Kornblith PL. Plasma fibronectin in patients with brain tumors. Neurosurgery 1985; 16:161–165.

203. Sawaya R, Mandybur T, Ormsby I, Tew JM. Antifibrinolytic therapy of experimentally grown malignant brain tumors. J Neurosurg 1986; 64:263–268.

204. Sawaya R, Highsmith R. Plasminogen activator activity and molecular weight patterns in human brain tumors. J Neurosurg 1988; 68:73–79.

205. Sawaya R, Zuccarello M, Highsmith R. Alpha-1-antitrysin in human brain tumors. J Neurosurg 1987; 67:258–262.

206. Scharrer I, Hubner H. Studies of fibrinolysis in patients with metastasizing malignomas and in patients with non-metastasizing cerebral tumors. Verh Stsch Ges Inn Med 1977; 83:1144–1148.

207. Schnebli HP, Burger MM. Selective inhibition of growth of transformed cells by protease inhibitors. Proc Natl Acad Sci USA 1972; 69:3825–3827.

208. Schultz OT. Sudden death due to hemorrhage into silent cerebral gliomas. Am J Surg 1935; 30:148–153.

209. Seifert SC, Gelehrter TD. Mechanism of dexamethasone inhibition of plasminogen activator in rat hepatoma cells. Proc Natl Acad Sci USA 1978; 75:6130–6133.

210. Senger DR, Galli SF, Dvorak AM, Perruzzi CA, Harvey VS, Dvorak HF. Tumor cells secrete a vascular permeability factor that promotes accumulation of ascites fluid. Science 1983; 219:983–985.

211. Shapiro WR. Treatment of neuroectodermal brain tumors. Ann Neurol 1982; 12:231–237.

212. Sherry S, Alkjaersig N, Fletcher AP. Assay of urokinase preparations with the synthetic substrate acetyl-l-lysine methyl ester. J Lab Clin Med 1964; 64:145–154.

213. Siddiqi TS, Buchheit WA. Disseminated intravascular coagulation. A complication of 1,3-bis(2-chlorethyl)-nitrosourea therapy. Surg Neurol 1983; 19:154–155.

214. Sjoberg HE, Blomback, Granberg PO. Thromboembolic complications,

heparin treatment and increase in coagulation factors in Cushing's syndrome. Acta Med Scand 1976; 199:95–98.

215. Smokovitis A, Astrup T. Plasminogen activator activity and plasmin inhibition in nerves. Haemostasis 1983; 13:136–144.

216. Soberano ME, Ong EB, Johnson AJ, Levy S, Schoellmann G. Purification and characterization of two forms of urokinase. Biochim Biophys Acta 1976; 445:763–767.

217. Soreq H, Miskin R. Plasminogen activator in the rodent brain. Brain Res 1981; 216:361–374.

218. Sottrup-Jensen L, Petersen TE, Magnnsson S. In: Atlas of Protein Sequence and Structure. (Suppl) 3 1978; 5:91.

219. Stalder M, Hauert J, Kruithof EK, Bachmann F. Release of vascular plasminogen activator (v-PA) after venous stasis. Electrophoretic and zymographic analysis of free and complexed v-PA. Thromb Haemost 1983; 50:56.

220. Stead N, Kaplan AP, Rosenberg RD. Inhibition of activated factor XII by antithrombin-heparin cofactor. J Biol Chem 1976; 251:6481–6488.

221. Stein-Werblowsky R. On the prevention of haematogenous tumor metastases in rats. The role of proteinase inhibitor Trasylol. J Cancer Res Clin Oncol 1980; 97:129–135.

222. Strickland S, Reich E, Sherman M. Plasminogen activator in early embryogenesis. Enzyme production by trophoblast and partial endoderm. Cell 1976; 9:231–240.

223. Sueishi K, Nanno S, Tanaka K. Permeability enhancing and chemotactic activities of lower molecular weight degradation products of human fibrinogen. Thromb Haemost 1981; 45:90–94.

224. Svanberg L, Astedt B, Kullander S. On radiation-decreased fibrinolytic activity of vessel walls. Acta Obstet Gynecol Scand 1976; 55:49–51.

225. Symon L, Mohanty S. Haemorrhage in pituitary tumours. Acta Neurochir 1982; 65:41–49.

226. Thornes RD. Adjuvant therapy of cancer via the cellular immune mechanism or fibrin by induced fibrinolysis and oral anticoagulants. Cancer 1975; 35:91–97.

227. Thorsen S, Glas-Greenwalt P, Astrup T. Differences in the binding to fibrin of urokinase and tissue plasminogen activator. Thromb Diath Haemorrh 1972; 28:65–74.

228. Thorsen T. Association of plasminogen activator activity and steroid receptors in human breast cancer. Eur J Cancer Clin Oncol 1982; 18:129–132.

229. Tillet WS, Garner RL. The fibrinolytic activity of hemolytic streptococci. J Exp Med 1933; 58:485–495.

230. Tilka-Rudman L, Ledinski G. The help of coagulation tests in preventing thromboembolisms in neurosurgical patients. Lij Vjes 1976; 98:601–603.

231. Todd AS. The histological localization of fibrinolysin activator. J Clin Pathol 1959; 78:281–283.

232. Tovi D, Pandolfi M, Astedt B. Local haemostasis in brain tumours. Experientia 1975; 31:977–978.

233. Tucker WS, Kirsch WM, Martinez-Hernandez A, Fink LM. In vitro plas-

minogen activator activity in human brain tumors. Cancer Res 1978; 38:297–302.

234. Turner GA, Weiss L. Analysis of aprotinin-induced enhancement of metastasis of Lewis lung tumors in mice. Cancer Res 1981; 41:2576–2580.

235. Turpie AGG, Delmore T, Hirsh J, Hull R, Genton E, Hiscoe C, Gent M. Prevention of venous thrombosis by intermittent sequential calf compression in patients with intracranial disease. Thromb Res 1979; 15:611–616.

236. Twining S, Brecher AS. Large scale separation of protease inhibitors from malignant human breast tissue. Mol Cell Biochem 1977; 18:101–107.

237. Tyler HM, Lack CH. A tissue fibrin-stabilizing factor and fibrinolytic inhibition. Nature 1964; 202:114–115.

238. Unkeless JC, Gordon S, Reich E. Secretion of plasminogen activator by stimulated macrophages. J Exp Med 1974; 139:834–850.

239. Unkeless JC, Tobia A, Ossowski L, Quigley JP, Rifkin DB, Reich E. An enzymatic function associated with transformation of fibroblasts by oncogenic viruses. J Exp Med 1973; 137:85–111.

240. Unterberg A, Baethmann AJ. The kallikrein-kinin system as mediator in vasogenic brain edema. J Neurosurg 1984; 61:87–96.

241. Vallandares JB, Hankinson J. Incidence of lower extremity deep vein thrombosis in neurosurgical patients. Neurosurgery 1980; 6:138–141.

242. Van Der Sande JJ, Veltkamp JJ, Bouwhuis-Hoogerwerf ML. Hemostasis and intracranial surgery. J Neurosurg 1983; 58:693–698.

243. Vardi Y, Treifler M, Schujman E, Loewenthal M. Diffuse intravascular clotting associated with a primary brain tumor. J Neurol Neurosurg Psychiatr 1974; 37:987–990.

244. Verheijen JH, Chang GTG, Mullaart E. Inhibition of extrinsic (tissuetype) plasminogen activator in plasma. Thromb Haemost 1983; 50:294.

245. Vermylen JG, Chamone DAF. The role of the fibrinolytic system in thromboembolism. Prog Cardiovas Dis 1979; 21:255–266.

246. Vetterlein D, Young PL, Bell TE, Roblin R. Immunological characterization of multiple molecular weight forms of human cell plasminogen activators. J Biol Chem 1979; 254:575–578.

247. Von Ardenne M, Chaplain RA. The inhibitory effect of α–2–macroglobulin on tumour growth. Specialia 1973; 15:1271–1272.

248. Wainberg A, Israel E, Margolese RG. Further studies on the mitogenic and immune-modulating effects of plasminogen activator. Pathology 1982; 45:715–720.

249. Wakai S, Yamakawa K, Manaka S, Takakura K. Spontaneous intracranial hemorrhage caused by brain tumor. Its incidence and clinical significance. Neurosurgery 1982; 10:437–444.

250. Wallen P. Biochemistry of plasminogen. In: Fibrinolysis. Kline DL, Reddy KNN, eds. Boca Raton, FL, CRC Press, 1980; pp. 1–25.

251. Wallen P, Kok P, Ranby M. The tissue activator of plasminogen in regulatory enzymes and their control. Magnusson S, Ottesen M, Foltman B, Dano K, Neurath H, eds. Oxford, Pergamon Press 1978; pp. 127–135.

252. Wallen P, Pohl G, Bergsdorf N, Ranby M, Jornvall H. Purification and

characterization of a melanoma cell plasminogen activator. Eur J Biochem 1983; 132:681–686.

253. Wallen P, Wiman B. Characterization of human plasminogen. I. On the relationship between different molecular forms of plasminogen demonstrated in plasma and found in purified preparations. Biochim Biophys Acta 1970; 221:20–30.

254. Weick JK. Intravascular coagulation in cancer. Semin Oncol 1978; 5:203–211.

255. Weinstein ZR, Downey EF. Spontaneous hemorrhage in medulloblastomas. Am J Neurol 1983; 4:986–988.

256. Weiss JF, Morantz RA, Bradley WP, Chretien PB. Serum acute-phase proteins and immunoglobulins in patients with gliomas. Cancer Res 1979; 39:542–544.

257. Wetzel N, Anderson MC, Shields TW. Pulmonary embolism as a cause of death in the neurosurgical patient. J Neurosurg 1960; 17:664–668.

258. Whur P, Robson RT, Payne NE. Effect of a protease inhibitor on the adhesion of Ehrlich cells to host cells in vivo. Br J Cancer 1973; 28:417–428.

259. Wilson EL, Dowdle E. Plasminogen activator secretion by normal and neoplastic human tissues cultured in vitro. In: Regulatory Proteolytic Enzymes and Their Inhibitors. Magnusson S, Ottesen M, Dano K, Neurath H, eds. New York, Pergamon Press, 1977; pp. 151–161.

260. Wilson EL, Dowdle E. Secretion of plasminogen activator by normal reactive and neoplastic human tissues cultured in vitro. Int J Cancer 1978; 22:390–399.

261. Wilson EL, Becker LB, Hoal EG, Dowdle EB. Molecular species of plasminogen activators secreted by normal and neoplastic human cells. Cancer Res 1980; 40:933–938.

262. Wilson EL, Jacobs P, Dowdle EB. The effects of dexamethasone and tetradecanoyl phorbol acetate on plasminogen activator release by human acute myeloid leukemia cells. Blood 1983; 61:561–567.

263. Wilson EL, Jacobs P, Dowdle EB. The secretion of plasminogen activators by human myeloid leukemic cells in vitro. Blood 1983; 61:568–574.

264. Wiman B. Biochemistry of the plasminogen to plasmin conversion. In: Fibrinolysis: Current Fundamental and Clinical Aspects. Gafney JJ, Balkuv-Ulutin S, eds. London, Academic Press, 1978; pp. 47–60.

265. Wiman B, Chmielewska J. A novel fast inhibitor to tissue plasminogen activator inplasma which may be of great pathophysiological significance. Scand J Clin Lab Invest 1985; 45:43–47.

266. Wiman B, Chmielewska J, Ranby M. Inactivation of tissue plasminogen activator in plasma. Demonstration of a complex with a new rapid inhibitor. J Biol Chem 1984; 259:3644–3647.

267. Wiman B, Collen D. Molecular mechanism of physiological fibrinolysis. Nature 1978; 272:549–550.

268. Wiman B, Collen D. On the kinetics of the reaction between human antiplasmin and plasmin. Eur J Biochem 1978; 84:573–578.

269. Wiman B, Collen D. Purification and characterization of human anti-

plasmin, the fast-acting plasmin inhibitor in plasma. Eur J Biochem 1977; 78:19–26.
270. Wiman B, Mellbring G, Randy M. Plasminogen activator release during venous stasis and exercise as determined by a new specific assay. Clin Chim Acta 1983; 127:279–288.
271. Wiman B, Wallen P. The specific interaction between plasminogen and fibrin. A physiological role of the lysine binding site in plasminogen. Thromb Res 1977; 10:213–222.
272. Yonemitsu T, Niizuma H, Kodama N, Fujiwara S, Suzuki J. Acoustic neurinoma presenting as subarachnoid hemorrhage. Surg Neurol 1983; 20:125–130.
273. Yoshimura S, Tamaoki N, Ueyama Y, Hata J. Plasma protein production by human tumors xenotransplanted in nude mice. Cancer Res 1978; 38:3474–3478.
274. Zanker KS, Stavrou D, Osterkamp U, Wriedt-Lubbe I, Blumel G. Fibrinolysis induced by rat glioma cells. J Neurol Sci 1978; 38:67–75.
275. Zanker KS, Stavrou D, Blumel G. Fibrin degradation produced by glioma cell-associated fibrinolysis and the partial inhibition of cell growth and migration in tissue culture. Cell Mol Biol 1980; 25:387–394.
276. Zimmerman RA, Bilaniuk LT. Computed tomography of acute intra-tumoral hemorrhage. Neuroradiology 1980; 135:355–359.
277. Zuccarello M, Sawaya R, Ray M. Immunohistochemical demonstration of alpha–1-proteinase inhibitor in brain tumors. Cancer 1987; 60:804–809.

6

Oncogenes, Growth Factors, and Brain Tumors

*Marius Maxwell and
Peter McL. Black*

Cancer is a disease in which one or a few cells of the body are released from their normally strict growth control and proliferate to form a tumor. The last few years have seen quantum advances in the understanding of the regulation of cellular proliferation. Subtle genetic differences between neoplastic cells and their normal counterparts have been discovered, shedding new light on malignant change. The fundamental role played by growth factors in controlling the normal proliferation of cells is well-established and their corresponding genes have been characterized. In addition to these genes, many genes capable of inducing a transformed phenotype have been identified. It is now becoming clear that these two families of genes are almost identical.

Before techniques for comparing the DNA of normal and neoplastic cells recently became available, the genetic material of tumor viruses was studied as a model system. Of these, the acutely transforming retroviruses, or RNA tumor viruses, rapidly induce tumors in animals and man (in the case of the human immunodeficiency viruses, HIV) and neoplastic transformation of cells in tissue culture. The first to be discovered was the Rous sarcoma virus, which was hypothesized to exist by Peyton Rous who, in 1911, found that a cell-free filtrate from a chicken sarcoma could induce the formation of a

From: Kornblith PL, Walker MD (editors). Advances in Neuro-Oncology. Futura Publishing Company, Inc., Mount Kisco, NY, © 1988.

159

pathologically identical lesion when innoculated into a normal fowl.[1] Retroviruses are unusual in that their genetic material resides on two strands of RNA instead of double-helical DNA. The impasse reached in trying to understand how the RNA of the virus could integrate into and influence the DNA of its host was solved by the discovery of the enzyme reverse transcriptase by Baltimore and Temin in 1970.[2,3] Through the action of reverse transcriptase, a double-stranded sequence of complementary DNA is synthesized and integrated into the host genome.

The basic retroviral genome has the following regions: the *gag* gene, which encodes the core proteins of the virus; the *pol* gene, which codes for reverse transcriptase; and the *env* gene, which codes for the viral envelope glycoproteins. In addition to these genes, retroviruses contain specific repetitious nucleotide sequences at each end of their genome, called long terminal repeats (LTRs). These contain promotor and enhancer sequences which drive transcription of the integrated, or proviral, genome. None of the protein products of *gag*, *pol*, or *env* are able to transform cells, and nontransforming retroviruses (which contain only this complement of genes) do not induce tumors. When the genome of RSV was compared with that of nontransforming retroviruses, an additional nucleotide sequence was found. This sequence was called a viral oncogene, v-*src*, and was found to encode a protein, pp60^{src}, responsible for the transforming property of RSV. Confirmation of this function was provided by the discovery that different mutated RSV strains existed, some transforming and others nontransforming. Those RSV strains that had intact v-*src* genes were transforming, whereas those possessing a complement of only *gag*, *pol* and *env* genes were not.

Twenty such retroviral oncogenes, designated v-*onc*, have been discovered and have contributed greatly to the understanding of neoplastic growth (Table 1).

Much excitement was generated by the discovery, in 1976, of sequences nearly identical with those of viral oncogenes in the genomes of all vertebrate and many invertebrate cells.[4] These genes were called cellular, or proto-oncogenes (c-*onc*). The evolutionary ubiquity of these cellular oncogenes found in such phylogenetically distinct organisms as *Drosophilia* implies a vital role in the control of cellular growth and development.

It is now recognized that retroviruses have captured cellular oncogenes transducing or structurally altering them in the process. The activated oncogene then directs the synthesis of qualitatively or

Table 1

Well-Characterized Transforming Retroviruses, Their Oncogenes, and Oncogene Products

Oncogene	Retrovirus	Tumor	Subcellular Localization of Product	Properties
abl	Abelson murine leukemia virus	Lymphoid leukemia	Plasma membrane	Protein tyrosine kinase
*erb*A	Avian erythroblastosis virus	Sarcoma, leukemia	Cytoplasm, nucleus	Thyroid hormone receptor
*erb*B	Avian erythroblastosis virus	Sarcoma, leukemia	Plasma membrane	Protein tyrosine kinase; truncated form of EGF receptor
fms	McDonough feline sarcoma virus	Sarcoma	Plasma membrane	Protein tyrosine kinase; mutated form of CSF-1 receptor
fos	FBJ and FBR murine osteoviruses	Osteosarcoma	Nucleus	Binds DNA
mos	Moloney murine sarcoma virus	Sarcoma	Cytoplasm	Protein serine-threonine kinase
myc	Avian myelocytomatosis virus	Lymphomas, sarcomas leukemias	Nucleus	Binds DNA
Ha-*ras*	Harvey murine sarcoma virus	Sarcoma, erythroleukemia	Plasma membrane	Binds ATP
Ki-*ras*	Kirsten murine sarcoma virus	Sarcoma	Plasma membrane	Protein serine-threonine kinase binds ATP
ros	UR2 avian sarcoma virus	Sarcoma	Plasma membrane	Protein tyrosine kinase; truncated receptor (?)
sis	Simian sarcoma virus	Sarcoma	Secreted	Corresponds to B-chain of PDGF
src	Rous sarcoma virus	Sarcoma	Plasma membrane	Protein tyrosine kinase

quantitatively abnormal proteins that effect neoplastic transformation. The cellular origin of viral oncogenes is implied by their structure.

Cellular oncogenes contain intervening sequences, or introns, between their coding sequences, or exons. The introns are spliced out during the formation of mature messenger RNA (mRNA). Viral oncogenes, however, consist of a continuous uninterrupted sequence of exons. This absence of introns is most likely due to the recombinational events with host mRNA, which led to the integration of the cellular oncogene into the viral genome.

Two reasons may account for the tumorigenicity of transduced retroviral oncogenes, despite their apparently harmless cellular origin. In the first instance, structural changes in the transduced genes may alter the function of the proteins they encode. A second reason for the oncogenicity of viral oncogenes may be found in the retroviral LTRs also incorporated into the host genome. The powerful proviral promoter-enhancer sequences causing high expression of a structurally normal gene may lead to neoplastic transformation.

Evidence for the direct involvement of cellular oncogenes in cancer has been gleaned largely by the use of gene-transfer, or transfection, studies. Cells transformed to a neoplastic phenotype display in vitro growth characteristics which differ markedly from those of normal cells growing in culture. Normal cells grow as a monolayer and exhibit contact inhibition, ceasing to proliferate further upon contact with their neighbors. This behavior is lost in neoplastic transformation, when the cells clump into small mounds called foci. Focus-formation was initially studied in virally infected cells, until it was discovered that viral DNA could transform cells after being introduced to the cells in the form of a co-precipitate with calcium phosphate. In 1981, Weinberg and his co-workers found that DNA from the EJ/24 human bladder carcinoma cell line induced focus-formation when transfected into mouse fibroblast NIH 3T3 cells.[5,6] Subsequent cloning and identification of a gene contained within the bladder carcinoma DNA extracted from foci of transformed NIH 3T3 fibroblasts found it to be c-Ha-*ras*, the cellular homologue of v-Ha-*ras*, the transforming viral oncogene of the Harvey murine sarcoma virus. Nucleotide sequence comparison between the activated c-Ha-*ras* and its normal homology showed the difference to be a point mutation causing a single amino acid substitution in the gene product.[7–9]

Concurrent investigations were underway trying to identify the intracellular and biochemical functions of viral oncogenic and, thus, proto-oncogenic products.

In 1978, the protein product pp60[src] of the acutely transforming RSV gene v-*src* was found to engender a protein kinase activity catalyzing the addition of a phosphate group to various cytoplasmic proteins.[10,11] Protein phosphorylation has been implicated in many vital steps in intracellular signal transduction pathways. In addition, it was subsequently found that the v-*src* protein kinase is tyrosine-specific, as opposed to all hitherto characterized protein kinases. As is now known, tyrosine-specific protein kinases account for less than 0.1% of intracellular kinases, the great majority phosphorylate serine or threonine residues. This protein tyrosine kinase activity, also found in the c-*src* protein product, has since been found in a whole family of retroviral oncogenes.[12] The first evidence, albeit indirect, unifying the two fields of oncogenes and growth factors was soon to follow.

Epidermal growth factor (EGF) is a single chain polypeptide comprised of 53 amino acids and defined by its ability to increase mitotic rate in epidermal cells. First extracted and purified from murine submaxillary salivary glands by Stanley Cohen in 1962, it was shown to bind to specific cell membrane receptors (EGF-R) in responsive cells.[13] The discovery that the v-*src* product was a protein tyrosine kinase prompted the suggestion that the phosphorylation of tyrosine residues of cellular proteins is vital for cell division in general, and viral transforming kinases may be related to normal kinases involved in cell regulation. Pursuing this lead, Cohen and his co-workers demonstrated in 1980 that the EGF receptor membrane glycoprotein possesses EGF-dependent tyrosine kimase activity.[14]

Further evidence linking growth factors to tumorigenesis arose from the finding that retrovirally transformed cell lines secrete factors able to temporarily transform normal fibroblasts.[15] The fact that transformed cell lines were able to grow in media containing low concentrations of serum growth factors was already well-established. The identification of transforming growth factors (TGFs) secreted by tumor cells led Sporn and Todaro to hypothesize that secretion of growth factors by a cell resulting in autostimulation may underlie the transformed phenotype characteristic of cancer cells.[16] This was termed the "autocrine hypothesis." It is now four years since the demonstration of the relationship between v-*sis*, the oncogene of the acutely transforming simian sarcoma virus (SSV), and platelet-derived growth factor (PDGF) provided the first direct confirmation that an oncogene encodes a molecule involved in growth control. The v-*sis* oncogene provides the transforming potential enabling the SSV to induce a variety of gliomas and sarcomas in monkeys and to transform fibroblasts in vitro. Subsequent nucleotide sequence determination showed that the v-*sis* oncogene product p28[sis] is virtually identical to the B chain of PDGF, a potent dimeric growth factor for fibroblasts and other mesenchymal tissues.[17,18] It now seems that the c-*sis* proto-oncogene, on chromosome 22, was captured by the retroviral genome.

The intracellular synthesis of PDGF-like proteins has been described in cultures of human glioblastoma cells.[19] The presence of these proteins has been correlated with the presence of a c-*sis* mRNA species transcribed by the human c-*sis* locus. Expression of the c-*sis* gene and synthesis of PDGF have only been shown to occur in permanent glioma cell lines. The activity of c-*sis* in primary tumors remains to be demonstrated. PDGF receptors have been found by ligand binding and affinity labeling techniques on some classes of glial cells. Although glial cells mount a mitogenic response to PDGF, no definite physiological role for PDGF has been demonstrated in the central nervous system.

Close on the heels of this signal discovery came a similar finding linking another oncogene product to a growth factor. Sequence analysis of the oncogene, v-*erb*-B, of the avian erythroblastosis virus, revealed it to be a truncated version of the EGF receptor.[20] As shall be seen, the v-*erb*-B protein encodes a membrane glycoprotein receptor lacking an extracellular, ligand-binding domain. This is thought to result in high constitutive activity independent of growth factor stimulation. The normal EGF-R encoded by c-*erbB*, has been shown to be overexpressed in 40% of human glial tumors. These glial tumors overexpressing EGF-R also have amplified and rearranged copies of the c-*erb*-B gene.[21] A selective growth advantage may be conferred on the transformed glia by amplification of c-*erb*-B which encodes the EGF-R. Alternatively, since EGF is present at low concentration, an increase in the number of EGF-R would confer a growth advantage on such cells. A third possibility would be that cells with heightened c-*erb*-B expression would respond in an autocrine fashion to secretion of TGF-α, a close homologue of EGF. Such amplified cellular genes are frequently manifested as one of two cytologically recognizable forms: double minute chromosomes or homogenously staining regions.

Although both the presence of EGF receptors on cells of the central nervous system (CNS) and their EGF-stimulated proliferation and differentiation has been demonstrated, the question of whether EGF plays a normal functional role in the CNS remains to be elucidated. Adamson and co-workers have studied the temporal variation of mouse brain EGF-R, finding a sharp increase early in gestation, implying a developmental role for EGF in the nervous system.[22] EGF levels in the adult brain are low but the peptide has been localized to a variety of structures including the pallidum.

Recently, a novel transforming gene was identified through transfection studies with DNA from chemically induced rat neuroblastomas and glioblastomas.[23] This gene, called c-*neu* (c-*erb*-B2), has been shown to be related to, but distinct from, the c-*erb*-B proto-oncogene. The c-*neu* gene encodes a member of the tyrosine kinase family, a transmembrane glycoprotein with features of a cellular receptor for an as yet unidentified ligand. The c-*neu* oncogene is amplified in 40% of breast cancer patients. In a similar fashion to c-*erb*-B, c-*fms* the proto-oncogene of the v-*fms* oncogene of the McDonough feline sarcoma virus has been shown to bear close homology to the macrophage-colony-stimulating factor receptor (CSF–1R).[24]

The human c-*ros*-1 gene is the cellular analogue of v-*ros*, the transforming gene of the avian UR2 retrovirus.[25] c-*ros*-1 encodes a tyrosine kinase with a potential transmembrane domain, displaying the structure of a growth factor receptor. c-*ros*-1 has been found to be expressed in astrocytoma and glioblastoma cells at levels ranging from 10 to 200 messenger molecules per cell.[26] c-*ros*-1 was either not expressed or expressed only at low levels in a variety of either brain and systemic tumor cell lines.

Recently, a novel gene termed *gli* has been found to be amplified in two gliomas: in one 50-fold, and in the other 10-fold.[27] Work to characterize this gene is presently being undertaken. It is apparent that a given tumor is probably induced by oncogene-activation events.

Almost 40 oncogenes and proto-oncogenes have now been identified, making it apparent that, in principle, any gene encoding a growth factor, a receptor and intracellular signaling molecule, or a transcription-regulating protein may be considered a proto-oncogene. Analysis of many tumors has revealed structural changes in proto-oncogenes, be they amplifications, translocations, or point mutations, further implicating proto-oncogenes in the progression to tumorigenesis (Table 2).

The discovery of oncogenes has provided functional clues for the roles of gross chromosomal rearrangements in tumorigenesis. The

Table 2
Proto-Oncogenes Implicated in the Tumorigenesis
of Human Cancer

Neoplasm	Proto-Oncogene	Lesion
Chronic myelogenous leukemia	c-*abl*	Translocation
Glioblastoma	c-*erb*B	Amplification
Burkitt's lymphoma	c-*myc*	Translocation
Breast cancer	c-*neu*	Amplification
Small cell lung carcinoma	L-*myc*	Amplification
Neuroblastoma	N-*myc*	Amplification
Bladder carcinoma	Ha-*ras*	Point mutation
Colon carcinoma	Ki-*ras*	Point mutation

cellular oncogene c-*myc* is present on the long arm of chromosome 8 on band 8q24. This is the precise site involved in the 8–14 translocation characteristic of Burkitt's lymphoma. This and other rearrangements found in Burkitt's lymphoma (2–8,8–22) approximate the c-*myc* locus with the immunoglobulin heavy or light chain loci. It is generally agreed that the c-*myc* gene's transciptional activity has been brought under the control of the powerful heavy and light immunoglobulin promoter-enhancer sequences, resulting in the higher expression of c-*myc* in RNA.[28,29] The mechanism of c-*myc* activation is now known to be more complicated than this, perhaps involving increased stability of mRNA.

Ninety percent of patients with chronic myelocytic leukemia (CML) display a simple reciprocal translocation between the long arms of chromosomes 9 and 22.[30] The resultant chromosomes are known as the 22q- (the Philadelphia chromosome) and the 9q+ derivative. The cellular oncogene c-*abl*, present on 9q34, is fused with a recently identified locus called the breakpoint cluster region (*bcr*). The resulting locus encodes a mutated chimeric protein with heightened enzymatic activity.[31] These discoveries are gratifying since they provide a molecular explanation of the first chromosomal translocation to be identified in a human malignancy.[32]

Of the characterized oncogene products, many biochemical functions have been implicated. In most cases, oncogenes have been found to short-circuit the actions of growth factors by encoding proteins that mimic such factors or their receptors by acting on an intracellular growth control pathway.[33] As has been seen, the best characterized serve as growth factors (c-*sis*) or mutated growth factor receptors (c-*erb-B*, c-*fms*, c-*neu*). Those proteins with tyrosine-kinase activity (c-*src*, c-*erb-B*, c-*abl*, c-*fms*, c-*ros*) remain enigmatic since some are found on cell membranes, while others reside in the cytoplasm and others in the nucleus. A central issue in understanding how growth factors stimulate cellular proliferation is that of sigmal transduction. The binding of growth factor ligands to their cell surface receptors induces physiological changes within seconds, changes in gene expression within minutes, and DNA synthesis within hours. A gulf still remains in the identification of those intracellular events bridging the receipt of mitogenic signals at the cell membrane and resultant DNA replication in the nucleus.

Current knowledge may be reviewed with reference to the binding of PDGF to its receptor, PDGF-R, which displays tyrosine kinase activity. Two of the most rapid responses following PDGF-R stimulation are a rise in intracellular pH and an increase in intracellular Ca^{++} concentration. PDGF, together with other mitogens whose receptors are tyrosine kinases, induce rapid turnover of phosphatidylinositol (PI), a second messenger.[34] This entails the phosphorylation of PI to PIP_2, which is then hydrolyzed by phospholipase C to diacylglycerol (DAG) and inositol triphosphate (IP_3) IP_3 mobilizes Ca^{++} and DAG is a potent activator of the Ca^{++}-sensitive, phospholipid-dependent protein kinase C. Activation of protein kinase C may represent an important molecular link in the sequence of events following binding of mitogenic factors to their receptors. Its substrates are many and include EGF-R, interleukin-2, pp60[*src*], the glucose transporter, phospholipase C, and the Na^+/H^+ antiport system.[35]

Another family of molecules which has been implicated in signal transduction is the G-protein family. Binding of GTP activates G-proteins to interact with various other proteins. Circumstantial evidence implies that the phospholipase C responsible for PI turnover is coupled to receptors via GTP-binding G-proteins. The homologies between the GTP-binding and GTPase activities of the p21 protein of the *ras* oncogenes and G-proteins have suggested a coupling role for the p21 *ras* proteins.

Stimulation of mitogenesis of cultured cells by a variety of growth factors has been shown to lead to the induction of expression of two nuclear proto-oncogenes, c-*fos* and c-*myc*.[36–38] Much research is being directed towards unravelling the influence these gene products may have on transcription and replication of DNA. Increased expression of c-*myc*, together with amplification and rearrangement, has been reported for one glioblastoma.[39] Schwab et al. have identified the amplified presence of an oncogene, related to c-*myc*, in human neuroblastoma cell lines.[40] They have called it N-*myc*. There is a striking positive correlation between genomic amplification of N-*myc* and early tumor progression subsequent to dingnosis.[41]

Transformation of cells in vitro with oncogenes has been a powerful technique for studying the molecular basis of cancer. Since such systems are oversimplified, much research is being directed towards factors controlling the function of genetically engineered oncogenes in vivo within transgenic mice. Transgenic mice may be defined as mice in which the genome of each cell contains specific DNA sequences that were microinjected during early embryogenesis. The introduction of oncogenes expressed from tissue-specific promoters into the germ-line of mice enables tissue-specific effects to be studied. Hyperplasia of all cells experiencing oncogene expression occurs, although tumors arise as rare clonal outgrowths, probably as a result of secondary events—further evidence that cancer is a multistep process. Transgenic mice bearing c-*fos* develop bone tumors; those with c-*myc* develop mammary tumors or B-cell lymphomas, depending on the specific regulatory region; and those carrying c-*ras* develop pancreatic tumors.[42–44] These studies have illustrated how inherited abnormalities of proto-oncogenes might contribute to tumorigenesis.

Much evidence has accumulated to suggest that another class of genes acts in a "recessive" manner in tumorigenesis. This is in distinction to the "dominant" activities of the aforementioned classical oncogenes as measured, for example, by transfection assays.

The possibility that malignant tumors may arise as a result of recessive mutations emerged from cell fusion studies of normal and neoplastic cells, which were found to suppress the neoplastic phenotype.[45,46] The suppressive influence of the normal cells has been proposed to result from the pairing of normal chromosomes with neoplastic partners bearing recessive mutations.

By the use of both enzymatic markers and karyotypic studies, further evidence for the presence of recessive genetic mutations underlying some cancers has been obtained. By their absence, they are thought to remove regulatory influences on cell growth and possibly unveil potential oncogenes. These "recessive" or "anti-oncogenes" provide a link to hereditary cancers, including retinoblastomas, meningiomas, acoustic neuromas, osteosarcomas, and Wilms tumors (nephroblastomas). Through their homozygosity at a gene locus, these neoplasms may lack a vital gene and gene product. The retinoblastoma gene, isolated a year ago, has now been sequenced, providing valuable insights into why it fails to function in some patients.[47]

Retinoblastoma is the most common eye tumor of children, occurring with an incidence of one in 20,000. It occurs in two forms: one sporadic nonhereditary form characterized by a single unilateral tumor, and the other which is inherited in an autosomally dominant fashion with an early age of onset and multiple tumor foci.[48] In this study, Knudson hypothesized that, although the genetic events were the same in the two forms of tumor, one of the alleles was mutated or lost at the germline stage in the heritable form. The homologous allelic locus on the normal chromosome would then be inactivated by a subsequent event leading to tumor formation. In sporadic forms of the disease, both alleles would have to be inactivated by two distinct events.

This model has been substantiated by karyotypic investigations, a study of a linked enzyme polymorphism (esterase D) and analysis of DNA restriction fragment length polymorphisms (RFLPs).[49-51] The locus determining retinoblastoma susceptibility, *Rb*, maps to chromosome 13q14, along with the esterase D gene. This *Rb* locus was further implicated in cases of heritable retinoblastoma by visible deletions of this region and by reduced esterase D activity.[51] The *Rb* gene has now been sequenced showing abnormal transcription in six out of six retinoblastomas studied. This included undetectable *Rb* mRNA and aberrant *Rb* mRNA.

In contrast, full-length *Rb* mRNA was isolated from human fetal retina and placenta. Sequencing of the *Rb* gene predicts a protein product that could well be a nucleic acid-binding protein. It may be that two forms of genetic lesions cause cancer: one is tumorigenic if it produces an active product and the other is tumorigenic if it does not. The *Rb* gene causes cancer by its absence rather than by its presence. A cell bearing one copy of the *Rb* gene is normal; one that is homozygous for deletions or mutations is cancerous. The *Rb* gene is thought to encode a normal cellular protein that may be involved in keeping cell growth in check.

The *Rb* gene may be active in other tumors. Osteosarcomas are common secondary tumors in patients with the heritable form of retinoblastoma. Homozygous deletions of the *Rb* locus, 13q14, have been reported to occur in osteosarcomas.[52] This suggests a common tumorigenic mechanism for these two distinct neoplasms.

Such recessive mutations have also been implicated in the case of tumors arising in bilateral acoustic neurofibromatosis (BANF).

Acoustic neuromas, neurofibromas, and meningiomas have been shown to lose alleles from chromosome 22, suggesting a common oncogenic mechanism.[53]

The active gene locus has been narrowed down to band 22q11, which has been shown to be deleted in many of the tumors. By analogy with the retinoblastoma model, these could inactivate a tumor suppressor gene.

Von Recklinghausen neurofibromatosis (VRNF) has an incidence of one in 3,000 and is one of the most frequent Mendelian disorders of man.[54] Associated nervous system tumors include neurofibromas and optic gliomas. The VRNF gene has been shown to be linked to the locus encoding the nerve growth factor (NGF) receptor on the long arm of chromosome 17.[55] However, the appearance of recombination events between the two loci argues against the NGF receptor gene being primarily responsible for this disease.

The molecular events causing the growth of new blood vessels or angiogenesis have recently been discerned as contributing to the understanding of how tumors influence their blood supply to meet their needs. In 1794, John Hunter hypothesized that blood vessels respond to the body's requirements and grow in length and diameter as and when required to do so.[56] In 1907, Goldmann further suggested that solid tumors produce a substance that stimulates the growth of new blood vessels from their host, a theme that has since been echoed by others.[57]

In 1971, Folkman demonstrated that the growth of a solid tumor beyond the size of a few millimeters in diameter is dependent upon the proliferation of new blood vessels from adjacent tissue.[58] Furthermore, he showed that extracts of solid tumors contain a diffusable substance that can induce neurovascularization in rat fascia and in the chorioallantoic membrane of chicks and cornea of rabbits. This process of generating new capillary blood vessels is termed *angiogenesis* and leads to neurovascularization, which occurs in several normal and pathological situations such as placental growth, embryogenesis, wound healing, diabetes, arthritis, psoriasis, and myocardial infarction.[59]

Glioblastomas are markedly heterogenous and are, by definition, characterized by rich neovascularization. By employing the chick chorioallantoic membrane assay, many groups have demonstrated the presence of a tumor angiogenesis factor (TAF) in the supernatants of cultured gliomas.[60-62] Many angiogenic growth factors have now been identified. Angiogenin, the first to be isolated, is a single chain basic protein.[63] Its gene has now been cloned, as have those of other angiogenic growth factors, including basic fibroblast growth factor (bFGF), transforming growth factor alpha (TGF-α), and endothelial cell growth factor (ECGF), a precursor of acidic FGF (aFGF-α).[65,66]

Libermann et al. have shown that human glioma cell lines express the gene encoding ECGF or aFGF and produce an ECGF-like polypeptide.[66] Furthermore, human glioma cells possess specific ECGF receptors and are mitogenically stimulated by administration of this peptide. The authors have proposed two actions for glioma-derived ECGF: an autocrine mechanism of glial cell stimulation and a paracrine stimulation of endothelial cell proliferation leading to neurovasculatization of the glioma.

Conclusion

The last decade has seen the discovery of the importance of oncogenes in human cancers, revealing the fundamental differences between normal and neoplastic cells. It is now agreed that the mutation of normal genes to form oncogenes causes the genesis of human tumors. Genetic lesions involving proto-oncogenes, identified through retroviral transduction, have been shown to encode aberrant proteins whose normal homologs are actively involved in growth control.

The importance of oncogenes for the transformed phenotype can be determined by experimentally blocking their action. Suppression of the neoplastic phenotype of cells carrying activated *neu* and *ras* genes has been achieved through the use of antibodies raised against their protein products.[67,68]

In the case of anti-oncogenes, replacement of genes inactivated by recessive mutations may also restore the normal phenotype. This may be tested directly when the *Rb* gene product is synthesized. Towards this end, it has been shown that the microinjection of a normal chromosone 11 into a Wilms' tumor cell line, associated with the deletion of 11p13, controls its tumorigenic expression.[69] Because of the virtual identity between oncogenes and normal genes, the likelihood that therapies taking advantage of this difference will emerge is small. This difference may be as subtle as a change in the expression of a gene or a variation in its sequence.

While the differences between a normal protein product and an oncogenic product may be minute, it would seem that the best chance for effective chemotherapy would be to recognize a difference between normal and neoplastic cells at this level. Such drugs capable of attacking biochemical and structural properties of oncogenic proteins would differ fundamentally from current antineoplastic agents, which target general properties of cancer cells such as their higher mitotic index. Further problems may arise through the appearance of new oncogenes in a tumor, allowing clonal selection of drug-resistant cells to occur.

Although therapeutic modalities arising from oncogene research are a long way off, improved diagnosis and prognosis of morphological types of cancer is in the offing. As has been seen, a multiplicity of oncogenes may act in a variety of molecular mechanisms in a given tumor and may underscore different pathological subtypes or grades. Precise molecular diagnosis, using DNA hybridization probes or monoclonal antibodies, is now an attainable goal and has now been employed in neuroblastomas and breast carcinomas.

As has been seen, the oncogene N-*myc* is present in multiple copies in some human neuroblastomas, its degree of amplification correlating with the stage of disease. Neuroblastomas are pathologically staged as follows: stage I is a tumor confined to the structure of origin; stage IV is a primary tumor that has metastasized widely.

Seeger found that N-*myc* amplification is an independent prognostic index and that the more copies of N-*myc* that are present in cancer cells, the worse the prognosis.[41] Indeed, patients with stage II neuroblastoma but with N-*myc* amplification had prognoses of stage III and IV patients, indicating that N-*myc* amplification is an even better predictor of survival time than pathological staging.

The oncogene c-*neu* has been found to be amplified in 40% of patients with breast carcinomas.[70] The *neu* amplification is a better prognostic indicator than hormone receptor status, patient age, positive lymph nodes, and size of tumor.

It can only be hoped that as the genome of the cancer cell is further unravelled, new anti-cancer therapies will emerge.

REFERENCES

1. Rous P. Transmission of a malignant new growth by means of a cell-free filtrate. J Am Med Assoc 1911; 56:198.
2. Baltimore D. Viral RNA-dependent DNA polymerase. Nature 1970; 226:1209–1211.
3. Temin HN, Mizutani S. RNA-dependent DNA polymerase in virion of Rous sarcoma virus. Nature 1970; 226:1211–1213.

4. Stehelin D, Varmus HE, Bishop JM. DNA related to the transforming gene(s) of avian sarcoma viruses is present in normal avian DNA. Nature 1976; 260:170–173.

5. Murray MJ, Shilo B-Z, Shih C, et al. Three different human tumor cell lines contain different oncogenes. Cell 1981; 25:355–361.

6. Krontiris TG, Cooper GM. Transforming activity of human tumor DNAs. Proc Natl Acad Sci USA 1981; 78:1181–1184.

7. Tabin CJ, Bradley SM, Bargmann CI, et al. Mechanism of activation of a human oncogene. Nature 1982; 300:143–149.

8. Taparowsky E, Suard Y, Fasano O, et al. Activation of the T24 bladder carcinoma transforming gene is linked to a single amino acid change. Nature 1982; 300:782–785.

9. Reddy EP, Reynolds RK, Santos E, et al. A point mutation is responsible for the acquisition of transforming properties by the T24 human bladder carcinoma oncogene. Nature 1982; 300:149–152.

10. Collett MS, Erikson WL. Protein kinase activity associated with the avian sarcoma virus *src* gene product. Proc Natl Acad Sci USA 1978; 75:2021–2024.

11. Levinson AD, Oppermann H, Levintow L, et al. Evidence that the transforming gene of avian sarcoma virus encodes a protein kinase associated with a phosphoprotein. Cell 1978; 15:561–572.

12. Hunter T, Cooper JA. Protein-tyrosine kinases. Annu Rev Biochem 1985; 54:897–930.

13. Cohen S. Isolation of a mouse submaxillary gland protein accelerating incisor eruption and eyelid opening in the newborn animal. J Biol Chem 1962; 237:1555–1562.

14. Ushiro H, Takai K, Narumiya S, et al. Isolation and reconstitution of two electron transfer components of tryptophan side chain oxidase. J Biol Chem 1979; 254:11794–11797.

15. de Larco JE, Todaro GJ. Growth factors from murine sarcoma virus-transformed cells. Proc Natl Acad Sci USA 1978; 75:4001–4005.

16. Sporn MB, Todaro GJ. Autocrine secretion and malignant transformation of cells. N Engl J Med 1980; 303:878–880.

17. Waterfield MD, Scrace GT, Whittle N, et al. Platelet-derived growth factor is structurally related to the putative transforming protein p^{28sis} of simian sarcoma virus. Nature 1983; 304:35–39.

18. Doolittle RF, Hunkapiller MW, Hood LE, et al. Simian sarcoma virus *onc* gene, v-*sis*, is derived from the gene (or genes) encoding a platelet-derived growth factor. Science 1983; 221:275–277.

19. Pantazis P, Pelicci PG, Dalla-Favera K. Synthesis and secretion of proteins resembling platelet-derived growth factor by human glioblastoma and fibrosarcoma cells in culture. Proc Natl Acad Sci USA 1985; 82:2404–2408.

20. Downward J, Yarden Y, Mayes E, et al. Close similarity of epidermal growth factor receptor and v-*erb*-B oncogene protein sequences. Nature 1984; 307:521–527.

21. Libermann TA, Nusbaum HR, Razon N, et al. Amplification, enhanced expression and possible rearrangement of EGF receptor gene in primary human brain tumors of glial origin. Nature 1985; 313:144–147.

22. Adamson ED, Meek J. The ontogeny of epidermal growth factor receptors during mouse development. Dev Biol 1984; 103:62–70.
23. Schechter Al, Stern DF, Vaidyanathan L, et al. The *neu* oncogene: an *erb*-B-related gene encoding a 185,000-M_r tumour antigen. Nature 1984; 319:513–516.
24. Sherr CJ, Rettenmier CW, Sacca R, et al. The c-*fms* proto-oncogene product is related to the receptor for the mononuclear phagocyte growth factor, CSF–1. Cell 1985; 41:665–676.
25. Neckameyer WS, Wang LH. Nucleotide sequence of avian sarcoma virus UR2 and comparison of its transforming gene with other members of the tyrosine protein kinase oncogene family. J Virol 1985; 53:879–884.
26. Birchmeier C, Young D, Wigler M. Characterization of two new human oncogenes. Cold Spring Harbor Symposia 1986; 21:993–1000.
27. Kinzler KW, Bigner SH, Bigner DD, et al. Identification of an amplified, highly expressed gene in a human glioma. Science 1987; 236:70–73.
28. Dalla-Favera R, Bregni M, Erikson J, et al. Human c-*myc onc* gene is located on the region of chromosome 8 that is translocated in Burkitt lymphoma cells. Proc Natl Acad Sci USA 1982; 82:7824–7827.
29. Thub R, Moulding C, Battey J, et al. Activation and somatic mutation of the translocated c-*myc* gene in Burkitt lymphoma cells. Cell 1984; 36:339–348.
30. Shitivelman E, Lifshitz B, Gale RP, et al. Fused transcript of *abl* and *bcr* genes in chronic myelogenous leukaemia. Nature 1985; 315:551–554.
31. Ben-Neriah Y, Daley GQ, Mes-Masson AM, et al. The chronic myelogenous leukemia-specific P210 protein is the product of the *bcr/abl* hybrid gene. Science 1986; 233:212–214.
32. Nowell PC, Hungerford DA. A minute chromosome in human chronic granulocytic leukemia (abst). Science 1960; 132:1497.
33. Bishop JM. The molecular genetics of cancer. Science 1987; 235:305–311.
34. Berridge MJ, Irvine RF. Inositol triphosphate, a novel second messenger in cellular signal transduction. Nature 1984; 312:315–320.
35. Hunter T. Phosphorylation in signal transmission and transformation. In: Oncogenes and Growth Control (Kahn P, Graf T, eds). New York, Springer-Verlag, 1986; pp. 138–147.
36. Muller R, Bravo R, Burckhardt G. Induction of c-*fos* gene and protein by growth factors precedes activation of c-*myc*. Nature 1984; 312:716–720.
37. Kelly K, Cochran RH, Stiles CD, et al. Cell-specific regulation of the C-*myc* gene by lymphocyte mitogens and platelet-derived growth factor. Cell 1983; 35:603–610.
38. Kruijer W, Cooper JA, Hunter T, et al. Platelet-derived growth factor induces rapid but transient expression of the c-*fos* gene and protein. Nature 1984; 312:711–716.
39. Trent J, Meltzer P, Rosenblum M, et al. Evidence for rearrangement, amplification, and expression of c-*myc* in a human glioblastoma. Proc Natl Acad Sci USA 1986; 83:470–473.
40. Schwab M, Alitalo K, Klempnauer K-H, et al. Amplified DNA with limited homology to *myc* cellular oncogene is shared by human neuroblastoma cell lines and a neuroblastoma tumour. Nature 1983; 35:359–367.

41. Seeger RC, Brodeur GM, Sather H, et al. Association of multiple copies of the N-*myc* oncogene with rapid progression of neuroblastomas. N Engl J Med 1985; 313:1111–1116.
42. Stewart TA, Pattengal PK, Leder P. Spontaneous mammary adenocarcinomas in transgenic mice that carry and express MTV/*myc* fusion genes. Cell 1983; 38:603–610.
43. Adams JM, Narris AW, Pinkert CA, et al. The c-*myc* oncogene driven by immunoglobulin enhancers induces lymphoid malignancy in transgenic mice. Nature 1985; 318:533–538.
44. Quaife CJ, Pinkert CA, Ornitz DM, et al. Pancreatic neoplasia induced by *ras* expression in acinar cells of transgenic mice. Cell 1987; 48:1023–1034.
45. Harris H, Miller OJ, Klein G, et al. Suppression of malignancy by cell fusion. Nature 1969; 223:363–368.
46. Stanbridge EJ, Der CJ, Doersen CJ, et al. Human cell hybrids: analysis of transformation and tumorigenicity. Science 1982; 215:252–259.
47. Lee W-H, Bookstein R, Hong F, et al. Human retinoblastoma susceptibility gene: cloning, identification, and sequence. Science 1987; 235:1394–1399.
48. Knudson AG Jr. Mutation and cancer: statistical study of retinoblastoma. Proc Natl Acad Sci USA 1971; 68:820–823.
49. Sparkes RS, Murphree AL, Lingua RW, et al. Gene for hereditary retinoblastoma assigned to human chromosome 13 by linkage to esterase D. Science 1983; 219:971–973.
50. Benedict WF, Murphree AL, Banerjee A, et al. Patient with 13 chromosome deletion: evidence that the retinoblastoma gene is a recessive cancer gene. Science 1983; 219:973–975.
51. Cavenee WK, Hansen MF, Nordenskjold M, et al. Genetic origin of mutations predisposiag to retinoblastoma. Science 1985; 228:501–503.
52. Hansen MF, Koufos A, Gallie BL, et al. Osteosarcoma and retinoblastoma: a shared chromosome mechanism revealing recessive predisposition. Proc Natl Acad Sci USA 1985; 82:6216–6220.
53. Seizinger BR, Rouleau G, Ozelius LJ, et al. Common pathogenic mechanism for three tumor types in bilateral acoustic neurofibromatosis. Science 1987; 236:317–319.
54. Crowe FW. A clinical, pathological, and genetic study of multiple neurofibromatosis. Springfield, Illinois, Charles C Thomas, 1956.
55. Seizinger BR, Rouleau GA, Ozelius LJ, et al. Genetic linkage of von Recklinghausen neurofibromatosis to the nerve growth factor receptor gene. Cell 1987; 49:589–594.
56. Hunter J. A treatise on the blood, inflammation and gunshot wounds. London, AG Nichols, 1794.
57. Goldmann E. The growth of malignant disease in man and the lower animals, with a special reference to the vascular system. Lancet 1907; 1236–1240.
58. Folkman J, Merler E, Abernathy C, et al. Isolation of a tumor factor responsible for angiogenesis. J Exp Med 1971; 133:275–288.
59. Fenselau A. Tumor angiogenesis oncology overview. National Cancer Institute, Bethesda, 1983.

60. Klagsbrun M, Knighton D, Folkman J. Tumor angiogenesis activity in cells grown in tissue culture. Cancer Res 1976; 36:110–114.
61. Kelly PJ, Suddith RL, Hutchinson HT, et al. Endothelial growth factor present in tissue culture of CNS tumors. J Neurosurg 1976; 44:342–346.
62. Matsuno H. Tumor angiogenesis factor (TAF) in cultured cells derived central nervous system tumors in humans. Neurol Med Chir (Tokyo) 1981; 21:765–773.
63. Fett JW, Strydom DJ, Lobb RR, et al. Lysozyme: a major secretory product of a human colon carcinoma cell line. J Biochem 1985; 24:965–975.
64. Abraham JA, Mergia A, Whang JL, et al. Nucleotide sequence of a bovine clone encoding the angiogenic protein, basic fibroblast growth factor. Science 1986; 233:545–548.
65. Jaye M, Howk R, Burgess W, et al. Human endothelial cell growth factor: cloning nucleotide sequence, and chromosome localization. Science 1986; 233:541–551.
66. Libermann TA, Friesal R, Jaye M, et al. An angiogenic growth factor is expressed in human glioma cells. EMBO 6.: 6:1627–1632, 1987.
67. Feramisco JR, Clark R, Wong G, et al. Transient reversion of *ras* oncogene-induced cell transformation by antibodies specific for amino acid 12 of *ras* protein. Nature 1985; 314:639–642.
68. Drebin JA, Link VC, Stern DF, et al. Down-modulation of an oncogene protein product and reversion of the transformed phenotype by monoclonal antibodies. Cell 1985; 41:695–706.
69. Weissman BE, Saxon PJ, Pasquale SR, et al. Introduction of a normal human chromosome 11 into a Wilms' tumor cell line controls its tumorigenic expression. Science 1987; 236:175–180.
70. Slamon DJ, Wong SG, Levin WJ, et al. Human breast cancer: correlation of relapse and survival with amplification of the HER-2/*neu* oncogene. Science 1987; 235:177–182.

7

Viruses and Central Nervous System Tumors

Jacob R. Rachlin and George J. Dohrmann, III

The relationship between viruses and cancer has been the subject of intensive research for the last two decades. Initial work was designed to generate animal models for various types of tumors. More recent investigations have centered on the possible role of oncogenic viruses as etiologic agents in human cancers, the use of oncogenic viruses to study molecular mechanisms involved in cell transformation, and the maintenance of the transformed state. In this chapter, the animal models of virally induced central nervous system (CNS) tumors will be reviewed, the evidence suggesting a possible role for papovaviruses in human CNS tumors will be presented, and possible future areas of investigation will be discussed.

History

The Rous sarcoma virus (RSV), discovered in 1912, was the first recognized oncogenic virus. In 1936, avian sarcoma virus (ASV) was found to produce sarcomas in 75% of 3–5-month-old chickens inoculated intracranially with the virus.[1] In 1964, Rabotti and Raine produced gliomas in newborn Syrian hamsters by direct intracerebral inoculation of the Schmidt-Ruppian strain of ASV.[2] Since that time, a number of deoxyribonucleic acid (DNA) and ribonucleic acid (RNA)

From: Kornblith PL, Walker MD (editors). Advances in Neuro-Oncology. Futura Publishing Company, Inc., Mount Kisco, NY, © 1988.

viruses have been found to produce CNS tumors in experimental animals (Table 1).

Most virus-induced intracranial tumors are produced following direct intracranial inoculation of high titers of virus into neonatal animals. Adult animals have been much less susceptible to viral tumor induction. Fewer tumors are formed, and they occur with a much longer latency. Several explanations are possible for the age dependence of tumor formation. The central nervous system of fetal or neonatal animals provides a unique environment for an oncogenic virus. Many viruses require specific membrane receptors in order to successfully infect a cell. These receptors may only be present on fetal cells, or may be present in higher concentrations on fetal cells. The virus is susceptible to the immune system until it has managed to enter a cell. A fetal or neonatal animal may have an incompetent immune system which is incapable of identifying and destroying an oncogenic virus. Finally, most oncogenic viruses must insert a copy of their DNA or RNA into the DNA of a host cell to transform that cell. The CNS of a fetal or neonatal animal provides a large number of rapidly dividing cells that are constantly involved with DNA synthesis. These cells may be better targets for DNA integration by an oncogenic virus.

The use of direct intracerebral inoculation of virus may introduce other artifacts into animal models of viral-induced CNS tumors. It was initially thought that inoculation of a small volume of virus was a relatively innocuous procedure. Mims found that pressures of 200–300 cm of H_2O were required to inoculate 0.03 ml intracranially into an adult mouse.[3] Because of the great pressures used, most of the inoculum passes into the ventricles rather than remaining in nervous tissue. Walsh suggested that the tendency of some viruses to produce ependymomas or choroid plexus papillomas may be due to this tendency of virus inoculated into the cerebral hemispheres to largely end up in the ventricles.[4] The virus would then have the greatest likelihood of coming into contact with and transforming cells of the ependyma and choroid plexus. Thus, the type of tumor produced may have more to do with the route of administration than any actual biological property of the virus itself.

Cell Transformation

The DNA and RNA tumor viruses use significantly different strategies to transform cells. The DNA tumor viruses are usually lytic

Table 1
Animal Models of Viral-Induced CNS Tumors*

Virus	Animals	Tumors Induced
RNA Viruses		
Avian sarcoma virus (ASV)	Syrian hamster, rabbit, mouse, guinea pig, rat monkey, cat, dog	Anaplastic astrocytoma ependymoma glioblastoma
Murine sarcoma virus (MSV)	Syrian hamster, rat	Gemistocytic astrocytoma glioblastoma, oligodendroglioma
Simian sarcoma virus (SSV)	Marmoset	Glioblastoma
DNA Viruses		
Adenovirus type 12	Syrian hamster, mouse	Undifferentiated neuroectodermal tumors
Simian adenovirus (SA-7)	Syrian hamster	Primitive, neuroectodermal tumors, glioblastoma, choroid plexus carcinoma
Simian adenovirus (SA-20)	Syrian hamster	Undifferentiated neuroectodermal tumors
Avian adenovirus (CELO)	Syrian hamster	Ependymoma
Sv_{40}	Syrian hamster, mastomys	Ependymoma, choroid plexus papilloma
BK	Syrian hamster	Ependymoma, choroid plexus papilloma
SV_{40} (PML)	Syrian hamster	Choroid plexus papilloma
JC	Syrian hamster, rat, owl monkey	Pineocytomas, glioblastomas, ependymoma, primitive neuroectodermal tumors

* Adapted from Walsh et al., 1982.[4]

in their natural host. In the lytic cycle, the virus infects the cell and monopolizes cellular metabolism to replicate viral DNA and produce viral proteins. Viral particles are assembled within the cell. The lytic cycle ends with cell lysis (a terminal event for the host cell) and the release of progeny virus. The DNA tumor viruses are only capable of transforming nonpermissive cells. The viruses are not capable of completing the lytic cycle (or producing progeny) in a nonpermissive cell. The virus will initially infect the cell, and several of the early proteins will be translated. However, not all the viral proteins are made, and progeny are not assembled. The early viral proteins frequently induce DNA synthesis in the host cell, and help integrate the viral DNA into the host cell DNA. In the vast majority of cells, the viral DNA is not stably integrated into the host cell DNA, and only a temporary or abortive transformation takes place. In a small number of cells, the viral DNA may be stably integrated in the host cell DNA, and the cell permanently transformed. These cells will now carry a portion of the viral genome stably integrated into their DNA and several of the viral antigens may be present in the nucleus. The transformed cells will not produce infectious virus. However, the virus may be rescued from these cells if the transformed cells are fused with permissive cells which allow for viral replication.

The RNA viruses which are oncogenic for the CNS are all retroviruses. Retroviruses contain high molecular weight RNA and reverse transcriptase. The reverse transcriptase is capable of making DNA transcripts of the viral RNA. The RNA tumor viruses reproduce by budding from the cell membrane. Thus, permissive cells are not killed by viral replication. These viruses are capable of producing progeny virus and transforming a permissive cell concurrently. A retrovirus usually infects a cell by fusion with the cell membrane. The viral RNA and reverse transcriptase are then transported to the cell nucleus. Initially, the reverse transcriptase makes a DNA copy of the viral RNA. A second complementary strand of DNA is then made. This double-stranded DNA is then integrated into the host cell DNA. The viral RNA and proteins can be then synthesized by cellular enzymes. In permissive cells, integration of the viral-encoded DNA may lead to production of progeny virus, transformation, or both.

The different mechanisms used by DNA and RNA tumor viruses to transform cells have important implications. The DNA tumor viruses can only transform nonpermissive cells that do not allow viral replication. Thus, in most animal models $>10^6$ particles of DNA tumor virus are required to initiate a single focus of transformation.

Since the RNA tumor viruses are capable of transforming and reproducing in the same permissive cell, they are significantly more efficient at tumor induction. The permissive cells are constantly producing progency virus which are capable of transforming other cells. However, this greater efficiency is lost when the RNA virus is placed into a nonpermissive host cell (a cell which does not allow viral replication). Other factors may also affect the efficiency of transformation. Each type of virus is made up of subtypes called *strains*. Strains may differ significantly in their efficiency of cell transformation. Host cells may vary in their rate of DNA synthesis, rate of division, or efficiency of DNA repair. Cells that are dividing and undergoing rapid cell division, or are unable to effectively repair DNA damage, are more susceptible to transformation by DNA and RNA tumor viruses.

RNA Tumor Viruses

All RNA viruses known to induce CNS tumors in animals are retroviruses. They contain two molecules of single-stranded RNA, banded into a 70S RNA, and reverse transcriptase. The most important neuro-oncogenic RNA viruses are ASV, murine sarcoma virus (MSV), and simian sarcoma virus (SSV). The ASV-induced astrocytoma is the most widely used of these tumor models. Multiple strains of the virus produce anaplastic astrocytomas and other glial tumors following intracerebral inoculation. The model developed by Bigner et al, in the neonatal rat is particularly useful because tumors occur in almost 100% of the animals, and survival is highly reproducible.[5] These tumors have been used for multiple trials of chemotherapeutic agents. The possible effect of immunotherapy against these tumors has not been thoroughly investigated. Tumor induction by ASV was reported to be inhibited by the concurrent administration of a wall preparation from bacillus Calmette-Guerin (BCG).[6]

The MSV and SSV tumor models are less frequently used. The Maloney and Kirsten strains of MSV produce a variety of glial tumors in rats, while the Harvey strain produces only sarcomas. No infectious viruses are seen in these tumors, and survival is usually 4–5 weeks. These tumors are characterized by intense vascular proliferation. It is unclear whether this is true endothelial proliferation, or a sarcomatous element of the tumor. SSV produced glioblastomas in six of 10 marmosets following intracerebral inoculation of neonatal animals.

These tumors appeared with long latencies, up to 26 months. The virus could be recovered from the tumors.

DNA Tumor Viruses

The papovaviruses and adenoviruses have been shown to induce CNS tumors in experimental animals. The major adenoviruses used include human adenovirus type 12, simian adenovirus strains 7 (SA-7) and 20 (SA-20), and the avian adenovirus (CELO). Adenovirus type 12 produces a wide variety of primitive neuroectodermal tumors in hamsters and mice. The type of tumor produced frequently depends on the site of inoculation. SA-20 induces undifferentiated neuroectodermal tumors in hamsters.

The papovaviruses have been divided into two genera: the polyoma viruses and the papilloma viruses. The papilloma viruses can be distinguished from the polyoma viruses by virtue of their larger size (55 nm in diameter versus 45 nm), and larger nucleic acid molecules (5×10^6 daltons versus 3.6×10^6 daltons). The papilloma viruses are very difficult to grow in tissue culture and have not been demonstrated to be oncogenic for CNS tissues.

The polyomaviruses include polyoma, originally isolated from mice,[7] simian virus 40 (SV_{40}) found in cultures of monkey kidney cells,[8] and three viruses isolated from humans, JC, BK, and SV_{40} (PML) which are closely related to SV_{40}. JC virus and SV_{40} (PML) were isolated from the brains of immunosuppressed patients with progressive multifocal leukoencephalopathy (PML);[9,10] and BK virus was isolated from the urine of immunosuppressed individuals.[11]

All polyoma viruses have been shown to induce CNS tumors in laboratory animals. These animal models generally involve the inoculation of very high titers of purified virus (10^8–10^{10} plaque-forming units) directly into the cerebral hemisphere of neonatal Syrian hamsters, mastomys, or athymic mice. After 4–6 months, the animals begin to develop a variety of neurological signs. One or more intracranial tumors can then be found. The viral DNA and large T antigen can always be demonstrated in the tumor cells. Inoculation with SV_{40} usually results in the formation of malignant ependymomas or choroid plexus papillomas.[12–18] Similar tumors are produced by inoculation with BK.[19–25]

A much wider variety of tumors has been found following intracerebral inoculation with JC virus. JC induces ependymomas, medulloblastomas, glioblastomas, and pineoblastomas.[26,27] In addition, one study has been done involving the intracerebral inoculation of owl monkeys with JC virus. After 16 and 25 months, a glioblastoma and a malignant glial tumor with some neuronal differentiation were found.[28]

Walsh postulated that all the tumors induced by intracerebral inoculation with polyoma viruses should really be regarded as primitive neuroectodermal tumors.[4] They all display monotonous arrays of small, poorly differentiated cells that occur in uniform sheets. Cellular pleomorphism, bizarre mitotic figures, and high nuclear to cytoplasmic ratio were common. Subarachnoid spread was seen in many of the cases. True rosettes, Homer-Wright rosettes, and papillary fronds were occasionally seen.

Viral-derived tumor antigens can be demonstrated by immunocytochemistry in these viral-induced tumors. There is a good deal of cross-reactivity between antisera raised to the large T antigen of each of the polyoma viruses.[29] Large T antigen has been localized to the nuclei of SV_{40},[30–32] polyoma,[33–35] and JC[30] transformed glial cells. Small t antigen is seen only in the cytoplasm. Capsid antigens are not found in transformed cells.[36] Viral DNA can also be found integrated into the tumor cell DNA using the DNA hybridization technique of Southern.[37] The Southern blot has been used to demonstrate the presence of SV_{40},[38,39] BK,[40] and JC[41] viral sequences integrated into the genome of viral-induced tumors.

Following the development of the animal models of viral-induced tumors, a number of investigators have attempted to associate the papovaviruses with human CNS tumors. The first efforts were largely epidemiological. The early Salk vaccines used from 1954 to 1963 were grown on rhesus monkey kidney cells. Since SV_{40} is endogenous to monkey kidneys, and the formalin process used to inactivate the poliovirus has little effect on SV_{40}, tens of millions of people were inoculated with infectious SV_{40}.[42] Fraumeni et al. reported mortality rates for all neoplasms other than leukemia which developed in children under 1 year of age in a hospital-based population. They found a 20% increase in 1956 over that seen in 1955, 1957, and 1958, and attributed this increase in tumors to the use of SV_{40} contaminated vaccines.[43,44] However, it is difficult to accept this conclusion because the Salk vaccine was not widely used until 1956.

Innis compared the rates of vaccination of 816 children who developed malignancies between 1958 and 1963 with age- and sex-matched children who did not develop tumors. He found that 88%

of the children with malignancies had been exposed to the contaminated vaccine, but only 81% of the matched controls had been immunized.[45] Stewart and Hewitt conducted a similar study and found no differences in vaccination rate between children with tumors and matched controls.[46]

Heinoen et al. studied the outcome of the 50,897 pregnancies that occurred between 1959 and 1966.[47] They compared the malignancy rate in the first four years of life among 18,324 children whose mothers received the potentially contaminated vaccine during pregnancy and children born to mothers who were not vaccinated during pregnancy. The overall malignancy rate was 7.6/10,000 in the children exposed to the contaminated vaccine in utero, and only 3.1/10,000 in the children whose mothers were not vaccinated. This difference in this malignancy rate between those exposed and not exposed to the contaminated vaccine is significant at the $p < 0.05$ level. The difference in the overall malignancy rate was almost completely accounted for by the difference in the rate of neural tumors. Seven of the 14 tumors that appeared in the vaccine-exposed children were of neuronal derivation, but only one of the 10 in the control group was of neural derivation.

Farwell et al., using records of the Connecticut Tumor Registry, identified 120 children born between 1956 and 1962 who subsequently developed CNS tumors.[48] They compared the rate of in utero exposure to the SV_{40}-contaminated vaccine between 40 of the children who developed CNS tumors and 80 age- and sex-matched controls who did not develop tumors. It was found that 37% of the children with CNS tumors had been exposed to SV_{40}, but only 21% of those without tumors had been exposed. This evidence is suggestive, but not statistically significant ($p = 0.15$). However, the difference is significant if one looks at medulloblastomas, one of the primitive neuroectodermal tumors produced in animals by the JC virus. Ten of 15 (67%) of those children with medulloblastomas had been exposed to the contaminated vaccine in utero. This difference in rates of exposure is significant at the $p < 0.01$ level.

An animal model of transplacental transmission of SV_{40} in a nonpermissive host was recently developed.[49] Inoculation of 10^7 plaque-forming units of SV_{40} into pregnant hamsters (a host in whom the virus cannot replicate), during the 8th and 12th day of gestation produced subcutaneous tumors in offspring 4 to 10 months after birth (Table 2). These tumors contained SV_{40} T antigen and SV_{40} DNA was integrated into tumor cell DNA. Lower doses of virus or the same

Table 2

In Utero Induction of Tumors in Syrian Hamsters with Papovavirus

Day of Gestation Inoculated	Dose of SV_{40} (PFU)	Tumors Months 1–5	Tumors Months 6–10	Total Tumors
4	10^7	0/19	0/19	12 dead at 4 weeks
8	10^7	7/24	6/24	13/24 (54)%
12	10^7	6/30	7/30	13/30 (43%)
4	10^5	0/22	0/22	0/22
8	10^5	0/29	0/29	0/29
12	10^5	0/16	0/16	0/16
4	10^3	0/20	0/20	0/20
8	10^3	0/19	0/19	0/19
12	10^3	0/17	0/17	0/17
4	Control	0/23	0/23	0/23
8	Control	0/31	0/31	0/31
12	Control	0/26	0/26	0/26

amount inoculated later in gestation had no effect. None of the inoculated mothers showed any effect of the virus. These findings demonstrate that SV_{40} can cross the placenta of a nonpermissive host and induce tumors in susceptible offspring.

"Dot blot" DNA hybridizations were recently done with tumor specimens from children identified in the epidemiologic study of Farwell et al.[50] The results are summarized in Table 3. In the group of children whose mothers did not receive the SV_{40}-contaminated vaccine, one of four gliomas (25%) and one of five medulloblastomas (20%) had DNA sequences homologous to SV_{40}. Ten tumors were examined from children whose mothers received the SV_{40}-contaminated polio vaccine during pregnancy. One of the six gliomas (16%) in this group had DNA sequences homologous to SV_{40}. Three of four (75%) of the medulloblastomas which appeared in children whose mothers received the SV_{40}-contaminated polio vaccine during pregnancy were found to have DNA sequences homologous to SV_{40} in the tumor cell DNA. This high incidence of SV_{40}-like sequences in these medulloblastomas correlates very well with the epidemiological information.

PML is a rare demyelinating condition that is a result of JC virus infection in immunosuppressed individuals.[9] Two changes are seen when the PML plaques are examined histologically. The first is an

Table 3

Childhood Brain Tumors from the Connecticut Tumor Registry
Examined for the Presence of DNA Sequences Homologous to
SV_{40} Viral DNA

Tissue	No. Examined	No. with Positive Hybrids
Mother vaccinated*—Child medulloblastoma	4	3
Mother vaccinated*—Child glioma	6	1
Mother not vaccinated**—Child medulloblastoma	5	1
Mother not vaccinated**—Child glioma	4	1

* Mother vaccinated = mother inoculated with SV_{40}-contaminated polio vaccine during pregnancy.
** Mother not vaccinated = mother not inoculated with SV_{40}-contaminated polio vaccine

extensive lytic infection of oligodendrocytes, with intranuclear viral inclusions. The second is the appearance of many bizarre astrocytes and mitotic figures in the area at the periphery of the PML plaque. These atypical astrocytes greatly resemble those seen in malignant astrocytomas. Castigne et al. reported multiple small gliomas arising in areas of demyelination in a case of PML. However, they were unable to demonstrate large T antigen in the nuclei of tumor cells.[51] Watanabe and Preskorn hypothesized that JC virus is capable of a lytic infection or abortive transformation of human glial cells.[52] The plaques of demyelination in PML represent areas of lytic infection, while the atypical astrocytes are a result of abortive transformation.

Most of the adult population has circulating antibodies against the capsid antigens of papovaviruses. Serum antibodies have been found against BK virus in 83% of the general population over 10 years of age[53] and antibodies against JC virus have been found in 65% of those over 14 years of age.[54] No illnesses are associated with the appearance of these antibodies. Anti-large T antibodies have been difficult to identify in human sera. They are not found in the sera of patients with PML, or proven cases of infection with other papovaviruses.[51] However, this may be explained by the fact that most of the people with PML or other papovavirus infections are immunosuppressed, and may be incapable of mounting a significant response to any viral infection. The sera of 72 patients with brain tumors have been examined for anti-T antibodies; only three were positive for anti-papovavirus-T antibody.[55,56]

Three hundred thirty-six intracranial tumors have been examined for the presence of papovavirus large T antigen using various immunocytochemical techniques. Specific anti-serum can be raised against SV_{40}, JC, or BK large T antigen in tumor-bearing animals and applied to cryostat sections of human brain tumors. Intranuclear staining specific for large T antigen was seen in only 36 of the tumors examined. These included 32 meningiomas,[57–60] an ependymoma,[61] a glioblastoma[58] and a "reticulum cell sarcoma."[62] These results are very difficult to explain. Conflicting results were reported when tumors were examined by multiple investigators. Meningiomas that are not true CNS tumors and have never been prduced by papovaviruses in experimental animals are the tumors most frequently reported to contain large T antigen. This may be due to a problem with the specificity of the antisera used, or a cellular protein may be present in meningiomas which has significant homology with large T antigen. There may be several explanations for the negative results with the true CNS tumors. The large T antigen may be expressed by few cells or at very low levels so that immunofluorescence techniques most commonly used were not sufficiently sensitive. Another possibility is that the human tumors may not be producing a complete large T antigen. Rundell et al. described a mutant strain of SV_{40} which produced a truncated large T antigen that was only 33 kilodaltons in molecular weight.[63] Antisera raised against a wild type large T antigen might not recognize a markedly altered protein.

Only two investigators have reported the isolation of a papovavirus from a human intracranial tumor. Takemoto et al. isolated a mutant strain of BK virus from a "reticulum cell sarcoma" which developed in a child with Wiskott-Aldrich syndrome.[62] The virus was rescued by co-cultivation with permissive VERO monkey kidney cells. It was found to be defective in the region which codes for small t antigen. Scherneck et al. reported the isolation of an SV_{40}-like virus from a glioblastoma multiforme following fusion with permissive CV-1 monkey cells.[58] The rescued viruses may be laboratory contaminants or endogenous in the permissive cell. In addition, even if the rescued viruses are not contaminants, it is uncertain whether tumor cells became infected with papovaviruses after transformation, or whether the virus played some part in the transformation of the cell.

The most sensitive means of identifying viruses associated with human tumors is through the use of DNA/DNA hybridization techniques. A number of investigators have used various papovavirus DNA probes in hybridization experiments with DNA from human intracranial tumors. A total of 13 CNS tumors have been reported to contain DNA sequences homologous to BK virus.[40,64–66] These studies have several technical problems. All of them, with the exception of Pater et al., were done with liquid hybridization techniques which cannot differentiate integrated viral DNA sequences from episomal contaminants. None of them used normal brain tissue and other viral DNA probes as controls. Several investigators reported conflicting results when examining the same cell lines.

Barbanti-Brodano et al. recently examined 40 human brain tumors and five specimens of normal human brain for DNA sequences homologous to BK virus. They found 12 of the tumors had DNA sequences homologous to BK. The viral DNA was episomal and was present in a low copy number (0.2–2 genomes per cell). No sequences homologous to BK were found in the normal brain. A virus very similar to BK was rescued from two of the tumors. This BK variant was found to have an insertion in the early region of the genome.[67]

Two investigators have performed hybridization experiments using SV_{40} DNA as a probe for human intracranial tumors. Meinke et al. found sequences homologous to SV_{40} in one of seven glioblastoma multiforme using a liquid hybridization technique. No control tissues or probes were reported.[68] Ibelgaufts and Jones examined 32 brain tumors for SV_{40} RNA using an in situ technique with 5 mm thick frozen sections. Thirty-four percent of these tumors were found to contain SV_{40} RNA.[69] The same 32 tumors were examined with an identical technique using adenovirus DNA as a probe. Adenovirus-related RNA sequences were found in 62% of the tumors examined.[70] Neither of the techniques used in these two studies is capable of distinguishing integrated viral DNA sequences from contaminants or episomal DNA.

Southern blot hybridizations were done with an SV_{40} probe utilizing control tissues and probes in one study.[71] A total of 30 specimens were examined (Table 4) including nine meningiomas, seven intermediate to high grade astrocytomas, six tumors metastatic to the brain, one schwannoma, and seven non-neoplastic partial lobectomy specimens removed to control seizures. DNA sequences homologous to SV_{40} were not identified in the schwannoma, metastatic tumors, or non-neoplastic brain. Two of the meningiomas and two astrocytomas were found to have DNA sequences homologous to SV_{40}. These tumors contained high molecular weight DNA sequences

Table 4

Human Tissues Examined by Southern Blot
Hybridization for the Presence of DNA
Sequences Homologous to SV_{40} Viral DNA

Tissues	No. Examined	No. With Positive Hybrids
Meningioma	9	2
Glioma	7	2
Metastatic	6	0
Schwannoma	1	0
Normal (nontumor)	7	0

homologous to SV_{40} following digestion of total tumor DNA with endonucleases that cut the SV_{40} viral genome. This indicates that the sequences homologous to the virus were integrated into the host cell DNA.

The presence of viral DNA or viral antigens within a tumor is not conclusive evidence that a particular virus caused that tumor. A tumor is usually only clinically apparent long after the initial transforming event. When examining specimens from human tumors, it is impossible to determine if an oncogenic virus was present at the time of transformation or merely infected previously transformed cells. Many patients harboring malignancies are known to have depressed immune systems, which may make them more susceptible to viral infection or reactivation of a latent infection. The virus may be present at the time of transformation, but only serve to make the cell more susceptible to transformation by another agent. No single piece of evidence can conclusively demonstrate that viruses are etiologic agents for human CNS tumors. Nonetheless, much recent work has made a strong argument for the possible role of papovaviruses in the formation of human CNS tumors.

Summary

Many experimental models of DNA and RNA virus-induced CNS tumors have been developed. These models have proved valuable in the evaluation of various forms of therapy. The possible role of these viruses as etiologic agents for human tumors is under investigation. The most thoroughly studied neuro-oncogenic viruses are the papovaviruses. JC virus induces glial tumors in owl monkeys. Epidemiologic studies have associated in utero exposure to SV_{40}-contaminated polio vaccines with an increased incidence of CNS tumors. SV_{40} and BK DNA sequences and T antigen have been found in a number of CNS tumors. This evidence suggests a possible role for the papovaviruses in the production of human CNS tumors.

Most carcinogens are also mutagens capable of producing changes in cellular DNA. The molecular events involved in the transformation of a cell may be common to many carcinogens. The greatest value of animal models of virus-induced CNS tumors may be in elucidating some of these basic molecular events. The oncogenic viruses contain a small number of genes and proteins. The interaction of these genes and proteins with normal cellular genes and proteins may yield important information in the understanding of molecular events involved in cell transformation in the CNS.

REFERENCES

1. Vasquez-Lopez E. Sarcomas following intracerebral inoculation with an Avian sarcoma virus. Am J Cancer 1936; 26:29–55.
2. Rabotti GF, Raine WA. Brain tumors induced in hamsters inoculated intracerebrally at birth with Rous Sarcoma virus. Nature 1964; 204:898–899.
3. Mims CA. Intracerebral injections and the growth of viruses in the mouse brain. Br J Exp Pathol 1960; 41:52–59.
4. Walsh JW, Zimmer SG, Perdue ML. Role of viruses in the induction of primary intracranial tumors. Neurosurg 1982; 10:643–662.
5. Bigner DD, Pegram CN. Virus-induced experimental brain tumors and putative association of viruses with human brain tumors: A review. In: Advances in Neurology, Vol. 15. New York, Raven Press, 1976; pp. 57–83.
6. Walker JS, Bigner DD. Virus induced brain tumors. in Neurosurgery. New York, McGraw-Hill, 1985; pp. 522–525.
7. Gross L. Oncogenic viruses. in Oncogenic Viruses, 2nd. Ed. Oxford, Pergamon, 1970; pp. 1–34.
8. Sweet BH, Hilleman MR. The vacuolating virus SV40. Proc Soc Exp Biol Med 1960; 105:420–427.
9. Padgett BL, Walker DL, ZuRhein GM, Echroade RJ, Desse BH. Cultivation of papova-like virus from human brain with progressive multifocal leukoencephalopathy. Lancet 1971; 1:1257–1260.
10. Weiner LP, Herndon RM, Narayan O, Johnson RT, Shah K, Rubinstein LJ, Preziozi TJ, Conley FK. Isolation of virus related to SV40 from pa-

tients with progressive multifocal leukoencephalopathy. N Engl J Med 1972; 286:385–390.

11. Gardner SD, Field AM, Coleman DV, Hulme B. New human papovavirus (BK) isolated from urine after renal transplantation. Lancet 1971; 1:1253–1257.

12. Duffel D, Hinzell R, Nelson E. Neoplasms in hamsters induced by simian virus 40. Am J Pathol 1964; 45:59–73.

13. Eddy BE. Tumors produced in hamsters by SV40. Fed Proc 1962; 21:930–935.

14. Ikuta F, Ogawa H, Kumanishi T. Experimental DNA virus-induced brain tumors. In: Proceedings VIIth International Congress of Neuropathology. Amsterdam, Excerpta Medica, 1965; pp. 453–460.

15. Gerber P, Kirschstein R. Biological properties of ribonucleic acid from virulent and attenuated poliovirus. J Exp Med 1960; 111:525–532.

16. Rabson AS, O'Conor GT, Kirschstein RL, Branigan WJ. Papillary ependymomas produced in Rattus natalensis inoculated with vacuolating virus (SV40). J Natl Cancer Inst 1962; 29:765–787.

17. Unterharnschiedt F, Bonin O, Schmidt K, Schmidt I. Die pathomorphologie von virusinduzierten (SV40) neoplasminen bei neugeborenen goldhamstern. Acta Neuropathol (Berlin) 1964; 3:362–371.

18. Wilkins RH, Odom CL. Attempted induction of gliomas utilizing simian virus 40. Arch Neurol 1965; 13:149–153.

19. Corallini A, Barbanti-Brodano G, Bartolini W, Nenci I, Cassai E, Tapieri M, Portalini M, Borgatti M. High incidence of ependymomas induced by BK virus, a human papovavirus. J Natl Cancer Inst 1977; 59:1561–1564.

20. Costa J, Yee C, Talka TS, Rabeson AS. Hamster ependymomas produced by intracerebral inoculation of human papovavirus (MMV). J Natl Cancer Inst 1976; 56:863–864.

21. Greenlee JE, Narayan O, Johnson RT, Herndon RM. Induction of brain tumors in hamsters with BK virus, a human papovavirus. Lab Invest 1977; 36:636–641.

22. Tsuboi M, Moriya Y, Tabuchi K, Nishimoto A. Electron microscopic features of brain tumor induced in hamster by BK virus, a human papovavirus. Acta Med Okayama 1979; 33:423–430.

23. Uchida S, Watanbe S, Aizawa T, Furuno A, Muto T. Polyoncogenicity and insulinoma-inducing ability of BK virus, a human papovavirus, in Syrian golden hamsters. J Natl Cancer Inst 1979; 63:119–126.

24. Becker LE, Narayan O, Johnson RT. Studies of papovavirus tumor antigen in experimental and human cerebral neoplasms. Can J Neuro Sci 1976; 3:105–109.

25. Narayan O, Weiner LP. Biological properties of two strains of simian virus 40 isolated from patients with progressive multifocal leukoencephalopathy. Infect Immunol 1974; 10:173–179.

26. Padgett BL, Walker DL, ZuRhein GM, Varakis JN. Differential neuro-oncogenicity of strains of JC virus, a human polyoma virus, in newborn Syrian hamsters. Cancer Res 1977; 37:718–720.

27. Walker DL, Padgett BL, ZuRhein GM, Albert AE, Marsh RF. Human papovavirus JC: induction of brain tumors in hamsters. Science 1973; 181:674–676.

28. London WT, Houff SA, Madden DL, Fucillo DA, Gravell M, Wallen WC, Palmer AE, Sever JC, Padgett BL, Walker DL, ZuRhein GM, Ohashi T. Brain tumors in owl monkeys inoculated with a human polyoma virus (JC virus). Science 1978; 201:1246–1249.
29. Beth E, Cikes M, Schloen L, diMayorca G, Giraldo G. Interspecies-, species- and type specific T antigenic determinants of human papovavirus (JC and BK) and of simian virus 40. Int J Cancer 1977; 20:551–559.
30. Frisque RJ, Rifkin DB, Walker DL. Transformation of primary hamster brain cells with JC virus and its DNA. J Virol 1980; 35:265–269.
31. Shein HM. Transformation of astrocytes and destruction of spongioblasts induced by a simian tumor virus (SV40) in cultures of human fetal neuroglia. J Neuropathy Exp Neurol 1967; 26:60–76.
32. Shein HM. Neoplastic transformation induced by simian virus 40 in Syrian hamster neurological and meningeal cell cultures. Arch Ges Virusforsch 1968; 22:122–142.
33. deMicco C, Triplier MF, Hassoun J, Lipcey C, Meyer G, Toga M. Neoplastic transformation of hamster brain cells in vitro by polyoma virus. Int J Cancer 1978; 21:516–522.
34. Shein HM. Neoplastic transformation of hamster astrocytes and choroid plexus cells in culture by polyoma virus. J Neuropathol Exp Neurol 1970; 29:70–88.
35. Tanaka R, Sekiguchi K, Veki K, Gilden DH, Koprowski H. Morphological studies of hamster brain cells transformed in vitro by a human papovavirus, BK. Acta Neuropathol (Berlin) 1978; 41:236–239.
36. Howley PM. Molecular biology of SV40 and the human polyomaviruses BK and JC. In: Viral Oncology. New York, Raven Press, 1980; pp. 489–550.
37. Southern EM. Detection of specific sequences among sequences separated by gel electropheresis. J Mol Biol 1975; 98:503–517.
38. Botcham M, Stringer J, Mitchinson T, Sambrook J. Integration and excision of SV40 DNA from the chromosome of a transformed cell. Cell 1980; 20:143–152.
39. Ketner G, Kelly TJ Jr. Integrated simian virus 40 sequences in transformed cell DNA: Analysis using restriction endonucleases. Proc Nat Acad Sci USA 1976; 73:1102–1106.
40. Wold WSM, Mackey JK, Brackman HK, Takemori N, Ridgen P, Green M. Analysis of human tumors and malignant cell lines for BK virus specific DNA sequences. Proc Nat Acad Sci USA 1978; 75:454–458.
41. Wold WSM, Green M, Mackey JM, Martin JD, Padgett BL, Walker DL. Integration pattern of human JC virus sequences in two clones of a cell line established from a JC virus-induced hamster brain tumor. J Virol 1980; 33:1225–1228.
42. Shah KV, Nathanson M. Human exposure to SV40: review and comment. Am J Epidemiol 1976; 103:1–12.
43. Fraumeni JF, Ederer F, Miller RW. An evaluation of the carcinogenicity of simian virus 40 in man. JAMA 1963; 185:713–718.
44. Fraumeni JF, Stark CR, Gold E. Simian virus 40 in polio vaccine: follow-up of newborn recipients. Science 1970; 167:59–60.

45. Innis MD. Oncogenesis and poliomyelitis vaccine. Nature 1968; 219:972–973.
46. Stewart AM, Hewitt D. Aetiology of childhood leukemia. Lancet 1965; 2:789–790.
47. Heinoen OP, Shapiro S, Monson RR, Hartz SC, Rosenberg L, Slone D. Immunization during pregnancy against poliomyelitis and influenza in relation to childhood malignancy. Int J Epidemiol 1973; 2:229–235.
48. Farwell JR, Dohrmann GJ, Marnell LD, Meigs JW. Effect of SV40-contaminated polio vaccine on the incidence and type of CNS neoplasms in children: a population-based study. Trans Am Neurol Assoc 1979; 104:261–263.
49. Rachlin JR, Wollmann RW, Dohrmann GJ. (in press) Lab Invest 1988.
50. Dohrmann GJ, Rachlin JR, Wollmann RW. (submitted for publication)
51. Castigne P, Rondot P, Escourolle R, Ribedeau Dumas JC, Cathala F, Hauw JJ. Leucoencephalopathie multifocale progresive et gliomas multiples. Rev Neurol (Paris) 1974; 130:379–392.
52. Watanabe I, Preskorn SH. Virus cell interaction in oligodendroglia, asroglia, and phagocyte in progressive multifocal leukoencephalopathy. Acta Neuropathol (Berlin) 1976; 36:101–115.
53. Gardner SD. Prevalence in England of antibody to human polyomavirus (BK). Br Med J 1973; 1:77–78.
54. Padgett BL, Walker DL. Prevalence of antibodies in human sera against JC virus, an isolate from a case of progressive multifocal leukoencephalopathy. J Infect Dis 1973; 127:467–470.
55. Costa J, Yee C, Rabson AS. Absence of papovavirus T antibody in patients with malignancies. Lancet 1977; 2:709.
56. Corallini A, Barbanti-Brodano G, Portalini M, Balboni PG, Grossi MP, Possati L, Honorati C, LaPlaca M, Mazzoni M, Caputo A, Veronesi U, Orefice S, Cardinali G. Antibodies to BK virus strucutral and tumor antigens in human sera from normal persons and from patients with various diseases, including neoplasia. Infect Immunol 1976; 13:1684–1691.
57. Geissler E, Scherneck S, Waehite H, Zimmerman W, Luebbe W, Krause H, Theile M, Herolk HJ, Rudolph M, Weickmann M, Nisch G. Further studies on the relationship of SV40-like viruses to human tumors. Cold Spring Harbor Symp Quant Biol 1980; 44:31–39.
58. Scherneck S, Rudolph M, Geissler E, Vogel F, Lubbe L, Waehite H, Nisch G, Weickmann F, Zimmerman W. Isolation of an SV40 like papovavirus from a human glioblastoma. Int J Cancer 1979; 24:523–531.
59. Weiss AF, Portmann R, Fischer H, Simon H, Zang KD. Simian virus 40 related antigens in three human meningiomas with defined chromosome loss. Proc Nat Acad Sci USA 1975; 72:609–613.
60. Zang KD, May G, Fischer H. Expression of SV40 related T antigen in cell cultures of human meningiomas. Naturwissen Schaften 1979; 66:59.
61. Tabuchi K, Kirsch WM, Low M, Gaskin D, Buskirk JV, Shane M. Screening of human brain tumors for SV40 related T antigen. Int J Cancer 1978; 21:12–17.
62. Takemoto KK, Rabson AS, Mullarkey MF, Balese RM, Garon CF, Nelson D. Isolation of papovavirus from brain tumor and urine of a patient with Wiskott-Aldrich syndrome. J Nat Cancer Inst 1974; 53:1205–1207.

63. Rundell K, Collins JK, Tegtmeyer P, Oxer HL, Lai CJ, Nathans D. Identification of Simian virus 40 protein A. Am J Virol 1977; 21:636–646.
64. Fiori M, DiMayorca G. Occurrence of BK virus DNA in DNA obtained from certain human tumors. Proc Nat Acad Sci USA 1976; 73:4662–4666.
65. Israel MA, Martin MA, Takemoto KK, Howley PM, Aaronson SA, Solomon D, Khoury G. Evaluation of normal and neoplastic human tissue for BK virus. Virology 1978; 90:187–196.
66. Pater MM, Pater A, Fiori M, Slota J, DiMayorca G. BK virus DNA sequences in human tumors and normal tissues and cell lines. Cold Spring Harbor Conf Cell Proliferation 1980; 7:329–341.
67. Barbanti-Brodano G, Silini E, Mottes M, Milinesi G, Pagani M, Reshligan P, Cerna G, Corrallini A. DNA probes to evaluate the possible association of papovaviruses with human tumors. In: Monoclonals and DNA Probes in Diagnostic and Preventative Medicine. New York, Raven Press, 1987; pp. 147–155.
68. Meinke W, Boldstein DA, Smith RA. Simian virus 40 related DNA sequences in a human brain tumor. Neurology (New York) 1979; 29:1590–1594.
69. Ibelgaufts H, Jones KW. Papovavirus related RNA sequences in human neurogenic tumors. Acta Neuropathol (Berlin) 1982; 56:118–122.
70. Ibelgaufts H, Jones KW, Maitland N, Shaw JF. Adenovirus related RNA sequences in human neurogenic tumors. Acta Neuropathol (Berlin) 1982; 56:113–117.
71. Rachlin JR, Wollmann RW, Dohrmann GJ. SV40 viral DNA in human CNS tumors. J Neuropathol Exptl Neurol 1984; 43:301.

Section II
Approaches to Brain Tumor Diagnosis

Introduction

The diagnosis of brain tumors has been revolutionized by the CT scan. Whereas prior to CT tedious and dangerous pneumoencephalography, ventriculography, and angiography were required, now CT scans can safely and accurately tell the clinician whether there is an intracranial mass and where it is located in a 3-dimensional fashion. It is still difficult to tell exactly the nature of the tumor, its growth rate, its probable biology, and its degree of neoplastic activity.

Certain newer diagnostic technics offer hope of moving diagnosis forward even further. MRI (NMR) is a remarkable new technique which gives anatomical detail and allows visualization of areas poorly seen on the CT scan. Without contrast agents, MRI does have limits in distinguishing tumor from peritumoral edema in certain gliomas but can delineate tumors in the brain stem and posterior fossa extremely well. Also, the safety of the MRI allows for the first time serial and even weekly follow-up of tumor patients and can provide enough data points to assess growth rates.

PET scanning is wonderfully applicable to the study of brain tumor patients. It allows one to see the actual metabolic rate of a tumor, the response to therapy, and may enable us to predict biological behavior with greater precision.

The promise of monoclonal antibodies as a diagnostic reagent lies in their potential for specificity. The ability to recognize a specific protein moeity and then to image that recognition process with isotopes offers a really striking approach to diagnostic specificity.

Studies of the CSF in brain tumors have been considered as an old and somewhat outdated technique; however, there are some new wrinkles to this classic approach worthy of appreciation. The ability to grow cells from the CSF is, in particular, a valuable adjunct for determining whether a tumor which sheds cells into the CSF pathways is continuing to do so after treatment, thereby allowing physicians to quantitate the responses to therapy.

Although the diagnosis of brain tumors has already advanced significantly, these contributions offer a vision of areas yet to be explored and new data likely to become available to aid in tumor diagnosis.

8

Brain Imaging in the Diagnosis of Intracranial Neoplasms

Nicholas J. Patronas, William D. Moore, and Dieter R. Schellinger

The radiological evaluation of neoplastic processes involving the central nervous system has evolved significantly in the recent past. Due to advances in the treatment of CNS diseases which have occurred during the last few decades, the need for early and accurate detection of CNS neoplasms becomes obvious. Simple localization of a lesion is no longer sufficient to design a therapeutic regimen. Additional information regarding the extent of the lesion and its relationship to adjacent structures becomes necessary. Furthermore, histological characterization and evaluation of the biological behavior of brain tumors is desirable and possible with current imaging techniques.

In response to these demands, classic neurodiagnostic modalities (skull radiography and pneumoencephalography) have been completely abandoned while the role of others such as arteriography has been diminished considerably. With the tremendous expansion in computer technology, newer imaging devices have been developed which dramatically improve our diagnostic capabilities. These include computed tomography (CT), magnetic resonance imaging (MRI), and positron emission tomography (PET).

From: Kornblith PL, Walker MD (editors). Advances in Neuro-Oncology. Futura Publishing Company, Inc., Mount Kisco, NY, © 1988.

Due to the number and complexity of diagnostic tests that we now have in our armamentarium, it is necessary for the clinician to understand and utilize the different types of information each of these tests will provide. With this knowledge, a diagnostic plan that will provide the maximum useful information with the least cost and discomfort to the patient can be developed.

In this chapter, we will outline the contributions made by MRI and PET in tumor imaging and will discuss the role of these two modalities relative to that of CT in evaluating these patients.

Magnetic Resonance Imaging

Theoretical Considerations: Methodology

Magnetic resonance imaging is a relatively new technique that has been used for the evaluation of various organ systems and has been found to be particularly useful for the central nervous system. This method does not utilize x-rays or radioactive materials and in that respect becomes an attractive alternative to CT and PET. Additionally, MRI routinely acquires images in three planes directly rather than by reconstruction of data acquired in a single plane; consequently, there is no loss of resolution or anatomic information.

MRI utilizes radiowave pulses which penetrate the body and interact with the nuclei of certain atoms which are naturally present in the tissues. To date, the nucleus of the hydrogen atom, the proton, has been used almost exclusively in the production of the MR image and in the following discussion we will be referring to this atomic particle. MR images have also been generated using the nucleus of sodium which may, in the future, open new avenues of investigation in the study of central nervous system diseases, particularly neoplasms.

The nucleus of the hydrogen atom is composed of a single proton possessing a rotational movement called "spin." Since protons are charged particles, their rotation creates a small magnetic field in their immediate environment which causes them to behave as small bar magnets. If spinning protons are placed in a strong static magnetic field, as exists in an MR scanner, they will align themselves along the lines of the externally applied field. This process is known as magnetization. MR scanning is a gross imaging phenomenon which does not directly measure each individual proton but rather measures their behavior in aggregate. This summation of the effects of many millions of protons is expressed with a mathematical term called the "net magnetization vector" which is graphically represented by an arrow (i.e., a "vector" quantity with magnitude and direction) aligned with the direction of the external field.

Once magnetization is achieved, one can produce the magnetic resonance phenomenon by irradiating the protons with radiofrequency (RF) pulses. The frequency of these pulses must be chosen properly for magnetic resonance to occur. This specific frequency, called the Larmor frequency, depends on the nature of the atom and also on the strength of the static magnetic field. During the application of the RF pulses, the protons acquire energy, causing the net magnetization vector to deviate from its equilibrium position aligned with the external field. The RF pulses are characterized by the degree of deviation of the magnetization vector they produce. The commonly used RF pulses are 90° which deviates the vector by 90° from the direction of the static magnetic field and 180° which inverts the vector to the opposite position. After being excited with RF pulses, the protons return to the lower energy state and emit an RF signal which can be measured and localized in space. This allows the production of images reflecting the relative concentration of hydrogen nuclei in the various tissues.

Two other nuclear magnetic phenomena, the relaxation times T1 and T2, have been used to produce MR images which in practice were found to be superior to the proton MRI. The relaxation time T1 is the time needed for the magnetization vector to return to its original position after it is displaced by an RF pulse. In other words, T1 represents a measurement of the rapidity with which the displaced protons lose their excess energy to their environment (Fig. 1). The relaxation time T1 is influenced by the temperature of the sample and the molecular structure in which the hydrogen is incorporated. Assuming that the temperature is constant, liquids with the hydrogen incorporated in the water molecule will have long T1 values whereas body tissues, with the hydrogen bound in larger molecules, will have short T1 values. Similarly, cancer cells or edematous body tissues, both of which have increased water content, have longer T1 values than normal. In the T2 relaxation process, no energy is transferred to the environment, but there is an exchange of energy from one nucleus to another. The T2 relaxation time is measured when the magnetization vector, under the influence of an RF pulse, is flipped 90° from its original vertical position and begins to resonate on a

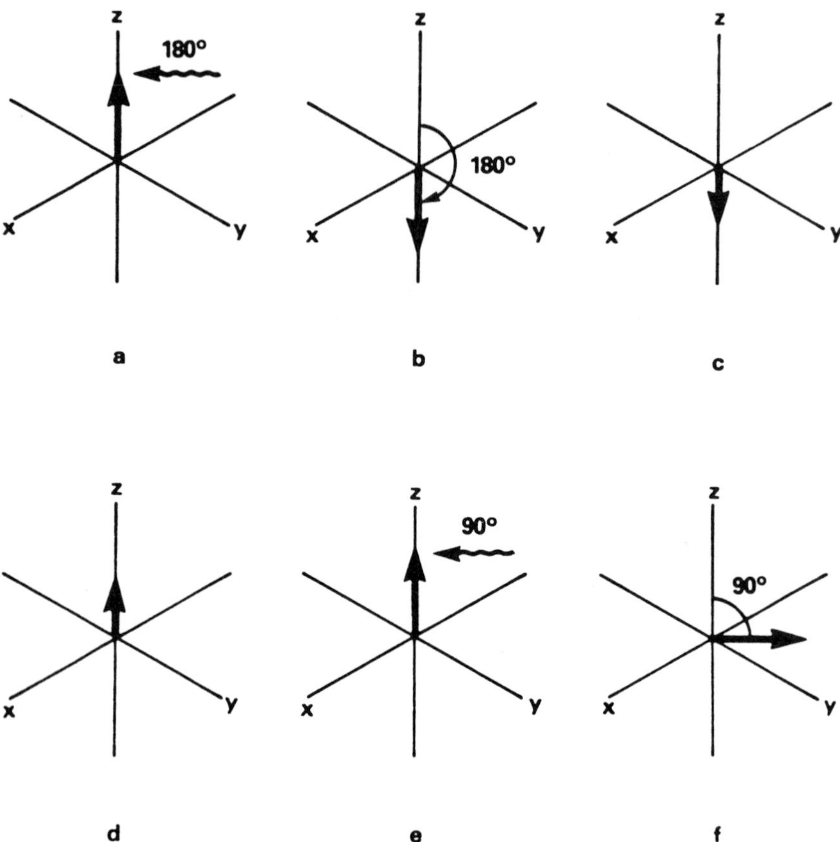

Figure 1. Schematic presentation of relaxation time T1. In a, the net magnetization vector points upwards, while a 180° pulse is applied. In b, the net magnetization vector has been displaced to a diametrically opposite position where the individual protons possess extra energy. Several milliseconds later in c, part of this energy has been released to the environment and although the vector remains inverted, its magnitude is now smaller. In d, most of the originally inverted proton bar magnets have been given up their extra energy and point upward. Complete recovery has not been accomplished as yet and the magnitude of the vector is still shorted than that of its original alignment. In e, all extra energy of the protons has been given up to the environment and the magnitude of the vector has reached its maximum value. At this point, a 90° pulse is applied to displace the vector onto the x,y plane where the signal is measured (f). The time required for the vector to return from the position b to the position e is the relaxation time T1.

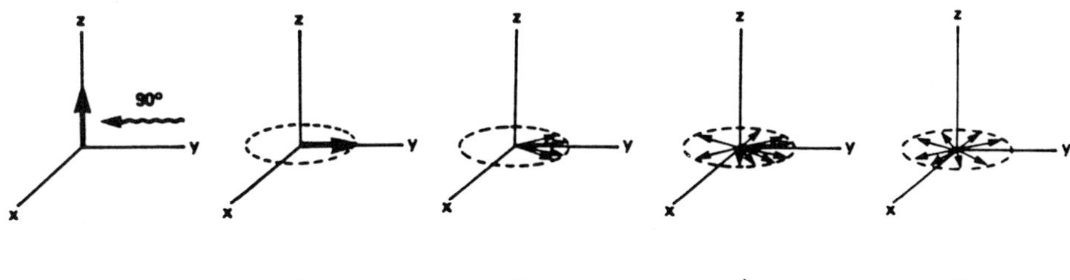

Figure 2. Schematic presentation of relaxation time T2. In a, the magnetization vector is pointing upward while a 90° pulse is applied. In b, the magnetization vector has been flipped onto the x,y plane, and temporarily, the individual proton bar magnets rotate synchronously. At this point, all protons are said to be in phase and the MR signal has its maximum value. Soon after, c and d, due to the inhomogeneity of the magnetic fields and also due to the interactions between the individual protons, rotate at different frequencies as they gradually lose their energy. This dephasing process is accompanied by a decrease in the intensity of the MR signal. When complete disorganization of the rotational movement has taken place (e), the MR signal is zero. The time required for the complete dephasing of the rotating protons is the relaxation time T2.

plane (x,y) that is perpendicular to the vertical axis (z). Momentarily, all resonating protons are in phase and the generated MR signal has its maximum amplitude. The signal intensity will immediately start to diminish as the various protons rotate at different speeds and will gradually fade to become zero. The time required for this complete loss of coherence of the rotating protons, which coincides with the time required for the total disappearance of the MR signal, is the T2 relaxation time (Fig. 2). The rate at which this signal decays depends on two factors: (1) nonuniformities in the static magnetic field, and (2) the intrinsic magnetic interactions between nearby nuclei. The inhomogeneity of the static magnetic field is a mechanical imperfection and is, therefore, present in every experimental setting. The intrinsic magnetic interactions vary with the molecular size. Thus in small molecules such as H_2O, the interactions between neighboring nuclei are fewer, and the T2 is relatively long as opposed to larger molecules in which the T2 values are shorter. The T2 values in biological tissues are always shorter than T1, although in liquid the T2 value can equal but never exceed, the T1 value. Therefore, it is apparent that the molecular structure in the body tissues modifies greatly the T1 and the T2 values, thus creating a sensitive scale which can be used to discriminate one tissue from the other.

By proper choice of pulse sequences, images can be produced in which the signal intensity (high signal intensity is bright; low signal intensity is dark) is predominantly dependent upon differences in T1, T2, or a combination of both. In clinical MR, the terms T1 weighted or T2 weighted have emerged and are useful in the choice of scanning techniques and interpretation of images. T1 weighted images provide anatomical detail because the brain parenchyma and cerebrospinal fluid (CSF) differ markedly on T1. Most pathologies affect T2, and therefore, the T2 weighted pulse sequences produce images sensitive to pathology. One drawback of MRI is that most pathological processes affect both T1 and T2 in a similar fashion, prolonging both. Hence, the abnormal signal intensities seen in the images are infrequently histologically specific, and the diagnosis rests primarily on distribution and morphology.

One of the most commonly used T1 weighted techniques is called "inversion recovery." To perform an inversion recovery (IR) scan, two pulses are applied. The first is a pulse of 180° that inverts the magnetization vector to the opposite position. In this new position, protons possess extra energy which is gradually released to the environment as the magnetization vector returns to its original position. After waiting a certain period of time, another pulse of 90° is applied to displace the magnetization vector onto the x,y plane where the intensity of the MR signal is measured. The time period between the 180° and the 90° pulse is called inversion time (TI) and is usually between 100 and 600 milliseconds (msec). During inversion recovery scanning, the scheme of pulse sequences already described is constantly repeated, and the time interval between two consecutive repetitions is called repetition time (TR) which usually varies from 1,000 to 2,500 msec (Fig. 3). On inversion recovery images, CSF is black while cerebral and cerebellar cortex as well as the basal ganglia are gray. The white matter is bright.

The second scanning technique is called "spin echo" and can be either T1 weighted or T2 weighted. When a spin echo technique is used, initially a 90° pulse is applied. After waiting a certain period called "echo time" (TE), which usually ranges from 15 to 120 msec, the signal is measured. Commonly a 180° pulse is inserted midway to correct for inhomogeneity of the field. This pulse sequence is then repeated, and the time interval between two consecutive repetitions is the TR (Fig. 4). In order to obtain T1 weighted spin echo images

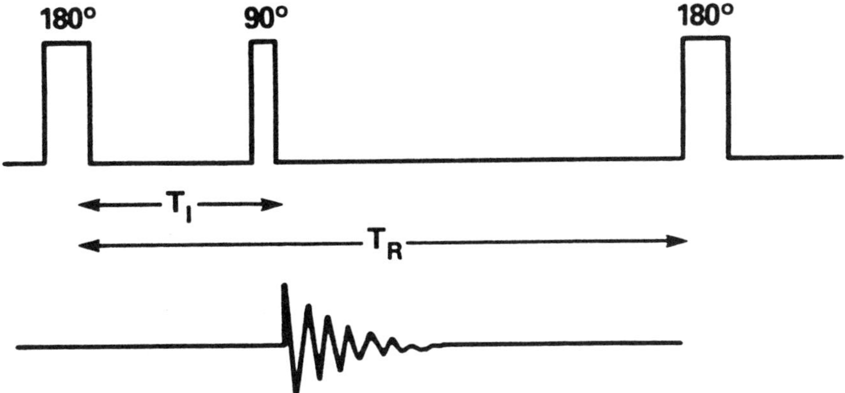

Figure 3. Pulse sequence inversion recovery. Initially, a 180° pulse is applied displacing the net magnetization vector to a diametrically opposite position. After a period of time (TI-time of inversion), a 90° pulse displaces the vector onto the x,y plane where the signal is measured. The TI can be between 100 and 600 msec. Then the same pulse sequence is repeated. The time between two consecutive 180° pulses is called repetition time (TR), and it usually varies between 1,000 and 2,500 msec.

the interval TE as well as the repetition time must be short (TE 15–26 msec, TR 300–700 msec). The appearance of the T1 weighted spin echo images is similar to that of inversion recovery. The only difference is that the contrast between gray and white matter is less sharp with this technique.

Two different pulse sequences are used for T2 weighted spin echo images. The first is with a TE of 25–40 msec and TR 1,500–2,500 msec and the second with TE 80–120 msec and TR 2,000–3,000 msec. In the former, which is moderately T2 weighted and is also called a proton density image, the cortex and basal ganglia are bright gray while the white matter is dark gray. The CSF spaces present with brightness similar to that of white matter or slightly less depending on the values of TE and TR. This technique is preferable for lesions adjacent to cavities containing fluid such as the ventricles because it can easily separate one from the other and still show the T2 effect on pathology. On the latter, known as heavily T2 weighted technique, both cortex and white matter appear as shades of darker gray but CSF becomes white. Some neural structures (globus pallidus, red nucleus, and substantial nigra) appear very dark due to normal iron deposition in their parenchyma (Fig. 5).[1–6]

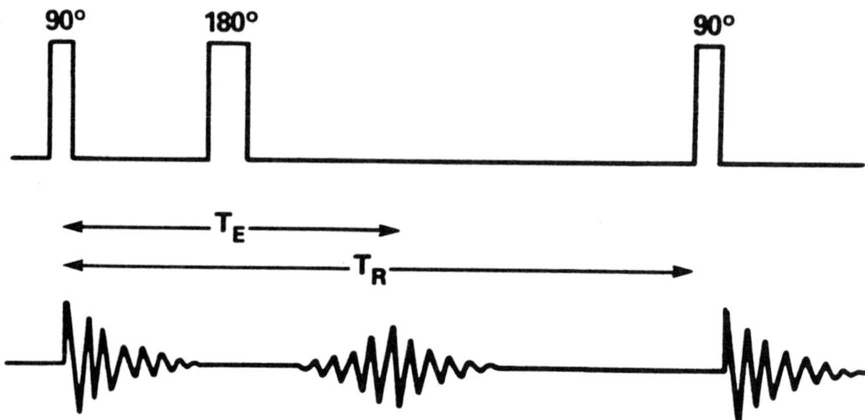

Figure 4. Pulse sequences in spin-echo. Initially, a 90° pulse is applied, displacing the net magnetization vector onto the x,y plane. A period of time, which varies between 13 and 55 msec, is allowed to elapse and a 180° pulse is applied. After waiting for an identical period of time, the MR signal is measured. The period from the 90° pulse to the time the MR signal is measured is called echo time (TE). Repetition time (TR) is the time between two consecutive 90° pulses.

As with CT scanning, MRI can be performed after intravenous administration of contrast material. These compounds improve the sensitivity and specificity of the method and increase the diagnostic value of the MR images. Unlike the iodinated contrast for CT which alters the radiodensity of tissues by absorbing the x-rays, contrast agents for MRI alter the relaxation times T1 and T2 by changing the local magnetic environment of the signal-producing hydrogen nuclei. The majority of such MR contrast agents are paramagnetic substances which intrinsically possess a magnetic moment due to the presence of an unpaired particle. An unpaired proton, neutron, or electron can produce this phenomenon, but the effect with unpaired electrons is greatest.

A substance which has been found to show strong paramagnetic effects while being relatively nontoxic is gadolinium bound to diethylenetriamine pentaacetic acid (Gd-DTPA).[6-9]

Gd-DTPA has been studied as an intravenous contrast agent for central nervous system imaging and has been shown to be useful in a variety of brain lesions. Doses as small as 0.1 millimole/kilogram (mmol/kg) were used and no short-term side effects were noted. The

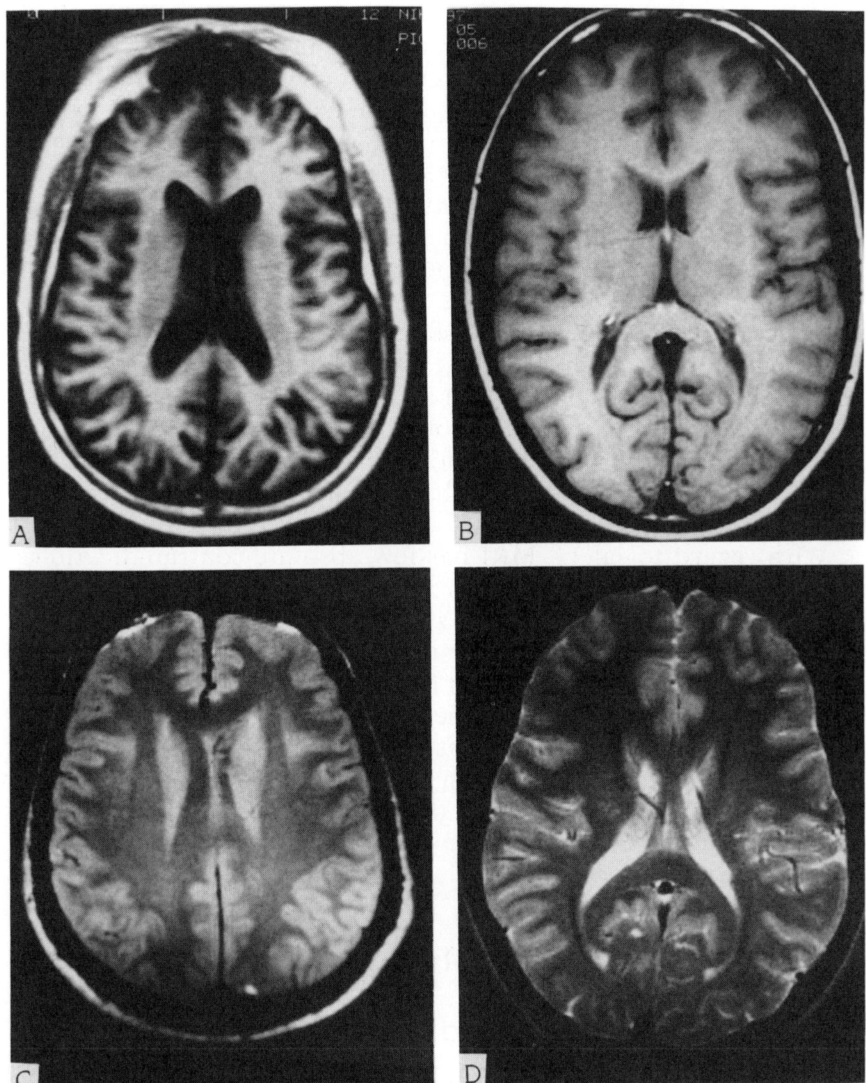

Figure 5. Brain images with various pulse sequences. A. Inversion recovery image TI = 600 msec TR = 2,500 msec. B. Spin echo—T1 weighted TE = 25 msec TR = 550 msec. C. Spin echo—proton density—intermediate TE = 25 msec TR = 2500 msec. D. Spin echo—T2 weighted TE = 90 msec TR = 2,500 msec.

evidence produced thus far suggests that this compound is less toxic than iodinated contrast materials by a factor of ten. Research in developing other MR contrast agents continues. Efforts are also underway to combine paramagnetic elements with substances such as monoclonal antibodies, hormones and metabolites in order to provide more specific information in future images.

Finally, another adjunct to MRI scanning is the utilization of surface coils. These are devices that are placed on the surface of the area to be examined to receive the emitted RF signals. In the conventional design of the MR scanner, the receiver coil is incorporated into the transmitter coil that sends the original radiofrequency pulse into the body. In scanning with surface coils, the received MR signals are stronger and the signal-to-noise ratio is increased. Consequently, one can perform scans with thinner slices while improving the spatial resolution. Thin slices with improved spatial resolution (3–5 mm) result in increased sensitivity which is particularly desirable in the study of small structures such as the optic nerve, the pituitary gland, and the spinal corrd.[10–12]

With regard to safety, MRI has few absolute contraindications; patients with cardiac pacemakers, ferromagnetic aneurysm clips or metallic objects inside the orbits should not be scanned. A number of physical limitations to MRI scanning have been noted particularly in acutely ill patients, patients on life support and patients with severe claustrophobia or marked obesity.[13]

Despite these minor difficulties, the popularity of MRI is increasing rapidly. The improved sensitivity, the multiplanar image availability, the lack of ionizing radiation, the promise of spectroscopy and the continuing evolution of new advances makes MRI even more promising in the near future.

Positron Emission Tomography (PET)

Theoretical Considerations and Methodology

Positron emission tomography utilizes radio-isotopes which decay by positron emission. These include: carbon 11, nitrogen 13, oxygen 15, fluorine 18, gallium 68, and rubidium 82. With the exception of oxygen 15 which is given immediately upon production by inhalation, the remaining isotopes are incorporated into naturally occurring biomolecules and administered either by inhalation or by intravenous injection to study the metabolic pathways of these substances. As the radioactive compound decays in the tissues positrons are emitted to its environment. Each positron collides with an electron which results in the annihilation of their mass and the production of two gamma rays (photons) that travel in opposite directions with an energy of 511 kV. During scanning, these rays are detected externally by a number of phosphor crystals placed circumferentially around the body in the PET scanner. As the gamma rays strike the crystals, light is generated which is converted by photomultiplier tubes to electrical signals. These signals are processed by computer to reconstruct transaxial images.[14,15] Thus PET images depict the relative distribution and concentration of the radioactive material in the tissues. Normal PET images of brain show a homogeneous ribbon of increased activity in the periphery representing the higher metabolic activity of the gray matter neurons. Similar increased activity is noted in the insular cortex and the basal ganglia. The white matter is relatively hypometabolic due to the fact that it is mainly composed of neuronal axons and glial cells. No metabolic activity is present in the ventricular system, the margin of which is not clearly defined from the adjacent white matter (Fig. 6).

Among the various positron-emitting isotopes, fluorine 18 has been used most widely in PET scanning to measure brain glucose metabolism. The theoretical basis of this method has been established by Sokoloff et al.[16] who performed autoradiographic studies using an analogue of glucose (deoxyglucose) labeled with carbon 14 to measure the rate of glucose consumption in the brain of rats. Deoxyglucose (DG) differs from glucose only in the replacement of a hydroxyl group on the second carbon atom; however, both share similar chemical and physiological properties. Thus, deoxyglucose is transported between blood and brain tissue by the same saturable carrier that transports glucose.[17,18] Inside the cell deoxyglucose competes with glucose for hexokinase which catalyzes a phosphorylation reaction resulting in the formation of deoxyglucose–6-phosphate ($DG–6-PO_4$) and glucose–6-phosphate, respectively. The latter continues its normal glycolytic pathway to form water and carbon dioxide. The phosphorylated deoxylglucose, on the other hand, is not a substrate for further reactions and its metabolic processing is temporarily interrupted. The $DG–6-PO_4$ cannot cross the cell membrane easily and the reverse reaction of dephosphorylation is very slow, therefore the compound is trapped intracellularly. Thus, the concentration of $DG–6-PO_4$ in

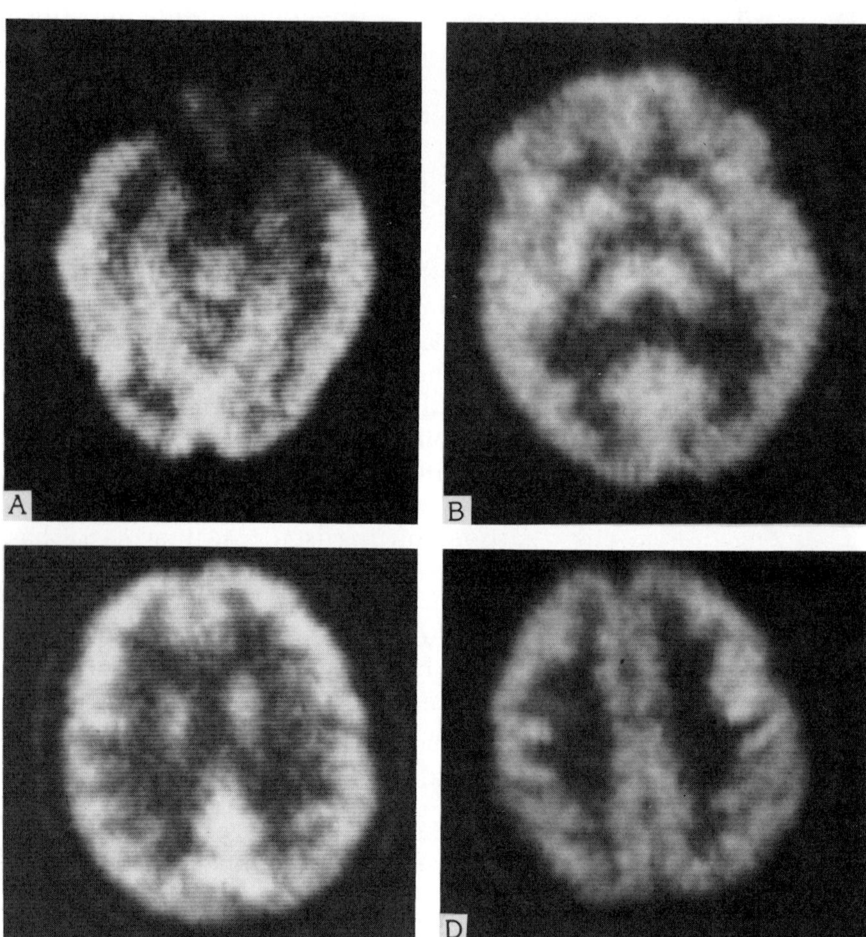

Figure 6. Four consecutive PET-FDG images showing a ribbon of increased activity in the cerebral cortex. Increased activity is also seen in the gray matter of basal ganglia.

the cells increases gradually until, in about 30–45 minutes, it reaches a plateau after which it remains unchanged for approximately 1 hour.

Using the above concepts, Sokoloff and co-workers developed a compartmental model that described the behavior of DG in tissues. From this model, a mathematical formula was derived which takes into consideration the transport rate constants of glucose and deoxyglucose and allows actual quantitative calculation of glucose consumption. Since carbon 14-labeled deoxyglucose is not a gamma emitter and cannot be used in in vivo imaging studies, another step was essential. This was made by Ido[19] who replaced the hydrogen from the second carbon atom of the DG molecule with fluorine 18. The new compound called fluorodeoxyglucose (FDG) also has chemical properties similar to glucose and was found to be suitable for use in humans.

Using the FDG-PET scanning method, a number of investigators have studied in vivo cerebral glucose consumption.[20,21] The original mathematical model of Sokoloff was modified by Huang, Phelps, and co-workers[22,23] who measured the transport rate constants of FDG in human experiments. This newer model takes into consideration the possible dephosphorylation reactions of FDG. In these studies, normal values of glucose utilization were established for gray and white matter in men and were found to be 7.30 ± 1.18 and 3.41 ± 0.65 mg/min per 100 g of brain tissue, respectively. Thus our ability to measure regional glucose utilization by tissues in vivo opened new horizons in medical imaging. This is particularly true in the central nervous system which derives most of its energy from glucose. Measurement of cerebral glucose metabolism utilizing PET allows evaluation of cerebral function in various physiological and pathological states.

During PET scanning, the patient's head is placed in the center of the scanner just as with CT. The eyes are patched and the ears are plugged to minimize stimulation. Injection of FDG is given intravenously in one hand, while from a vein of the other hand blood samples are withdrawn for determination of FDG and glucose concentration in the plasma during the scanning period. An optimal dose of FDG is 5 mCi, although adequate studies can be obtained with a dose as little as 2 mCi. Scans are performed after the initial 45–50 minute period of FDG trapping. Ten-millimeter thick slices are usually obtained although thinner slices are possible. The spatial resolution of most modern scanners is 6–7 mm which is adequate to study most macroscopically visible brain lesions.[24]

A number of brain PET studies have been done utilizing carbon

11 as a tracer. Carbon 11 has a half-life of 20 minutes. Therefore, a cyclotron for its production and a means of synthesizing the compound whose metabolic path is to investigated must be available at the site of such studies. Carbon 11-labeled deoxyglucose was used to evaluate cerebral glucose metabolism and confirmed the observations made with FDG.[25] Studies of protein synthesis in brain have been conducted by labeling essential amino acids such as leucine and more commonly methionine with carbon 11. Both L and D stereoisomers were used and brain activity was measured with a PET scanner. These studies have shown that only the L enantiomer participates in protein synthesis. The stereospecificity in methionine and leucine incorporation indicates that this process is governed not by passive diffusion but rather by a facilitated transport.[26-30]

Carbon 11 has also been used to label polyamines which are believed to be biochemical markers of malignancy. PET scan studies with carbon 11-labeled putrescine, a polyamine, were carried out to detect cerebral tumors and evaluate their metabolic characteristics.[31]

Quantitative measurement of regional cerebral blood flow and brain oxygen metabolism have been successful in man using oxygen 15 and PET scanning. These studies are based on the fact that inhalation of molecular oxygen 15 or oxygen 15-labeled carbon dioxide results in production of radioactive water in the pulmonary capillaries. From the lungs, the radioactive water reaches the brain where a state of dynamic equilibrium is attained within three half-lives of continuous inhalation (6 minutes). PET scans are performed during equilibrium when the arrival of oxygen 15 to brain is balanced by its washout and the rate of radioactive decay. Blood samples are obtained throughout the experimental period to measure the blood plasma activity, the hematocrit, the arterial PO_2, PCO_2, and pH. A mathematical formula that takes into consideration these data as well as the measured brain activity by the scanner gives the cerebral blood flow expressed in ml/100 g/min. Dividing the cerebral activity during oxygen inhalation by that during carbon dioxide inhalation we obtain a measurement of oxygen extraction (OE). The cerebral metabolic rate (CMRO) for oxygen can be derived by multiplying CBF with OE and that with the total blood oxygen content. Using this method Frackowiak et al. found the CMRO to be 5.88 ± 0.59 ml/100 ml/min for the gray matter and 1.81 ± 0.22 ml/100 ml/min for the white matter.[32,33]

Cerebral Gliomas

Tumor Detection

Until recently, CT scanning, with a sensitivity approaching 90%, was the primary modality used to detect intracranial tumors. False negative results usually occur in small nonenhancing tumors located near a dense bony surface. Computer artifacts caused by hardening of the x-ray beam as it passes through these bony structures are primarily responsible for this less than optimal sensitivity. Locations where this problem is encountered more often include the high convexity of the cerebral hemispheres, the temporal lobes, and the brain stem.

The first indication that magnetic resonance could be used in the detection of tumors was made by Damadian who in 1971[34] observed that tumor cells in vitro have prolonged T1 and T2 values when compared to normal cells. This prolongation of relaxation times is not specific for neoplastic cells, as other types of non-neoplastic cells demonstrate the same increase. Nevertheless, by exploiting this difference in relaxation times MR exquisitely demonstrates cerebral lesions regardless of etiology. Among the different MR imaging techniques that are utilized, the T2 weighted pulse sequences are advantageous because the contrast between neoplastic and normal tissues is more distinct. When these techniques are used, the sensitivity of MR in detecting cerebral tumors approaches 100% (Fig. 7). The contrast between neoplastic and normal tissues is less impressive on T1 weighted pulse sequences. This method becomes valuable only when used in conjunction with intravenous administration of Gd-DTPA and in lesions with disrupted BBB. Under these circumstances, Gd-DTPA diffuses into the interstitial space of the tumor and increases the signal intensity dramatically (Fig. 8). Therefore, this method which requires one-third of the time needed for a T2 weighted technique demonstrates sharp contrast between tumor and normal brain.[35–40]

Sodium MR images have been used experimentally in the detection of cerebral neoplasms, but due to a number of technical problems which still remain unresolved, this method has not been adopted for routine use. Although the concentration of intracellular sodium increases dramatically in malignant cells, this information is not presented in the images because both intracellular and extracellular so-

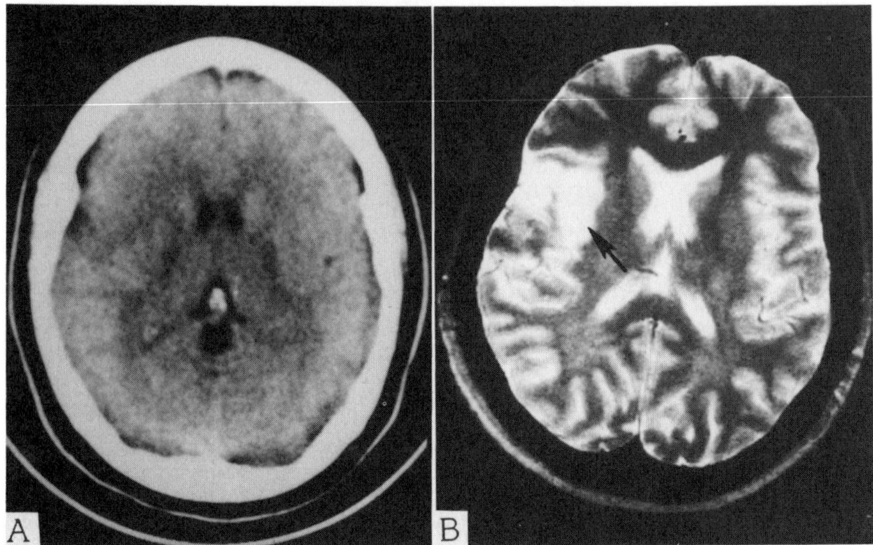

Figure 7. Glioma of the right insula and adjacent temporal lobe. CT scan of the brain (A) failed to demonstrate any abnormality. A T2 weighted MRI scan at the same level (B) showed an abnormal area of increased intensity which was proven to represent an astrocytoma grade II (arrow).

dium are imaged. Consequently, the sodium MR images of brain tumors have failed to separate the actual lesion from the edematous surrounding brain parenchyma. In addition, a certain amount of the intracellular sodium is not detected with the imaging methods currently used due to great variations of the chemical environment within the cytoplasm.[41,42]

The utility of PET scanning in tumor detection has not been evaluated thoroughly in comparative studies. It is well recognized, however, that the sensitivity of PET with its relatively poor spatial resolution would be inferior to both CT and MRI. Because of this poor resolution, small low grade gliomas confined to the white matter or high grade gliomas localized in the cortex may escape detection because the metabolic activity of the tumor does not differ appreciably from that of the host tissue. This does not occur commonly since most gliomas are invasive and do not respect the anatomic boundaries of the gray-white matter junction. In the experience of the authors, the PET-FDG method will demonstrate the lesion in the majority of cases.

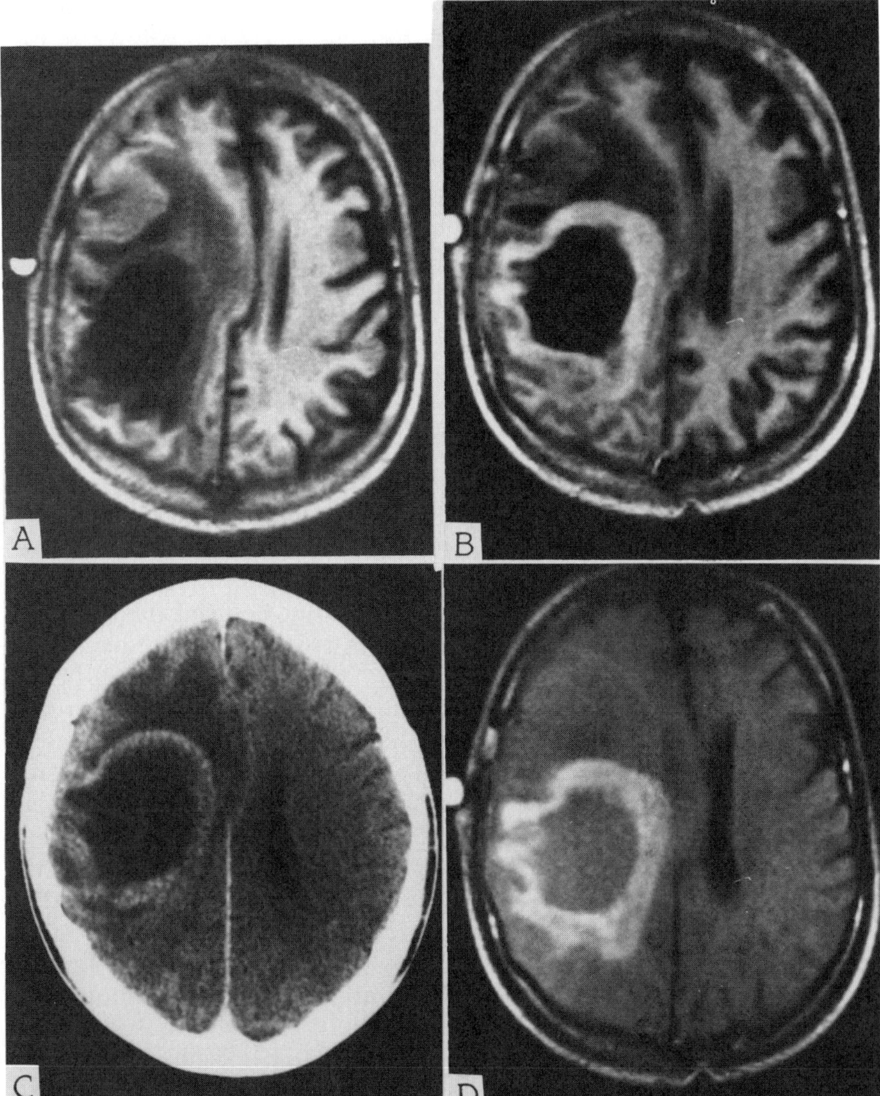

Figure 8. Glioblastoma of the right frontoparietal lobe. A. Precontrast inversion recovery MRI scan demonstrates a cavity mass surrounded by edema. B. Post Gd-DTPA inversion recovery MRI scan shows enhancement in the viable portion of the tumor. C. Enhanced CT scan reveals the same abnormality. D. Spin-echo T1 weighted technique with Gd-DTPA shows increased degree of enhancement on the MRI compared to CT.

Tumor detection can be achieved by depicting disruptions of the BBB in cerebral gliomas using gallium 68 EDTA or rubidium 82. Early studies have shown isotope localization in the tumor area even in cases that demonstrated lack of enhancement on CT with iodinated compounds.[29,43-45] Since the number of studies with this method is small, the issue of the best way to explore the BBB changes in tumors remains unresolved. Although it may be true that smaller amounts of positron-emitting isotopes are needed to show increased activity in the tumor parenchyma, the relatively poor spatial resolution of the PET scanner as compared with the CT may be enough to offset these gains.

Histologic Characterization

From the early experience in MRI, it became obvious that this method is unreliable in histological characterization of cerebral tumors. Indeed, published data have shown that there is considerable overlap of the T1 and T2 values in benign and malignant tissues.[46] Since the absolute values of T1 and T2 cannot be used for this purpose, new emphasis was placed on depicting tumor BBB changes with intravenous administration of Gd-DTPA.[47-50] In a recent report, it was noted that while all high grade gliomas show intense enhancement with Gd-DTPA, the low grade gliomas demonstrated either complete lack of enhancement or mild increase in their signal intensity. This latter subgroup may be of interest in an attempt to determine whether subtle disruptions of the BBB are accompanied by a higher rate of malignant transformation[51] (see Fig. 12). PET with FDG has been shown to be a reasonably accurate method of evaluating the histologic grade and hence the biologic behavior of cerebral gliomas. The theoretical basis of these studies is well established. It is known that normal tissues in the presence of adequate oxygen metabolize glucose via the Krebs cycle to water and carbon dioxide. Neoplastic cells, on the other hand, exhibit a high rate of anaerobic glycolysis. This mode of glycolysis is, from the energy point of view, an inefficient method of glucose utilization. Malignant tumors that have lost the ability of oxidative metabolism consume relatively larger amounts of glucose than normal tissues. Clinical confirmation of the above was obtained by Di Chiro et al.[52] who found positive correlations between the rate of glycolysis and the grade of malignancy in primary cerebral tumors. These investigators showed that the average rate of

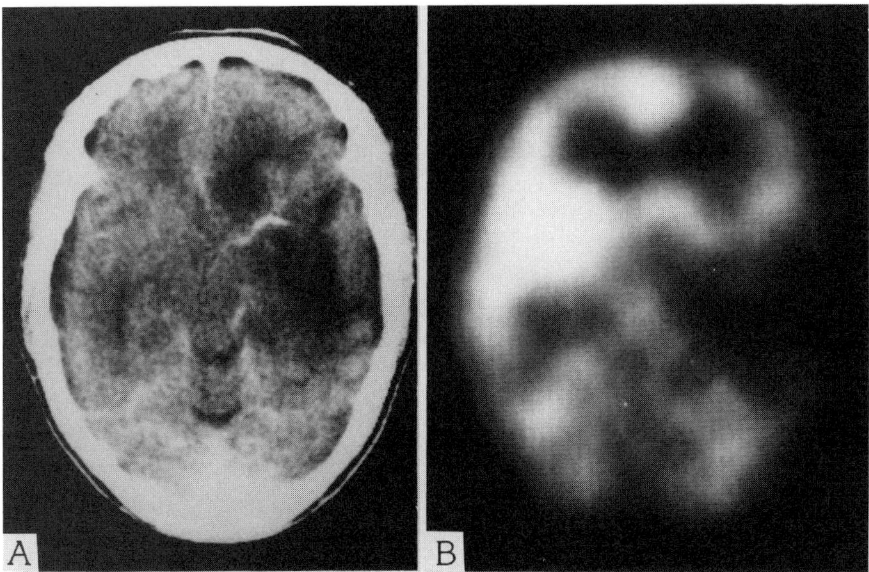

Figure 9. Low grade glioma. A. Post-contrast CT showing a hypodense mass in the left temporal lobe. B. PET-FDG scan shows the mass to be hypometabolic.

glucose utilization in 13 low grade gliomas was 4.0 ± 1.8 mg/100 g per minute (Fig. 9), while in 10 other patients with high grade gliomas the rate of glucose utilization was 7.4 ± 3.5 mg/100 g per minute (Fig. 10). This hypermetabolism of the most malignant tumors is an intrinsic property of neoplastic cells and is not related to breakdown of the BBB[53] (Fig. 11). Other investigators have confirmed the correlation between rate of glucose utilization and tumor grade in cerebral gliomas using not only FDG but carbon 11-labeled deoxyglucose as well.[29,31] Yamagushi et al. recently reported that the increase in FDG uptake observed in high grade gliomas actually is a reflection of the hexokinase activity. This activity is also increased in nonglial tumors such as hemangioblastomas, pituitary adenomas, meningiomas and metastatic lesions.[54]

When numerical values for the rate of glucose consumption are used to assess the biological behavior of a cerebral tumor, one must be careful to avoid errors inherent to the technique. These errors are generally sampling errors caused by tumor location. For example, a low grade glioma in the cortex will have a higher absolute rate of

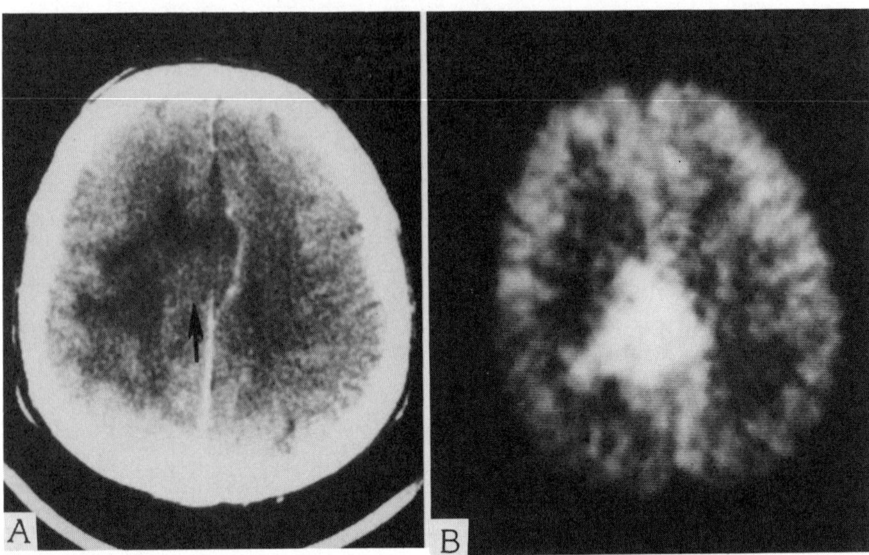

Figure 10. High grade glioma. A post-infusion CT scan of the brain (A) showing a hypodense abnormality in the right frontal and parietal lobe. This represents edema adjacent to a mass in the parietal region (arrow). The mass is isodense to the normal brain paranchyma and can be easily missed. PET scan with FDG (B) demonstrates the mass to be hypermetabolic in spite of the fact that the BBB was not disrupted. This abnormality was proven to be a high grade glioma.

glucose utilization than the same type of tumor in the white matter. This occurs because infiltrative tumors do not entirely replace the neuronal population in regions where they grow. Therefore, the measured metabolic rates represent average values of tumor cells and normal or nearly normal neurons. These values can be meaningful only when compared to normal cortex in a comparable region of the opposite hemisphere. Similarly, when a high grade glioma is located in the white matter, its calculated numerical metabolic value is contaminated by computer sampling from the normally hypometabolic environment. These artificially lower metabolic values should be compared to a comparable region of the opposite hemisphere. One needs to remember that these tumors originate from glial cells which are normally hypometabolic and any unusual activity within the white matter should be viewed with suspicion. Finally, another com-

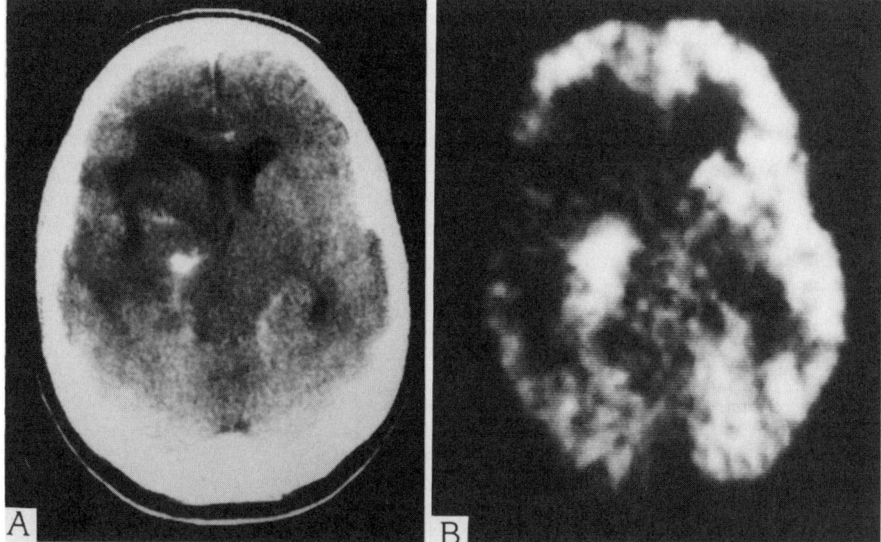

Figure 11. Oligodendroglioma with malignant characteristics. Post-contrast CT of the brain (A) shows a mass in the right temporal lobe invading the centrosylvial region. The hyperdense focus on the medial aspect of the mass represents calcification since it was also present on the preinfusion scan. PET-FDG scan of the same area (B) demonstrates increased metabolic activity in the region of calcification indicative of malignant degeneration. Also note depressed glucose utilization in the cortex overlying the lesion. A biopsy on the superficial layers of the right temporal lobe showed a mixed-type glioma that included oligodendrocytes. The hyperactive area was not biopsied. Patient had rapid clinical deterioration and died a few months later.

mon problem apt to cause confusion in histologic characterization of these tumors arises when we evaluate the metabolic rates of tumors with a large necrotic center and a thin peripheral rim of viable tumor. The measured activity in these cases is grossly underestimated since the necrotic tissues have zero metabolism. A more accurate presentation of the facts could be obtained if one corrects for the percentage of viable tumor that is included in the measured samples. All the above problems need to be addressed when interpreting PET scan images so that errors can be avoided and the true biological behavior of cerebral neoplasms can be determined accurately.

It is well established that glioblastomas originate in previously low grade gliomas which have undergone malignant transformation.

This change may not be visualized on CT which relies on BBB breakdown. PET scans will reveal which portion of the tumor has the highest metabolic activity and direct the surgeon to the most appropriate area for needle biospy (Fig. 10).

In addition to PET-FDG studies, gliomas have also been evaluated with oxygen 15 using the steady-state inhalation technique. Although the blood flow to the tumor was comparable to normal cortex, the O_2 consumption was depressed even in patients who had increased glucose utilization by the tumors. These findings support the concept that anerobic glycolysis is an important energy source in tumors.[55-57]

Secondary Brain Changes

The brain adjacent to the tumor parenchyma is affected by compression, edema, and tumor invasion. When CT was first used for routine evaluation of patients with suspected cerebral neoplasms, physicians became aware of the true extent of these abnormalities. It was more fully appreciated that excessive fluid escaping from the intravascular compartment diffuses into the interstitial space of the surrounding brain in the form of edema. This fluid spreads along the white matter fibers, reaching areas remote from the tumor site, exaggerating the mass effect produced by the neoplastic process itself. It was also noted that the amount of edema was proportional to the tumor size and grade. Clear separation of tumor from the edematous adjacent brain is impossible in low grade gliomas because the radiographic density of both is equally decreased with respect to normal brain. In the case of enhancing high grade tumors it was originally thought that tumor margins could be defined well by CT. Recent pathological reports though showed that tumor spread beyond the borders of enhancement.[58] MRI, due to its superior sensitivity, is more accurate in depicting the presence and extent of edema. T2 weighted techniques are superior for this purpose. Separation of tumor from adjacent edematous brain is also problematic on MRI. On the T2 weighted images, both appear hyperintense although the signal from the tumor is somewhat lower than that of the edema. On the post Gd-DTPA T1 weighted images, high grade gliomas show enhancement in the tumor parenchyma (Fig. 12). Unfortunately as on CT, this simply represents the tumor area in which the BBB is disrupted and not the entire extent of the neoplastic process. This unenhancing area was proven to be neoplastic unequivocally with stereo-

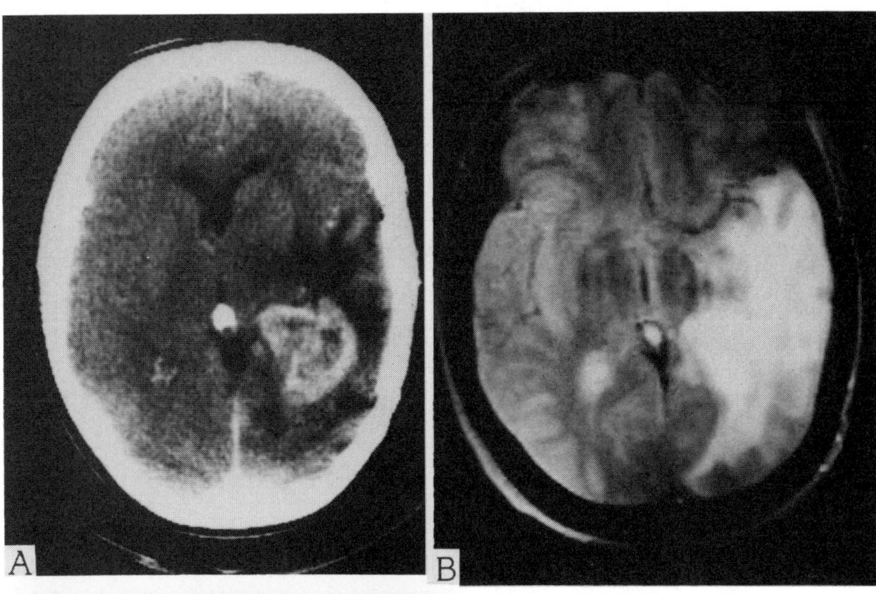

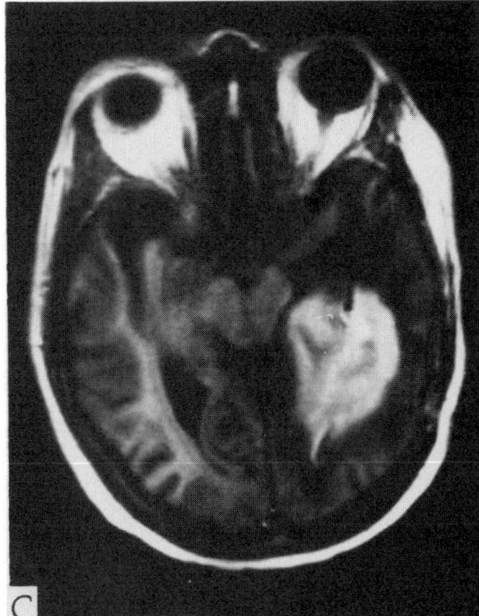

Figure 12. Glioblastoma of the left temporal lobe. Post-contrast CT scan of brain (A) showing an enhancing mass in the left temporal lobe. The hypodense area anterior to the mass represents edema. On the T2 weighted MRI (B), the mass cannot be separated from the edematous brain, both appearing hyperintense. On (C) the inversion recovery image (TI: 600 msec; TR: 2,000 msec) demonstrates obvious enhancement of the mass. The extent to the neoplastic process appears to be somewhat larger than that shown on CT.

tactic biopsy of the edematous peritumoral regions which showed no evidence of tumor invasion on CT or MRI.[59-61]

PET scans with FDG have shown rather impressive metabolic changes in brain tissue adjacent to neoplastic lesions. Thus, in a recent study by DeLapaz et al.,[62] 92% of patients with such lesions demonstrated suppression of gray matter glucose utilization ranging from 8% to 64% (mean 30%). In 32% of these cases, the regions of metabolic suppression corresponded to edematous hypodense gray matter seen on CT scans. In 34%, the metabolic suppression involved peritumoral gray matter regions with normal CT attenuation, and in 26%, regions of FDG suppression corresponded to gray matter structures that were spatially remote from the mass lesion. The degree of metabolic suppression was most strongly correlated with the presence of gray matter hypodensity due to edema and with the total volume of the lesion (tumor-plus-edema). This suggests that mechanical compression of white matter fibers or myelin destruction suppresses the metabolism of the neurons in areas of brain where these axons originate (Fig. 11). Furthermore, the fact that FDG suppression was noted in brain regions remote from the tumor suggests that transneural interactions are important mechanisms for this type of metabolic suppression. Tumors in the motor strip region have been noted to produce metabolic suppression in the ipsilateral thalamus, and conversely, tumors in the thalamus cause decrease activity in the ipsilateral cerebral cortex and in the opposite cerebellum.[63] These secondary effects of brain neoplasms on seemingly normal brain have not been shown by any other modality. However, they are clearly important in evaluating and understanding the clinical presentation since not uncommonly symptoms are produced from areas remote to the pathology. A very good example of remote metabolic suppression producing symptoms related to decreased neuronal function was recently demonstrated in patients with cerebral tumors presenting with homonymous visual defects. These patients had tumors in the parietal, temporal, and suprasellar regions which involved either directly or indirectly the retrochiasmatic optic pathways. The primary visual cortex in the occipital lobes was normal on CT while PET scan with FDG showed decreased activity in the occipital cortex on the same side as the tumor and contralateral to the field defect offering an explanation for the patient's symptoms.[64]

In attempting to separate tumor from edema, PET scan images are subjected to the same limitations mentioned with CT and MRI. However, we have seen a number of cases with aggressive high grade gliomas infiltrating areas remote from the original tumor, such as the ventricular walls or the brain stem which demonstrated increased activity on PET. Lack of adequate contrast enhancement failed to document these lesions on CT, while on MRI, these abnormalities, although present, were falsely mistaken as edema. Finally, when compression phenomena are being evaluated, CT scans and MRI, with a superior spatial resolution, are preferable to PET.

Post-Treatment Brain Changes

CT has been the study of choice in the immediate postoperative period. The presence of edema, transfalcial or transtentorial herniation, and compression of vital structures such as the brain stem are well appreciated by CT. Furthermore, hemorrhage at the surgical site or arterial occlusions causing ischemic infarctions can be shown easily on CT scans. Post-contrast CT is used to demonstrate the amount of unresected tumor. However, surgical trauma may increase the area of enhancement causing overestimation, while steroid medication, which repairs the disrupted BBB, causes underestimation of the amount of residual tumor.

MRI is a somewhat cumbersome procedure and may not be practical in very ill patients during the early postoperative period. This technique provides most of the information obtained by CT, it has an edge in depicting edema, but it is inferior to CT in showing acute hemorrhage. The role of MRI is more valuable and by far superior to CT in the later stages of the disease when the first brain abnormalities appear as a result of radiation therapy. Post-radiation-induced brain lesions affect the white matter and present as abnormal foci of increased intensity on the T2 weighted images (Fig. 13). In more severe cases, these lesions are confluent, extending in wide regions of the white matter producing a scalloped configuration at the junction of the gray-white matter where the signal is more intense. The time interval between completion of radiation therapy and development of these lesions varies widely from a few months to several years. These changes are encountered more commonly in older patients in whom associated vascular insufficiency may play a contributing role. The underlying defect responsible for these lesions is believed to be demyelination, microvascular occlusion and blood-brain barrier breakdown producing edema.[65,66]

Besides radiation, white matter abnormalities have developed

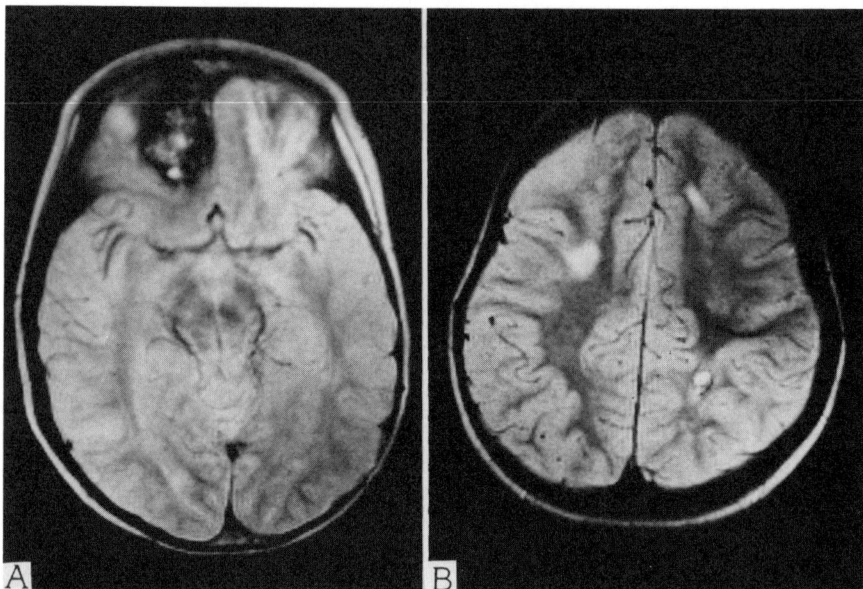

Figure 13. Post-radiation cerebral lesions in a child with cerebellar medulloblastoma. A moderately T2 weighted image (TE: 35 sec; TR: 2,000 msec) shows a heterogeneous lesion in the right frontal lobe which represents radionecrosis (A). The hypointensity in the periphery of this lesion most likely represents hemosiderin deposits from old hemorrhage. The hyperintense center is due to tissue necrosis with cystic changes in gliosis. In (B), there are three hyperintense lesions in the white matter representing focal areas of leukomalasia which developed several months after completion of radiation treatments. These latter abnormalities were not visible on CT.

following intracarotid infusion of chemotherapeutic agents such as BCNU or *cis*-platinum.[67] These lesions appear within days or weeks after the treatment and progress rapidly, involving the white matter of the exposed hemisphere. Both the rapidity and severity of involvement suggest that myelin is sensitive to such treatment. Indeed, while the white matter lesions in these patients are best shown on the MRI scan, the gray matter metabolic abnormalities are very extensive and demonstrated clearly the PET-FDG method[68] (Fig. 14).

Brain irradiation and chemotherapy produce not only structural but also metabolic changes. Ito et al.,[69] measuring glucose utilization with ^{14}C-deoxyglucose and autoradiography in irradiated rats, documented metabolic abnormalities. These investigators showed that

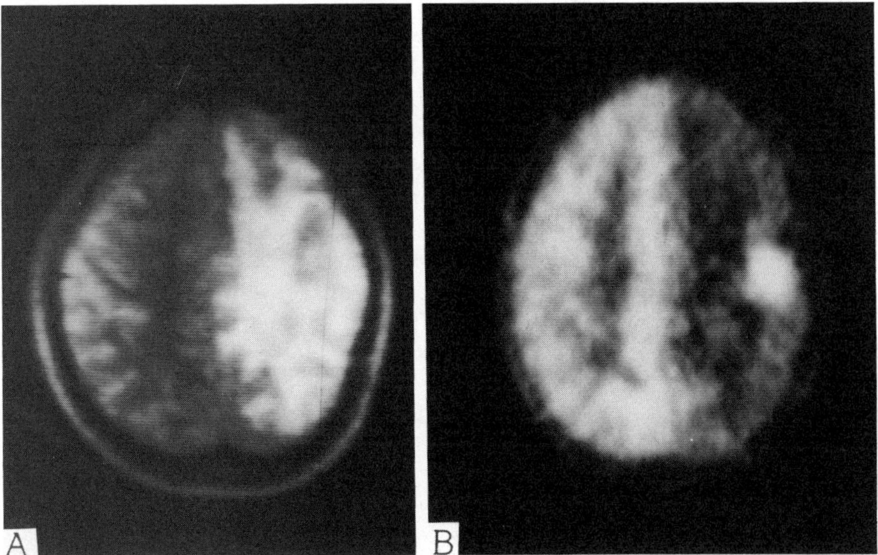

Figure 14. Post-BCNU infusion for treatment of glioma in the left cerebral hemisphere. (A) MRI T2 weighted image demonstrates diffuse increased signal in the entire hemisphere involving both gray and white matter. (B) PET-FDG shows decrease metabolic activity in the left cerebrum with a focus of increased activity which represents persistent tumor.

animals receiving 1,500 rads demonstrated decreased values of glucose utilization 4 days and 4 weeks post-treatment as compared to nonirradiated controls. The differences, ranging from 17% to 45%, were generally larger in the animals studied 4 weeks after exposure to radiation. Both gray and white matter structures were affected. In patients with acute lymphocytic leukemia, cerebral glucose metabolism was shown to be diminished immediately after intravenous injections of high dose methotrexate. PET scans with FDG in these patients showed an approximately 20% reduction in brain glucose utilization.[70] These findings suggest that the PET-FDG method is sensitive enough to detect early neurotoxicity after such treatments. Many months or a few years following treatment for intracranial tumors, patients develop diffuse and/or focal atrophic changes which are shown equally well by CT and MRI. Additionally, dystrophic calcifications can develop in the tumor bed in patients after brain irradiation. Calcifications are often found in children who receive radiation to the brain. These calcifications are in normal structures at the junction of gray and white matter and in the basal ganglia. In general, calcific abnormalities are best shown by CT.

Another interesting complication occurring as a result of radiation therapy of is that of radionecrosis. This complication, having a peak incidence about 24 months after treatment, presents with breakdown of tissue leading to cavitation. There is also injury to the integrity of the wall of the vessels resulting in intravascular thrombosis. The BBB is invariably disrupted allowing excessive amounts of fluid to extravasate into the interstitial space producing extra mass. The combined effect of tissue destruction and extra mass manifests itself clinically by exacerbation of symptoms which raises the question of recurrent tumor. CT and MRI are incapable of establishing the diagnosis, since both demonstrate an irregular cavity, contrast enhancement, and edema. These findings as well as the clinical pre-

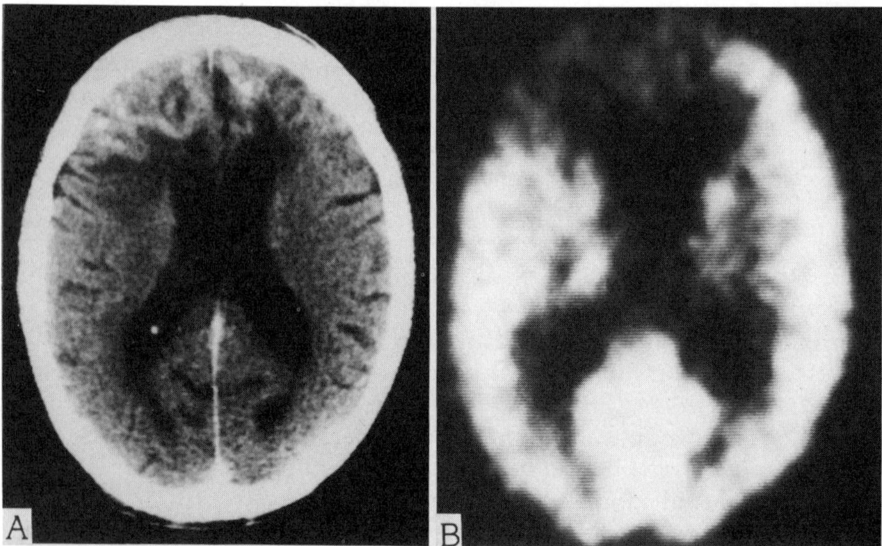

Figure 15. Post-radiation necrosis. A post-infusion CT (A) shows an irregular enhancing lesion in the right frontal lobe. A similar but smaller abnormality is noted in the medial aspect of the left frontal lobe. This patient had previously been irradiated for cerebral tumor. The question raised at this time is whether the abnormalities in the frontal lobes represent recurrent tumor. The decreased metabolic activity seen on the PET-FDG scan (B) in the same area indicates that the lesion is due to post-radiation necrosis.

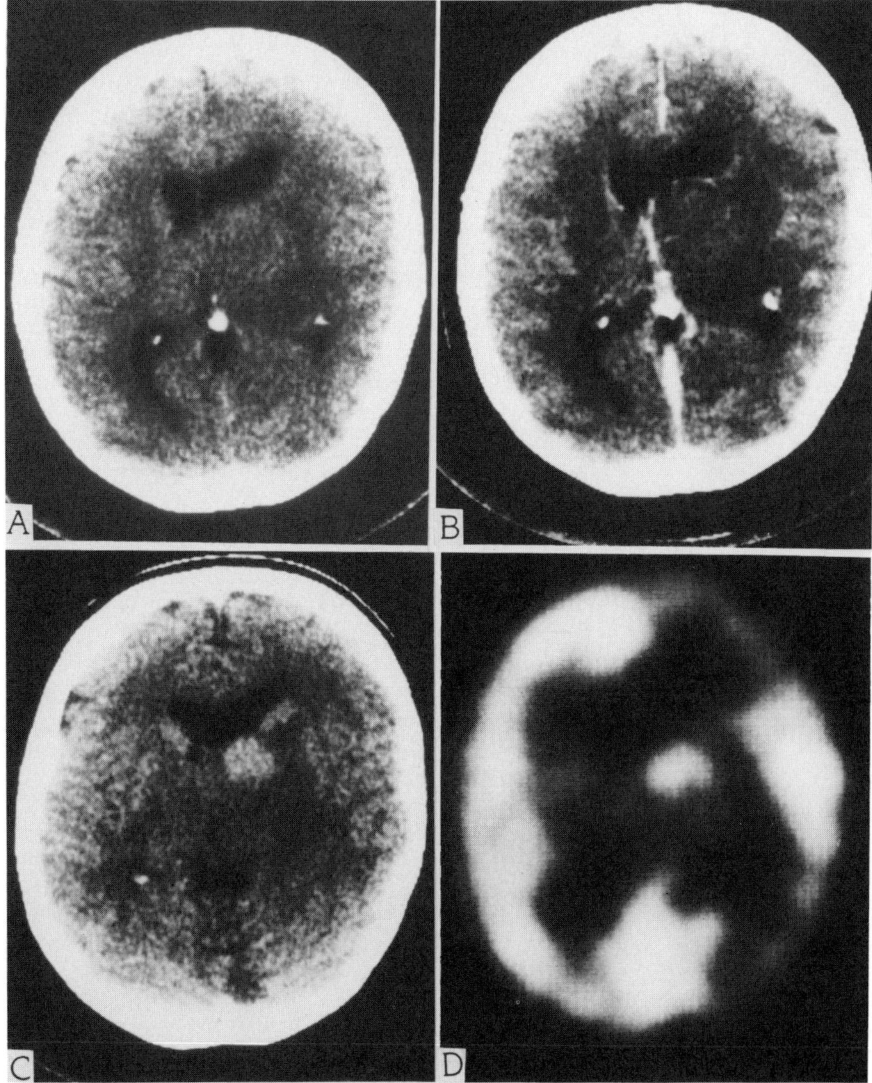

Figure 16. Gliomas responding unfavorably to treatment. Precontrast CT scan (A) on a patient with high grade glioma in the left basal ganglia. No contrast enhancement was noted on the post-infusion scan (B). After radiation a precontrast CT (C) showed the tumor to be hyperdense, due to deposition of calcium in its parenchyma. PET-FDG scan (D) at the same time demonstrates increased glucose consumption. Patient had poor clinical course which was correctly predicted by the findings of the PET-FDG scan.

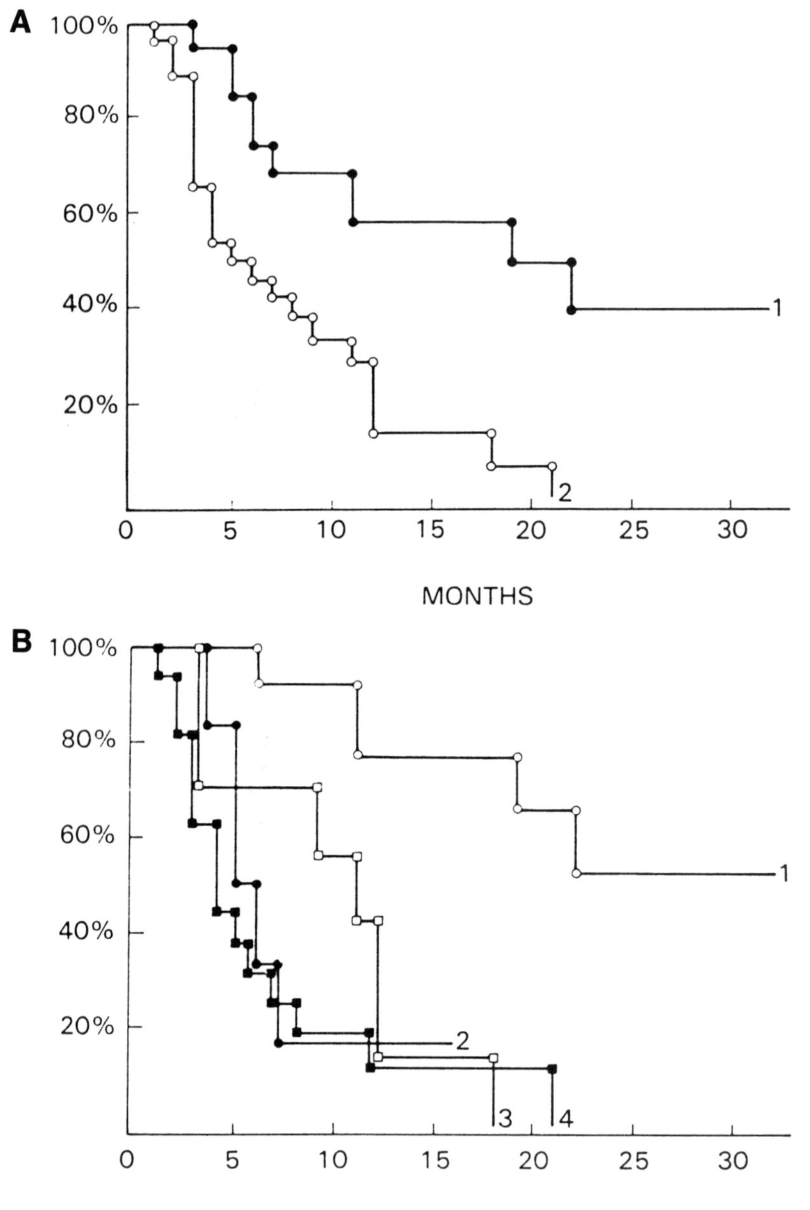

Figure 17. A. Survival time related to tumor grade. Plot 1 (closed circles) is for patients with histologically verified grade III astrocytomas. Plot 2 (open

sentation are identical in tumor recurrence and radionecrosis. PET scan with FDG has been established as the best method to solve this dilemma—showing increased metabolic activity is in the former and hypometabolism in the latter[71,72] (Fig. 15).

The PET-FDG method is useful in assessing tumor response to treatments. An illustrative example is presented in Figure 16. In the original post-contrast CT, a mass in the left caudate nucleus demonstrates no enhancement. A few months after radiation, dystrophic calcifications are seen in its parenchyma presenting an identical image on the pre- and post-contrast scans. No contrast enhancement was noted and the presence of calcifications may lead to the erroneous assumption of satisfactory response to treatment. A PET scan at the same time showed increased metabolic activity in the tumor area, indicative of a poor prognosis.

Regardless of the treatment given, PET with FDG is useful as a prognostic test in patients with high grade cerebral gliomas. In a group of 45 patients with grade III or IV astrocytomas, the mean survival in those with tumors exhibiting high glucose utilization was 5 months, whereas survival in those with gliomas showing lower utilization was 19 months (Fig. 17A). Glucose utilization of the tumor was measured and compared to the utilization of the normal opposite hemisphere. A metabolic ratio was then established. When the ratio was greater than 1.4 the estimated probability of survival decreased significantly. The relationship between tumoral metabolic activity and length of survival was maintained regardless of histologic grade (III or IV) (Fig. 17B) and regardless of tumor location.[73]

Extra-Axial Tumors

Intracranial tumors originating outside the brain parenchyma such as meningiomas and neurinomas are routinely evaluated by CT.

---

circles) is for patients with grade IV tumors. The latter group has shorter survival times. B. Survival time related to glucose utilization (GU) ratio and tumor grade. Plot 1 (open circles) is for patients with grade III astrocytomas and a GU ratio ≤1.4:1. Plot 2 (closed circles) is for patients with grade III astrocytomas and a GU ratio >1.4:1. Plot 3 (open squares) is for patients with grade IV astrocytomas and a GU ratio ≤1.4:1. Plot 4 (closed squares) is for patients with Grade IV astrocytomas and a GU ratio >1.4:1. Patients with GU ratios >1.4:1 have very short survival times regardless of whether the tumor is grade III or grade IV. Thus, the GU ratio is a stronger prognostic factor than histological grading in these tumors.

Diagnostic features characterizing meningiomas include psammomatous calcifications, hyperostotic bone changes, and homogeneous enhancement after intravenous contrast injection. The configuration of these types of tumors is also characteristic: they demonstrate a flat surface of meningeal attachment and a convex medial border displacing the adjacent brain. The overall sensitivity of CT has been reported to be as high as 96%.[74]

In studying meningiomas with MRI, several problems are encountered. The bone abnormalities of the skull and the calcifications in the tumor parenchyma, so obvious and often diagnostic on CT images, are not demonstrated on MRI. Also, the signal intensity of the tumor on the T1 and T2 images is similar to that of the gray matter and therefore there is no contrast between tumor and brain in the majority of cases. On rare occasions, meningiomas will show increased signal and appear bright on T2 weighted techniques. Until recently, the diagnosis of meningiomas on MRI was based primarily on secondary findings such as the presence of mass effect and edema in the underlying compressed brain. These abnormalities, however, may be absent or very subtle when the tumor size is small and the sensitivity of MRI in the diagnosis of meningiomas is unsatisfactory. For this reason, post Gd-DTPA MR scans have been performed in an effort to improve tumor detection. Early published data using this technique indicate that there is enhancement in the tumor parenchyma which in certain cases may be more intense than that achieved with iodine on CT (Fig. 18). At this point of development, it appears that the diagnostic yield of post-contrast MRI and CT is comparable.[75-77] On the question of tissue characterization, the value of both methods is limited. The enhancing features of both benign and malignant meningiomas are identical. It is the configuration of the malignant meningiomas that can suggest their aggressive nature on CT or MRI scans. This type of tumor was shown to have a broad and irregular surface of attachment and demonstrate more than one focus of nodularity on its surface.

As has been shown with gliomas, an increase in the amount of glucose utilization in meningiomas is also an indication of malignancy[78] (Fig. 19). Involvement of the leptomeninges by metastatic neoplasms represents another diagnostic challenge. This complication occurs more often than can be demonstrated using any imaging modality. Consecutive CT or MR scans will show gradual or very subtle enlargement of the ventricles. This finding is nonspecific although it occurs in a majority of patients if enough time elapses.

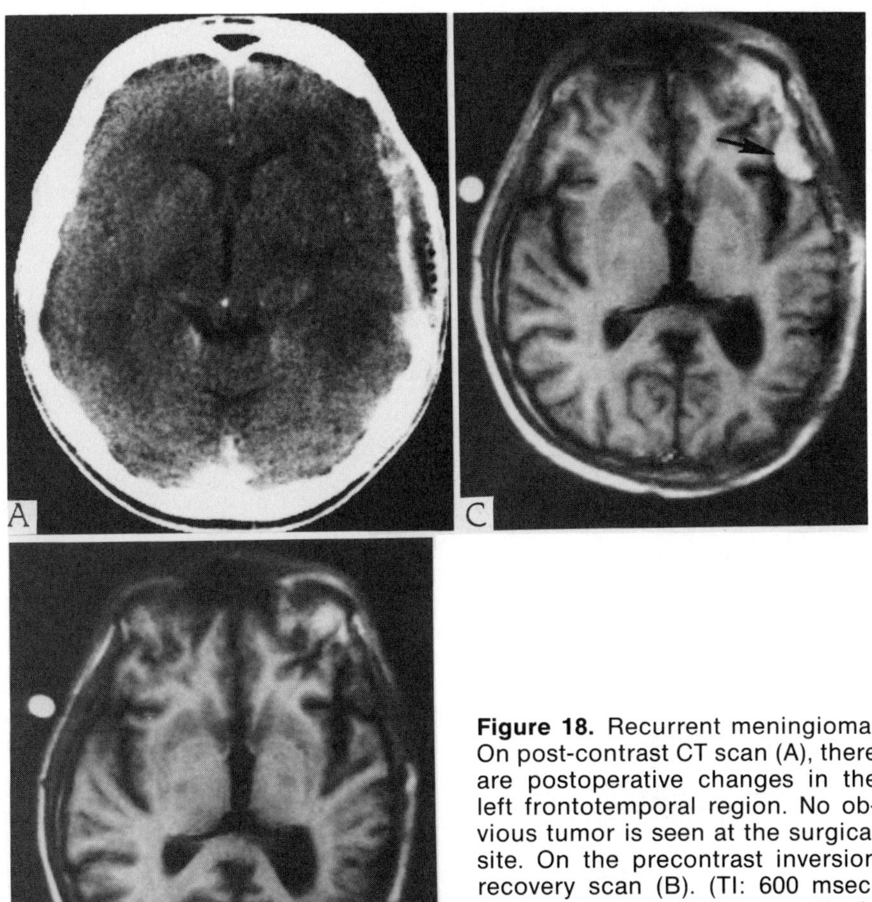

Figure 18. Recurrent meningioma. On post-contrast CT scan (A), there are postoperative changes in the left frontotemporal region. No obvious tumor is seen at the surgical site. On the precontrast inversion recovery scan (B). (TI: 600 msec; TR: 2,000 msec), no abnormality is present. On the post-Gd-DTPA inversion recovery scan (C), there is intense enhancement at the surgical site (arrow) which was proven to be a recurrent meningioma.

In approximately 35% of these patients post-contrast CT scans will reveal enhancement of the leptomeninges. This occurs only in cases in which neoplastic cells have formed relatively thick layers of meningeal infiltration. Since a certain degree of leptomengeal enhancement is present normally, distinction from that occuring in meningeal carcinomatosis is often difficult.[79] Comparative studies of CT

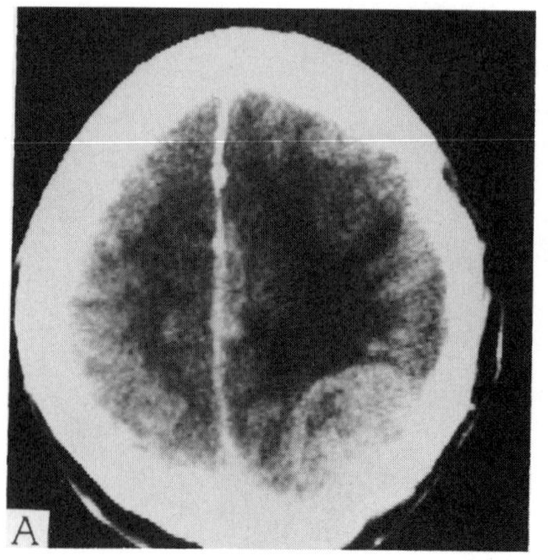
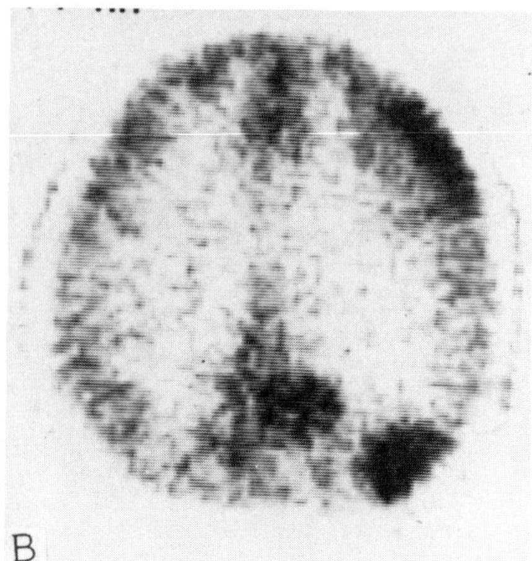
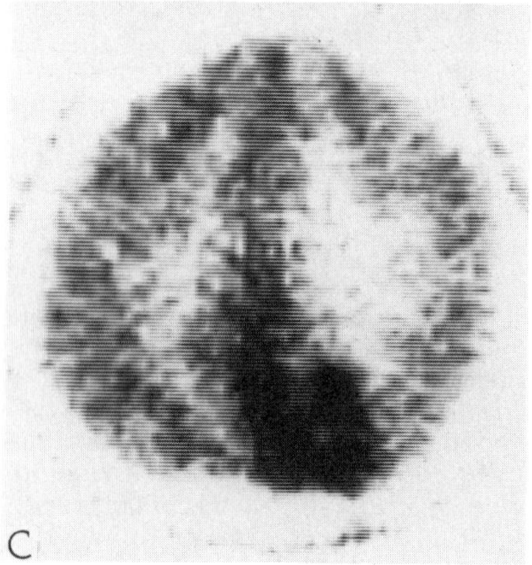

Figure 19. Recurrent meningioma evaluated by CT and PET-FDG. A. Post-contrast CT showing an enhancing extraaxial mass consistent with meningioma. B & C. PET-FDG axial images showing two hypermetabolic masses in the left post-parietal region. A third lesion is seen in left frontal region. All three abnormalities were proven to represent malignant meningioma recurrencies.

and MRI to evaluate their efficacy are not available at this time. Animal experiments, however, have shown that the sensitivity of MRI with Gd-DTPA may improve our current diagnostic capabilities in this entity.[80]

Neurinomas represent the second most common type of extraaxial tumor that is easily diagnosed using imaging techniques. The most common neurinomas are tumors of the 8th nerve. These tumors originate from the intracanalicular portion of the 8th nerve and as they grow, they erode the bony canal and project into the cerebellar pontine angle (CP) cistern.

Tumors that have reached the CP angle and measure more than 5 mm in diameter can be detected in the majority of cases on post-contrast CT scans. However, it is not uncommon for small tumors to be missed on routine CT due to artifacts caused by the marked density of the petrous bone. If the tumor is entirely intracanalicular, it cannot be resolved by CT. In such cases, if the diagnosis is strongly supported by clinical data, indirect evidence of an 8th nerve tumor is sought utilizing air cisternography. This technique, which requires lumbar puncture and injection of air into the subarachnoid space, can readily exclude the presence of an acoustic neuroma if the CT images show air in the canal. However, air cisternography can be unsuccessful due to technical problems which may lead to both false negative and false positive results.[81]

MRI of the internal auditory canal is performed using T1 and T2 weighted techniques in axial and coronal planes. The absence of signal from bone allows exquisite visualization of the 8th nerve and therefore MRI is much more sensitive to early lesions than CT. Since focal enlargement of the 8th nerve is an anatomic finding, T1 weighted images are more sensitive than T2 weighted images in which the nerves and the CSF are isointense and therefore cannot be separated.[82-84] It is this earlier detection capability that has made MRI the procedure of choice since the surgical outcome depends on tumor size.

When neurinomas are very large, they obliterate the subarachnoid space of the CP angle and may compress the brain stem or the cerebellum. On the T1 weighted images, they appear hypointense with respect to adjacent structures, and hyperintense on the T2 technique. On post-contrast MR and CT scans, acoustic neurinomas enhance intensely but are better delineated on MRI. With recent technological improvements using surface coils and Gd-DTPA, it has been shown that this enhancement occurs in the intracanalicular tumors as well which improves further the sensitivity of this method (Fig. 20).

Fifth nerve neurinomas originate in the region of Meckle's cave and expand both posterolaterally toward the CP angle and anteriorly towards the parasellar region. The primary differential feature which distinguishes these from acoustic neuromas is the fact that the IAC is intact in a fifth nerve tumor. CT differentiation of a fifth nerve neurinoma from a meningioma is problematic since they have almost identical density and enhancement characteristics. MRI utilizing T2 weighted images resolves this dilemma since the meningioma follows

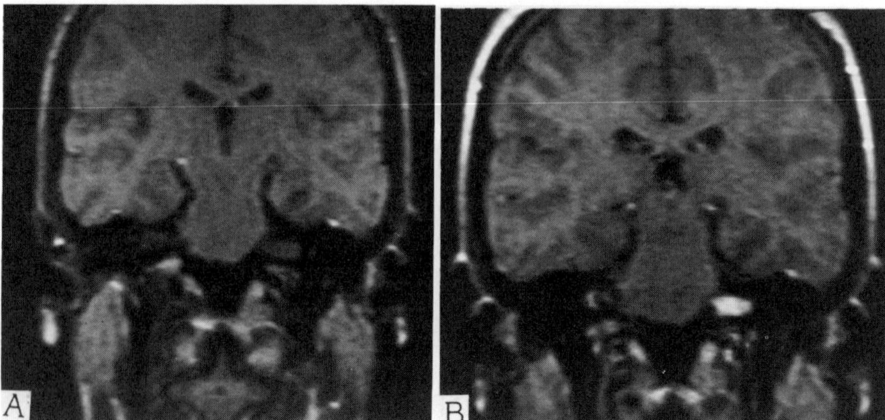

Figure 20. Intracanalicular acoustic neurinoma. Coronal section in the region of the internal auditory canal (IAC) using T1 weighted spin echo technique (A) TE 2.6 msec TR 550 msec). There is borderline enlargement of the left acoustic nerve. On the post-Gd-DTPA scan (B) using the exact same technique, there is intense enhancement inside the IAC indicating the presence of intracanalicular neurinoma.

the gray matter in signal intensity while the neurinoma is hyperintense. Neurinomas and meningiomas enhance identically with Gd-DTPA. The post Gd-DTPA T1 weighted images with their fine anatomic detail which is acquired in three planes are helpful in surgical planning.

Finally, neurinomas of the jugular fossa, usually arising from the ninth nerve, may be difficult to detect on CT when they grow outside of the cranial cavity since there is no contrast between the tumors and the soft tissues adjacent to the skull. MRI with T2 weighted pulse sequences and particularly inversion recovery images with a TI 100 msec and TR 1,500 msec will demonstrate these lesions as a high signal area separating them from the adjacent soft tissues and vessels. Commonly, these tumors also extend into the posterior fossa where they are easily detected by CT or MRI. In fact, bone destruction is better evaluated by CT. From the overall experience gained thus far, it appears that although tumor detection may not be a serious problem with either modality, the multiplanar capabilities of MRI and the superior definition of the extracranial component of the tumor make this method preferable to CT for treatment planning.

Optic gliomas are tumors of the optic chiasm that compress and

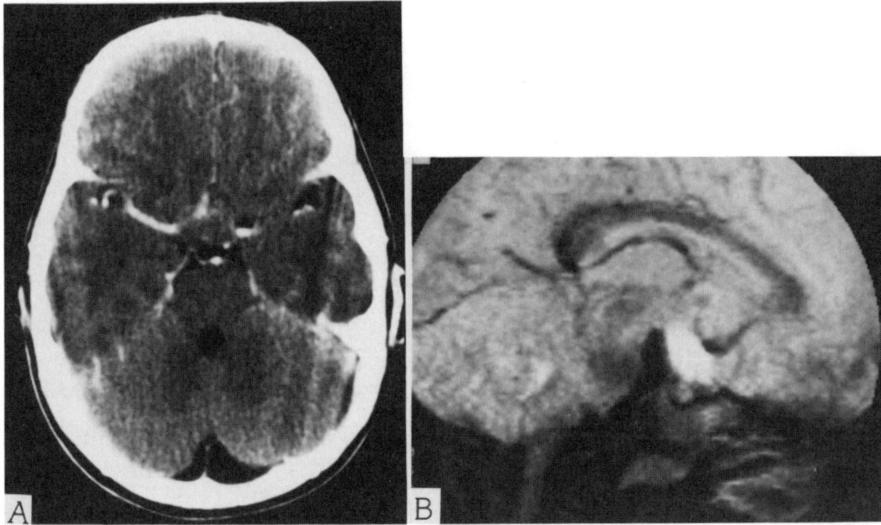

Figure 21. Optic glioma. A. Post-contrast CT shows enlargement of the optic chiasm. Since no contrast enhancement is present, exact tumor margins cannot be derived. B. T2 weighted sagittal MRI scan show the same lesion which presents increased signal. There is good definition of the mass from the adjacent hypothalamus.

often invade the adjacent brain substance along the optic tracts. These tumors are routinely visible on CT and many of them enhance in a variable pattern with intravenous contrast material. Some optic gliomas do not enhance at all or their enhancement does not extend throughout the tumor parenchyma. Consequently, the tumor margins are not well defined. With MRI using T2 weighted techniques, optic gliomas are hyperintense and often extend beyond the enhancing margins of the CT scans (Fig. 21). This demonstrates accurately the extent of the tumor and the degree of brain invasion.[85] This additional information can be used for treatment planning and in assessing tumor growth and response to treatment. T1 weighted sagittal images are useful in delineating the tumor from CSF spaces in the suprasellar region. This information is important in distinguishing optic gliomas from other hypothalamic lesions such as teratomas, cysts, and hamartomas, all of which, if the development in children, may present clinically with precocious puberty.

An additional fairly common mass which occurs in the same area

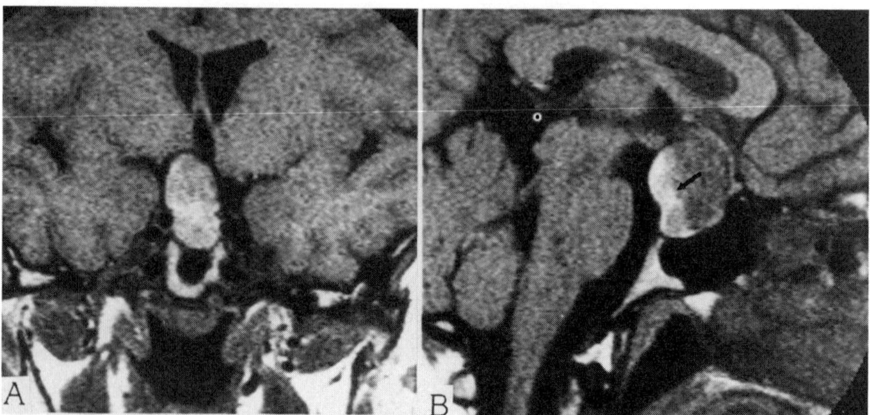

Figure 22. Craniopharyngioma. A & B. Coronal and sagittal T1 weighted images showing a large mass in the sella and suprasellar regions compressing the optic chiasm. The high signal intensity area seen within the mass (arrow) represents either hemorrhage or fat.

is the craniopharyngioma. These tumors are frequently calcified and exhibit cystic changes. They compress the hypothalamus, the optic nerve, and also extend inferiorly, eroding the floor of the sella. CT has routinely demonstrated these lesions with a very high sensitivity and specificity due to the very characteristic appearance. MRI, although equally sensitive, is not as specific because it is unable to demonstrate calcifications. This technique, however, will more accurately demonstrate hemorrhage into the cystic component which commonly is responsible for acute exacerbation of symptoms (Fig. 22).

In addition, MRI which is sensitive in the depiction of fat, can identify cholesterol in the fluid component. Since it has been established that spillage of this fluid into the subarachnoid space can cause a chemical meningitis, it will be interesting to determine if MRI can identify the chemical composition of the cyst and predict which patients are at risk to develop this complication.

Pituitary Adenomas

CT revolutionized the diagnosis and follow-up of pituitary adenomas. Pituitary adenomas are categorized on the basis of size as being microadenomas (less than 10 mm) or macroadenomas (greater than 10 mm).

Macroadenomas, with extension upward into the suprasellar cistern, downward into the sphenoid sinus, or laterally into the cavernous sinus, are well evaluated with axial and direct coronal MR and CT scans. It appears that both modalities are satisfactory in depicting the exact size of the tumor and its relationship to the adjacent structures; however, MRI is superior in three areas. The first is evaluation of the degree of carotid artery compression since the flow void of the vessel is well contrasted against the adjacent tumor. Second, hemorrhagic elements of the tumor which present with increase in signal on T1 are well seen, a finding rarely demonstrated by CT. Evidence of hemorrhage is useful in the evaluation of patients with sudden deterioration of vision which may result from hemorrhagic expansion of the tumor. Third, the three-dimensional presentation of these tumors is helpful in designing surgical therapy.[86,87]

The diagnostic contribution of PET in macroadenomas is somewhat limited. PET-FDG studies have shown increased glucose utilization by the adenoma; however, close correlation between glucose consumption and pituitary function or tumor growth has not been established (Fig. 23). More promising results have been obtained with functional studies of adenoma metabolism. Bergstrom et al. used L- and D-methionine in patients harboring hormonally active adenomas (prolactinomas) and in patients with adenomas lacking hormonal production (null cell adenomas). When D-methionine was injected, there was rapid initial uptake of the isotope by the tumor tissue which was followed by equilibration between the tissue and the plasma radioactivity. This indicates that there is no participation of D-methionine in protein synthesis. When L-methionine was used, there was gradual accumulation of this amino acid and the ratio of tissue to plasma activity increased linearly with time over a period of 60 minutes. In the prolactinomas, the isotope accumulation was three times higher in the tumors than in cerebellum.[88] In the null cell adenomas, the ratio was 2.8. When the amino acid metabolism was compared before and after bromocriptine treatment, the prolactinomas showed a decrease ranging from 40% to 70% in isotope concentration, whereas the null cell adenomas showed no effect.[89,90] These findings point to the potential use of PET in monitoring the results of treatment in these groups of patients. Additionally, PET scans have been used in patients with pituitary prolactinomas after intravenous administration of ^{11}C-labeled dopamine-D_2 antagonists

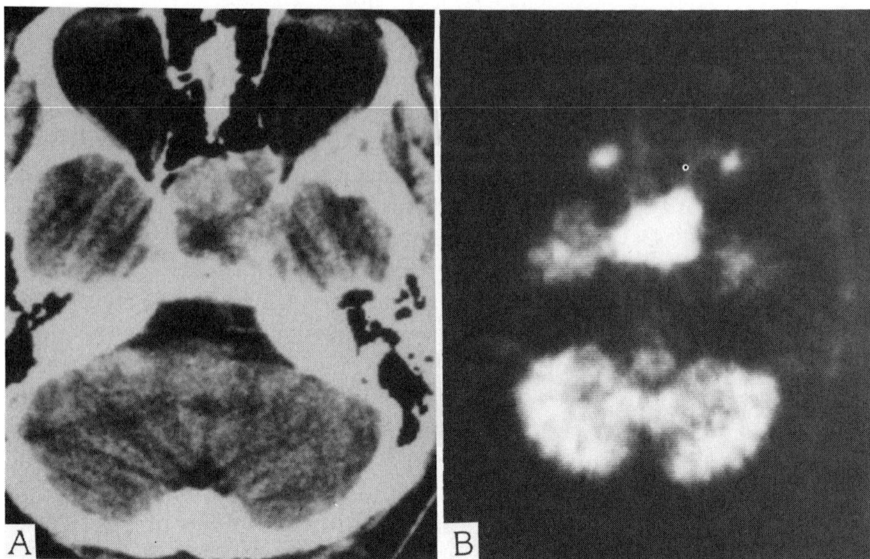

Figure 23. Pituitary macroadenoma. A. CT scan with contrast showing a large adenoma extending into the sphenoid sinus. B. PET-FDG showing the adenoma to be hypermetabolic.

(N-methylspiperone and raclopride). Marked tracer uptake proportional to the serum prolactin level was found in active prolactinomas. Minimal uptake was noted in nonsecreting adenomas. In a few patients, PET scans were repeated after the administration of haloperidol which protects the D_2 receptors. This caused marked suppression of uptake in those with actively secreting tumors while what uptake there was in the nonsecreting patients was not changed. The above results would indicate that assessment of the dopamine-D_2 receptors in prolactinomas should influence our choice of treatment because adenomas with high amounts of receptors are, in most cases, effectively treated with dopamine agonists like bromocriptine.[91]

A more challenging task from the diagnostic point of view is the detection of microadenomas. The most common of these include prolactinomas and ACTH-secreting adenomas. Prolactinomas are usually treated medically while those that secrete ACTH are treated by resection of the portion of the gland that contains the microadenoma preserving enough pituitary gland to prevent hypopituitarism. Therefore, it is imperative to demonstrate the exact size and location of the lesion.

Contrast-enhanced, direct coronal CT images with 1.5 mm slice thickness may reveal a focal area of hypodensity within the normally enhancing gland. The majority of microadenomas enhance homogeneously with the remaining pituitary gland and cannot be detected directly. Consequently, a number of secondary signs are employed to increase the diagnostic yield. These include (1) absolute height measurements, (2) focal convexity of the superior portion of the gland, (3) the midline position of the pituitary stalk and the vascular tuft, both of which are displaced away from the side of a microadenoma, and (4) focal bony changes in the floor of the sella. These secondary signs are less reliable and contribute to both false positive and false negative results. The reported incidence of detection using any of the above criteria in patients with ACTH-secreting microadenomas is approximately 30% and in prolactinomas it has been reported as high as 87%.[92,93]

Because of these deficiencies, in patients contemplating surgery, petrosal venous sampling has been developed as an additional diagnostic tool. Selective catherization of both petrosal sinuses is accomplished via the femoral vein and venous samples are obtained and assessed for hormonal activity. Differential values indicate the site of the lesion and provide a high diagnostic yield.[94]

In MRI, the detection of microadenomas requires surface coils and 3 mm coronal and sagittal sections. More recently, intravenous Gd-DTPA has been used. On unenhanced T1 weighted images, cystic microadenomas will demonstrate a focal area of decreased signal. On the T2 weighted images, the same abnormalility will present as an area of increased signal. On enhanced T1 and T2 weighted images, Gd-DTPA diffuses into the cystic component and causes dramatic signal increase on both techniques (Fig. 24). However, the majority of microadenomas which are solid appear isointense with the pituitary parenchyma; consequently, the diagnostic yield of unenhanced MRI is equivalent to contrast-enhanced CT. After Gd-DTPA, the normal gland enhances intensely while the adenoma, if solid, will remain hypointense (Fig. 25). Preliminary results indicate that post Gd-DTPA MRI will improve the yield significantly, making contrast-enhanced MRI the most rewarding modality.[95,96]

The posterior pituitary displays a focal area of increased signal intensity on T1 weighted images in the vast majority of normal patients if appropriate techniques are utilized. On sagittal sections, it

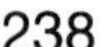

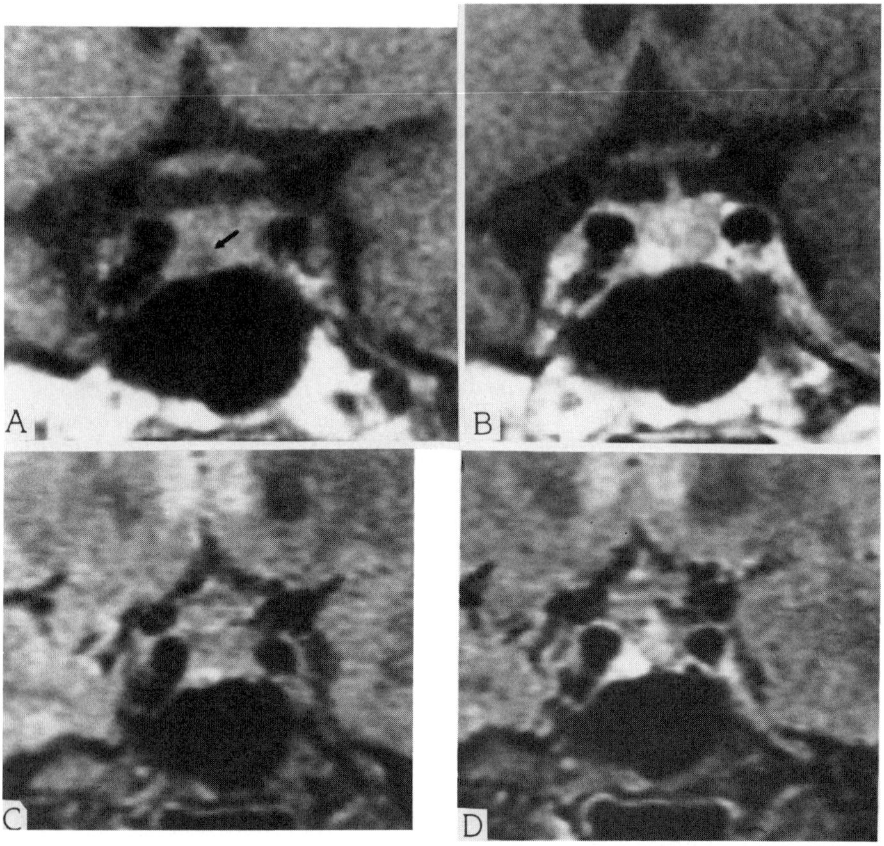

Figure 24. ACTH-secreting cystic microadenoma. A. Pre-Gd-DTPA T1 weighted image showing a small rounded hyperintense lesion in the right half of the gland (arrow). B. Pre-Gd-DTPA T2 weighted image showing increased signal at the same site findings consistent with a cystic lesion. C & D. Post-Gd-DTPA T1 weighted (C) and T2 weighted (D) images, showing marked increase in signal intensity due to concentration of the contrast in the cystic adenoma.

is seen just anterior to the dorsum sella while on the coronal sections, it is at the midline.[97]

The increased signal is believed to be due to the elevated lipids in the secretory granules in the axons in the hypothalamohypophyseal tract. Displacement of the posterior lobe off of the midline can

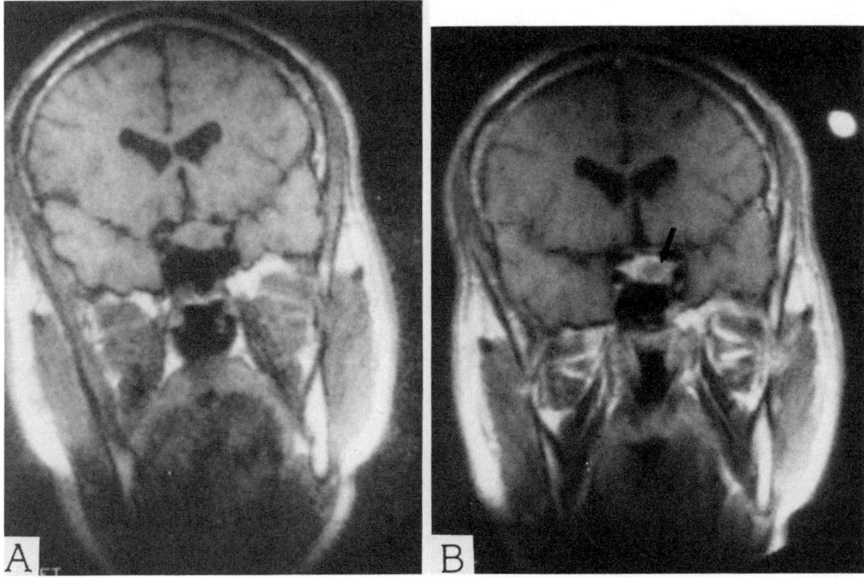

Figure 25. Solid ACTH-secreting microadenoma. A. Pre-Gd-DTPA T1 weighted MRI scan showing no definite focal abnormalities. B. Post-Gd-DTPA T1 weighted image showing a focal area of decreased intensity in the left half of the gland (arrow) while the remaining gland shows intense signal due to enhancement by Gd-DTPA.

serve as an additional secondary sign of a microadenoma in the anterior pituitary. Complete obliteration of the posterior lobe signal is found in the majority of macroadenomas and also in lesions of the hypothalamus such as teratomas, germinomas, and histiocytosis, which invade the pituitary stalk.[98] Finally, disruption of the stalk by trauma causes disappearance of this signal. All of these abnormalities can present clinically with diabetes insipidus. Therefore, MRI is the best method available to evaluate this entity.

Metastatic Brain Tumors

Clinical studies have shown that both the length and quality of life are improved when solitary metastatic deposits are surgically removed.[99] Therefore, it is essential that such a lesion be detected at

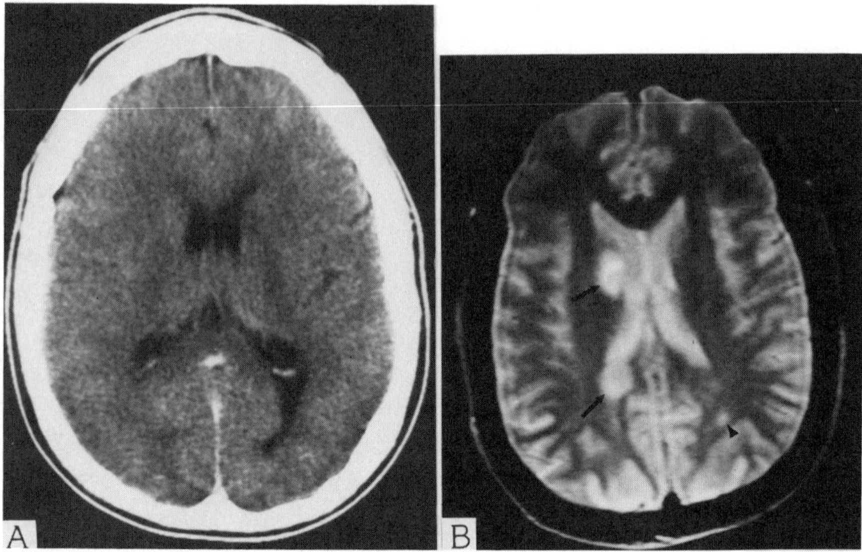

Figure 26. Metastatic tumors missed by CT. A. Post-infusions CT section failing to demonstrate any abnormality. B. T2 weighted image through the same region showing two abnormal areas of increased signal in the right hemisphere (arrows). A third probable lesion is present in the left parietal region (arrow head). Stereotactic biopsy of one of them revealed metastatic lymphoma.

the earliest possible stage. The high incidence of metastatic brain disease in certain types of malignant tumors is well recognized, although some of these may be clinically silent.

Contrast-enhanced CT will demonstrate a lesion in a majority of patients with neurologic deficits; however, a second, smaller lesion may be inapparent. Identification of all lesions is vital because treatment choices are based on the number of lesions present. CT which is insensitive to small tumors is unsatisfactory as a screening test in asymptomatic patients. MRI scans, on the other hand, are far more sensitive in detecting such tumors (Fig. 26). Besides the inherent superior contrast resolution of MRI, the detection of these tumors is facilitated by the fact that the tumor and the surrounding edema produce similar increased intensity. On T2 weighted images, this summation effect causes an apparent increase in tumor size, thereby improving detectibility. Furthermore, post Gd-DTPA T1 weighted images show intense enhancement of metastatic tumors which is more obvious than the enhancement accomplished with iodinated compounds on CT. It has also been shown to be more sensitive than T2 weighted images in determining the precise number of lesions. Clearly, MRI is preferable to CT for screening, for staging and for choosing the appropriate therapy in these patients. As for histologic characterization, neither CT nor MRI are reliable.[100,101] Occasionally, a suggestion of tumor histology can be obtained by increased signal on T1. This often occurs in melanomas due to hemorrhage or the presence of melanin, a paramagnetic substance containing a stable free radical with an unpaired electron. Other tumors with a tendency to hemorrhage when they metastasize to the brain include choriocarcinoma, hypernephroma, and thyroid.

Conclusion

It is rapidly becoming clear that as the technology surrounding MRI evolves towards the ability to obtain thinner slices with shorter scan time, MRI will replace CT in the evaluation of brain tumors. PET scanning will also continue to evolve and will assume a more important role in staging various lesions and in post-treatment follow-up.

CT, which appears to have reached a plateau in development will continue to be utilized for some time, particularly in very ill patients; however, its role in neurodiagnosis is expected to diminish gradually.

REFERENCES

1. Pykett IL, Newsome JH, Buonanno FS, Brady TJ, Goldman MR, et al. Nuclear magnetic resonance: Principles of nuclear manetic resonance imaging. Radiology 1982; 143:157–168.
2. Partain CL, Price RR, Patton JA, Stephens WH, Price AC, et al. Nuclear magnetic resonance imaging. Radiographics 1984; 4:5–25.
3. Harms SE, Morgan TJ, Yamanashi WS, Harle TS, Dodd GD. Principles of nuclear magnetic resonance imaging. Radiographics 1984; 4:26–43.
4. Pavlicek W, Modic M, Weinstein M. Pulse sequence and significance. Radiographics 1984; 4:49–65.
5. Jones JP, Partain CL, Mitchell MR, et al. Principles of magnetic resonance. In: Magnetic Resonance Annual 1985, Dressel HY, ed., New York, Raven Press, 1985; pp 71–112.
6. Caille M, Lemanceau B, Bonneman B. Gadolinium as a contrast agent for NMR. AJNR 1983; 4:1041–1042.
7. Brasch RC, Weinmann HJ, Wesbey GE. Contrast-enhanced NMR im-

aging: animal studies using gadolinium-DTPA complex. AJR 1984; 142:619–624.

8. Gadian DG, Payne JA, Bryant DJ, Young IR, Carr DH, et al. Gadolinium-TPA as a contrast agent in MR imaging: Theoretical projections and practical observations. J Comput Assist Tomogr 1985; 9(2):242–251.

9. Wolf GL, Burnett KR, Goldstein EJ, Joseph PM. Contrast agents for magnetic resonance imaging. In: Magnetic Resonance Annual 1985, Dressel HY (ed.), New York, Raven Press, 1985; pp. 247.

10. Axel L. Surface coil magnetic resonance imaging. J Comput Assist Tomogr 1984; 8(3):381–384.

11. Bydder GM, Butsen PC, Harman RR, Gilderdale DJ, Young IR. Technical note. Use of spherical receiver coils in MR imaging of the brain. J Comput Assist Tomogr 1985; 9(2):413–414.

12. Malko JA, McClees EC, Braun IF, Davis PC, Hoffman JC. A Flexible mercury-filled surface coil for MR imaging. AJNR 1986; 7:246–247.

13. Budinger TF, Cullander C. Health hazards in nuclear magnetic resonance in vivo studies. Radiographics 1984; 4:74.

14. Raichle ME, Welch MJ, Grubb RL, Higgins CS, Ter-Pogossian MM, et al. Measurement of regional substrate utilization rates by emission tomography. Science 1978; 199:968–987.

15. Ter-Pogossian MM, Raichle ME, Sobel DE. Positron emission tomography. Sci Am 1980; 243:170–181.

16. Sokoloff L, Reivich M, Kennedy C, Des Rosiers MH, Patlak CS, et al. The [14C] deoxyglucose method for the measurement of local cerebral glucose utilization: theory, procedure, and normal values in the conscious and anesthetized albino rat. J Neurochem 1977; 28:897–916.

17. Oldendorf WH. Brain uptake of radiolabeled aminoacids, amines, and hexoses after arterial injection. Am J Physiol 1971; 221:1629–1639.

18. Horton RW, Meldrun BS, Bachelard HS. Enzymic and cerebral metabolic effects of 2-deoxy-D-glucose. J Neurochem 1973; 21:507–520.

19. Ido T, Wan CN, Fowler JS, Wolf AP. Fluorination with F_2, a convenient synthesis of 2-deoxy-D-fluoro-D-glucose. J Org Chem 1977; 42:2341–2342.

20. Reivich M, Kuhl D, Wolf A, Greenberg J, Phelps M, et al. The [18F]fluorodeoxyglucose method for the measurement of local cerebral glucose utilization in man. Circ Res 1979; 44:127–137.

21. Kuhl DE, Phelps ME, Hoffman EJ, Robinson GD, MacDonald NS. Initial clinical experience with (F–18)-deoxy-D-glucose for determination of local cerebral glucose utilization by emission computed tomography. In: Cerebral Function, Metabolism, and Circulation, Ingvar DH, Lassen NA, eds., Copenhagen, Munksgaard, 1977; pp. 192–193.

22. Huang SC, Phelps ME, Hoffman EJ, Sideris K, Selin CJ, et al. Noninvasive determination of local cerebral metabolic rate of glucose in man. Am J Physiol 1980; 238:E69–82.

23. Phelps ME, Hugan SC, Hoffman EJ, Selin C, Sokoloff L, et al. Tomographic measurement of local cerebral glucose metabolic rate in humans with (F–18)2-fluoro–2-deoxy-D-glucose: Validation of method. Ann Neurol 1979; 6:371–388.

24. Brooks RA, Sank VJ, Faiauf WS, Leighton SB, Cascio HE, et al. Design

considerations for positron emission tomography. IEEE Trans Biomed Eng BME 1981; 28:158–177.

25. Reivich M, Alavi A, Wolf A, et al. Use of 2-deoxy-D-[1–[11]C]-glucose for the determination of local cerebral glucose metabolism in humans: Variation within and between subjects. J Cereb Blood Flow Metab 1982; 2:307–319.

26. Bustany P, Henry JH, Soussaline F, Comar D. Brain protein synthesis in normal and demented patients. A study by positron emission tomography with [11]C Methionine. In: Functional Radionuclide Imaging of the Brain, Magstretta PL, New York, Raven Press, pp. 321–328.

27. Bergstrom M, Collins JP, Ehrin E, Ericson K, Eriksson L, et al. Discrepancies in brain tumor extent as shown by computed tomography and positron emission tomography using [^{68}Ga] EDTA, ^{11}C] glucose and ^{11}C] methionine. J Comput Assist Tomogr 1983; 7:1062–1066.

28. Lundqvist H, Stalnacke CG, Langstrom B, Jones B. Labeled metabolites in plasma after intravenous administration of [[11]CH$_3$]–1-Methionine. In: The Metabolism of the Human Studied with Positron Emission Tomography, Greitz T, et al., eds. New York, Raven Press, 1985.

29. Ericson K, Lilja A, Bergstrom M, Collins VP, Eriksson L, et al. Positron emission tomography with (^{11}C]Methyl)-L-Methionine, ^{11}C]D-glucose, [^{68}Ga]-EDTA in supratentorial tumors. J Comput Assist Tomogr 1985; 9(4):683–689.

30. Bergstrom M, Ericson K, Hagenfeldt L, Mosskin M, von Holst H, et al. PET study of methionine accumulation in glioma and normal brain tissue: competition with branched chain amino acids. J Comput Assist Tomogr 1987; 11(2):208–213.

31. Hiesiger E, Fowler JS, Wolf AP, Logan J, Brodie JD, et al. Serial PET studies of human cerebral malignancy with ^{11}C]putrescine and ^{11}C]2-deoxy-D-glucose. J Nucl Med 1987; 28:1251–1261.

32. Jones T, Chesler DA, Ter-Pogossian MM. The continuous inhalation of oxygen–15 for assessing regional oxygen extraction in the brain of man. Br J Radiol 1976; 49:339–343.

33. Frackowiak R, Lenzi G, Jones T, et al. Quantitative measurement of regional cerebral blood flow and oxygen metabolism in man using [15]O and positron emission-tomography: Theory, procedure and normal values. J Comput Assist Tomogr 1980; 4:727–736.

34. Damadian R. Tumor detection by nuclear magnetic resonance. Science 1971; 171:1151–1153.

35. Claussen C, Laniado M, Schorner W, Niendorf HP, Weinmann HJ, et al. Gadolinium-DTPA in MR imaging of glioblastomas and intracranial metastases. AJNR 1985; 6:669–674.

36. Graif M, Bydder GM, Steiner RE, Niendorf P, Thomas DG, et al. Contrast-enhanced MR imaging of malignant brain tumors. AJNR 1985; 6:855–862.

37. Felix R, Schorner W, Laniado M, Niendorf HP, Claussen C, et al. Brain tumors: MR imaging with gadolinium-DTPA. Radiology 1985; 156:681–688.

38. Graif M, Bydder GM, et al. Contrast-enhanced MR imaging of malignant brain tumors. AJNR 1985; 6:855–862.

39. Brantawadzki M, Berry I, Osaki L, Brasch R, Murovic J, et al. Gd-DTPA in clinical MR of the brain: 1. Intra-axial lesions. AJNR 1986; 7:781–788.
40. Earnest F, Kelly PJ, Scheithauer BW, Kall BA, Cascino TL, et al. Cerebral astrocytomas: histopathologic correlation of MR and CT contrast enhancement with stereotactic biopsy. Radiology 1988; 166:823–827.
41. Hilal SK, Maudsley A, Ra JB, Simon HE, Roschmann P, Wittekoek S, Cho ZH. Mun SK. In vivo NMR Imaging of sodium 23 in the human head. J Comput Assist Tomogr 1985; 9(1):17.
42. Turnski PA, Houston LW, Perman WH, Hald JK, Turski D, et al. Experimental and human brain neoplasms: Detection with in vivo sodium MR imaging. Radiology 1987; 163:245–249.
43. Jarden JO, Dhawan V, Kearfott KJ, Rottenberg DA. Measurement of brain/tumor capillary permeability using ^{82}Rb and positron emission tomography. Ann Neurol 1984; 16:131.
44. Yen CK, Budinger TF. Evaluation of blood-brain barrier permeability changes in rhesus monkeys and man using ^{82}Rb and positron emission tomography. J Comput Assist Tomogr 1981; 5(6):792–799.
45. Illsen HW, Sato M, Pawlik G, Herholz K, Wienhard K, et al. (^{68}Ga)-EDTA positron emission tomography in the diagnosis of brain tumors. Neuroradiology 1984; 26:393–398.
46. Komiyama M, Yagura H, Baba M, Yasui T, Hakuba A, et al. MR imaging: Posibility of tissue characterization of brain tumors using T1 and T2 values. AJNR 1987; 8:65–70.
47. Carr DH, Bydder GM, Brown J, Weinmann HJ, Speck U, et al. Intravenous chelated gadolinium as a contrast agent in NMR imaging of cerebral tumors. Lancet 1984; I:484.
48. Carr DH, Brown J, Bydder GM, Steiner RE, Weinmann HJ, et al. Gadolinium-ETPA as a contrast agent in MRI: initial clinical experience in 20 patients. AJR 1984; 143:215–224.
49. Felix R, Schorner W, Laniado M, Neindorf HP, Claussen C, et al. Brain tumors: MR imaging with gadolinium-ETPA. Radiology 1985; 156:681–688.
50. Brantawadzki M, Berry I, Osaki L, Brasch R, Murovic J, et al. Gd-DTPA in clinical MR of the brain: 1. Intraaxial lesions. AJNR 1986; 7:781–788.
51. Graif M, Bydder GM, Steiner RE, Niendorg P, Thomas DG, et al. Contrast-enhanced MR imaging of malignant brain tumors. AJNR 1985; 6:855–862.
52. Di Chiro G, DeLapaz RL, Brooks RA, Sokoloff L, Kornblith PL, et al. Glucose utilization of cerebral gliomas measured by (^{18}F) fluorodeoxyglucose and positron emission tomography. Neurol 1982; 32:1323–1329.
53. Patronas NJ, Brooks RA, DeLapaz RL, Smith BH, Kornblith PL, et al. Glycolytic rate (PET) and contrast enhancement (CT) in human cerebral gliomas. AJR 1983; 4:533–535.
54. Yamagushi T, Sasaki II, Ogawa T, Mineura K, Uemura K, et al. Relation between tissue nature and (^{18}F) fluorodeoxyglucose kinetics evaluated

by dynamic positron emission tomography in human brain. Acta Radiol (suppl) 1986; 369:415–418.

55. Ito M, Lammertsma AA, Wise RJS, Bernardi S, Frackowiak RJS, et al. Measurement of regional cerebral blood flow and oxygen utilization in patients with cerebral tumours using ^{15}O and positron emission tomography: analytical techniques and preliminary results. Neuroradiology 1982; 23:63–74.

56. Rhodes CG, Wise RJS, Gibbs JM, Frackowiak RJS, Hatazawa J, et al. In vivo disturbance of the oxidative metabolism of glucose in human cerebral gliomas. Ann Neurol 1983; 14:614–626.

57. Lammertsma AA, Wise RJS, Cox TCS, Thomas DGT, Jones T. Measurement of blood flow, oxygen utilisation, oxygen extraction ratio, and fractional blood volume in human brain tumours and surrounding oedematous tissue. Br J Radiol 1985; 58:725–734.

58. Lilja A, Bergstrom K, Spannare B, Olsson Y. Reliability of computed tomography in assessing histopathological features of malignant supratentorial gliomas. J Comput Assist Tomogr 1981; 5:625–636.

59. Kelly PJ, Earnest F, Kall BA, Goerss SJ, Scheithauer B. Surgical options for patients with deep-seated brain tumors: computerssisted stereotactic biopsy. Mayo Clin Proc 1985; 60: 223–229.

60. Le Bas JF, Leviel JL, Decorps M, Benabid AL. NMR relaxation times from serial stereotactic biopsies in human brain tumors. J Comput Assist Tomogr 1984; 8(6): 1048–1057.

61. Earnest F, Kelly PJ, Scheithauer BW, Kall BA, Casino TL, et al. Cerebral astrocytomas: Histopathologic correlation of MR and CT contrast enhancement with stereotactic biopsy. Radiology 1988; 166:823–827.

62. DeLaPaz RL, Patronas NJ, Brooks RA, Smith BH, Kornblith PL, et al. A positron emission tomography (PET) study of suppression of glucose utilization in cerebral gray matter associated with brain tumor. AJNR 1983; 826–829.

63. Patronas NJ, Di Chiro G, Smith BH, DeLaPaz R, Brooks RA, et al. Cerebellar glucose metabolism in supratentorial tumors. Brain Res 1984; 291:93–101.

64. Fishbein DS, Chrousos GA, Di Chiro G, Wayner RE, Patronas NJ, et al. Glucose utilization of unstimulated visual cortex following extraoccipital interpretations of the visual pathways: a positron emission tomography study. Arch Ophthal J Clin Neuropathol 1987; 7(2):63–68.

65. Dooms GC, Hecht S, Brantawadzki M, Berthiaume Y, Norman D, et al. Brain radiation lesions: MR imaging. Radiology 1986; 158:149–155.

66. Tsuruda JS, Kortman KE, Bradley WG, Wheeler DC, Dalsem WV, et al. Radiation effects on cerebral white matter: MR evaluation. AJNR 1987; 8:431–437.

67. Kleinschmidt-DeMasters BK. Intracarotid BCNU leukoencephalopathy. Cancer 1986; 57:1276–1280.

68. Di Chiro G, Oldfield E, Wright DC, De Michele D, Katz DA, et al. Cerebral necrosis after radiotherapy and/or intraarterial chemotherapy for brain tumors: PET and neuropathologic studies. AJNR 1987; 8:1083–1091.

69. Ito M, Patronas NJ, Di Chiro G, Mansi L, Kennedy C. Effect of moderate

level x-radiation to brain cerebral glucose utilization. J Comput Assist Tomogr 1986; 10(4):584–588.

70. Shishido F, Uemura K, Komatsu K, Inugami A, Ogawa T, et al. Cerebral glucose metabolic change after high-de methotrexate treatment in patients with acute lymphocytic leukemia. Acta Radiologica 1986; (Suppl 369) 422–425.

71. Patronas NJ, Di Chiro G, Brooks RA, De LaPaz RL, Kornblith PL, et al. Nuclear Medicine. Work in progress: [18F] fluorodeoxyglucose and positron emission tomography in the evaluation of radiation necrosis of the brain. Radiology 1982; 144:885–889.

72. Doyle WK, Budinger TF, Valk PE, Levin VA, Gutin PH. Differentiation of cerebral radiation necrosis from tumor recurrence by [18F]FDG and 82Rb positron emission tomography. J Comput Assist Tomogr 1987; 11(4):563–570.

73. Patronas NJ, Di Chiro G, Kufta C, Bairamian D, Kornblith PL, et al. Prediction of survical in glioma patients by means of positron emission tomography. J Neurosurg 1985; 62:816–822.

74. New PFJ, Aronow S, Hesselink JR. National Cancer Institute Study: Evaluation of computed tomography in the diagnosis of intracranial neoplasms. Radiology 1980; 136:665–675.

75. Berry I, Brant-Zawadzki M, Osaki L, Brasch R, Murovic J, Newton TH. Gd-DTPA in clinical MR of the brain: 2. Extraaxial lesions and normal structures. AJNR 1986; 7:789–793.

76. Mikhael MA, Ciric IS, Wolff AP. Differentiation of cerebellopontine angel neuromas and meningiomas with MR imaging. J Comput Assist Tomogr 1985; 9(5):852–856.

77. Haughton VM, Rimm AA, Czervionke LF, Breger RK, Fisher ME, Sensitivity of Gd-DTPA-enhanced MR imaging of benign extraaxial tumors. Radiology 1988; 166:829–833.

78. Di Chiro G, Hatazawa J, Katz DA, Rizzoli HV, De Michele DJ. Glucose utilization by intracranial meningiomas as an index of tumor agressivity and probability of recurrence: A PET study. Radiology 1987; 164:521–526.

79. Lee YY, Glass JP, Goeffray A, Wallace S. Cranial computed tomographic abnormalities in leptomeningeal metastasis. AJNR 1984; 5:559–563.

80. Frank JA, Girton M, Dwyer AJ, Wright DC, Cohen PJ, et al. Gadolinium-DTPA enhanced MRI in the detection of meningeal carcinomatosis in the VX2 rabbit tumor model. Radiology 1988; 167:825–829.

81. Kricheff II, Pinto RS, Bergeron RT, Cohen N. Air CT cisternography and canalography for small acoustic neuromas. AJNR 1980; 1:57–63.

82. Enzmann DR, O'Donohue J. Optimizing MR imaging for detecting small tumors in the cerebellopontine angle and internal auditory canal. AJNR 1987; 8:99–106.

83. Daniels DL, Millen SJ, Meyer GA, Pojunas KW, Kilgore DP, et al. MR detection of tumor in internal auditory canal. AJNR 1987; 8:249–252.

84. Mikhael MA, Ciric IS, Wolff AP. MR diagnosis of acoustic neuromas. J Comput Assist Tomogr 1987; 11(2):232–235.

85. Patronas, NJ, Dwyer AJ, Papathanasiou M, Schiebler ML, Schellinger

D. Contributions of magnetic resonance imaging in the evaluation of optic gliomas. Surg Neurol 1987; 28:367–371.

86. Lee BCP, Deck MDF. Sellar and juxtasellar lesion detection with MR. Radiology 1985; 157:143–147.

87. Davis PC, Hoffman JC, Spencer T, Tindall GT, Braun IF. MR imaging of pituitary adenoma: CT, clinical, and surgical correlation. AJNR 1987; 8:107–112.

88. Bergstrom M, Muhr C, Lundberg PO, Bergstrom K, Lundqvist H, et al. Amino acid distribution and metabolism in pituitary adenomas using positron emission tomography with D-[^{11}C]methionine and L-^{11}C]methionine. J Comput Assist Tomogr 1987; 11(3):384–389.

89. Bergstrom M, Muhr C, Lundberg PO, Bergstrom K, Lundqvist H, et al. Amino acid metabolism in pituitary adenomas. Acta Radiol 1986; (suppl) 369:412–413.

90. Bergstrom M, Muhr C, Lundberg PO, Bergstrom K, Gee AD, et al. Rapid decrease in amino acid metabolism in prolactin-secreting pituitary adenomas after bromocriptine treatment: A PET study. J Comput Assist Tomogr 1987; 11(5):815–819.

91. Muhr C, Bergstrom M, Lundberg PO, Bergstrom K, Langstrom B. In vivo measurement of dopamine receptors in pituitary adenomas using positron emission tomography. Acta Radiol 1986; (suppl.) 369:406–408.

92. Saris SC, Patronas NJ, Doppman JL, Loriaux DL, Cutler GB, et al. Cushing syndrome: pituitary CT scanning. Radiology 1987; 162:775–777.

93. Marcovitz S, Wee R, Chan J, Hardy J. Diagnostic accuracy of preoperative CT scanning of pituitary prolactinomas. AJNR 1988; 9:13–17.

94. Oldfield EH, Chrousos GP, Schulte HM, et al. Preoperative lateralization of ACTH secreting pituitary microadenomas by bilateral and simultaneous inferior petrosal venous sinus sampling. N Engl J Med 1985; 312:100–103.

95. Dwyer AJ, Frank JA, Doppman JL, Oldfield EH, Hickey AM, et al. Pituitary adenomas in patients with Cushing disease: Initial experience with Gd-DTPA-enhanced MR imaging. Radiology 1987; 163:421–426.

96. Davis PC, Hoffman JC, Malko JA, Tindall GT, Takei Y, et al. Gadolinium-DTPA and MR imaging of pituitary adenoma: A preliminary report. AJNR 1987; 8:817–823.

97. Fujisawa I, Asato R, Nishimura K, Togashi K, Itoh K, et al. Anterior and posterior lobes of the pituitary gland assessment by 1.5 T MR imaging. J Comput Assist Tomogr 1987; 11(2):214–220.

98. Fujisawa I, Nishimura K, Asato R, Togashi K, Itoh K, et al. Posterior lobe of the pituitary in diabetes insipidus: MR findings. J Cat 1987; 11(2):221–225.

99. Golicich JH, Sundaresan N, Thaler HT. Surgical treatment of simple brain metastasis. J Neurosurg 1980; 53:63–67.

100. Lee BCP, Kneeland JB, Cahill PT, Deck MD. MR recognition of supratentorial tumors. AJNR 1985; 6:871–878.

101. Claussen C, Laniado M, Schorner W, Niendorf HP, Weinmann HJ, et al. Gadolinium-ETPA in MR imaging of glioblastomas and intracranial metastases. AJNR 1985; 6:669–674.

9

Monoclonal Antibodies in the Diagnosis and Therapy of Brain Tumors

J. Behnke, H.B. Coakham, J.P. Mach, S. Carrel, and N. de Tribolet

Introduction

The technique for making monoclonal antibodies developed by Köhler and Milstein[1] provides the possibility of producing homogenous and pure antibodies against unique antigenic determinants in high amounts and of reproducible quality. A number of monoclonal antibodies are reactive with gliomas, allowing the identification of three different groups of markers.

The first is called *glioma associated*, because the antigens that belong to this group are expressed by most gliomas. BF7 and GE2 belong to this group.[2] These monoclonal antibodies were raised against an established human glioma cell line and are reactive in antibody binding radioimmunoassay with most of the glioma cell lines tested. BF7 and GE2 are not specific for gliomas, because a reactivity was found also to some of the tested schwannoma, melanoma, meningioma cell lines and, in addition, GE2 also bound to one of the three tested medulloblastoma cell lines.[3-5] In immunohistochemistry, astrocytes, in both the grey and the white matter of normal brain, are stained,[6] although less intensely than malignant or reactive

From: Kornblith PL, Walker MD (editors). Advances in Neuro-Oncology. Futura Publishing Company, Inc., Mount Kisco, NY, © 1988.

astrocytes. Certain dendritic cells of normal spleen and normal thymus are positive for GE2 and BF7 in immunohistochemistry.[6] The glioma mesenchymal extracellular matrix (GMEM) antigen also belongs in the first group. It is localized on the basement membranes of glioblastomas and associated with proliferative endothelium and hyperplastic vessels. It is defined by the monoclonal antibody 81C6.[7] In antibody binding radioimmunoassay, it has been shown that GMEM antigen is present on most glioma and fibroblast cell lines and on some of the tested neuroblastoma, sarcoma, and melanoma cell lines. Immunohistology shows binding to fetal and adult spleen, liver, and adult kidney. Wikstrand et al.[8] have described a monoclonal antibody 2F3, which is only reactive with gliomas and fetal skin fibroblasts.

The second group of markers represents *common neuroectodermal antigens* expressed by gliomas. Antibodies such as MeI-5, MeI-14, Me3-TB7, Me4-F8, and Me5-D5[9,10] were raised against membrane-enriched fractions from two melanoma cell lines and react in antibody binding radioimmunoassay not only with a large number of melanoma cell lines but also with other neuroectodermal tumors. Herlyn et al.[11] have defined neuroectodermal antigens with the monoclonal antibodies 19-19 and Nu4B. The spectrum of reactivity in antibody binding radioimmunoassay includes a wide range of melanoma and glioma cell lines, and antibody Nu4B also reacts with one of four tested fibroblast cell lines. UJ13A is an antibody against a shared neuroectodermal antigen recognizing all neuroectodermal tumors except melanomas and is also reactive with normal brain. It was raised after immunization with human fetal brain.[12] M19 characterizes a heat labile molecule present on a portion of melanomas, astrocytomas, epithelial cancers, normal fibroblasts and kidney.[13] In the same fusion as the former one, Q24 was raised, which has a reactivity spectrum similar to M19, but also reacts with fetal brain, liver, and fibroblasts. Thus the defined antigen belongs to a subpopulation of the group II markers, to the *shared neuroectodermal-oncofetal markers*, which are shared neuroectodermal tumor antigens also detected on human fetal tissue including the fetal CNS and lymphoid system.[14] 4C7, 5B7[8] 4D2, 7H10,[15] and UJ1814[16] characterize antigens of this group as well as antibodies raised by Liao et al.[17] and Seeger et al.[18] A shared neuroectodermal-oncofetal marker is also detected by CG12,[2] an antibody which was raised in the same fusion as in group I BF7 and GE2 antigens.

The last group includes *shared nervous system-lymphoid cell mark-*

ers. Normal brain cells and tumors of neuroectodermal origin express lymphoid differentiation antigens. Examples are the observed cross-reactivity between T cells and Purkinje neurons with the antibody UCHT1[19] and the presence of other hematopoetic cell type markers on ectodermally derived tumor cells.[20] The expression of two well-defined lymphoid differentiation antigens has been demonstrated on glioma cells:

• Common acute lymphoblastic leukemia antigen (CALLA) could be shown to be present on a broad panel of gliomas with an anti-CALLA-antiserum[21] and with anti-CALLA monoclonal antibodies N2A12[22] and J-5.[23]
• HLA-DR is present on a spectrum of glioma cells as it could be shown by means of the monoclonal antibody D1-12.[21] HLA-DR could be demonstrated also on reactive astrocytes in normal brain.[24] Thy-1, a human T cell associated antigen, is expressed on cell surfaces of neuronal and glial cells[25] and on neuroblastoma, glioma, and teratoma cells.[26] PI153/3, a monoclonal antibody which reacts with neuroectodermally derived tumors and fetal brain,[27] identifies a cell surface determinant shared by common acute lymphoblastic leukemias and B lineage cells.[28]

This introduction encompasses only a selection of some monoclonal antibodies reacting with gliomas and some of them may play a role in the diagnosis and treatment of gliomas.

Pharmacokinetics of Monoclonal Antibodies

From the injection to the binding of an antibody, some transport steps are interposed in which the delivery of the antibody to the tumor can be hindered. By intravenous administration, the antibody is diluted into the vascular system and can there be bound to pre-existing anti-mouse IgG or target tumor antigens shedded into the circulation. Primus et al.,[29,30] using goat antiserum against carcinoembryonic antigen (CEA), have demonstrated that CEA as well as human anti-goat antibodies can form complexes with radiolabeled anti-CEA antiserum, which do not seem to disturb the radioimmunodetection. Mach et al.[31] have observed that among patients with positive results in radioimmunodetection, using radiolabeled goat antibodies against CEA, some had high levels of circulating CEA, which obviously did not prevent the antibody localization. Larson et al.,[32] imaging melanomas with radiolabeled monoclonal antibodies, have demonstrated antibodies against mouse IgG in the sera of patients after they had intravenously received unlabeled mouse IgG. These patients cleared the labeled antibody much more rapidly into the liver and the tumor uptake was reduced. Besides this more rapid clearance, one could also expect a serum sickness when large quantities of antibodies are infused into a patient possessing pre-existing anti-species immunoglobulins. Davies et al.[33] have reported on the presence of anti-mouse immunoglobulin in a patient who was scheduled for radioimmunolocalization. The pharmacokinetics of the injected monoclonal antibody in this patient did not significantly differ from the other 10 patients studied. All these results concerning the possible significance of pre-existing anti-species antibody or shedded tumor antigens are not homogenous and may differ depending on the type and malignancy of the tumor, the individuality of the patient, and the monoclonal antibody.

Further important points influencing the antibody delivery to the tumor are the blood flow through the tumor and the transfer of the antibody through the blood-brain barrier. The delivery of the antibody could be partially or completely blocked by a low blood flow. Blasberg et al.[34,35] have analyzed the regional blood flow in experimentally induced brain tumors and have found that the blood flow is variable within a tumor: lower in the center and higher in the periphery, very low in necrotic regions. The range of blood flow increases with the size of the tumor and the mean blood flow is a bit higher in small tumors than in larger tumors. The blood flow in the adjacent brain is lower than in the same anatomic region of the contralateral hemisphere, but is higher than in the tumor periphery. In the same model, Blasberg et al.[36] have examined the blood-to-tissue transport rate, which is influenced by the regional blood flow, the vascular permeability for the substance, the extent of vascularization and the extracellular fluid circulation. They have found that the mean rate for intracerebral gliomas is only two-fold higher than in the corresponding region of the contralateral site. The blood-to-tumor transport rate does not correlate with the localization, size, or histological classification of the tumor. These results indicate that the breakdown of the blood-brain barrier with the increased vascular permeability in brain tumors[37–39] does not necessarily lead to a free exchange between blood and brain tumor.

Supposing that the antibody has overcome all the limitations for its delivery and has specifically bound to the target antigen on the tumor cell surface, other events can occur which have not been observed in brain tumor models but which could prevent the desired antibody-mediated action in patients. Froese et al.[40] have observed an accelerated clearance rate of radioactivity from tumors after administration of a radiolabeled goat antitumor membrane antiserum into tumor-bearing mice. In vitro, they have confirmed the existence of an accelerated antibody metabolism in the presence of tumor cells due to an enzymatic degradation of cell-bound antibody.[41] Modulation of the surface antigen by the target cell after binding of the antibody is another mechanism by which a target cell can escape antibody-mediated effects. Pesando et al.[42] have demonstrated the modulation of CALLA by monoclonal antibody J5 by means of which the antigen is rapidly internalized and degraded. The antibody induces this antigenic modulation rapidly after addition to CALLA positive cell lines.[43] After modulation, there is a specific loss of antigen and antibody from the surface and the cells develop resistance to lysis with rabbit complement. The process is temperature-dependent and CALLA can be re-expressed after transfer into antibody-free medium.

Therapeutic Applications

Monoclonal antibodies could theoretically be used for glioma therapy by exerting a direct cytotoxic effect after binding to the target antigen.

Some monoclonal antibodies have been shown to have an antitumor effect.[44,54] A good correlation has been found between the in vivo antitumor effect and the in vitro antibody-dependent macrophage-mediated cytotoxicity, and macrophages are therefore believed to play an important role in the observed in vivo tumoricidal effect of these antibodies.[45,53] In the system of Seto et al.,[53] in which tumor cells pretreated with a monoclonal antibody were injected into syngenic mice, IgG2a showed the best suppression of tumor growth followed by IgG2b and IgG1 antibodies whereas IgM, IgG3, and IgA antibodies failed to show any significant effect. Concerning solid tumor systems, the antitumor effect of some monoclonal antibodies could be shown for colorectal carcinoma xenografted into nude mice,[44] for rat sarcomata xenografted into athymic rats,[53] and for nude mice bearing human melanoma cells.[52] Clinical studies exist only with patients suffering from leukemias or lymphomas.[46,47,49] B-cell lymphomas or leukemias present the possibility of studying the direct effect of monoclonal antibodies because each B-cell tumor expresses surface immunoglobulins that are monoclonal, and the idiotype of each lymphoma clone may be considered as a tumor-specific antigen, an ideal condition which does not exist in such heterogenous solid tumors as human gliomas.

Despite high complement-mediated cytotoxic titers, IgM does not show any antitumor activity by itself.[51] IgM-idiotypic monoclonal antibodies directed against tumor cells could be selectively activated for rendering macrophages tumoricidal when bound to the immunomodulating agent muramyldipeptide,[55] an example for the use of monoclonal antibodies as carrier of so-called "biological response modifiers." In this way, macrophages that infiltrate human brain tumors[56,57] could be stimulated to act against tumor cells without systemic effects. A further example of a monoclonal antibody conjugated with immunomodulating agents is the coupling to alpha-interferon,[58,59] with resulting natural killer cell activation.

Monoclonal Antibodies as Carriers of Plant and Bacterial Toxins

Abrin, ricin, and modeccin are related toxins which bind to similar glycoprotein cell surface receptors, enter the cell, and inhibit the protein synthesis. The binding to the surface receptor is mediated by binding of one unit, the B-chain, following which the toxic A-subunit enters the cell and exerts the toxic effect. The diphtheria toxin acts in a similar way. If the whole toxin is bound to an antibody, there is still an unspecific cytotoxicity due to binding of the B-subunit. This can be circumvented by conjugating only the toxic A-unit with the antibody which takes the place of B-subunit in the action of the toxin[60] or by using the whole toxin and saturating the galactose binding sites in the B-subunit with lactose.[61] The plant lectin gelonin has also a ribosomal inactivating activity like the A-unit or the above-mentioned toxins but lacks a B-subunit cell receptor binding site so that it can directly be bound to the antibody for an antibody-specific action. Immunotoxins—as these hybrid molecules of antibodies and toxins are called—develop specific cytotoxic effects to the target cells and fail to have any effect against cells not carrying the target antigen since the binding to a target is the precondition for any cytotoxic event. They have been used in in vitro systems against normal and neoplastic murine B-cells,[62] normal and neoplastic T cells,[61,63] against CALLA positive cells,[64] and against colorectal carcinoma cells.[65] Thorpe et al.[66] have conjugated gelonin with the monoclonal anti-Thy1.1 antibody and injected this conjugate into T-cell deprived mice bearing a Thy1.1 expressing lymphoma graft and could show a significantly prolonged survival of these mice. In another in vivo system, tumor cells could be removed from infiltrated murine bone marrow.[67] Cells treated this way were able to repopulate the hematopoetic system of lethally irradiated mice, the majority of which remained free of tumor. These trials with these well-acting conjugates have been performed in vitro or in nude mice and mostly concern lymphatic antigens. There are no corresponding trials with glioma cell lines or glioma xenografts, probably because of a lack of suitable antibodies and the heterogeneity of these tumors.

Monoclonal Antibodies as Carriers of Chemotherapeutic Agents

One disadvantage of conventional chemotherapy is the side effect to the whole nontumor-proliferating system. The idea of the antibody-drug conjugate is to achieve high drug delivery on the tumor target cell and to reduce the toxic effect on normal cells. The effectiveness of the drug-antibody or drug-carrier antibody conjugate is dependent upon the reactivity of the chemotherapeutic drug against the tumor cells, upon the specificity and affinity of the antibody, and upon the preservation of these features in the conjugate. Ford et al.[68] have demonstrated that the drug conjugation does not impair the antibody targeting in patients with metastatic carcinoma using radiolabeled vindesin-anti-CEA conjugate injected into patients for immunolocalizing studies. Uadia et al.[69] have shown in vitro that human melanoma cells M21 take up more methotrexate conjugated to a monoclonal antibody directed against human melanoma cells than methotrexate bound to rabbit anti-melanoma IgG absorbed with human red blood cells. The net uptake of methotrexate conjugated to polyclonal anti-melanoma antibody was better than that of free methotrexate or methothrexate linked to irrelevant immunoglobulin. Pimm et al.[70] have described the in vivo effect of an adriamycin-monoclonal antibody conjugate effective against rat mammary carcinoma cells. They have demonstrated the specific uptake of the antibody by rat carcinoma and when conjugated to adriamycin, the significantly retarded growth of the tumor and prolonged survival intumor-bearing rats at 1/25th of the effective dose of the free drug. Treatment with adriamycin mixed with the antibody or adriamycin conjugated to normal immunoglobulin did not significantly reduce the tumor growth. No such study has been carried out in comparable brain-tumor systems.

Radioimmunolocalization

Monoclonal antibodies can act as carriers for radionuclides. The radiolabeling of antibodies directed against tumor antigens and the radioimmunodetection by means of external scanning or direct measurement of radioactivity in the tumor and different tissues of nude mice is a prerequisite for estimating the enrichment of the antibody in the tumor.

The paired-label technique described by Pressman et al.[71] permits direct measurement of the intratumoral enrichment of the tumor-directed antibody due to its binding to the target antigen over the nonspecific accumulation. It allows, by help of a localization index[72] or a specificity index,[73] definition of specific antibody uptake and excludes factors such as vascularity, necrosis, extracellular space,[72] in vivo radiolysis, binding through the Fc-portion,[74] and uptake into the reticuloendothelial system since these factors apply equally to the control antibody and to the tumor-directed antibody. Pressman et al.[75] have demonstrated the localization of radiolabeled anti-mouse-Wagner-sarcoma antiserum in the tumor but also in the liver and kidney of tumor-bearing mice. Since it was possible in vitro to partially separate tumor-localizing antiserum from kidney- and liver-localizing antiserum, this phenomenon was not only caused by antiserum enrichment due to the previously mentioned mechanism but also by cross-reactivities due to unspecificity of the antibody.

Using the paired-label technique, Pressman et al.[71] could demonstrate a specific antibody uptake in lymphosarcomas grafted into rats. They radiolabeled the globulin fraction of the antiserum with one isotope (iodine-131) and the globulin fraction of normal serum with another isotope. The two preparations were simultaneously injected into tumor-bearing rats. By this technique, it has been found that the antiserum uptake in the tumor is not uniform and differs from one area to the other. Mach et al.[73] could show, with the nude mice model bearing human colon carcinoma grafts, that goat antiserum against the CEA was enriched up to nine times higher in the tumor than in the liver, whereas the activity of the labeled control-IgG was never found to be more than 2.3 times higher in the tumor than in the liver.

Moshakis et al.[76] injected ^{125}I-labeled monoclonal antibody binding to germ cell tumor membrane and ^{131}I-labeled control IgG into immunosuppressed mice bearing xenografts of several types of germ cell tumors. On the autoradiography, the antibody was mostly seen in areas of high vascularity, whereas no localization occurred with radiolabeled normal IgG. In experiments[72] with the same model, they have demonstrated that it is possible, using the paired label method, to show an enrichment of specific antibody in the xenografted tumors due to its binding to tumor antigen because the uptake of the antibody by the tumor was higher than in blood or normal tissue, a condition which was not observed for the normal IgG or an indifferent monoclonal antibody. Furthermore, the localization of the radiolabeled-specific antibody could be blocked by an excess of unlabeled antibody and no localization could be shown for nongerm-cell tumor xenografts. Among normal organs, the liver had the highest uptake of specific antibody, whereas muscle and intestine had the lowest. When examining the antibody clearance, the decrease of the specific antibody was slower in the tumor than in blood or normal tissue, whereas the IgG behaved indifferently and the concentration in tumors and other tissues was always lower than in blood. The localization to the tumor increased with decreasing weight of the tumor. The same observation was made by Buchegger et al.,[77] who have worked with nude mice bearing human colon carcinoma grafts and have examined the localization of monoclonal antibody against CEA obtaining a 7- to 15-fold higher tumor antibody uptake than in the whole mouse with specificity indices of localization of 3.4 to 6.8 at day 4–5 after injection. Epenetos et al.[78] have observed an increasing nonspecific uptake proportionally to the size of the tumor in a nude mouse model, using a monoclonal antibody against an epithelial cell antigenic determinant, an epithelial proliferating antigen. This increasing nonspecific uptake may be one reason for the better antibody localization in smaller-sized tumors, but this fact may also be related to the blood supply of the surrounding tissue which has also been observed by Epenetos et al.[78] as an important factor for the degree of antibody uptake. Ballou et al.[79] have obtained similar results by comparing the localization of ^{131}I-labeled monoclonal antibodies against murine teratocarcinoma. Pictures were taken after subsequent injection of ^{123}I-labeled control IgG and a mixture of both into teratocarcinoma-bearing mice.

Because of the high immunogenicity and the delayed clearance of whole antibodies as described by Smith et al.[80] and because of the direct binding of the whole antibody to complement and Fc receptor-bearing cells such as macrophages and hepatocytes (Hopf et al.[74]), several researchers have compared the distribution and elimination of whole radiolabeled antibodies, F(ab')2-fragments and Fab-fragments. Buchegger et al.[77] have obtained in the nude mouse model, using the F(ab')2-fragments, specificity indices ranging between 5.3 and 8.2 at day 3 and, using the Fab-fragments, between 12 and 19 at day 2 to 3. With double label studies in human colon carcinoma xenografted into hamsters and using monoclonal antibodies against CEA and its fragments F(ab')2 and Fab as well as control radiolabeled monoclonal IgG with its corresponding fragments, Wahl et al.[81] have demonstrated that radiolabeled F(ab')2-fragments are better suitable for scintigraphy than radiolabeled Fab or whole antibody, because the images obtained with the F(ab')2-fragments delineated the tumor earlier and with less background radioactivity than intact antibody at comparable time points. Herlyn et al.[82] have obtained similar results in immunosuppressed mice xenografted with human colon carcinoma, using radiolabeled whole antibody and F(ab')2-fragments binding to human tumors of the gastrointestinal tract. F(ab')2-fragments are cleared faster from the tumors, therefore the dose of F(ab')2-fragments has to be larger. However, even with a larger dose, the total radiation exposure would be less than with radiolabeled whole antibody, because of the faster clearance.[81] Images with Fab-fragments are not satisfactory.[81] The tumor as well as the whole body, especially the kidney, were visualized. The lower molecular weight and rapid in vivo deiodination could be the reason for this rapid clearance. Two days after injection, most of the Fab was excreted with only low tumor uptake.

Goldman et al.[83] have worked with nude mice bearing xenografts of human neuroblastoma and radiolabeled anti-neuroectodermal monoclonal antibody UJ13A. They did not apply the paired-label method but injected a radiolabeled irrelevent IgG into animals of a tumor-bearing control group. In the xenografted mouse, there was a 4 to 23 times greater uptake of the antibody than in blood 5 to 6 days after injection, whereas in the control group no uptake could be shown. Stavrou et al.[84] have demonstrated localization of a monoclonal antibody raised against membrane components of an experimental rat glioma using as control radiolabeled irrelevant IgG injected into a group of tumor-bearing mice. The tumor was detectable 2 days after injection of the radiolabeled antibody and the results obtained by external scanning of both groups together with the tissue counting of the activity indicate an antibody uptake due to its specificity.

Bourdon et al.[85] have radiolabeled the antiglioma monoclonal antibody 81C6[7] which defines a GMEM antigen. They have shown in paired-label analysis that the monoclonal antibody localizes due to its specificity in two GMEM antigen expressing gliomas which were xenografted subcutaneously and intracranially into athymic mice. There were peak levels of antibody uptake in subcutaneous as well as in intracranial xenografts 1 to 2 days after injection of the antibody and the levels were held for the next 5 to 7 days. In the tissue autoradiography of the subcutaneous xenograft, the distribution of the antibody corresponded to the extracellular stroma in the tumor like the distribution of the GMEM antigen demonstrated in PAP stainings of frozen sections. Furthermore, the antibody could be eluted as a single peak. The localization could be inhibited by infusion of unlabeled monoclonal antibody. Comparing the localization and imaging properties of radiolabeled 81C6 with radiolabeled unspecific control monoclonal antibodies in athymic rats intracranially inoculated with a human glioma cell line, Bullard et al.[86] have shown that 81C6 is significantly better for imaging small and intermediate-sized tumors than control antibody. Large tumors were visualized by both antibodies, but higher quality scans were obtained earlier and more frequently with the specific antibody. The levels of the unspecific antibody in the tumor were significantly higher than in normal brain but also significantly lower than those achieved with the specific antibody. These experimental data provide evidence that in immunosuppressed mouse or rat, the localization of antitumor antibody is possible, that this localization is demonstrable and can be differentiated from unspecific accumulation.

Clinical experiments for the radioimmunodetection of gliomas in patients began early[87–89] with ^{125}I-radiolabeled anti-glioma antiserum. Fe, ^{131}I-albumin, or globulin were taken as controls. The excision of the glioma was performed 3 to 5 days after intracarotid application of the radiolabeled antiserum and control. Autoradiography[89] showed a close relationship between the distribution of the ^{125}I-labeled anti-glioma antiserum and the tumor cell distribution and this localization was distinct from the pictures obtained with the control. In two of five cases, Day et al.[87] obtained clear evidence of radiolocalization by external scanning and autoradiography after surgery, and two cases were borderline. Two decades later, Phillips et al.[90,91] have published results indicating that they could localize a human glioma in one patient by means of radiolabeled human monoclonal antibodies raised after hybridization of the patient's intratumoral lymphocytes with a human myeloma cell line. With the labeled monoclonal anti-neuroectodermal antibody UJ13A,[12] Goldman et al.[83] successfully demonstrated the primary tumor after 24 hours and improved clarity by taking the scans 3 days later in six of nine patients with histologically confirmed neuroblastoma. Localization in the brain was not demonstrable because of the blood-brain barrier, although the antibody is known to be reactive with normal brain.[12] Although these results were promising, they failed to rule out unspecific localization.

Several studies have been done with radiolabeled antisera against different tumor antigens: for example, lymphoscintigraphic studies using radiolabeled anti-CEA antiserum,[92] radioimmunodetection of cancers with radiolabeled antiserum against alpha-fetoprotein,[93] radioimmunodetection of primary and metastatic ovarian cancers using radiolabeled antiserum against CEA.[94] These studies indicate that a truly tumor-specific antigen is not required for radioimmunolocalization. By means of radiolabeled antisera against CEA, carcinomas could be detected with a high true positive rate (ranging between 70% and 90%) and a high true negative rate (ranging between 83% and 100%) for different tumor types by external body scanning.[95] In these studies, only the external scanning with computer-assisted blood pool subtraction of 99m-technetium (^{99m}Tc) background activity were used.[96] These studies are more optimistic than those performed by Mach et al.,[31] using external scanning with the computerized substraction of the blood pool activity as well as a direct tissue counting by means of the double-label technique in some patients. Scans clearly revealed tumors in only 11 of 27 patients with carcinomas and doubtfully in eight further patients when interpreted by somebody who did not know the localization of the tumor. Despite the evidence of specific antibody-enrichment as obtained by the paired-label technique, they found that the total amount of specific antibody uptake was only 0.1% of the injected dose. They have obtained better results[97] with a monoclonal antibody against an antigen expressed by colorectal carcinomas: using the intact antibody, 51%

of the sites could be detected. The antibody concentration in the resected tumor was 3.6 to 6.3 times higher than in adjacent normal tissue with specificity indices ranging from 2.1 to 5.1 as estimated by means of tissue counting with the double label method.

Farrands et al.[98] have obtained similar optimistic results demonstrating tumor detection by external scanning in 10 of 11 patients. There was no intense localization of radioactivity in liver and spleen, which is surprising, since high unspecific uptake by the liver is the main problem in the nude mouse system.[72] Larson et al.[32] have imaged melanoma patients with ^{131}I-labeled monoclonal antibodies. Fifty percent of the activity carried by whole antibody was taken up by the liver. Mach et al.[31,99] have described a high nonspecific antibody uptake in the liver of patients without demonstrable liver metastases. Based on the experiences of using radiolabeled fragments in the nude mouse model,[77,81,82] some researchers have used radiolabeled F(ab')2-fragments in patients[97,99,100] and could confirm the results obtained in nude mice: F(ab')2-fragments localize faster in the tumor with less unspecific enrichment and slightly higher percentage of positive results. The clearance of Fab-fragments[32] was faster as compared to whole antibody (t1/2 for Fab: 20 min, t1/2 for 90% of the whole antibody: 31 hours). Chatal et al.,[100] detecting gastrointestinal cancers, obtained images with the sharpest contrast using whole antibody after 7 to 8 days and using F(ab')2-fragments after 4 to 5 days. Using F(ab')2-fragments, Mach et al. observed a decreased nonspecific uptake of radioactivity in the liver[99] and 61% positive results in the scans compared to 51% by using whole antibody.[97]

The immunolocalization studies on children with neuroblastoma had been preceded by similar work using nonhuman primates. These studies also showed that the radiolabeled antibody was unable to cross the normal blood-brain barrier. In the knowledge that the blood-brain barrier within cerebral tumors is disrupted,[37,38] the anti-neuroectodermal antibody UJ13A was used in a trial of radioimmunolocalization.[16] In 12 cases of cerebral tumors, the majority being astrocytomas grade III–IV, whole antibody was employed, labeled with 1 to 2 mCi of [131]I. Initial diagnosis had been made by CT scan and gamma scanning with ^{99m}Tc-glucoheptonate was carried out in order to assess the permeability of the blood-brain barrier. In most cases, positive scintigrams were obtained, highest levels of radionuclide uptake in tumor occurring between 4 and 24 hours, and tumor images being subjectively maximal at about 5 days (Fig. 1). Surgical

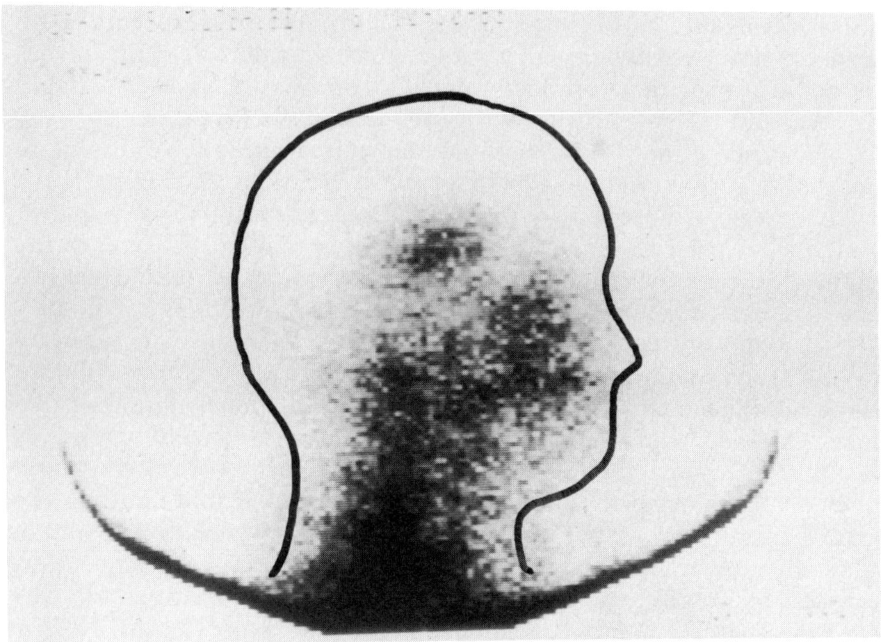

Figure 1. A right lateral scintigram of a patient with an anaplastic astrocytoma of the temporal region. This image was obtained 5 days after intravenous administration of 2 mCi ^{131}I labeled to monoclonal antibody UJ13A. In addition to the tumor image, a blood pool image of the face and neck is seen.

resection was carried out at an appropriate interval following intravenous injection of immunoconjugate, so that direct measurements of radioactivity in tumor and normal brain could be obtained. Using histological control, measurements were made from viable tumor, necrotic tumor, cyst fluid, and brain adjacent to tumor. Temporalis muscle and blood were also taken. Tumor to brain ratios of up to 16:1 were obtained but it must be noted that the normal brain was usually sufficiently close to tumor to be either infiltrated or edematous. The brain uptake of the ^{131}I-UJ13A in these samples was therefore higher than expected. In one case of long-standing oligo-astrocytoma, there had been recent clinical deterioration due to a small area of higher malignancy within the tumor. This region enhanced with intravenous contrast on CT scan and also took up technetium-glucoheptonate. However, uptake of the larger molecules of radiolabeled antibody in this region was minimal.[101] This variation in blood-brain barrier permeability, which is both regional and quantitative, has been previously described in animal models.[36,102]

The accessibility of brain tumor cells to intravenously administered radiolabeled antibody is unfortunately not good. In the above experiments, whole antibody was used and measurements on resected tumor showed that less than 0.005% of the injected dose was delivered to each gram of tumor. Unless major improvements can be made, this dose would be inadequate for antibody-guided radiation by the intravenous route. Another problem concerns the high level of control antibody which is found in the tumor. When a true antibody, distinctively labeled with ^{125}I is injected simultaneously with the ^{131}I-labeled experimental antibody, a large amount of nonspecific accumulation is found in viable tumor areas and also in necrosis and cyst fluid where levels of experimental and control antibody may be even higher.[103] This nonspecific pooling effect has been previously shown with albumin and is presumably a property of the interstitial space of gliomas. Also, immunoglobulin may be bound by the Fc receptors of benign or malignant astrocytes. Strategies for improving delivery of radiolabeled antibody to tumor cells will be discussed later.

Radiotherapy

Based on experience with immunodetection, some investigators have labeled monoclonal antibodies for therapeutic irradiation of human malignancies.[104–108] Courtenay-Luck et al.[107] have injected a radiolabeled monoclonal antibody against a tumor-associated antigen intrapleurally, intracardially, and intraperitoneally into patients with corresponding malignant effusions and could reveal regressions. An important point of this work is the administration of the radiolabeled antibody into the anatomical compartment involved by tumor thus circumventing all problems which exist when the radiolabeled antibody is given by the intravascular route. Coakham et al.[105] have used the same advantage with intrathecal application of a radiolabeled monoclonal antibody recognizing an oncofetal neuroblast antigen (UJ181.4) in a patient suffering from neoplastic meningitis due to a pineal carcinoma. Epenetos et al.[104] have treated a patient with recurrent grade IV glioma with an intracarotid infusion of a radiolabeled monoclonal antibody against epidermal growth factor receptor and blood group A antigen. This infusion was followed by clinical improvement and decreased tumor size and edema was shown by computerized tomography. After Jones et al.[106] had shown a tumoricidal effect of radiolabeled antibody defining a neuroectodermal antigen in nude mice xenografted with human neuroblastoma, Kemshead et al.[108] carried out a clinical study in which they tested the effect of monoclonal radiolabeled antibody in neuroblastoma patients and in two patients with neoplastic meningitis from neuroectodermally derived brain tumors. In the neuroblastoma patients as well as in the patients with the brain tumors, small tumor deposits were more responsive to therapy. In this study, the administration of the radiolabeled antibody to the brain tumor patients was performed intrathecally. Although isotope was seen in blood, there was no detectable liver and spleen uptake as demonstrated by scintigraphy.

Immunohistochemistry

Immunohistological techniques in brain tumor diagnosis have become well established.[109,110] Monoclonal antibodies have added an important new dimension to this technique. Certain hetero-antisera are highly specific and valuable in immunohistology but suffer from limitation of supply and batch-to-batch variation. However, a good monoclonal antibody can be distributed in virtually unlimited quantities to laboratories throughout the world thus permitting uniformity of results. Also, new antigens are continually being recognized by monoclonal antibodies as a result of being selected by the immune system of the immunized mouse. This avoids the biochemical purification of antigens necessary to produce a good specific antiserum.

Monoclonal antibodies now exist which can readily distinguish different cell types by recognizing differentiation antigens present in the cytoplasm on the cell surface. The application of these antibodies in diagnosis has recently been reviewed.[111] Using a large panel of monoclonal antibodies directed against differentiation antigens (such as glial fibrillary acidic protein, neuroectodermal antigens, and lymphoid differentiation antigens), against epithelial proliferation antigens and against oncofetal antigens, it is possible to give cerebral gliomas, medulloblastomas, neurinomas, meningiomas, metastatic carcinomas, and primary cerebral lymphomas, respectively, a characteristic picture of reactivities corresponding to their antigenic profiles.[112,113] Coakham et al.[112] recognized the most important advantage in the classification of neuroblastic and primitive tumors of childhood to be the differential diagnosis of secondary carcinomas and in classifying brain lymphomas, which significantly contributes to the final diagnosis in approximately 20% of cases.[113] The worth of using a panel of monoclonal antibodies for the differential diagnosis of lymphoblastomas and lymphoblastic disorders has been underlined by Kemshead et al.,[114] who examined bone marrow aspirates, tumor sections, and malignant effusions. Allan et al.[115] used a panel of monoclonal antibodies for classifying brain lymphomas. For the future, Coakham et al.[112] have considered a more biological classification of primary cerebral tumors by identifying antigenic phenotypes.

The application of this technique also helps to identify malignant cells in the cerebrospinal fluid.[112,113,116] Garson et al.[113] demonstrated the occurrence of malignant cells in the cerebrospinal fluid of 21 of 22 cases and were able to assign them to one of four categories: carcinoma, neuroectodermal tumor (excluding melanoma), melanoma, or lymphoma. Li et al.,[116] examining cerebrospinal fluid, established the diagnosis of B-cell non-Hodgkin's lymphoma in six of nine cases and could differentiate this diagnosis from a reactive lymphocytosis in the remaining three cases.

Preliminary Results Obtained with Monoclonal Antibody Mel-14

In the following, results are presented concerning the anti-melanoma antibody, MeI-14, which recognizes a neuroectodermal antigen present on the majority of gliomas. It was raised by Carrel et al.[9] after immunization of mice with a membrane-enriched fraction from the melanoma cell line Me-43 and following somatic cell fusion of their spleen cells with the mouse myeloma cell line P3-NSI/1Ag4. MeI-14, which is an IgG2 antibody,[117] has been shown to recognize a polypeptide with a molecular weight of 230.[118] It was positive in antibody binding radioimmunoassay for all 16 melanoma cell lines tested without any significant reactivity to 29 control non-melanoma cell lines.[9] In further studies,[5,10,117,118] it was found that MeI-14 also reacts with gliomas, neuroblastomas, and medulloblastomas. Forty-eight percent of the 45 glioma cell lines tested were found to be positive in antibody binding radioimmunoassay, as well as two of the three neuroblastoma and medulloblastoma cell lines tested.

One hundred thirty-two brain tumors have been tested in our laboratory for reactivity with MeI-14 in immunohistochemistry on frozen sections and using the avidin-biotin-immunoperoxidase method.[119] The brain tumors were obtained after surgical resection: 4 oligodendrogliomas; 16 grade I and II astrocytomas; 8 grade III astrocytomas; 35 glioblastomastomas, including 4 grade IV astrocytomas; 8 ependymomas and ependymoblastomas; 3 germinomas; 11 neurinomas; 24 meningiomas; 18 metastasis; and a mixed group, containing 1 foreign-body granuloma, 1 fibroma, 1 chordoma, 1 colloid cyst, and 1 craniopharyngioma. Very strikingly, MeI-14 binds to the endothelial cells within the tumors, whereas the vessels in three specimens of normal brain were negative. As shown in Fig. 2, more than 50% of all tumors have some endothelial cells binding MeI-14.

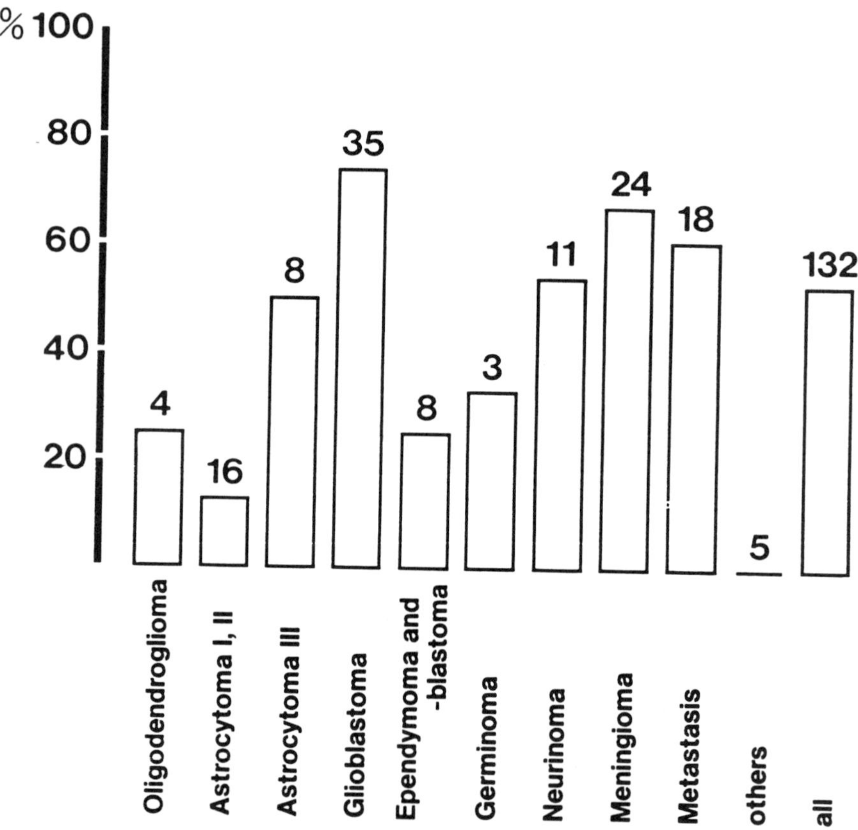

Figure 2. The number of tumors with Mel-14-positive endothelial cells (in %) according to histological diagnosis.

The highest number was found in the glioblastoma group with nearly 75%. As shown in Figure 3, vessels of glioblastomas contained the highest proportion of positive endothelial cells with a mean value of 80%. A positive correlation between the malignancy and the presence of positive endothelial cells within the glioma groups occurs in two respects: As shown in Figure 1, the number of positive tumors increases from low grade astrocytomas to grade III astrocytomas up to grade IV astrocytomas and glioblastomas. The same correlation is seen for the proportion of positive endothelial cells within the tumors of increasing degree of malignancy (Fig. 3). The high number of positive metastases (over 50%) and the high proportion of positive endothelial cells (65% in the group of the positive metastases and 40% for the whole group) is remarkable. Since meningiomas had a similar binding of MeI-14 as the group of metastases, this feature cannot be regarded as a general marker of malignancy.

These results are comparable to the results of Schreyer et al.,[6] who tested besides gliomas also normal brain, normal skin, normal spleen, and normal thymus. They observed that MeI-14 did not stain, or stained only very slightly, the blood vessels in the normal tissues.

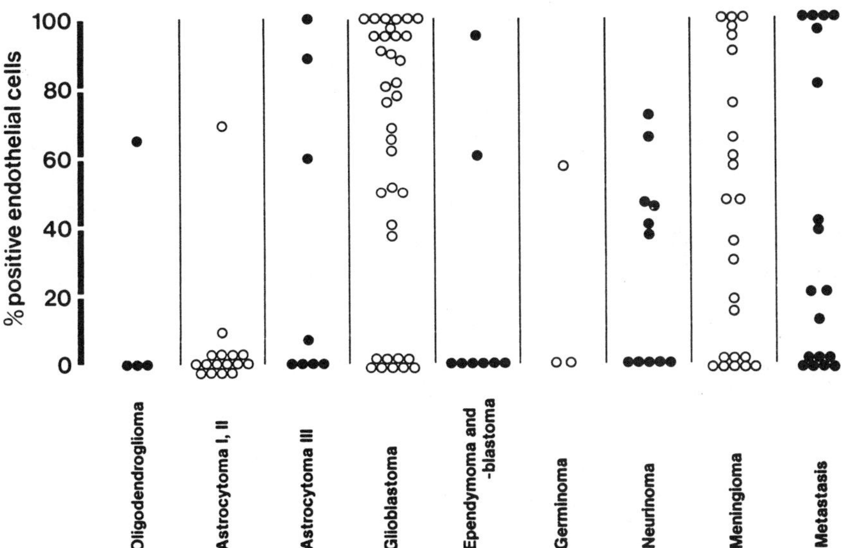

Figure 3. The number of Mel-14-positive endothelial cells (in %) according to histological diagnosis.

Wikstrand et al.[120] have radiolabeled MeI-14 with ^{125}I to study its immunolocalization in nude mice xenografted subcutaneously with human gliomas. Using the paired label method, they found evidence for specific uptake of MeI-14 into the tumor with specificity indices ranging from 2 to 5 relative to the blood pool activity.

The results of one case will now be presented. This patient was scheduled for surgical resection of a glioblastoma and preoperatively received radiolabeled monoclonal antibody MeI-14 for in vivo localization of the antibody in the tumor. F(ab')2-fragments of MeI-14 were labeled with ^{123}I and ^{125}I and as a control, F(ab')2-fragments of an irrelevant IgG were labeled with ^{131}I using the iodogen method[121,122] and filtered on a Sephadex-G-25 column equilibrated in pyrogen-free 0.15 M saline. The ^{123}I has a physical half-life of 13 hours and was used only for external scanning, whereas labeling with ^{125}I allows later in vitro measurement of radioactivity. The patient had no personal or family history of allergy and received 2 mg clemastine p.o. and 100 mg prednisolone i.v. 1 hour before the injection, and 400 mg perchlorate on the day of the injection. Ten drops of Lugol 5% iodine solution p.o. every day for 5 days beginning on the day before the injection were also given. The mixture of ^{125}I- and ^{123}I-labeled F(ab')2-fragments of MeI-14 and ^{131}I-F(ab')2-fragments of an irrelevant IgG was diluted in 100 ml 0.9% NaCl solution and injected intravenously over 30 minutes. The patient was tested by computerized tomoscintigraphy at 6 and 24 hours after injection. Three days after injection, the operation was performed. Activities of both isotopes ^{125}I and ^{131}I were counted at later time points in tumor and normal tissues. Tumor material was also used for immunohistochemistry with MeI-14 using the biotin-avidin-peroxidase method and also cultured in monolayer to obtain cells for the antibody binding radioimmunoassay with MeI-14. Cells were tested after the second passage at 6 weeks. Figure 4 shows vessels from the tumor region with typical positive endothelial cells. The endothelial cells were counted and more than 95% were found to bind MeI-14.

In the antibody binding radioimmunoassay, radiolabeled MeI-14 had an activity of 15 times the background activity resulting in a binding ratio of 15, which is considered to be strongly positive. The immunohistochemistry and the antibody binding radioimmunoassay indicate that MeI-14 binds in the tumor both to the endothelial cells and to the tumor cells.

The activities of ^{125}I ⟨=antibody F(ab')2⟩ per gram resected tumor and tissue specimen as well as the activities of ^{131}I ⟨=control

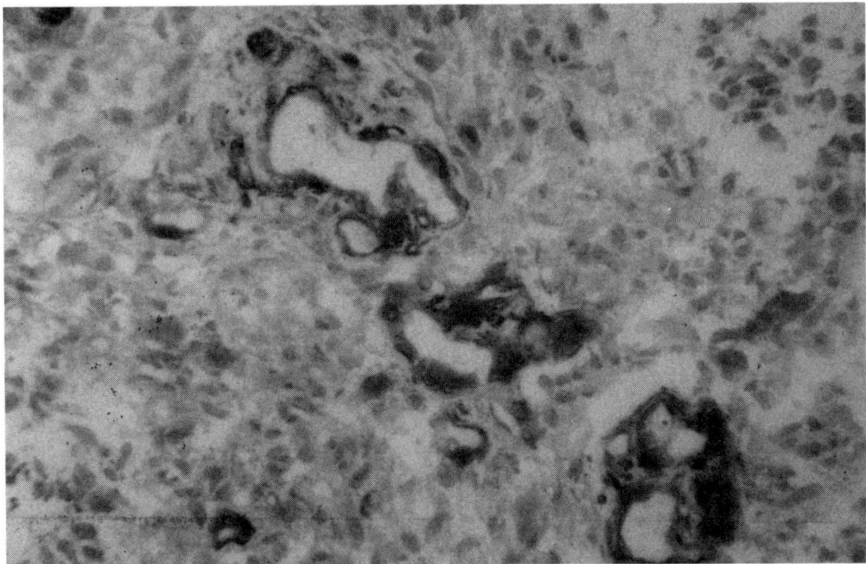

Figure 4. Immunohistological localization of the antigen recognized by monoclonal antibody Mel-14 on a cryostat section of a glioblastoma using avidin-biotin-peroxidase technique with aminocarbazole as chromogen and hematoxylin counter-staining. The endothelial cells of the tumor vessels are strongly positive. (Magnification ×100.)

F(ab')2⟩ per gram are represented in Figure 5. The activity of ^{125}I per gram resected tumor was 13.95 times higher than in resected normal brain, whereas for ^{131}I, it was 5.51 times higher in tumor than in normal brain, resulting in a specific index of localization of 2.53 (Fig. 6). The same ratios for tumor and blood gave values of 2.29 for ^{125}I and 0.42 for ^{131}I, resulting in a specificity index of 5.39. The values were obtained by taking the average of two different tumor specimens. Figure 7 shows the specificity indices for a tumor specimen which was rich in blood vessels. The tumor-to-brain ratio for the ^{125}I was 18.45 and for the ^{131}I was 5.87, resulting in a specificity index of 3.15. The increased antibody uptake of this vessel-rich tumor part is not due to higher blood content or accumulation of interstitial fluid in the tumor, because any increase of blood or serum in the tumor would also increase the accumulation of ^{131}I-bound activity, resulting in a lower specificity index. Whether the better values for the vessel-rich part are due to increased binding to the more numerous endo-

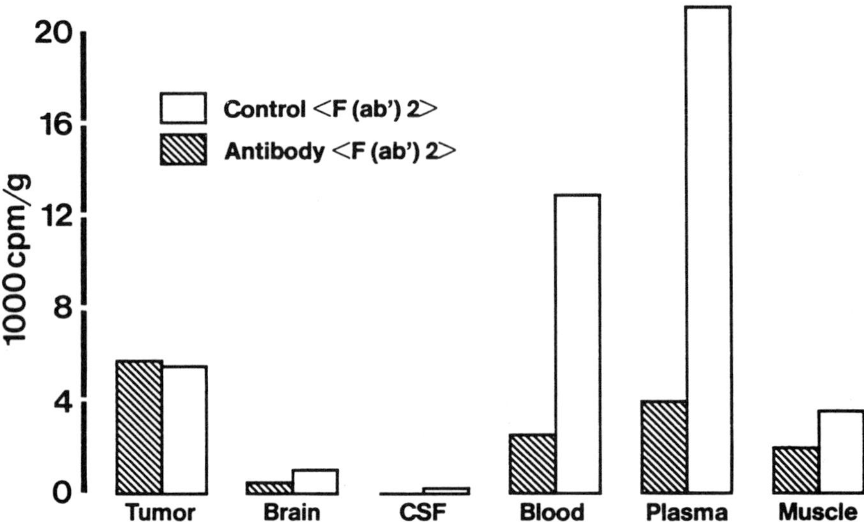

Figure 5. Activity of [125]I [F(ab')2-antibody] and of [131]I [F(ab')2-control] per gram of the tissue. The value for the tumor represents an average of two specimens.

thelial cells or to a better antibody clearance caused by a higher blood to tumor transport rate with following specific binding to tumor cells cannot be decided here. The results indicate that there is some accumulation of specific antibody and control antibody in the tumor but there also is a definitely higher uptake of the antibody due to its specificity. Despite these results, the external detection of tumor by tomoscintigraphy was difficult because of accumulation of antibody fragments in the skull.

Coakham et al. (manuscript in preparation) have used radiolabeled MeI-14 after radioimmunolocalization for treatment of one patient who was seriously ill with neoplastic meningitis due to a melanoma strongly positive for MeI-14 as shown by immunofluorescence and immunoperoxidase on a stereotactically guided biopsy. The therapeutic dose of 39.86 mCi, given by the intrathecal route, resulted in a marked clinical improvement and remission as could be documented by CT-scan.

Discussion

Immunolocalization can be improved in several different ways. Delivery of the immunoconjugate to brain tumor cells is a crucial

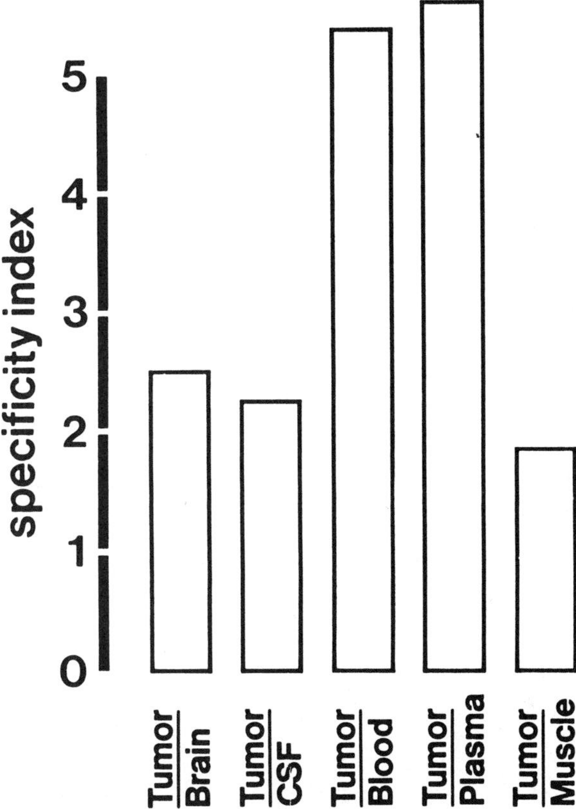

Figure 6. Specificity indices of the reported case. The values refer to an average of two tumor specimens.

aspect. Coakham and Kemshead's group[105,108] have chosen the intrathecal route, because brain tumor scintigraphy studies indicate that very low amounts of Ig given intravenously enter primary tumors of neuroectodermal origin. They proposed a ^{99m}Tc scan to document blood-brain barrier breakdown before immunolocalization. It is possible to open the blood-brain barrier with an intracarotid perfusion of 1.4 M mannitol or 1.6 M arabinose in immature Fischer-344 rats.[123] An enhanced methotrexate delivery to the CNS of normal rats and avian sarcoma virus-induced rat glioma could be shown after intracarotid hyperosmolar mannitol infusion.[124,125] Intracarotid perfusion with these hyperosmolar agents was required in Fischer-344 rats to disrupt the blood-brain barrier and to significantly elevate the brain

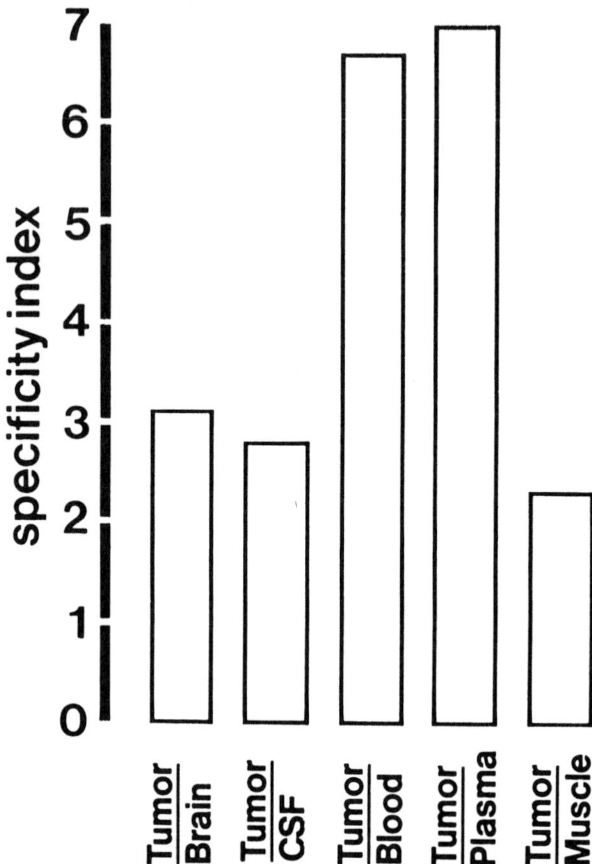

Figure 7. Specificity indices of the reported case. The values refer to the tumor specimen giving the highest antibody to control ratio of activity.

levels following intracarotid or intravenous administration of monoclonal antibodies.[126] No difference was seen between intracarotid and intravenous administration of monoclonal antibodies with or without disruption of the blood-brain barrier, but the interhemispheric level was dependent on the site of perfusion with the hyperosmolaric agent. Intracarotid hyperosmolar perfusion produced 450% to 500% ipsilateral increased brain-to-blood ratios of monoclonal antibody and 240% to 280% contralateral. The intravenous infusion of 1.4 M mannitol or 1.6 M arabinose did not lead to higher brain-to-blood levels of the monoclonal antibodies.

The tumor-to-blood ratio can also be increased by acceleration of the background clearance. A possibility for reducing the background activity would be to remove the "first" antibody, the monoclonal antitumor antibody, from the circulation and extravasal space. Trials have been performed with a second antibody either liposomally entrapped[127,128] or not,[129] binding to the first antibody and removing these antibodies which are not bound to the target antigen, resulting in an eight-fold increase of tumor-to-blood ratios.[130]

A method for obtaining better tumor-to-tissue ratios, especially for radioimmunodetection, is to use indium-111 labeled antibodies.[131–133] There is less background activity due to an increased blood clearance and a longer accumulation of the radiolabeled antibody in the tumor, probably due to its stability,[132] so that the tumor-to-tissue ratio is increased.[131] An important disadvantage is that the clearance of the indium-111-chelate-antibody mainly occurs in the liver, leading to a high accumulation of radioactivity there, lasting up to one week.[131] Other methods for obtaining good tumor-to-tissue ratios of monoclonal antibodies concern the monoclonal antibodies themselves. As mentioned above, Fab- and F(ab')2-fragments have been used to reduce immunogenicity of the foreign antibodies, to improve the kinetics,[80] and to prevent binding to complement and Fc-receptor-bearing cells.[74]

A better occupation of the tumor cell surface with antibodies can be achieved by combining different monoclonal antibodies binding to different tumor target antigens as demonstrated by Treleaven et al.[134] They coated neuroblastoma cells from bone marrow with a panel of six monoclonal antitumor antibodies. After binding to the tumor cells, the monoclonal antibodies were bound to polystyrene microspheres which contained magnetide and had been preincubated with anti-mouse IgG. In this way, the coated tumor cells could be successfully removed from the bone marrow by a magnet.

Chimeric monoclonal antibodies may provide perspectives in the use of monoclonal antibodies by producing molecules consisting of variable regions from a mouse monoclonal antibody joined to a different isotypic human constant region or by producing molecules consisting of two different variable regions resulting in an antibody with dual specificity. The first would imitate a human antibody and provide the advantage of low immunogenicity and flexibility in choosing the Fc-portion properly with its effector function. The production of chimeric antibodies has been done by chemical recombination,[135] hybrid hybridomas,[136] and by transfectomas, combining the recombinant DNA techniques and gene transfection.[137–139] The bispecific chimeric antibody is of interest because one antigenic site could bind to a tumor antigen and the other could mediate the desired interaction, binding to cytotoxic T cells, to a radiolabeled agent, to an antitumor drug, a toxin, or an immunomodulating agent. This could be mediated, for example, by a hapten which binds to the second antigenic site and is also a target for a second antibody which would bind the tumoricidal agent. Raso and Griffin,[140] who were able to demonstrate that antibodies with such dual specificity can mediate the action of ricin to a target cell, proposed a two-step protocol for the use of ricin. In the first step, the tumor-directed and ricin-binding bispecific antibody is infused until neoplastic cells are maximally saturated. After an interval permitting clearance of unbound antibody, ricin, ricin plus lactose, or free A-chain is given, which will be bound by the still free ricin-binding site on the coated target cell, resulting in the destruction of this cell.

Despite these recent technical advances, antibody specificity remains a problem. Until now, no truly tumor-specific monoclonal antibody has been found. Tumor-associated antigens mark the tumor cells of interest, but are also present on other types of tumor cells, on fetal cells, or on normal adult cells. Monoclonal antibodies of "relative specificity" or "operational specificity" against tumor-associated antigens can be raised. A monoclonal antibody against a tumor-associated antigen can only be operational if the tumor-associated antigen is present on the tumor cells in much higher amounts than on their normal counterparts. If the antigen is also present in high amounts in normal tissues, these tissues should not be within reach of the monoclonal antibody.

The search for more specific tumor antigens is continuing, one example being the epidermal growth factor receptor (EGF-R). The EGF-R-mediated mechanisms appear to play an important role in the growth of malignancies and EGF-R was found to be increased on tumor cell lines and tumors. It is present in human squamous carcinoma cell lines[141] and human mammary carcinoma cell lines.[142] Besides the increased expression on human cervical, ovarian and vulval carcinomas,[143] and human sarcomas,[144] it was found to be increased in human brain tumors.[145] High levels of EGF-R as evaluated by its autophosphorylation enzymatic activity were preferentially obtained in gliomas and meningiomas, whereas the two examined neuroblastomas and the brains of patients who had died from diseases not related to the CNS showed significantly lower EGF-R-kinase activity. Libermann et al.[146] could show that in brain tumors of glial origin with enhanced expression of EGF-R, the receptor genes are amplified. Monoclonal antibodies have been raised against EGF-R.[147,148] The determinant recognized by a group of these antibodies[148] has been identified as the blood group A determinant which is present on EGF-R of A431 cells, but is not expressed on EGF-R of other human cells. Epenetos et al.[104] have performed the irradiation of a brain glioma by intracarotid infusion of this radiolabeled monoclonal antibody. Since the patient had the blood group O, the monoclonal antibody was considered to be operationally specific.

Platelet-derived growth factor (PDGF) has been shown to be a stimulator of human glial cells[149,150] and release of an analog of PDGF by glioma cells could be demonstrated.[151] Specific receptors for PDGF have been found on glioma cells[152] and may be a suitable target for monoclonal antibodies.

REFERENCES

1. Köhler G, Milstein C. Continuous cultures of fused cells secreting antibody of predefined specificity. Nature 1975; 256:495–497.
2. Schnegg JF, Diserens AC, Carrel S, Accolla RS, de Tribolet N. Human glioma-associated antigens detected by monoclonal antibodies. Cancer Res 1981; 411:1209–1213.
3. De Tribolet N, Carrel S, Mach JP. Brain-tumor-associated antigens. In: Homburger F (ed). Prog Exp Tumor Res (Basel) 1984; 27:118–131.
4. De Muralt B, de Tribolet N, Diserens AC, Carrel S, Mach JP. Reactivity of antiglioma monoclonal antibodies for a large panel of cultured gliomas and other neuroectoderm derived tumors. Anticancer Res 1983; 3:1–6.
5. De Muralt B, de Tribolet N, Diserens AC, Stavrou D, Mach JP, Carrel S. Phenotyping of 60 cultured human gliomas and 34 other neuroectodermal tumors by means of monoclonal antibodies against glioma, melanoma and HLA-DR antigens. Eur J Cancer Clin Oncol 1985; 21:207–216.
6. Schreyer M, Hamou MF, Carrel S, Mach JP, de Tribolet N. Immunohistological localization of glioma- and melanoma-associated antigens with monoclonal antibodies. In: Staal GEJ, Veelen CWM (eds). Markers in Human Neuroectodermal Tumors. Boca Raton, Florida, CRC Press, 1986; pp. 53–62.
7. Bourdon MA, Wikstrand CJ, Furthmayr H, Matthews TJ, Bigner DD. Human glioma-mesenchymal extracellular matrix antigen defined by monoclonal antibody. Cancer Res 1983; 43:2796–2805.
8. Wikstrand CJ, Bigner SH, Bigner DD. Characterization of three restricted specific monoclonal antibodies raised against human glioma cell line D-54 MG. J Neuroimmunol 1984; 6:169–186.

9. Carrel S, Accolla RS, Carmagnola AL, Mach JP. Common human melanoma-associated antigen(s) detected by monoclonal and antibodies. Cancer Res 1980; 40:2523–2528.

10. Carrel S, de Tribolet N, Mach JP. Expression of neuroectodermal antigens common to melanomas, gliomas, and neuroblastomas. I. Identification by monoclonal anti-melanoma and anti-glioma antibodies. Acta Neuropathol (Berlin) 1982; 57:158–164.

11. Herlyn M, Clark WH, Mastrangelo MJ, DuPont Guerry IV, Elder DE, LaRossa D, Hamilton R, Bondi E, Tuthill R, Steplewski Z, Koprowski H. Specific immunoreactivity of hybridoma-secreted monoclonal anti-melanoma antibodies to cultured cells and freshly derived human cells. Cancer Res 1980; 40:3602–3609.

12. Allan PM, Garson JA, Harper EI, Asser U, Coakham HB, Brownell B, Kemshead JT. Biological characterization and clinical applications of a monoclonal antibody recognizing an antigen restricted to neuroectodermal tissues. Int J Cancer 1983; 31:591–598.

13. Dippold WG, Lloyd KO, Li LTC, Ikeda H, Oettgen HF, Old LJ. Cell surface antigens of human malignant melanoma: Definition of six antigenic systems with mouse monoclonal antibodies. Proc Natl Acad Sci USA 1980; 77:6114–6118.

14. Wikstrand CJ, Bigner DD. Use of monoclonal antibodies in neurobiology and neuro-oncology. In: Sell S, Reisfeld R (eds). Monoclonal Antibodies in Cancer. Clifton, Humana Press, 1985; pp. 365–397.

15. Wikstrand CJ, Bigner DD. Expression of human fetal brain antigens by human tumors of neuroectodermal origin as defined by monoclonal antibodies. Cancer Res 1982; 42:267–275.

16. Davies AG, Richardson RB, Bourne SP, Kemshead JT, Coakham HB. Immunolocalization of human brain tumors. In: Bleehen NM (ed). Tumours of the Brain. Berlin, Springer-Verlag, 1986; pp. 83–99.

17. Liao SK, Clarke BJ, Kwong PC, Brickenden A, Gallie BL, Dent PB. Common neuroectodermal antigens in human melanoma, neuroblatoma, retinoblastoma, glioblastoma and fetal brain revealed by hybridoma antibodies raised against melanoma cells. Eur J Immunol 1981; 11:450–454.

18. Seeger RC, Rosenblatt HM, Imai K, Ferrone S. Common antigenic determinants on human melanoma, glioma, neuroblastoma, and sarcoma cells defined with monoclonal antibodies. Cancer Res 1981; 41:2714–2717.

19. Garson JA, Beverley PCL, Coakham HB, Harper EI. Monoclonal antibodies against human T lymphocytes label Purkinje neurones of many species. Nature 1982; 298:375–377.

20. Kemshead JT, Fritschy J, Asser U, Sutherland R, Greaves MF. Monoclonal antibodies defining markers with apparent selectivity for particular haemopoietic cell types may also detect antigens on cells of neural crest origin. Hybridoma 1982; 1:109–123.

21. Carrel S, de Tribolet N, Gross N. Expression of HLA-DR and common acute lymphoblastic leukemia antigen on glioma cells. Eur J Immunol 1982; 12:354–357.

22. Carrel S, Heumann D, Sekaly RP, Zaech P, Buchegger F, Girardet C.

Characterization of a monoclonal antibody (A12) that defines a human acute lymphoblastic leukemia-associated differentiation antigen. Hybridoma 1983; 2:149–160.

23. Ritz J, Pesando JM, Notis-McConarty J, Lazarus H, Schlossman SF. A monoclonal antibody to human acute lymphoblastic leukemia antigen. Nature 1980; 283:583–585.

24. De Tribolet N, Hamou MF, Mach JP, Carrel S, Schreyer M. Demonstration of HLA-DR antigen in normal human brain. J Neurol Neurosurg Psychiatr 1984; 47:417–418.

25. Kemshead JT, Ritter MA, Cotmore SF, Greaves MF. Human Thy-1: Expression on the cell surface of neuronal and glial cells. Brain Res 1982; 236:451–461.

26. Seeger RC, Danon YL, Rayner SA, Hoover F. Definition of a Thy-1 determinant on human neuroblastoma, glioma, sarcoma, and teratoma cells with a monoclonal antibody. J Immunol 1982; 128:983–989.

27. Kennett RH, Gilbert F. Hybrid melanomas producing antibodies against a human neuroblastoma antigen present on fetal brain. Science 1979; 203:1120–1121.

28. Greaves MF, Verbi W, Kemshead J, Kennett R. A monoclonal antibody identifying a cell surface antigen shared by common acute lymphoblastic leukemias and B lineage cells. Blood 1980; 56:1141–1144.

29. Primus FJ, Bennett SJ, Kim EE, DeLand FH, Zahn MC, Goldenberg DM. Circulating immune complexes in cancer patients receiving goat radiolocalizing antibodies to carcinoembryonic antigen. Cancer Res 1980; 40:497–501.

30. Primus FJ, Goldenberg DM. Immunological considerations in the use of goat antibodies to carcinoembryonic antigen for the radioimmunodetection of cancer. Cancer Res 1980; 40:2976–2983.

31. Mach JP, Carrel S, Forni M, Ritschard J, Donath A, Alberto P. Tumor localization of radiolabeled antibodies against carcinoembryonic antigen in patients with carcinoma. N Engl J Med 1980; 303:5–10.

32. Larson SM, Brown JP, Wright PW, Carrasquillo JA, Hellström I, Hellström KE. Imaging of melanoma with ^{131}I-labeled monoclonal antibodies. J Nucl Med 1983; 24:123–129.

33. Davies AG, Bourne SP, Richardson RB, Czudek R, Wallington TB, Kemshead JT, Coakham HB. Pre-existing anti-mouse immunoglobulin in a patient receiving ^{131}I-murine monoclonal antibody for radioimmunolocalisation. Br J Cancer 1986; 53:289–292.

34. Blasberg RG, Kobayashi T, Horowitz M, Rice JM, Groothuis D, Molnar P, Fenstermacher JD. Regional blood flow in ethylnitrosurea-induced brain tumors. Ann Neurol 1983; 14:189–201.

35. Blasberg RG, Molnar P, Horowitz M, Kornblith P, Pleasants R, Fenstermacher J. Regional blood flow in RT-9 brain tumors. J Neurosurg 1983; 58:863–873.

36. Blasberg RG, Kobayashi T, Horowitz M, Rice JM, Groothuis D, Molnar P, Fenstermacher JD. Regional blood-to-tissue transport in ethylnitrosourea-induced brain tumors. Ann Neurol 1983; 14:202–215.

37. Groothuis DR, Fischer JM, Lapin G, Bigner, DD, Vick NA. Permeability

of different experimental brain tumor models to horseradish peroxidase. J Neuropathol Exp Neurol 1982; 41:164–185.

38. Groothuis DR, Vick NA. Brain tumors and the blood-brain barrier. Trends Neurosci 1982; 5:232–235.

39. Brightman MW, Klatzo I, Olsson Y, Reese TS. The blood-brain barrier to proteins under normal and pathological conditions. J Neurol Sci 1970; 10:215–239.

40. Froese G, Berczi I, Israels LG. Tumour cell-antibody interactions. I. In vivo experiments. Immunology 1982; 45:303–312.

41. Froese G, Berczi I, Israels LG. Tumour cell-antibody interactions. II. In vitro studies. Immunology 1982; 45:313–323.

42. Pesando JM, Ritz J, Lazarus H, Tomaselli KJ, Schlossman SF. Fate of a common acute lymphoblastic leukemia antigen during modulation by monoclonal antibody. J Immunol 1981; 126:540–544.

43. Ritz J, Pesando JM, Notis-McConarty J, Schlossman SF. Modulation of human acute lymphoblastic leukemia antigen induced by monoclonal antibody in vitro. J Immunol 1980; 125:1506–1514.

44. Herlyn DM, Steplewski Z, Herlyn MF, Koprowski H. Inhibition of growth of colorectal carcinoma in nude mice by monoclonal antibody. Cancer Res 1980; 40:717–721.

45. Herlyn D, Koprowski H. IgG2a monoclonal antibodies inhibit human tumor growth through interaction with effector cells. Proc Natl Acad Sci USA 1982; 79:4761–4765.

46. Nadler LM, Stashenko P, Hardy R, Kaplan WD, Button LN, Kufe DW, Antman KH, Schlossman SF. Serotherapy of a patient with a monoclonal antibody directed against a human lymphoma-associated antigen. Cancer Res 1980; 40:3147–3154.

47. Ritz J, Pesando JM, Sallan SE, Clavell LA, Notis-McConarty J, Rosenthal P, Schlossman SF. Serotherapy of acute lymphoblastic leukemia with monoclonal antibody. Blood 1981; 58:141–152.

48. Kirch ME, Hammerling U. Immunotherapy of murine leukemias by monoclonal antibody. I. Effect of passively administered antibody on growth of transplanted tumor cells. J Immunol 1981; 127:805–810.

49. Miller RA, Maloney DG, Warnke R, Levy R. Treatment of B-cell lymphoma with monoclonal anti-iodotype antibody. N Engl J Med 1982; 306:517–522.

50. Kennel SJ, Lankford T, Flynn KM. Therapy of a murine sarcoma using syngeneic monoclonal antibody. Cancer Res 1983; 43:2843–2848.

51. Ralph P, Nakoinz I. Cell-mediated lysis of tumor targets directed by murine monoclonal antibodies of IgM and all IgG isotypes. J Immunol 1983; 131:1028–1031.

52. Schulz G, Bumol TF, Reisfeld RA. Monoclonal antibody-directed effector cells selectively lyse human melanoma cells in vitro and in vivo. Proc Natl Acad Sci USA 1983; 80:5407–5411.

53. Seto M, Takahashi T, Nakamura S, Matsudaira Y, Nishizuka Y. In vivo antitumor effects of monoclonal antibodies with different immunoglobulin classes. Cancer Res 1983; 43:4768–4773.

54. North SM, Dean CJ: Monoclonal antibodies to rat sarcomata. II. A syn-

geneic IgG2b antibody with anti-tumor activity. Immunology 1983; 49:667–671.

55. Roche AC, Bailly P, Midoux P, Monsigny M. Selective macrophage activation by muramyldipeptide bound to monoclonal antibodies specific for mouse tumor cells. Cancer Immunol Immunother 1984; 18:155–159.

56. Morantz RA, Wood GW, Foster M, Clark M, Gollahon K. Macrophages in experimental and human brain tumors. Part 1: Studies of the macrophages content of experimental rat brain tumors of varying immunogenicity. J Neurosurg 1979; 50:298–304.

57. Morantz RA, Wood GW, Foster M, Clark M, Gollahon K. Macrophages in experimental and human brain tumors. Part 2: Studies of the macrophages content of human brain tumors. J Neurosurg 1979; 50:305–311.

58. Pelham JM, Gray JD, Flannery GR, Pimm MV, Baldwin RW. Interferon-alpha conjugation to human osteogenic sarcoma monoclonal antibody 791T/36. Cancer Immunol Immunother 1983; 15:210–216.

59. Flannery GR, Pelham JM, Gray JD, Baldwin RW. Immunomodulation: NK cells activated by interferon-conjugated monoclonal antibody against human osteosarcoma. Eur J Cancer Clin Oncol 1984; 20:791–798.

60. Raso V, Griffin T. Specific cytotoxicity of a human immunoglobulin-directed Fab'-ricin A chain conjugate. J Immunol 1980; 125:2610–2616.

61. Youle RJ, Neville DM. Anti-Thy 1.2 monoclonal antibody linked to ricin is a potent cell-type-specific toxin. Proc Natl Acad Sci USA 1980; 77:5483–5486.

62. Krolick KA, Villemez C, Isakson P, Uhr JW, Vitetta ES. Selective killing of normal or neoplastic B cells by antibodies coupled to the A chain of ricin. Proc Natl Acad Sci USA 1980; 77:5419–5423.

63. Blythman HE, Casellas P, Gros O, Gros P, Jansen FK, Paolucci F, Pau B, Vidal H. Immunotoxins: hybrid molecules of monoclonal antibodies and a toxin subunit specifically kill tumour cells. Nature 1981; 290:145–146.

64. Raso V, Ritz J, Basala M, Schlossman SF. Monoclonal antibody-ricin A chain conjugate selectively cytotoxic for cells bearing the common acute lymphoblastic leukemia antigen. Cancer Res 1982; 42:457–462.

65. Gilliland DG, Steplewski Z, Collier RJ, Mitchell KF, Chang TH, Koprowski H. Antibody-directed cytotoxic agents: Use of monoclonal antibody to direct the action of toxin A chains to colorectal carcinoma cells. Proc Natl Acad Sci USA 1980; 77:4539–4543.

66. Thorpe PE, Brown ANF, Ross WCJ, Cumber AJ, Detre SI, Edwards DC, Davies AJS, Stirpe F. Cytotoxicity acquired by conjugation of an anti-Thy1.1 monoclonal antibody and ribosome-inactivating protein, gelonin. Eur J Biochem 1981; 116:447–454.

67. Krolick KA, Uhr JW, Vitettra ES. Selective killing of leukemia cells by antibody-toxic conjugates: implications for autologous bone marrow transplantation. Nature 1982; 295:604–605.

68. Ford CHJ, Newman CE, Johnson JR, Woodhouse CS, Reeder TA, Rowland GF, Simmonds RG. Localisation and toxicity study of a vindesine-

anti-CEA conjugate in patients with advanced cancer. Br J Cancer 1983; 47:35–42.

69. Uadia P, Blair AH, Ghose T, Ferrone S. Uptake of methotrexate linked to polyclonal and monoclonal antimelanoma antibodies by a human melanoma cell line. J Natl Cancer Inst 1985; 74:29–35.

70. Pimm MV, Jones JA, Price MR, Middle JG, Embleton MJ, Baldwin RW. Tumour localization of monoclonal antibody against a rat mammary carcinoma and suppression of tumour growth with adriamycin-antibody conjugates. Cancer Immunol Immunother 1982; 12:125–134.

71. Pressman D, Day E, Blau M. The use of paired labeling in the determination of tumor-localizing antibodies. Cancer Res 1957; 17:845–850.

72. Moshakis V, McIlhinney RAJ, Raghavan D, Neville AM. Localization of human tumour xenografts after i.v. administration of radiolabelled monoclonal antibody. Br J Cancer 1981; 44:91–99.

73. Mach JP, Carrel S, Merenda C, Sordat B, Cerottini JC. In vivo localization of radiolabeled antibodies to carcinoembryonic antigen in human colon carcinoma grafted into nude mice. Natrure 1974; 248:704–706.

74. Hopf U, Meyer zum Büschenfelde KH, Dietrich MP. Demonstration of binding sites for IgG Fc and the third complement (C3) on isolated hepatocytes. J Immunol 1976; 117:639–645.

75. Pressman D, Korngold L. The in vivo localization of anti-Wagner osteogenic-sarcoma antibodies. Cancer 1953; 6:619–623.

76. Moshakis V, McIlhinney RAF, Neville AM. Cellular distribution of monoclonal antibody in human tumours after i.v. administration. Br J Cancer 1981; 44:663–669.

77. Buchegger F, Haskell CM, Schreyer M, Scazziga BR, Randin S, Carrel S, Mach JP. Radiolabeled fragments of monoclonal antibodies against carcinoembryonic antigen for localization of human colon carcinoma grafted into nude mice. J Exp Med 1983; 158:413–427.

78. Epenetos AA, Nimmon CC, Arklie J, Elliott AT, Hawkins LA, Knowles RW, Britton KE, Bodmer WF. Detection of human cancer in an animal model using radiolabeled tumour-associated monoclonal antibodies. Br J Cancer 1982; 46:1–8.

79. Ballou B, Levine G, Hakala TR, Solter D. Tumor location detected with radioactively labeled monoclonal antibody and external scintigraphy. Science 1979; 206:844–847.

80. Smith TW, Lloyd BL, Spicer N, Haber E. Immunogenicity and kinetics of distribution and elimination of sheep digoxin-specific IgG and Fab fragments in the rabbit and baboon. Clin Exp Immunol 1979; 36:384–396.

81. Wahl RL, Parker CW, Philpott GW. Improved radioimaging and tumor localization with monoclonal F(ab')2. J Nucl Med 1983; 24:316–325.

82. Herlyn D, Powe J, Alavi A, Mattis JA, Herlyn M, Ernst C, Vaum R, Koprowski H. Radioimmunodetection of human tumor xenografts by monoclonal antibodies. Cancer Res 1983; 43:2731–2735.

83. Goldman A, Vivian G, Gordon I, Prichard J, Kemshead J. Immunolocalization of neuroblastoma using radiolabeled monoclonal antibody UJ13A. J Pediatr 1984; 105:252–256.

84. Stavrou D, Mellert W, Bilzer T, Senekowitsch R, Keiditsch E, Mehraein P. Radioimmunodetection of gliomas by administration of radiolabeled monoclonal antibodies. Anticancer Res 1985; 5:147–156.
85. Bourdon MA, Coleman RE, Blasberg RG, Groothuis DR, Bigner DD. Monoclonal antibody localization in subcutaneous and intracranial human glioma xenografts: Paired-label and imaging analysis. Anticancer Res 1984; 4:133–140.
86. Bullard DE, Adams CJ, Coleman RE, Bigner DD. In vivo imaging of intracranial human glioma xenografts comparing specific with nonspecific radiolabeled monoclonal antibodies. J Neurosurg 1986 64:257–262.
87. Day ED, Mahaley MS, Woodhall B, Pircher F. Localization of purified ^{125}I-antitumor radioantibodies in human brain tumors. J Nucl Med 1964; 5:357–358.
88. Day ED, Lassiter S, Woodhall B, Mahaley JL, Mahaley MS. The localization of radioantibodies in human brain tumors. I. Preliminary exploration. Cancer Res 1965; 6:773–778.
89. Mahaley MS, Mahaley JL, Day ED. The localization of radioantibodies in human brain tumors. II. Radioautography. Cancer Res 1965; 25:779–793.
90. Phillips J, Sikora K, Watson JV. Localisation of glioma by human monoclonal antibody. Lancet 1982; 2:1214–1215.
91. Phillips J, Alderson T, Sikora K, Watson J. Localization of malignant glioma by a radiolabeled human monoclonal antibody. J Neurol Neurosurg Psychiatr 1983; 46:388–392.
92. DeLand FH, Kim EE, Goldenberg DM. Lymphoscintigraphy with radionuclide-labeled antibodies to carcinoembryonic antigen. Cancer Res 1980; 40:2997–3000.
93. Kim EE, DeLand FH, Nelson MO, Bennett S, Simmons G, Alpert E, Goldenberg DM. Radioimmunodetection of cancer with radiolabeled antibodies to alpha-fetoprotein. Cancer Res 1980; 40:3008–3012.
94. Van Nagell JR, Kim E, Casper S, Primus FJ, Bennett S, DeLand FH, Goldernberg DM. Radioimmunodetection of primary and metastatic ovarian cancer using radiolabeled antibodies to carcinoembryonic antigen. Cancer Res 1980; 40:502–506.
95. Goldenberg DM, Kim EE, DeLand FH, Bennett S, Primus FJ. Radioimmunodetection of cancer with radioactive antibodies to carcinoembryonic antigen. Cancer Res 1980; 40:2984–2992.
96. Goldenberg DM, DeLand F, Kim E, Bennett S, Primus FJ, van Nagell JR, Estes N, DeSimone P, Rayburn P. Use of radiolabeled antibodies to carcinoembryonic antigen for the detection and localization of diverse cancers by external photoscanning. N Engl J Med 1978; 298:1384–1388.
97. Mach JP, Chatal JF, Lumbroso JD, Buchegger F, Forni M, Ritschard J, Berche C, Douillard JY, Carrel S, Herlyn M, Steplewski Z, Korpowski H. Tumor localization in patients by radiolabeled monoclonal antibodies against colon carcinoma. Cancer Res 1983; 43:5593–5600.
98. Farrands PA, Perkins AC, Pimm MV, Hardy JD, Embleton MJ, Baldwin RW, Hardcastle JD. Radioimmunodetection of human colorectal cancers by anti-tumor monoclonal antibody. Lancet 1982; 2:397–400.

99. Mach JP, Forni M, Ritschard J, Buchegger F, Carrel S, Widgren S, Donath A, Alberto P. Use and limitations of radiolabeled anti-CEA antibodies and their fragments for photoscanning detection of human colorectal carcinomas. Oncodev Biol Med 1980; 1:49–69.

100. Chatal JF, Saccavini JC, Fumoleau P, Douillard JY, Curtet C, Kremer M, Le Mevel B, Koprowski H. Immunoscintigraphy of colon carcinoma. J Nucl Med 1984; 25:307–314.

101. Richardson RB, Davies AG, Bourne SP, Staddon GE, Jones D, Kemshead JT, Coakham HB. Radioimmunolocalization of primary cerebral tumours in humans. In: Walker M, Thomas DGT (eds). Biology of Brain Tumours. Amsterdam, Martinus Nijhoff (in press).

102. Giacomelli F, Wiener J, Spiro D. The cellular pathology of experimental hypertension. V. Increased permeability of cerebral arterial hypertension. Am J Pathol 1970; 59:133–160.

103. Richardson RB, Davies AG, Bourne SP, Staddon GE, Jones DE, Kemshead JT, Coakham HB. Radioimmunolocalization of human brain tumours: Biodistribution of radiolabeled monoclonal antibody UJ13A (in press).

104. Epenetos AA, Courtenay-Luck N, Pickering D, Hooker G, Durbin H, Lavender JP, McKenzie CG. Antibody-guided irradiation of brain glioma by arterial infusion of radioactive monoclonal antibody against epidermal growth factor receptor and blood group A antigen. Br Med J 1985; 290:1463–1466.

105. Coakham HB, Richardson RB, Bourne S, Davies AG, Kemshead JT. Antibody-guided radiolocalisation and therapy of neoplastic meningitis. Br J Cancer 1985; 52:655.

106. Jones DH, Goldman A, Gordon I, Pritchard J, Gregory BJ, Kemshead JT. Therapeutic application of a radiolabeled monoclonal antibody in nude mice xenografted with human neuroblastoma: Tumoricidal effects and distribution studies. Int J Cancer 1985; 35:715–720.

107. Courtenay-Luck N, Epenetos AA, Halnan KE, Hooker G, Hughes JMB, Krausz T, Lambert J, Lavender JP, MacGregor WG, McKenzie CJ, Munro A, Myers MJ, Orr JS, Pearse EE, Snook D, Webb B, Burchell J, Durbin H, Kemshead J, Taylor-Papadimitriou J. Antibody-guided irradiation of malignant lesions: Three cases illustrating a new method of treatment. Lancet 1984; 1:1441–1443.

108. Kemshead JT, Jones DH, Lashford L, Pritchard J, Gordon I, Breatnach F, Coakham HB. [131]I coupled to monoclonal antibodies as therapeutic agents for neuroectodermally derived tumors. Fact or fiction. Cancer Drug Delivery 1986; 3:25–43.

109. Eng L, Rubinstein LC. Contribution of immunohistochemistry to diagnostic problems of human cerebral tumors. J Histochem Cytochem 1978; 26:513–522.

110. Bonnin JM, Rubinstein LC. Immunohistochemistry of central nervous system tumors: Its contribution to neurosurgical diagnosis. J Neurosurg 1984; 60:1121–1133.

111. Coakham HB, Brownell DB. Monoclonal antibodies in the diagnosis of intracranial tumours and cerebrospinal fluid neoplasia. In: Cavanagh

J (ed). Recent Advances in Neuropathology, Vol. 3. Edinburgh, Churchill-Livingstone (in press).

112. Coakham HB, Garson JA, Brownell B, Kemshead JT. Monoclonal antibodies as reagents for brain tumour diagnosis: a review. J Roy Soc Med 1984; 77:780–787.

113. Garson JA, Coakham HB, Kemshead JT, Brownell B, Harper E, Allan P, Bourne S. The role of monoclonal antibodies in brain tumour diagnosis and cerebrospinal fluid (CSF) cytology. J Neuro-Oncol 1985; 3:165–171.

114. Kemshead JT, Goldman A, Fritschy J, Malpas JS, Pritchard J. Use of panels of monoclonal antibodies in the differential diagnosis of neuroblastoma and lymphoblastic disorders. Lancet 1983; 1:12–14.

115. Allan PM, Garson JA, Harper EI, Coakham HB, Brownell B. The classification of brain lymphoma using monoclonal antibodies. Neuropathol Appl Neurobiol 1983; 9:492–493.

116. Li CY, Witzig TE, Phyliky RL, Ziesmer SC, Yam LT. Diagnosis of B-cell non-Hodgkin's lymphoma of the central nervous system by immunocytochemical analysis of cerebrospinal fluid lymphocytes. Cancer 1986; 57:737–744.

117. Carrel S, de Tribolet N, Mach JP. Human melanoma- and glioma-associated antigen(s) identified by monoclonal antibodies. In: Busch H, Yeoman LC (eds). Methods in Cancer Research. Vol. XX, Tumor Markers. Orlando, Florida, Academic Press, 1982; pp. 317–354.

118. Carrel S, Schreyer M, Schmidt-Kessen A, Mach JP. Reactivity spectrum of 30 monoclonal antibodies to a panel of 28 melanoma and control cell lines. Hybridoma 1982; 1:387–397.

119. Guesdon JL, Ternynck T, Avrameas S. The use of avidin-biotin interaction in immunoenzymatic techniques. J Histochem Cytochem 1979; 27:1131–1139.

120. Wikstrand CJ, McLendon RE, Kemshead J, Coakham HB, Mach JP, Carrel S, de Tribolet N, Bullard DE, Bigner DD. Comparative localization of glioma reactive monoclonal antibodies in vivo in an athymic mouse human glioma xenograft model. J Neuroimmunol (in press).

121. Fraker PJ, Speck JC. Protein and cell membrane iodinations with a sparingly soluble chloramide, 1,3,4,6-tetrachloro-3a,6a-diphenylglycoluril. Biochem Biophys Res Comm 1978; 80:849–857.

122. Markwell MAK, Fox CF. Surface-specific iodination of membrane proteins of viruses and eucaryotic cells using 1,3,4,6-tetrachloro-3a,6a-diphenylglycoluril. Biochem 1978; 17:4807–4817.

123. Bullard DE, Bigner DD. Blood-brain barrier disruption in immature Fischer-344 rats. J Neurosurg 1984; 60:743–754.

124. Neuwelt EA, Barnett PA, Bigner DD, Frenkel EP, Effects of adrenal cortical steroids and osmotic blood-barrier opening on methotrexate delivery to gliomas in the rodent: The factor of the blood-brain barrier. Proc Natl Acad Sci USA 1982; 79:4420–4423.

125. Hasegawa H, Allen JC, Mehta BM, Shapiro WR, Posner JB. Enhancement of CNS penetration methotrexate by hyperosmolar intracarotid mannitol or carcinomatous meningitis. Neurology 1979; 29:1280–1286.

126. Bullard DE, Bourdon M, Bigner DD. Comparison of various methods

for delivering radiolabeled monoclonal antibody to normal rat brain. J Neurosurg 1984; 61:901–911.

127. Begent RHJ, Keep PA, Green AJ, Searle F, Bagshawe KD, Jewkes RF, Jones BE, Barratt GM, Ryman BE. Liposomally entrapped second antibody improves tumour imaging with radiolabeled (first) antitumour antibody. Lancet 1982; 2:739–742.

128. Begent RHJ, Green AJ, Keep PA, Bagshawe KD, Searle F, Jones BE, Jewkes RF, Ryman BE, Barratt GM. Liposomally entrapped second antibody. Lancet 1983; 1:1047–1048.

129. Bradwell AR, Vaughan A, Fairweather DS, Dykes PW. Improved radioimmunodetection of tumours using second antibody. Lancet 1983; 2:247.

130. Begent RHJ, Bagshawe KD. Clinical applications of radioimmunolocalisations. In: Baldwin RW, Byers VS. Monoclonal antibodies for cancer detection and therapy. London, Academic Press, Inc., 1985; pp. 181–200.

131. Fairweather DS, Bradwell AR, Dykes PW, Vaughan AT, Watson-James SF, Chandler S. Improved tumour localisation using indium-111 labelled antibodies. Br Med J 1983; 287:167–170.

132. Halpern SE, Hagan PL, Garver PR, Koziol JA, Chen AWN, Frincke JM, Bartholomew RM, David GS, Adams TH. Stability, characterization and kinetics of 111-indium-labeled monoclonal antitumor antibodies in normal animals and nude mouse-human tumor models. Cancer Res 1983; 43:5347–5355.

133. Rainsbury RM, Ott RJ, Westwood JH, Kalirai TS, Coombes RC, McCready VR, Neville AM, Gazet JC. Location of metastatic breast carcinoma by a monoclonal antibody chelate labelled with Indium-111. Lancet 1983; 2:934–938.

134. Treleaven JG, Gibson FM, Ugelstad J, Rembaum A, Philip T, Caine GD, Kemshead JT. Removal of neuroblastoma cells from bone marrow with monoclonal antibodies conjugated to magnetic microspheres. Lancet 1984; 1:70–73.

135. Brennan M, Davison PF, Paulus H. Preparation of bispecific antibodies by chemical recombination of monoclonal immunoglobulin G1 fragments. Science 1985; 229:81–83.

136. Milstein C, Cuello AC. Hybrid hybridomas and their use in the immunohistochemistry. Nature 1983; 305:537–540.

137. Neuberger MS, Williams GT, Fox RO. Recombinant antibodies possessing novel effector functions. Nature 1984; 312:604–608.

138. Neuberger MS, Williams GT, Mitchell EB, Jouhal SS, Flanangan JG, Rabbitts TH. A hapten-specific chimaeric IgE antibody with human physiological effector function. Nature 1985; 314:268–270.

139. Boulianne GL, Hozumi N, Shulman MJ. Production of functional chimaeric mouse/human antibody. Nature 1984; 312:643–646.

140. Raso V, Griffin T. Hybrid antibodies with dual specificity for the delivery of ricin to immunoglobulin-bearing target cells. Cancer Res 1981; 41:2073–2078.

141. Cowley GP, Smith JA, Gusterson BA. Increased EGF receptors on human squamous carcinoma cell lines. Br J Cancer 1986; 53:223–229.

142. Murphy LJ, Sutherland RL, Stead B, Murphy LC, Lazarus L. Progesting regulation of epidermal growth factor receptor in human mammary carcinoma cells. Cancer Res 1986; 46:728–734.
143. Gullick WJ, Marsden JJ, Whittle N, Ward B, Bobrow L, Waterfield MD. Expression of epidermal growth factor receptor on human cervical, ovarian, and vulval carcinomas. Cancer Res 1986; 46:285–292.
144. Gusterson B, Cowley G, McIlhinney J, Ozanne B, Fisher C, Reeves B. Evidence for increased epidermal growth factor receptors in human sarcomas. Int J Cancer 1985; 36:689–693.
145. Libermann TA, Razon N, Bartal AD, Yardan Y, Schlessinger J, Soreq H. Expression of epidermal growth factor receptors in human brain tumors. Cancer Res 1984; 44:753–760.
146. Libermann TA, Nusbaum HR, Razon N, Kris R, Lax I, Soreq H, Whittle N, Waterfield MD, Ullrich A, Schlessinger J. Amplification, enhanced expression and possible rearrangement of EGF receptor gene in primary human brain tumours of glial origin. Nature 1985; 313:144–147.
147. Waterfield MD, Mayes ELV, Stroobant P, Bennet PLP, Young S, Goodfellow PN, Banting GS, Ozanne B. A monoclonal antibody to the human epiderml growth factor receptor. J Cell Biochem 1982; 20:149–161.
148. Parker PJ, Young S, Gullick WJ, Mayes ELV, Bennett P, Waterfield MD. Monoclonal antibodies against the human epidermal growth factor receptor from A431 cells. J Biol Chem 1984; 259:9906–9912.
149. Heldin CH, Wasteson A, Westermark B. Growth of normal human glial cells in a defined medium containing platelet-derived growth factor. Proc Natl Acad Sci USA 1980; 77:6611–6615.
150. Pantazis P, Pelicci PG, Dalla-Favera R, Antoniades HN. Synthesis and secretion of proteins resembling platelet-derived growth factor by human glioblastoma and fibrosarcoma cells in culture. Proc Natl Acad Sci USA 1985; 82:2404–2408.
151. Nister M, Heldin CH, Wasteson A, Westermark B. A glioma-derived analog to platelet-derived growth factor: Demonstration of receptor competing activity and immunological cross-reactivity. Proc Natl Acad Sci USA 1984; 81:926–930.
152. Heldin CH, Westermark B, Wasteson A. Specific receptors for platelet-derived growth factor on cells derived from connective tissue and glia. Proc Natl Acad Sci USA 1981;3664–3668.

10

Cerebrospinal Fluid Studies in the Management of Brain Tumors

Marius Maxwell and Peter McL. Black

Cerebrospinal fluid (CSF) provides a bathing medium for the entire brain: through its continuity with interstitial fluid, it is in contact even with deep-seated tumors. Many investigators have therefore hoped that a study of CSF would lead to early detection of tumors within the central nervous system. They have used two general methods: a study of cells in CSF and a study of biochemical tumor markers.

The detection of malignant cells is of the greatest use in the diagnosis of tumors that involve the meninges or seed via the CSF. Of primary brain tumors, medulloblastomas most often fall into this category. For other tumors, CSF cytology may be useful in follow-up and determination of adjuvant therapy in circumstances where CSF can safely be sampled.

Recent research has also been directed toward the identification of tumor-specific markers that may help in diagnosing and monitoring the course of patients with brain tumors. As shall be seen, their lack of specificity with regard to pathological diagnosis hampers their use as diagnostic indices. The best-characterized CSF tumor markers may, however, be useful to monitor central nervous system (CNS) tumor progression and response to therapy.

From: Kornblith PL, Walker MD (editors). Advances in Neuro-Oncology. Futura Publishing Company, Inc., Mount Kisco, NY, © 1988.

Cerebrospinal Fluid Cytology

Since the occurrence of malignant cells in CSF was first reported by Dufour in 1904, the identification of malignant cells has been considered an accurate indicator of CNS involvement by tumor.[16] The detection rate of malignant cells in the face of known CNS malignancy is about 30%[22]; thus, CSF cytology is an accurate but not a very sensitive indicator of CNS neoplasia.

Normal CSF is crystal-clear and colorless and may contain from 1 to 5 lymphocytes per mm^3. Cells of many tissues line CSF pathways and may, therefore, also be normally present in CSF; these include ependymal cells arising from the ventricles and arachnoid cells from the arachnoid layer. The site of CSF collection influences the detection rate for malignant cells; the rate for lumbar puncture samples is less than that obtained with ventricular samples.[39] The volume of CSF obtained is also important in determining the rate of detection.

Malignant cells in CSF are recognized by irregularity of cellular and nuclear size and shape. They are foreign to their environment and have features typical of neoplastic cells, such as mitotic figures, multiple nucleoli, large cellular size, and a high nuclear-to-cytoplasmic ratio.[4] False positive tests may result from misinterpretation of normal cells; false negative tests may occur in lymphoma in which cells may be misinterpreted as normal lymphocytes.

A true positive CSF cytololgy implicates the presence of tumor cells in ventricular cavities or subarachnoid space. Malignant cells occur in the CSF most frequently as a result of diffuse and widespread seeding of the meninges by tumor and almost never due to entirely subpial parenchymal tumors. Glass et al. have suggested that positive cytology represents meningeal carcinomatosis with or without attendant parenchymal involvement until proven otherwise.[22] The clinical implication of a positive CSF cytology is therefore for neuraxis radiation or chemotherapy rather than ablative surgery.

It may be possible to increase the sensitivity of cytology tissue culture techniques. The most commonly employed techniques use air-dried cytocentrifuged preparations stained with either Romanowsky or Papanicolaou stains. Cells may also be efficiently concentrated by the use of Millipore or, more recently, Nucleopore and Gelman Metricel filters. Tissue culture techniques may add significantly to cytologic results. Black et al. reported on 35 cases of CNS malignancy and 74 control specimens incubated in tissue culture medium.[10] Using strict cytological criteria for malignant cells and evaluating cells in a "blinded" fashion, they examined CSF specimens 3 to 7 days after collection from lumbar puncture. 0.7 cc of CSF was cultured in a Leighton tube with 0.7 cc of F-10 nutrient medium with 10% fetal calf serum. Eight out of 35 patients with known CNS malignancy had positive cytology and 11 cases had equivocal characteristics of malignancy. By standard cytological techniques, four patients had malignant cells and four had equivocal cells. Thus, cell culture appeared to be superior to routine cytology, especially considering that less than 1 cc of CSF was necessary.

Most centers use direct CSF examination with or without cytocentrifuging for cytological diagnosis. The following will review the usefulness of CSF cytology in the diagnosis of meningeal carcinomatosis and various primary tumors, including medulloblastomas and glioblastomas.

CSF Cytology in Meningeal Carcinomatosis

Diffuse multifocal seeding of the subarachnoid space by tumor occurring alone or together with parenchymal involvement constitutes meningeal metastasis, carcinomatous meningitis, or meningeal carcinomatosis. The latter term was coined by Beerman in 1912 for the confusing spectrum of clinical signs, including cranial nerve palsies and seizures that accompany this condition.[8] Among patients with primary or metastatic CNS involvement by tumor, the incidence of parenchymal metastases far exceeds that of meningeal carcinomatosis, although the latter accounts for a higher detection rate by CSF cytology. In a study of over 2,000 cases of metastatic brain tumors, Gonzalez-Vitale and co-workers reported 18% with meningeal seeding, including 3% with only meningeal deposits.[23] Glass et al. reviewed 210 autopsied patients with metastatic CNS tumors. Of these, 9% were found to have dural metastases alone, 3% had leptomeningeal seeding, and 36% had involvement confined to the parenchyma. Sixteen percent found to have both meningeal and metastatic involvement. Fifty-nine percent of patients with leptomeningeal carcinomatosis had a positive cytology as opposed to 1% with strictly parenchymal neoplasms. They also found the degree of leptomeningeal involvement to correlate closely with cytological detection rates.

Systemic cancers accounting for the majority of cases of meningeal carcinomatosis include malignant melanoma and carcinoma of the lung, breast, and stomach. Of lung cancers, small cell neo-plasms or adenocarcinomas constitute the bulk of cases producing a positive CSF cytology. It has been estimated that up to 41% of patients with lung cancer have CNS metastases at postmortem.[1,19,21] Reported incidences of CNS metastasis for patients with breast carcinoma and melanoma are 20%[48] and 52%,[5] respectively.

Although gastric adenocarcinoma is a rare primary source of meningeal carcinomatosis, the great propensity to early metastases makes it and lung cancer leading candidates in cases of meningeal carcinomatosis of unknown origin. Of the rarer tumors known to involve the CNS, both retinoblastomas[37] and embryonal rhabdomyosarcomas possess a marked tendency for CNS metastasis. Meningeal carcinomatosis has a bleak prognostic outlook. In one series, 75% of patients died within 3 months of their first positive CSF cytological evaluation.[9]

The danger of CNS relapse is significant in patients who are in remission with systemic cancers because the brain is less open to chemotherapeutic agents than other parts of the body and is therefore especially prone to relapse of tumor. Planned lumbar punctures may provide an early sign of CNS tumor in these patients.

CSF Cytology in Primary Brain Tumors

Spiller, in 1907, is credited with the first account of a primary brain tumor extending to the meninges.[43] Views on the pathogenesis of malignant cells in CSF vary: some hold that this is invariably due to diffuse meningeal spread,[2] while others maintain that once an isolated tumor has breached the pia, it may exfoliate cells locally into the subarachnoid space or ventricular cavity.[12]

In their study of CSF cytology in CNS tumors, Balhuizen et al. found positive cytology to be diagnostic in 15% of all cases.[7] Two studies have extensively reviewed the incidence of meningeal spread for primary brain tumors determined at postmortem. Cairns and Russell reported that 36% of gliomas had meningeal spread.[11] In another study, the degree of meningeal spread was determined for 42 primary brain tumors.[38] Medulloblastomas accounted for 47% of cases of meningeal seeding, glioblastomas for 14%, ependymomas for 12%, oligodendrogliomas for 12%, astrocytomas for 7%, retinoblastomas for 5%, and pinealomas for 2%.

Medulloblastomas

Medulloblastomas are believed to arise from the fetal external granular cell layer of the cerebellum of children and young adults. Their proximity to CSF pathways accounts for their early spread into the fourth ventricle or subarachnoid space. Although CSF cytology might in theory be a good diagnostic test for their presence, a posterior fossa mass is a contraindication to lumbar puncture. The interpretation of positive postoperative CSF cytology is disputed; there may be a postoperative cellular reaction and surgery itself may release malignant cells into CSF. Balhuizen et al. reviewed CSF samples from 17 patients with medulloblastomas and found an overall positive cytology incidence of 28%,[7] reflecting an 11% rate for preoperative CSF samples and 91% for postoperative samples. These findings strongly support the view that surgery causes the shedding of neoplastic cells into the CSF.

Other Primary CNS Tumors

The value of CSF cytology is less clear in the case of gliomas. In a series of 122 glioma patients, positive preoperative cytology was obtained in 13%. A strong correlation existed between pathological grade and cytological diagnosis; however, grades I and II yielded a positive preoperative CSF cytology in 9% of cases and grades III and IV in 17%.[12] Similarly, for ependymomas, grades I and II produced positive results in 9% of cases and grades III and IV in 19%. Pineal germinomas have been reported to cause positive CSF cytologies in 25% to 100% of cases.[14] Due to their position, both choroid plexus papillomas and carcinomas invariably exfoliate cells into CSF.[1] Positive CSF cytologies have been reported to result from chordomas.[26]

Cerebrospinal Fluid Tumor Markers

Warburg, in 1930, found that neoplastic tissue was associated with increased rates of glycolysis.[46] It is now known that the glycolytic rate is proportional to the degree of differentiation of some tumors.[31,47] Differences in the constituents of such metabolic pathways may conceivably be employed as indices of neoplasia.

There has been an extensive search for substances acting as accurate markers of central nervous tumors. Such substances, present within the cerebrospinal fluid, would be expected to enable early diagnosis to be made with high specificity and to facilitate monitoring of tumor growth and regression in response to therapy. A perfect tumor marker would be elevated in all tumor-bearing patients and would be absent from the normal population. No such marker has hitherto been identified; the potential usefulness of many markers is tempered by their lack of specificity for brain tumors. The best characterized CSF tumor markers include the polyamines and the germ-cell markers, alpha fetoprotein (α-FP) and the beta subunit of human chorionic gonadotrophin (β-hCG). Other markers, less useful for the diagnosis of primary brain tumors, include carcinoembryonic antigen (CEA), β-glucuronidase, and deoxythymidine kinase.

The Polyamines

Increased intracellular concentrations of the polyamines spermine, spermidine, and putrescine occur in tissues with increased rates of cellular division and proliferation.[27,28] They are produced as by-products of cells undergoing ribonucleic acid (RNA) synthesis during the growth period, and elevated intracellular polyamine concentrations occur in neoplastic cells. Because of this, CSF polyamine levels have been used as markers for CNS tumors.

Spermidine has been reported to be increased in the CSF of patients with meningiomas.[20] It and other polyamines have been reported as elevated in patients harboring glial tumors but are unreliable for glial tumor diagnosis. CSF polyamines are very useful for following medulloblastomas. In their pilot study of 16 patients with medulloblastoma, Marton et al. found that CSF polyamine levels correlated with both the presence and regression of the tumor.[35] These findings were extended and confirmed by a subsequent study in which CSF polyamines were shown to detect early recurrence of medulloblastoma.[17,36] False positive results may be caused by meningitis, obstructive hydrocephalus, arteriovenous malformations, functional pituitary adenomas, and subarachnoid hemorrhage.[20]

Germ-Cell Tumor Markers

The spectrum of germ-cell tumors arising in the region of the pineal gland bears marked histological resemblance to that of the gonads and includes germinomas, mature teratomas, teratocarcinomas, embryonal carcinomas, yolk sac tumors, and choriocarcinomas. Ninety percent of patients with active nonseminomatous testicular tumors have elevated serum β-hCG and α-FP. Only 7.7% of patients with testicular seminomas show elevated serum β-hCG levels.[30]

A similar pattern of tumor marker expression is found in CNS germ-cell tumors. The usefulness of a particular germ-cell tumor marker in pathological diagnosis is limited somewhat by the pronounced histological heterogeneity of germ-cell tumors. The most valuable marker of pineal germinomas is β-hCG, though it is not invariably present. When elevated, β-hCG may be present in both plasma and CSF. Elevated β-hCG is classically associated with choriocarcinomatous elements and, more rarely, with syncytioblastic germinomas and embryonal carcinomas.[3,32] Graziano et al. reported a rise in both CSF and plasma β-hCG in a patient with a pineal embryonal cell carcinoma.[24] Pineal germinomas are not associated with raised α-FP concentrations. Increased CSF and serum α-FP have been reported in conjunction with a pineal endodermal sinus tumor.[33] Furthermore, Hasse et al. have ascribed the most important role of α-FP to be the detection of endodermal sinus tumors and embryonal carcinomas.[25]

β-Glucuronidase

β-Glucuronidase is a lysosomal enzyme normally found in central nervous tissue, but it is found in higher concentrations in choroid plexus and pia-arachnoid. Present in small amounts in CSF,[4] β-glucuronidase is mildly and nonspecifically increased in some primary brain tumors and meningitides.[6,34] Shuttleworth and co-workers have reported that a six- to tenfold increase in CSF β-glucuronidase is strongly indicative of meningeal dissemination of carcinoma, while low to intermediate levels are associated with meningitis.[42] Another study, by Schold et al., found that elevations by a factor of three times normal are highly suggestive of leptomeningeal carcinomatosis.[41] Elevations in CSF β-glucuronidase were highest in association with meningeal spread of breast, lung, and malignant melanoma metastases. Furthermore, CSF β-glucuronidase levels accurately parallel the clinical course following chemotherapy. β-Glucuronidase was found not to be an accurate index of leptomeningeal infiltration by lymphoma, metastases to brain parenchyma or spinal epidural space, or of primary brain tumors.

Carcinoembryonic Antigen

Perhaps the best characterized of all tumor markers, carcinoembryonic antigen (CEA) is a high molecular weight glycoprotein believed to be produced by neoplastic cells. Classically elevated in the serum of patients with colonic carcinoma, it also demonstrates an increase in association with tumors of breast, lung, ovaries, and pancreas.[15,29,40] Some controversy has centered on the question of whether normal subjects possess detectable amounts of CEA in CSF. Twijnstrom et al. have detected CEA in the CSF of most control subjects using a sensitive assay.[45] Other investigators have not detected it.[13,18] A blood-CSF threshold has been proposed to account for the appearance of CEA in CSF when plasma CEA exceeds 100 ng/ml in the presence of known CNS disease. Elevated CSF CEA levels are most indicative of leptomeningeal carcinomatosis especially arising from lung and breast, though not from lymphoma, and were seen to decline with successful therapy.[13,45] Patients with brain parenchymal metastases had elevated concentrations only in those cases with submeningeal or subependymal infiltration. Overall, however, CSF CEA assays possess a low sensitivity (31%) when used as an index of leptomeningeal carcinomatosis.[18] The determination of CSF CEA appears to be most valuable in those patients at risk from metastatic CNS disease, especially arising from breast and lung primaries.

REFERENCES

1. Aaronson SM, Garcia JH, Aronson BF. Metastatic neoplasms of the brain: their frequency in relation to age. Cancer 1964; 17:558–563.
2. Alass JP, Westlake PT. Malignant cells in cerebrospinal fluid and their clinical significance. In: Neurobiology of Cerebrospinal Fluid, Wood J, ed. New York, Plenum Press, 1983; pp. 411–425.
3. Allen JC, Nisselbaum J, Epstein F. Alpha-fetoprotein and human chorionic gonadotrophin determination in cerebrospinal fluid: an aid to the diagnosis and management of intracranial germ-cell tumors. J Neurosurg 1979; 51:368–374.
4. Allen N, Reagen E. β-Glucuronidase activity in cerebrospinal fluid. Arch Neurol 1964; 11:144–154.
5. Amer MH, Al-Saraf M, Baker LH, et al. Malignant melanoma and central

nervous system metastases: incidence diagnosis, treatment and survival. Cancer 1978; 42:660–668.

6. Anlyan A, Shaw A. β-Glucuronidase activity of spinal cord and ventricular fluids in humans. Cancer 1952; 5:578–580.
7. Balhuizen JC, Bots GT, Schaberg A, et al. Value of cerebrospinal fluid: cytology for the diagnosis of malignancies in the central nervous system. J Neurosurg 1978; 48:747–753.
8. Beerman WF. Meningeal carcinomatosis. JAMA 1912; 58:1437–1439.
9. Bigner SH, Johnson WW. The cytopathology of cerebrospinal fluid. II. Metastatic cancer, meningeal carcinomatosis and primary cerebral nervous system neoplasms. Acta Cytol 1981; 25:461–479.
10. Black PM, Callahan LV, Kornblith PL. Tissue cultures from cerebrospinal fluid specimens in the study of human brain tumors. J Neurosurg 1978; 49:697–704.
11. Cairns H, Russell DS. Intracranial and spinal metastases in gliomas of the brain. Brain 1931; 54:377–420.
12. Choi HH, Anderson PJ. Diagnostic cytology of cerebrospinal fluid by the cytocentrifuge method. Am J Clin Pathol 1979; 72:931–943.
13. Dearnaley DP, Patel S, Powles TJ, et al. Carcinoembryonic antigen estimation in cerebrospinal fluid in patients with metastatic breast cancer. Oncodev Biol Med 1981; 2:305–311.
14. DeGirolami U, Schmidek H. Clinicopathological study of 53 tumors of the pineal region. J Neurosurg 1973; 39:455–462.
15. Dhar P, Moore R, Zamcheck N. Carcinoembryonic antigen (CEA) in colonic cancer: use in pre- and postoperative diagnosis. JAMA 1972; 221:31–35.
16. Dufour H. Meningite sarcomateuse diffuse avec envaisement de la moelle et des racines: cytologie positive et speciale du liquide cephalorachidieu. Rev Neurol 1904; 12:104–106.
17. Edwards MS, Davis RL, Laurent JP. Tumor markers and cytological features of cerebrospinal fluid. Cancer 1985; 56:1773–1777.
18. Egan M, Lautenschleger JT, Coligan JE, et al. Radioimmune assay of carcinoembryonic antigen. Immunochemistry 1972; 9:289–299.
19. Fried BM, Buckley RC. Primary carcinoma of the lungs. IV. Intracranial metastases. Arch Pathol 1930; 9:483–527.
20. Fulton DS, Levin VA, Lubick WP, et al. Clinical correlations of cerebrospinal fluid polyamine levels. In: Neurobiology of the Cerebrospinal Fluid, Wood JH, ed. New York, Plenum Press, 1983; pp. 441–452.
21. Galluzi S, Payne PM. Brain metastases from primary bronchial carcinoma: a statistical study of 741 necropsies. Br J Cancer 1956; 10:408–414.
22. Glass JP, Melamed M, Chernik NL, et al. Malignant cells in cerebrospinal fluid (CSF): the meaning of a positive CSF cytology. Neurology 1979; 29:1369–1375.
23. Gonzalez-Vitale JC, Garcia-Bunuel R. Meningeal carcinomatosis. Cancer 1976; 37:2906–2911.
24. Graziano SL, Paolozzi FB, Rudolph AR, et al. Case report: mixed germ-cell tumor of the pineal region. J Neurosurg 1987; 66:300–304.
25. Hasse J, Nielson K. Value of tumor markers in the treatment of endo-

dermal sinus tumors and choriocarcinomas of the pineal region. Neurosurgery 1979; 5:485–488.

26. Heffelsinger MJ, Dahlin DC, MacCarty CS, et al. Chordomas and cartilaginous tumors of the skull base. Cancer 1973; 32:410–420.

27. Heby O, Marton LJ, Wilson CB. Polyamine metabolism in a rat brain tumor lines: its relationship to the growth rate. J Cell Physiol 1975; 86:511–522.

28. Heby O, Marton LJ, Zardi L. Accumulation of polyamines after stimulation of cellular proliferation in human diploid fibroblasts. In: The Cell Cycle in Malignancy and Immunity, Hampton JD, ed. Springfield, Virginia, National Technical Information Service, 1975; pp. 50–66.

29. Holyoke ED. Present and probable uses of CEA. Cancer 1975; 25:22–26.

30. Javadpur N. The role of biologic tumor markers in testicular cancer. Cancer 1980; 45:1755–1761.

31. Kornblith PL, Cummins CJ. Correlation of experimental and clinical studies of metabolism by PET scanning. Progr Exp Tumor Res 1984; 27:170–178.

32. Laidler P, Pander DJ. Pineal germinoma with syncytiotrophoblastic giant cells: a case with panhypopituitarism and isosexual pseudopuberty. Hum Pathol 1984; 15:285–287.

33. Lee SH, Sundararesan N, Jerels B. Endodermal sinus tumor of the pineal region: a case report. Neurosurgery 1978; 3:407–411.

34. Lehrer G. β-Glucuronidase in CSF of patients with diseases of the nervous system. Trans Am Neurol Assoc. 1963; 88:244–245.

35. Marton LJ, Edwards MS, Levin VA, et al. Predictive value of cerebrospinal fluid polyamines in medulloblastoma. Cancer Res 1979; 39:993–997.

36. Marton LJ, Edwards MS, Levin VA, et al. CSF polyamines: a new and important means of monitoring patients with medulloblastoma. Cancer 1981; 47:757–760.

37. Olson ME, Chernik NL, Posner JB. Infiltration of the leptomeninges by systemic cancer: a clinical and pathologic study. Arch Neurol 1974; 30:122–137.

38. Palmeteer FE, Kernohan JW. Meningeal gliomatosis: a study of forty-two cases. Arch Neurol Psych 1947; 57:593–616.

39. Posner J, Bigner DD, D'Angio GJ, et al. Subpanel on neoplasms. In: Report of the Panel on Stroke, Trauma, Regeneration and Neoplasms to the National Advisory Neurological and Communicative Disorders and Stroke Council. USDHEW, NIH; September 15, 1978; pp. 152–153.

40. Reynoso A, Chu T, Holyoke ED. CEA antigen in patients with different cancers. JAMA 1972; 220:361–365.

41. Schold SC, Wassertram WR, Fleischer M, et al. Cerebrospinal fluid biochemical markers of cerebral nervous system metastases. Ann Neurol 1980; 8:597–604.

42. Shuttleworth E, Allen N. Early differentiation of chronic meningitis by enzyme assay. Neurology (Minn.) 1968; 18:534–542.

43. Spiller WA. Gliomatosis of the pia and metastasis of glioma. Nerv Ment Dis 1907; 34:297–382.

44. Spriggs AI. Malignant cells in cerebrospinal fluid. J Clin Pathol 1954; 7:122–130.
45. Twijnstrom A, Nooyan WJ, van Zanten AP. Cerebrospinal fluid carcinoembryonic antigen in patients with metastatic and nonmetastatic neurological diseases. Arch Neurol 1986; 43:269–272.
46. Warburg O. The Metabolism of Tumors. London, Constable, 1930.
47. Weber G. Enzymology of cancer cells. N Engl J Med 1977; 296:486–492 (I); 541–551 (II).
48. Willis RA. One hundred sixty-two secondary tumors. In: Pathology of the Nervous System. Vol. II, Part 23, Minckler J, ed. New York, McGraw-Hill, 1971; pp. 2178–2196.

Section III
Therapeutic Modalities in Brain Tumors

General Introduction

Benign tumors of the brain and spinal cord have become, in large part, curable entities due to advances in microsurgical techniques, modern neuro-anesthesia, and earlier diagnosis with CT scan. Whereas some 30–40 years ago, even that most benign of tumors, the acoustic schwannoma, carried a higher intraoperative mortality rate, now most of the benign tumors can be removed safely and without recurrence. There are still instances of *en plaque* sphenoid wing meningiomas or atypical craniopharyngiomas which are hard to resect, but for the most part, benign tumors are a surgical problem in good control.

Surgery

The situation has not changed so cheerfully for malignant CNS tumors. The primary and secondary tumors of the CNS can be approached surgically, significant portions can often be removed but cures by surgery alone are rare.

The modern management of brain tumors has been improved by the development of image-guided stereotaxic surgery. These techniques make virtually any tumor accessible, at least for biopsy. There is minimal morbidity in using stereotactic approaches and the technology continues to be refined and applications expanded.

Radiotherapy

It was established over 10 years ago that radiation therapy did indeed have a significant role in extending survival of brain tumor patients. Although this modality had been in use for some time, it took a carefully controlled study to verify its value. At present, there are a variety of approaches to the radiation therapy of brain tumors and also an increased understanding of the biological variables which influence therapy. These biological issues are discussed initially and then the status of external beam radiation therapy of gliomas is updated. A new interest has arisen in the potential use of interstitial radiotherapy as a means of providing a higher dosage over a longer period than is possible with external beam approaches. This concept of placing radio-isotopes within the tumor mass has been greatly facilitated by advances in CT scan directed stereotactic surgery which permits accurate placement of the radioactive seeds and more precise prediction of the local dosage parameters. This "radiobrachytherapy" is described as what has now become, in many institutions, a part of the standard therapeutic armamentarium.

Chemotherapy

Although chemotherapy has played a major role in the management of many human cancers, its role in the treatment of malignant CNS tumors has not been dramatic. There is evidence that the nitrosourea compounds make a difference in survival, but no other class of agents has thus far had a large impact in management.

For these reasons, the section on chemotherapy starts with an update on the clinical trials but then focuses heavily on two approaches which are extremely promising for future work in chemotherapy. Three chapters are devoted to chemosensitivity testing and the cellular targets found in such studies. These targets include both DNA and also non-DNA related structures. The whole concept of chemotherapy at present does not adequately compensate for the marked heterogeneity of tumors nor the remarkable degree of resistance of these tumor cells to currently available agents. The use of individual custom-designed programs of chemotherapy based on drug sensitivity testing of the individual patient's tumor cells thus becomes very appealing. The techniques for chemosensitivity testing are now widely in use and should become part of the therapeutic armamentarium.

As was described earlier in Chapter 2, differentiation parameters are important in the study of human brain tumors, and in this therapeutic section our early insights into the therapeutic potential of such differentiating agents are explored. These agents offer the promise of a less toxic, more sustainable method for controlling tumor cell growth even without necessarily killing the cancerous cells.

Immunotherapy

There are many important observations which have been made in regard to the relation of the immune system of the glioma patient and its interaction with the tumor cells. In summary, it appears that patients with these tumors may have some direct impairment of their anti-tumor response. More specifically, it is evident that patients have a humoral response to their own gliomas when the tumors are of low grade, but that only 10% of patients have a significant cytotoxic response to their tumors when the tumors are of the higher grades. For obvious reasons, therefore, the absence of these immune responses is a poor prognostic sign. Similarly, cytotoxic cellular immune responses are lacking in virtually all of the malignant glioma patients.

A variety of approaches have been developed to try to circumvent these limitations of the immune system in combating gliomas. These have included vaccines, immunostimulants, and interferon. These studies have been of great interest. For this book, two of the most exciting new approaches have been chosen which show promise in overcoming the limits of immunotherapy.

The discovery that interleukin-2, a lymphokine, could cause a patient's own lymphocytes to become highly effective tumor-killing cells which spare normal cells while disposing of the cancerous cells has opened a new road to immunotherapy. Results in this work are quite preliminary in patients but show promise of a nontoxic and potentially effective therapy for certain types of tumors.

Another new and exciting approach uses the specificity and binding properties of monoclonal antibodies to allow them to serve as carriers for immunotoxins which are highly lethal to tumor cells when properly linked to antibodies. This work is still at an early stage and is described in its current development.

11

Image-Guided Stereotaxic Surgery in the Management of Brain Tumors

M. Peter Heilbrun

Introduction

Classical stereotaxic techniques have been used for years for accurate localization of paramedian brain structures. The most common application of the stereotaxic method was for placement of lesions in the thalamic region to treat movement disorders associated with Parkinson's disease. With the introduction of medication for the treatment of Parkinson's disease in the mid 1960's, the use of classical stereotaxy decreased.

Modern radiographic imaging with CT became widespread in this country by 1976. By 1979, as CT scanning revolutionized imaging of the brain, compatible stereotaxic methods were evolving.[1–5] Some systems were adaptations of classical stereotaxic instruments such as the systems of Leksell[6–8] and Reichert-Mundinger.[9–11]

In 1979, investigators at the University of Utah described a unique solution to (1) the transformation of two-dimensional CT scan coordinates into three-dimensional stereotaxic coordinates and (2) the derivation of a probe track direction and distance to any point within the brain, either deep or on the surface.[12] This latter solution was based on design considerations used in the development of the arm for the space shuttle.

From: Kornblith PL, Walker MD (editors). Advances in Neuro-Oncology. Futura Publishing Company, Inc., Mount Kisco, NY, © 1988.

The BRW (Brown-Roberts-Wells) image-guided stereotaxic system, named for the three investigators who developed it (Dr. Russell Brown, a medical student at the University of Utah, Dr. Theodore Roberts, Chairman of Neurosurgery at the University of Utah, and Trent Wells, an engineer with years of experience in design and manufacture of neurosurgical instruments, particularly stereotaxic systems), was introduced as a commercial stereotaxic system in 1981.[13–16] In 1983, Apuzzo and Heilbrun described preliminary experience with the BRW system in the management of lesions, predominantly tumors, at two institutions, the University of Utah and the University of Southern California Medical Center.[17,18] By mid 1984, the BRW system was being used in over 45 institutions. By June 1986, it was being used in over 200 institutions worldwide. Gildenberg recently reported a survey that showed a resurgence in stereotaxy related to brain tumor localization, with the BRW system the most commonly used stereotaxic system worldwide.[19]

Stereotaxy is rapidly becoming a neurosurgical standard for approach to CT-defined small intra-axial brain lesions.[20] Similar localization techniques for MRI and angiography are also available. Whereas the early methods allowed transformation of two-dimensional data to three-dimensional points in space, advanced microcomputer graphics now allow the transformation of volume arrays of two-dimensional data into three-dimensional stereotaxic volumes in space.

The accuracy of CT-guided stereotaxy in defining tumor position to obtain specimens of tissue has been widely reported.[5,11,17,18,20] Stereotaxic guidance is clearly the method of choice in the biopsy of small deep brain lesions. In addition, for moderate to large size intracranial lesions, the inherent precision of the stereotaxic technique allows approaches through smaller skull openings, which appear to reduce the morbidity associated with larger craniotomies necessitated by freehand approaches. In addition, stereotaxic localization enhances the neurosurgeon's intuitive three-dimensional conceptualization of intracranial structures, which may also enhance tactile requirements for meticulous neurosurgical technique. Stereotaxic localization can also provide important information for vascular structures so that general approaches which avoid them may be chosen and so that arteriovenous malformations can be more precisely managed.

Information provided by stereotaxic localization benefits surgical planning for many lesions regardless of size and depth. This chapter describes a 5-year experience in utilizing the BRW image-guided stereotaxic system—from the localization technique for closed biopsy to a system enhanced by a wide array of neurosurgical instruments.

Overview of System

The basic BRW guidance system consists of several components as follows:

The first component is an *aluminum head ring* which is fixed to the skull by the percutaneous fixation of four steel pins, each of which is carried by four carbon rods. The top surface of the head ring serves as the vertical reference plane (Fig. 1).

The second component is the *localizing picket fence* which establishes the reference plane. The localizing picket fence attaches to the head ring and provides the nine fiduciary points on the CT scan image from which the distance to any other point on an image slice can be computed (Fig. 2).

The third component is the *Epson HX2O microcomputer* which computes the two-dimensional image point coordinates of the CT

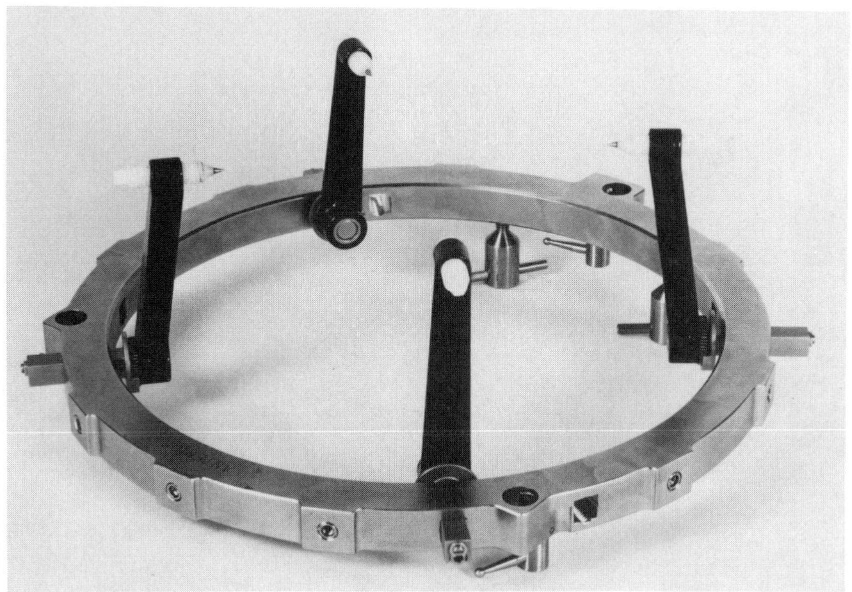

Figure 1. Head ring.

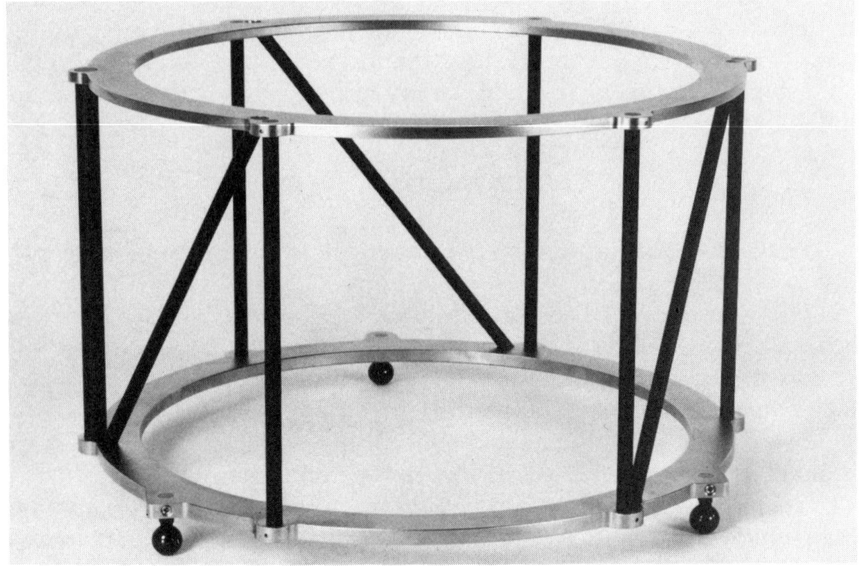

Figure 2. Localizing picket fence.

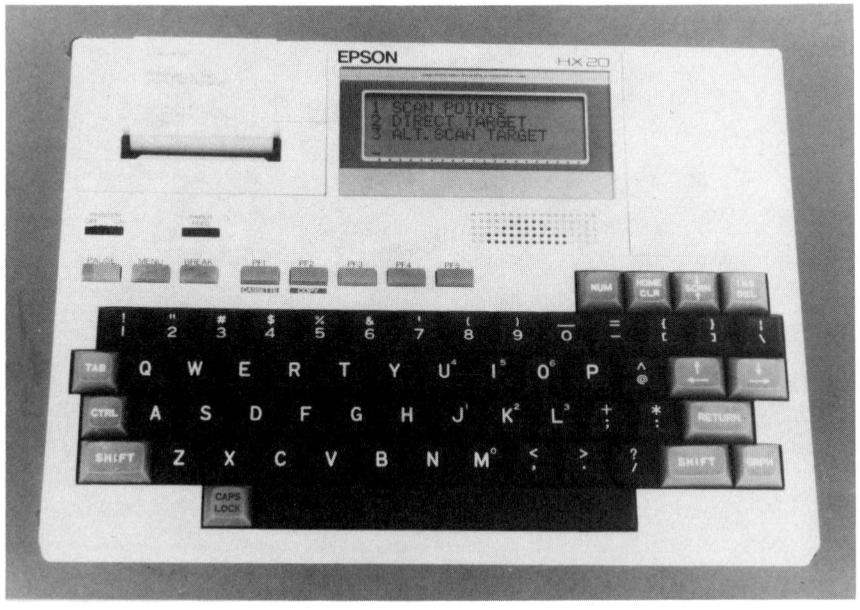

Figure 3. Epson HX–20 microcomputer.

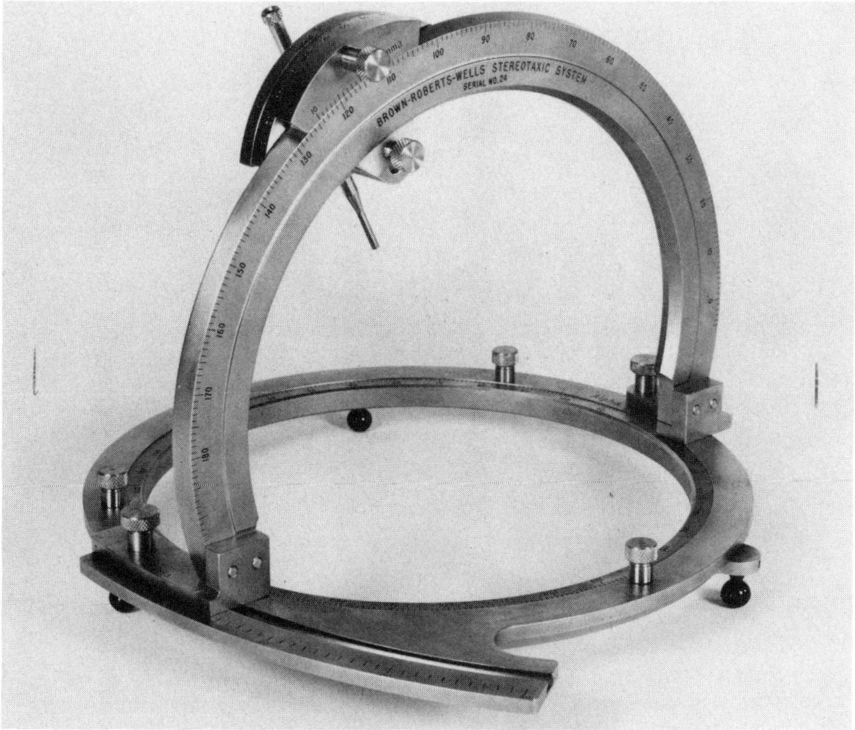

Figure 4. Arc guidance system.

scan to the three-dimensional BRW stereotaxic coordinate system and calculates the BRW arc settings and distances to the target (Fig. 3).

The fourth component is the *BRW arc system,* a unique combination of orthogonal rotations and pivots which allows the surgeon to connect an infinite number of skull entry points to target points within the geometry of the arc's sphere (Fig. 4).

The fifth component is the *phantom simulator* consisting of a second head ring, which is identical to the one fixed to the patient's skull. This second head ring sits on a base which holds a dummy point that can be moved in the AP, lateral, and vertical axes to any derived BRW stereotaxic coordinate (Fig. 5).

The sixth component is the *BRW floor stand,* which allows the use of standard ventriculography for functional neurosurgical targets

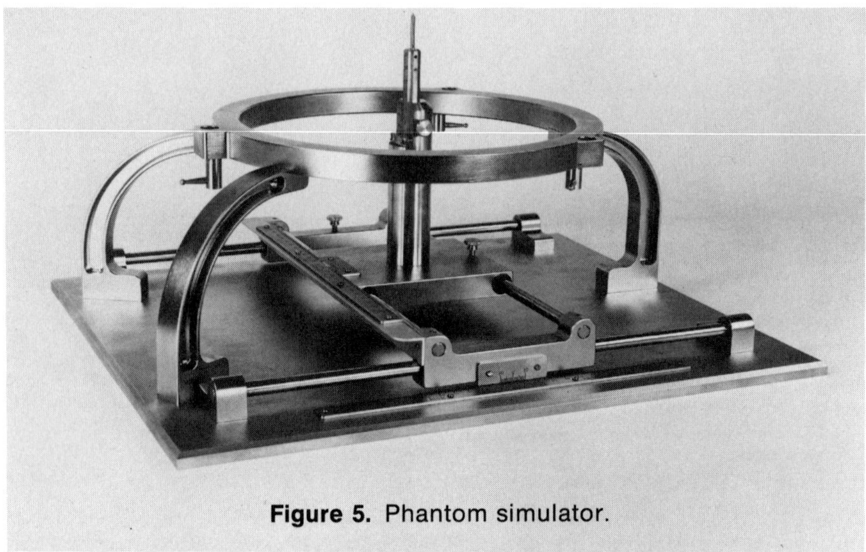

Figure 5. Phantom simulator.

by defining **BRW** coordinates with standard orthogonal AP and lateral radiographs (Fig. 6).

In addition, there are now a multitude of other adaptations to the system, allowing a diverse set of surgical applications from MRI and radiographic localization to computer-assisted laser resection of tumors.

System Independence

A unique BRW feature is its independent reference plane for transforming the two-dimensional data to a three-dimensional point. The head ring reference plane attaches to the patient's head and does not depend on the CT scanner for localizing computations. That is, no portion of the BRW stereotaxic frame attaches to the CT scanner table or gantry. So long as the CT scan image contains the lesion to be biopsied along with the fiduciary points of the nine localizing rods, a hand-held calculator or microcomputer can easily transform the two-dimensional CT scan data set to the three-dimensional BRW stereotaxic coordinate set. Since all patients undergoing stereotaxic biopsy have already had a CT scan for diagnosis, only 10 to 15 minutes of additional scanner time is required to collect the frame image data prior to the surgical procedure. Patient discomfort is minimized since

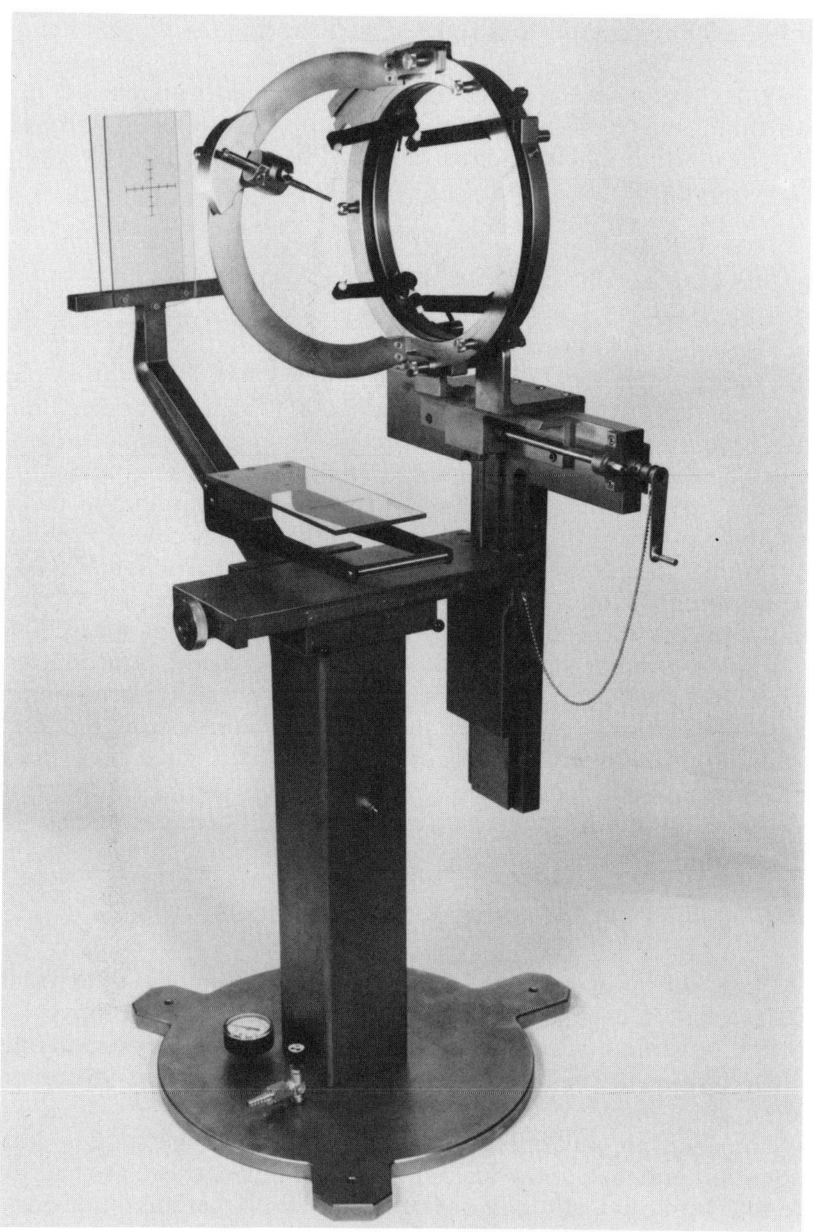

Figure 6. Floor stand with guidance arc and x-ray cassette holders.

rigid fixation to the table is unnecessary, and valuable scanner time is saved.

When the scan is completed, the patient is transported to the operating room, moved to the operating table, positioned with either the floor stand or the standard Mayfield head ring adapter, and the scalp is prepared for surgery.

Specific Localization Procedure

The localization procedure consists of fixing the head ring to the skull, using either local or general anesthesia. The localization picket fence is attached to the head ring and a CT scan is obtained of the brain image containing the target to be localized surrounded by the images of the nine localizer rods. The two-dimensional coordinates of each of these nine points and of the target are obtained through the cursor position program of the CT scanner console. In the operating room, these coordinates are entered into the Epson HX-20 microcomputer which calculates the three-dimensional BRW stereotaxic coordinates of the target from the two-dimensional CT scan data. Then the surgeon inputs chosen entry point coordinates or ranges, and the Epson computes the settings of the arc guidance system. These settings define a probe track and distance from a reference platform on the arc to the target. The simulator is used to verify in three-dimensional space the position of the BRW target coordinate and the accuracy of the arc settings and calculated distance.

General Considerations

Once the neurosurgeon decides upon stereotaxic localization, several strategies are available: (1) perform closed biopsy alone through twist drill or perforator openings, or (2) perform open biopsy followed by partial or complete resection through a small to moderate sized craniotomy or craniectomy.

The choice of an approach depends on several factors in addition to location and size of the lesion. Most obvious of these are the structure and apparent etiology of the lesion, i.e., whether the lesion appears circumscribed with a border or infiltrating without demarcation; whether it appears heterogeneous with cystic components and enhancing borders, and/or surrounding edema (e.g., a glioblastoma);

whether it appears homogeneous and of low density or homogeneous and of high density (e.g., a highly vascular lesion such as a metastatic tumor or a vascular angioma); whether there appears to be an associated mass effect on the surrounding brain with midline shifts, transtentorial herniation, or ventricular enlargement; and whether the lesion appears to be resectable.

Example of a Working Protocol

Under the University of Utah protocol, all intra-axial lesions with the exception of large life-threatening hematomas are managed with stereotaxic localization.

Biopsy Alone

The minority of lesions that are considered unresectable because of location, size, and/or appearance of infiltrative characteristics are usually considered for biopsy alone, provided that there are no characteristics suggesting that hemorrhage might be a problem and there is no significant mass effect suggesting that decompression should be considered. These cases are usually performed under local anesthesia with either a twist drill or perforator opening.

Small Craniotomy

The majority of lesions, however, fit into a category where there is a potential for partial or complete resection. These lesions are approached through a small craniotomy.

Anticipating Hemorrhage

Lesions with heterogeneous appearance on the CT scan, particularly those with cystic components and enhancing borders, carry a significant risk of hemorrhage. Biopsy, which attempts to minimize hemorrhage by targeting the central area of the lesion, will often obtain necrotic tissue or fluid that will be nondiagnostic even with cytology. In order to obtain an appropriate tissue diagnosis, these lesions must be biopsied at the enhancing border, thus increasing the risk of hemorrhage. The neurosurgeon must be prepared to open the biopsy instrument track to control the bleeding under direct vision in the event that it cannot be controlled with gentle irrigation through the biopsy cannula. Although this more extensive procedure can be done under local anesthesia, use of general anesthesia provides time-saving flexibility in the event of hemorrhage.

Avoiding Displacement

Of particular note are those lesions that are small, have the appearance on CT scan of being firm such that they might be displaced by standard biopsy instrumentation, or are either within or protruding into the ventricular system. These are best handled with a small craniotomy and a modified open approach.

Surgical Procedures

Closed Biopsy Through a Twist Drill or Perforator Opening

Opening the Skull

After the localization described above, the neurosurgeon is ready to make a scalp incision and a skull opening. In the case of a low density homogeneous lesion with little risk of hemorrhage, a twist drill opening is appropriate. With the arc in place, standard fittings are utilized. A $\frac{1}{4}$ inch drill bit for the twist drill allows the surgeon to visualize and open the dura and the cortex before advancing the biopsy instrument. Alternatively, a standard perforator opening can be made. The arc system can be pivoted or rotated to the side without breaking sterility. Once the perforator opening is completed and the dura and the cortex opened, the arc is moved back to the appropriate position.

Biopsy Procedure

Two types of instruments are commonly used: a side-cutting instrument provides a core of tissue 10 mm in length and 2 mm in diameter; if this does not obtain satisfactory tissue for diagnosis, a 2 mm cup forceps may be used. To use the cup forceps, a cannula containing an obturator is placed a few millimeters proximal to the target site. The obturator is removed and tissue specimens are obtained with the cup forceps, which fits through the cannula. Using these instruments, it is possible to obtain tissue at various points along the probe track. In some cases, multiple sampling is important in defining lesion borders.

If bleeding occurs following the biopsy, it is usually seen as a backflow of blood through the cannula of both instruments. A slow flow of blood is generally controlled with gentle irrigation through the cannula. However, if the bleeding does not stop quickly with irrigation, the twist drill opening must be enlarged to a small craniotomy for direct control.

In an attempt to develop a real-time monitor which might help in the recognition of significant hemorrhage, University of Utah neurosurgeons have placed a second slide onto the BRW arc and have attached an ultrasound probe which fits into a standard perforator opening. An ultrasound probe placed directly on the arc has the advantage of setting the ultrasound image plane automatically in the plane of the probe trajectory which contains the target.[21] Although this is a different orientation from the scan plane, as the probe passes to the target, it is possible to visualize changes in cyst size as fluid is removed as well as potential hemorrhage building into a mass. To date, this system has been used infrequently because of poor resolution of compatible ultrasound probes.

Open Biopsy and Resection Through Small Craniotomy

Both because of potential hemorrhage from heterogeneous lesions and for better transition from biopsy alone to combined stereotaxic localization, in most cases a small craniotomy will be the preferred skull opening. The localization technique is the same as for twist drill openings. Once the central point of the craniotomy opening is established stereotaxically, the arc system can be pivoted away or removed in order to utilize a craniotome unobstructed by the position of the arc. After the skull is opened, the arc system can be replaced.

At this point all of the alternatives for operative neurosurgical manipulation are available, beginning with placement of a biopsy instrument to obtain tissue for analysis.

If the biopsy area is to be inspected with an endoscope, a small cannula with an obturator large enough to accommodate a 7.5 mm diameter endoscope may be used. The initial probe track may be gradually dilated up to the appropriate diameter with soft probes, following which the endoscope is placed. Dilatation must be extremely gentle; otherwise the brain may be displaced and a false negative biopsy obtained. Although in low grade astrocytomas the transition from normal brain to tumor is not visible, in higher grade astrocytomas, particularly those with cysts, the endoscope can be useful. In such cases, biopsies can be obtained under direct vision and bleeding can generally be controlled with direct cauterization. In addition, both the argon and neodymium YAG lasers can be used through a fiber passed through the endoscope. If the opening to the lesion is to be more than 7.5 mm, the surgeon may prefer to make a cortical incision and to use standard retractor blades rather than a cylindrical cannula, as the blades provide better exposure and seem to result in less brain distortion. All standard retractor blades attach easily to either the head ring or arc or to special posts which fit into the system. Once the lesion is exposed, standard means of tumor resection can be accomplished.

Recently, University of Utah neurosurgeons have built special adapters to attach the operating microscope to the arc if magnification is necessary. In addition, these surgeons are trying CO_2 laser tumor resection, utilizing the Sharplan microscan attachment for manual definition of the tumor border and area of resection. They have also developed a computer software system which emulates the physician's console of the Siemens Somotome CT scanner. Presently this system is used to redefine tumor borders orthogonal to an identified probe track and to place parallel catheters and radiation sources for interstitial brachytherapy. This software system should enable automatic resection of tumors layer by layer along the probe track in a manner similar to that described by Kelly for a different stereotaxic system.[22,23]

Case Reports

CM

This 50-year-old white female presented two years prior to evaluation with olfactory hallucinations, lightheadedness, and a question of expressive aphasia. Studies, including CT scan, showed a heterogeneous lesion with an enhancing border in the right posterior frontal and anterior temporal regions, suggestive of either a tumor or an infarct. The patient was treated for seizures and a repeat CT scan several weeks later showed partial resolution of the lesion. The patient's neurologic deficit cleared and her seizures remained under satisfactory control for 15 months, then increased in frequency.

A repeat neurologic exam at that time was normal. CT scan demonstrated a larger lesion than was apparent on the second scan 15 months earlier, with diffuse infiltration of the brain on both sides of the sylvian fissure (Fig. 7). An MR image showed more intensive involvement of the right frontal and temporal lobes in both the T1 and T2 weighted pulse sequences (Fig. 8a,b).

It was elected to perform a closed biopsy without resection. Impedance measurement, as described by Tasker et al. to confirm the transition from the MRI abnormal area on the T2 weighted images to the tumor border as defined on CT, was utilized.[24] Specimens were obtained in the MRI T2 positive zone, at the CT-defined tumor

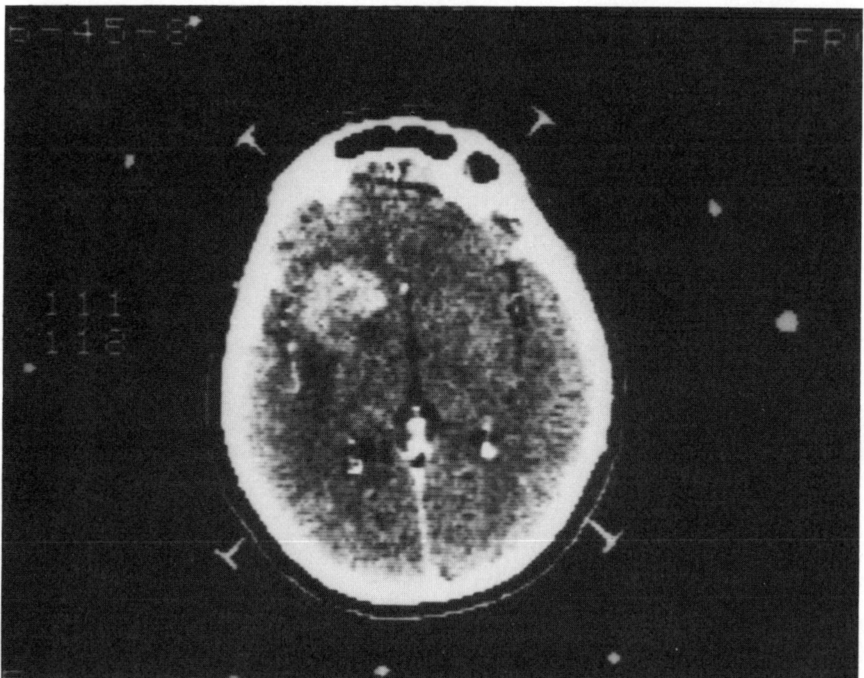

Figure 7. Stereotaxic localization CT scan demonstrating left posterior frontal lesion with target marked by cursor.

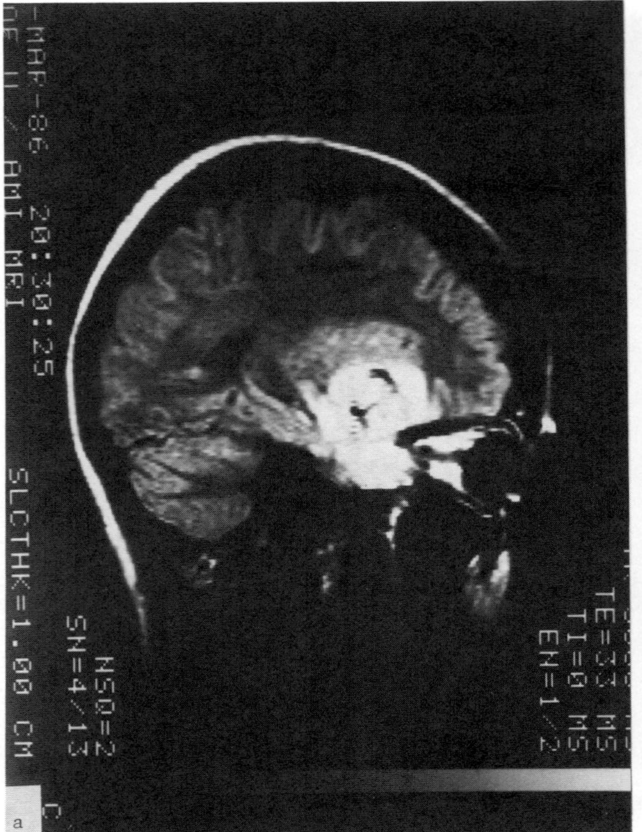
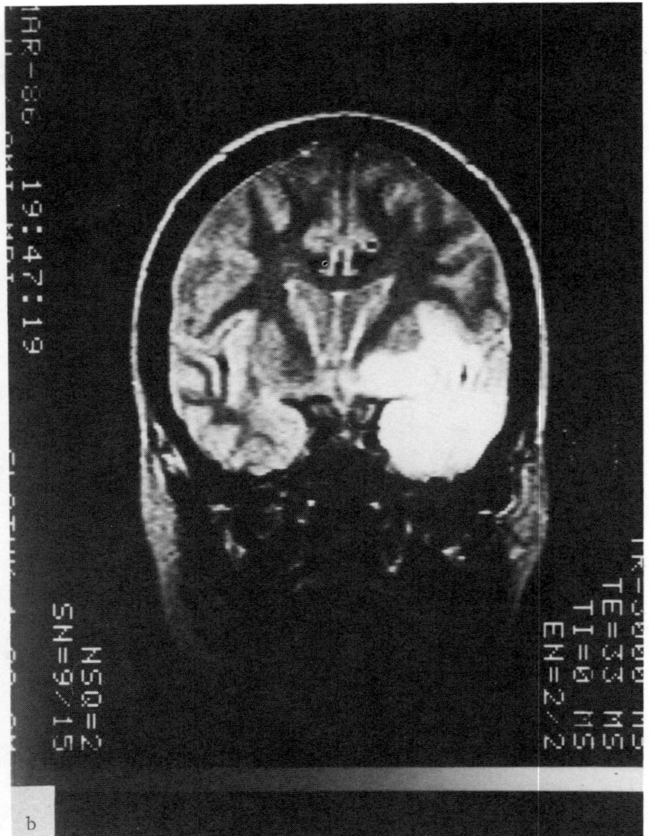

Figure 8a, b. Coronal and sagittal MR image showing diffuse infiltration of tumor surrounding the left proximal middle cerebral artery.

border, and within the CT-positive region. The CT target and border area showed anaplastic astrocytoma of class II as defined by Daumas-Duport and the MRI-positive area showed a few isolated tumor cells.[25] Impedance measures showed a differential of 130 ohms from normal tissue to the MRI-positive tissue and into the CT-positive area.

This technique of serial biopsy based on CT, MR imaging, and impedance measurement places this anaplastic astrocytoma lesion in the Daumas type II category, confirming the surgical opinion that biopsy for tissue diagnosis alone was appropriate. The stereotaxic analysis of the tissue confirmed that the tumor position on either side of the sylvian fissure coupled with extensive involvement of the white matter with isolated tumor cells precluded either debulking or complete resection. The patient was treated with external beam radiotherapy following the biopsy.

VS

This 39-year-old white female presented with a two-month history of headaches and a recent grand mal seizure. Neurologic exam was normal. A CT scan showed homogeneous low-density lesion in the dominant left frontal lobe extending posteriorly (Fig. 9). MRI was not available. Stereotaxic biopsy showed an anaplastic astrocytoma. The patient was treated with external beam radiotherapy. She had no significant neurologic symptoms or signs and her seizures remained satisfactorily controlled. Initial post-irradiation CT scans showed decrease in the area of the lesion. However, a CT scan 1 month later showed an enhancing area which persisted on subsequent CT and MR scans (Figs. 10, 11). Rebiopsy showed persistent tumor and was immediately followed by resection and interstitial brachytherapy with 125-iodine. The patient tolerated the procedure well without sustaining any new deficit. On examination, five months post resection and implant, the patient was seizure-free.

GM

This 22-year-old white male presented with progressive headaches and no neurologic symptoms. Progressive CT scans over several months showed an 8 mm low density lesion deep in the right frontal lobe (Fig. 12a,b). Because of the persistent headaches, it was elected

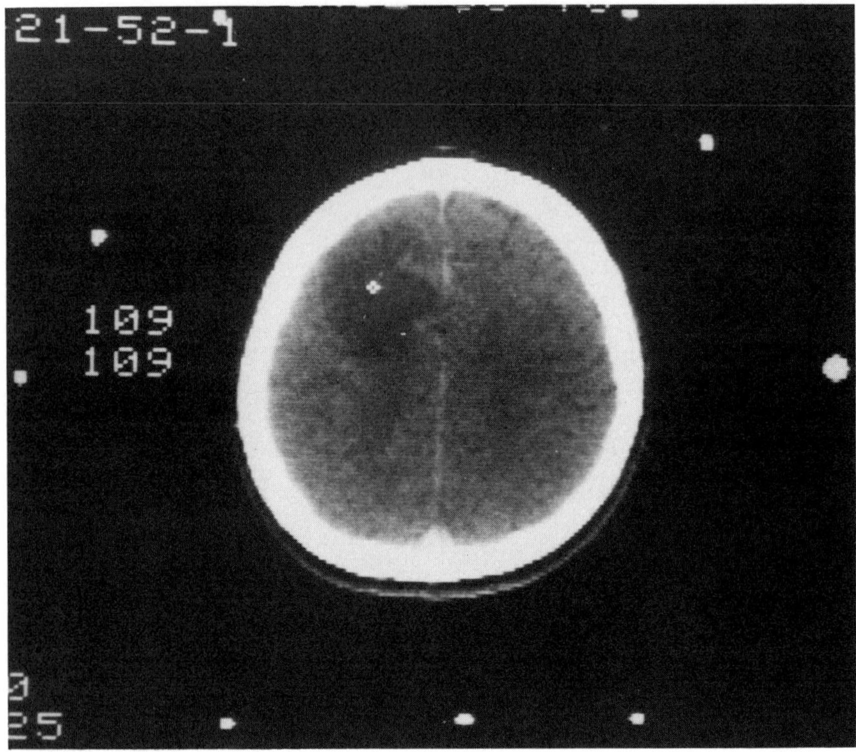

Figure 9. Stereotaxic localization CT scan showing target position within low density left frontal lesion.

to proceed with a stereotaxic biopsy and resection. Tissue showed a grade I astrocytoma of the protoplasmic type. Tissue was removed by closed suction. Postoperative CT scans showed a persistent defect. The headaches were decreased, but not eliminated.

Radiation therapy was deferred pending progression of symptoms or CT scan or MRI changes. Follow-up at 9 months showed no such changes.

Summary and Overview of the University of Utah Medical Center Cases

From 1979 through 1985, 180 stereotaxic localization procedures were performed at the University of Utah Medical Center and its

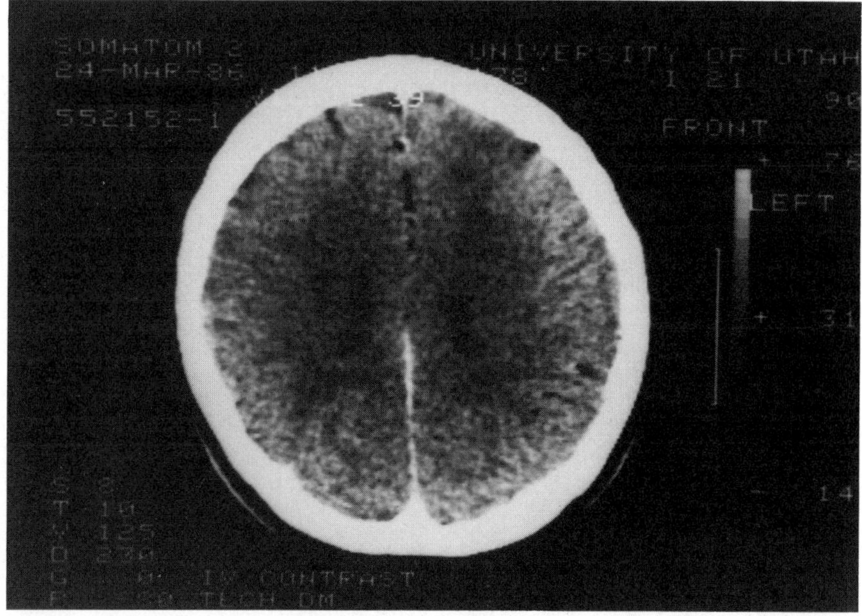

Figure 10. Post-biopsy and pre-resection CT scan showing smaller but persistent left frontal low density lesion.

affiliated hospitals (Fig. 13). By 1984, the majority of intra-axial brain lesions were approached utilizing stereotaxic localization. Moreover, interstitial brachytherapy has accounted for an increasing number of procedures over the past 2 years.

Generally, the majority of lesions were tumors, with the remainder consisting of infectious processes, vascular lesions, and degenerative lesions (Fig. 14). The category of nondiagnostic lesions was established for instances in which biopsy tissue at the target point was confirmed by postoperative CT, but nonetheless, microscopic exam revealed tissue that was either normal or otherwise unclassifiable. Seven of the 180 cases were classified as nondiagnostic.

Actual false negative biopsies occurred in an additional seven of the 180 cases. False negative biopsies occurred primarily in lesions that were relatively rigid compared to the normal brain. This disparity occasionally caused the target point to be displaced by blunt-ended biopsy instruments so that normal brain tissue was moved into and biopsied at the stereotaxically defined target. One false positive

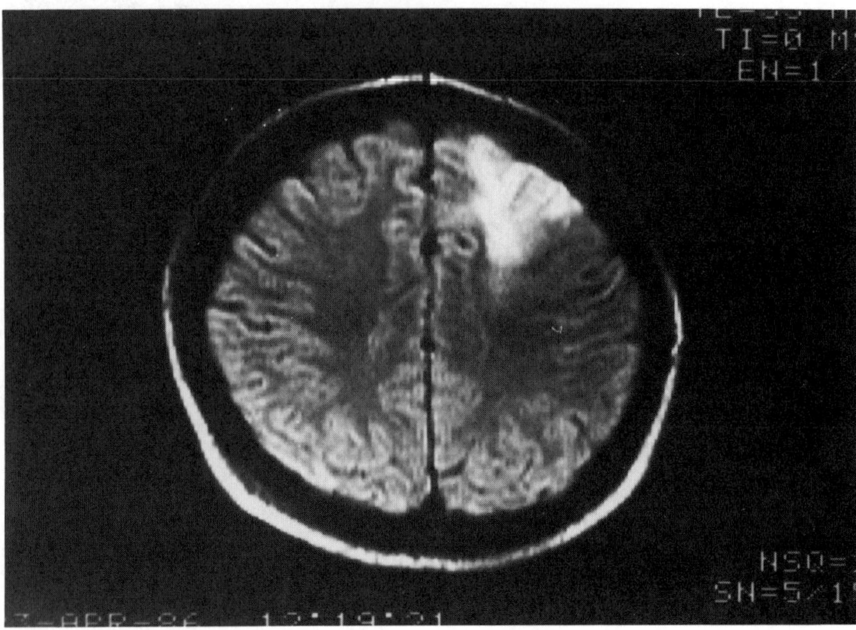

Figure 11. T2 weighted MR image showing enhanced signal which demarcates lesion better than CT scan.

biopsy occurred, also related to displacement of the lesion. The potential for target displacement is now addressed by minimally enlarging the probe track, so that the tissue lesion border or interface is exposed, and biopsy tissue can be obtained with direct visualization.

Serious complications included two deaths, both related to postbiopsy brain swelling associated with malignant tumors (Table 1). Hemorrhage into the lesion was ruled out in both cases. A third death occurred from hemorrhage into the tumor bed several days postop. Moderate morbidity resulting in hemiparesis occurred in one case when a clot evacuation followed by biopsy of the wall resulted in hemorrhage from an AVM not seen on preoperative angiography. One infection and one case of aseptic meningitis following a radiation implant occurred.

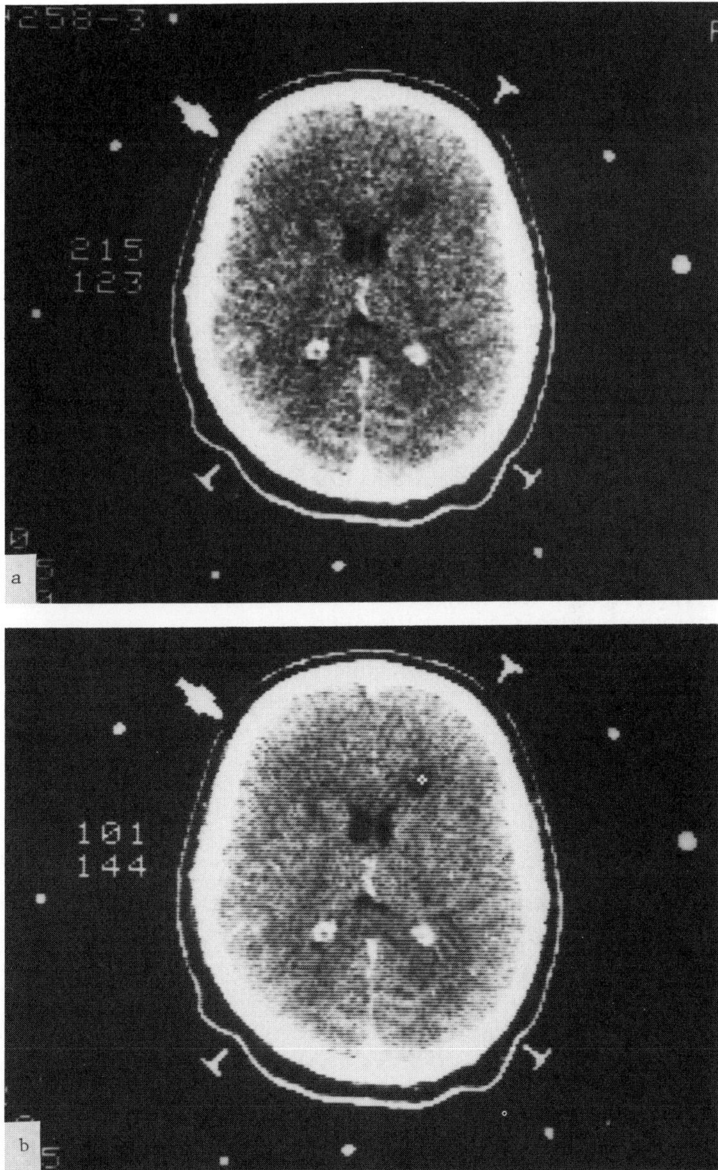

Figure 12a, b. Stereotaxic localization CT scan demonstrating low density right frontal lesion with target marked by cursor.

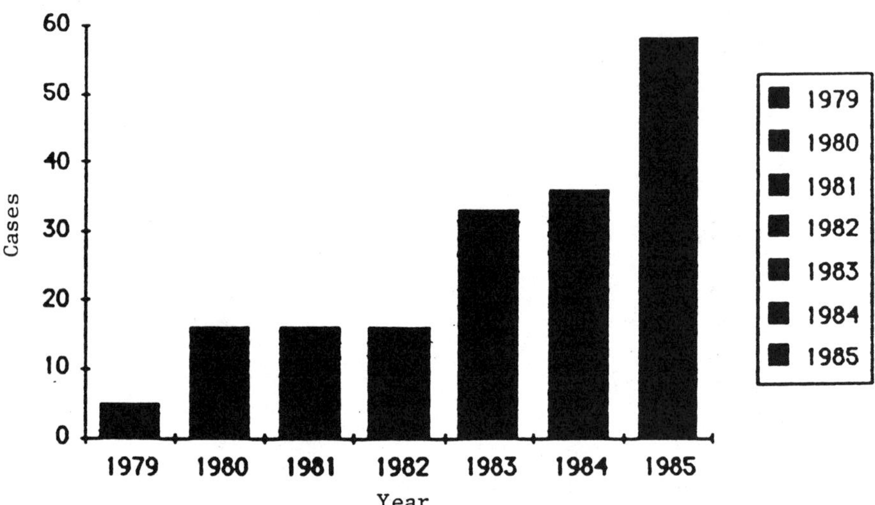

Figure 13. Image-guided stereotaxic cases performed annually at the University of Utah Medical Center 1979–1985.

Recent Advances: MRI Localization

Early experience suggests that structural detail is better on MRI than on CT images, particularly with T1 weighted images. Occasionally, lesions appear on T2 weighted images that are not seen on CT scans through the same region. In addition, MRI allows construction of MRI data into images in the coronal and sagittal as well as the axial planes. The versatility available with additional coronal and sagittal planes allows the operator to establish approaches that may better avoid structures such as the internal capsule.

In order to adapt the BRW system for MRI data, it was necessary to reconstruct the system from nonferrous materials which neither degrade nor distort the image. To date the MRI system has proven useful for localization of lesions in the brainstem and biopsy of lesions seen only on MRI. The MRI localization system can be combined with CT localization for comparison of images. Present limitations of the MRI system include the longer data acquisition time and the inability

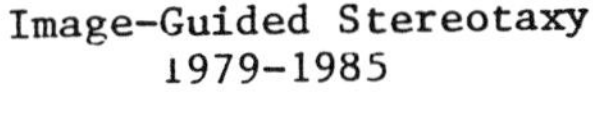

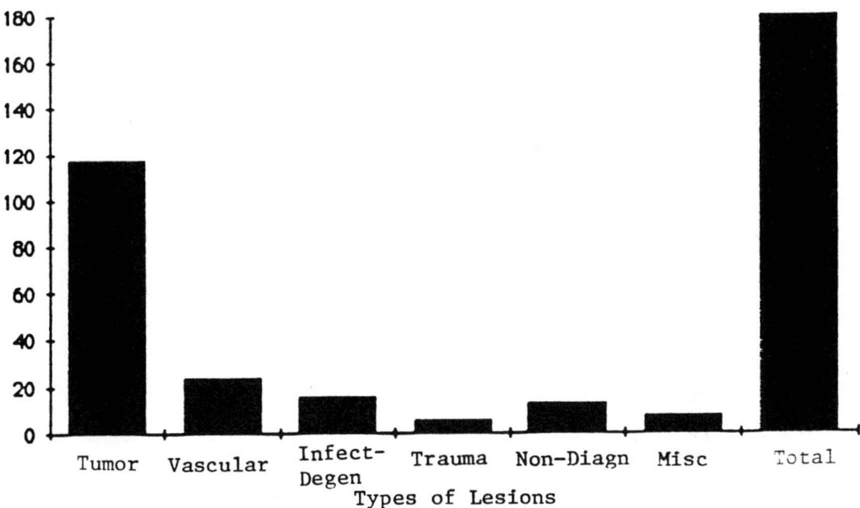

Figure 14. Categorization of cases treated with image-guided stereotaxy 1979–1986.

to use general anesthesia. However, in certain cases, MRI stereotaxic localization is essential.

Initial experience with a new BRW MRI localizer which allows localization of the target in all three planes has been reported previously.[26]

The Kelly Study

Recently, Kelly has described his experience with an independently designed system for utilizing combined CT and MRI stereotaxic biopsy to ascertain which combination of CT and MRI changes most accurately define the astrocytoma tumor border. Kelly obtains 1 cm long stereotaxic biopsies from a trajectory path which traverses the CT and MRI defined limits of the tumor. The important finding in this study was the presence of isolated tumor cells in the area of prolonged T2 signal outside of the CT defined tumor border in a high percentage of biopsies.[27]

Table 1
Image-Guided Stereotaxic Surgery: UUMC 1979–
1985 Complications (Total Cases, 180)

	Major *Tumor*	*Vascular*	*Total*
Death			
Swelling	2	0	2
Hemorrhage	1	0	1
Neurologic Deficit	1	1	2

	Minor
Wound infection	1
Post hematoma	1
Intraop hematoma	1
Postop seizures	1
Aseptic meningitis	1
CSF leak	1

	Summary	
Mortality	3/180	1.6%
Morbidity		
Major	2/180	1.1%
Minor	6/180	3.3%

This finding suggests that T2 weighted MR images detect larger areas of tumor involvement than CT scanning. Both CT perilesional hypodense areas and T2 weighted MR areas which have been considered to be due to surrounding edema associated with increased tissue water content also may contain isolated tumor cells.

This study of Kelly's demonstrates that, at least by histologic criteria, both CT perilesional hypodense areas and T2 weighted MR images with areas of prolonged signals, for the most part, are characterized by tumor infiltration with isolated tumor cells. In addition, this biopsy study seems to confirm the histologic classification of astrocytoma by the French neuropathologist, Daumas-Duport, which bases tumor malignancy on infiltrating characteristics as well as classic morphology. As surgeons combine image based stereotaxic biopsy with microscopic pathology to categorize astrocytoma malignancy, the Daumas-Duport type of histologic classification may be as important as classical morphology for treatment planning. The morphologic criteria for isolated tumor cells must also be confimed with appropriate immunohistochemical markers.

Summary

In summary, the use of image-guided stereotaxic localization, whether it be based on CT, MRI, or angiographic images alone or in combination, is becoming an essential step to define tumor distribution. The precision of the localization process has now been well demonstrated by several centers. In addition, Kelly's recent study suggesting that perilesional hypodense and T2 weighted images have isolated tumor cells further emphasizes the importance of stereotaxic localization in planning therapies comprised of regimens of surgical debulking, external beam and interstitial irradiation, and chemotherapy.

REFERENCES

1. Maroon JC, Bank WO, Drayer BP, et al. Intracranial biopsy assisted by computerized tomography. J Neurosurg 1977; 46:740–744.
2. Boethius J, Bergstrom M, Greitz T. Stereotaxic computerized tomography with a GE 8800 scanner. J Neurosurg 1980; 52:794–800.
3. Boethius J, Bergstrom M, Greitz T, Ribbe T. CT localization in stereotactic surgery. Appl Neurophysiol 1980; 43:164–169.
4. Perry JH, Rosenbaum AE, Lunsford LD, et al. Computed tomography-guided stereotactic surgery: Conception and development of a new stereotactic methodology. Neurosurgery 1980; 7:376–381.
5. Sheldon CH, McCann G, Jacques S, et al. Development of a computerized microstereotaxic method for localization and removal of minute CNS lesions under direct 3-D vision. J Neurosurg 1980; 52:21–27.
6. Bergstrom M, Greitz T, Steiner L. An approach to stereotaxic radiography. Acta Neurochir (Wein) 1980; 54:157–165.
7. Bergstrom M, Greitz T. Stereotaxic computed tomography. AJR 1976; 127:167–170.
8. Leksell L, Jernberg B. Stereotaxis and tomography: A technical note. Acta Neurochir (Wein) 1980; 52:1–7.
9. Birg W, Mundinger F, Klar M. A cumputer program system for stereotactic neurosurgery. Acta Neurochir (Wein) 1977; 24(Suppl):99–105.
10. Mundinger F, Birg W, Klar M. Computer-assisted stereotactic brain operations by means including computerized axial tomography. Appl Neurophysiol 1978; 41:169–182.
11. Ostertag CB, Mennel HD, Kiessline M. Stereotactic biopsy of brain tumors. Surg Neurol 1980; 14:275–283.

12. Brown RA. A computerized tomography-computer graphics approach to stereotaxic localization J. Neurosurg 1979; 50:715–720.
13. Brown RA. A stereotactic head frame for use with CT body scanners. Invest Radiol 1979; 14:300–304.
14. Brown RA, Roberts TS, Osborn AG. Simplified CT-guided stereotaxic biopsy. AJNR 1981; 2:181–184.
15. Brown RA, Roberts TS, Osborn AG. Stereotaxic frame and computer software for CT-directed neurosurgical localization. Invest Radiol 1980; 15:308–312.
16. Heilbrun MP, Roberts TS, Wells TH, et al. Technical manual: Brown-Roberts-Wells (BRW) CT stereotaxic guidance system. Burlington, Mass, Radionics Inc, 1982.
17. Heilbrun MP, Roberts TS, Apuzzo MLJ, et al. Preliminary experience with Brown-Roberts-Wells (BRW) computerized tomography stereotaxic guidance system. J. Neurosurg 1983; 59:217–222.
18. Apuzzo MLJ, Sabshin JK. Computed tomographic guidance stereotaxis in the management of intracranial mass lesions. Neurosurgery 1983; 12:277–284.
19. Gildenberg PL, Franklin P. Survey of CT-guided stereotaxic surgery. Appl Neurophysiol 1985; 48:477–480.
20. Kelly PJ, Earnest F, Kall BA, Goerss SJ, Scheithauer B. Surgical options for patients with deep-seated brain tumors: Computer assisted stereotactic biopsy. Mayo Clin Proc 1985; 60:223–229.
21. Chandler WF, Knake JE, McGillicuddy JE, Lillehel KO, Silver TM. Intraoperative use of real-time ultrasonography in neurosurgery. J Neurosurg 1982; 57:157–163.
22. Kelly PJ, Alker GJ. A method for stereotactic laser microsurgery in the treatment of deep-seated CNS neoplasms. Appl Neurophysiol 1980; 43–210–215.
23. Kelly PJ, Alker GJ, Goerss S. Computer-assisted stereotactic laser microsurgery for the treatment of intracranial neoplasms. Neurosurgery 1982; 10:324–331.
24. Tasker RR. Physiologic monitoring of stereotaxic biopsy. Appl Neurophysiol 1982; 10:324–331.
25. Daumas-Duport C, Monsaingeon V, Szenthe L, Szilka G. Serial stereotaxic biopsies. A double histologic code of gliomas according to malignancy and 3-D configuration as an aid to therapeutic decision and assessment of results. Appl Neurophysiol 1982; 45:431–437.
26. Heilbrun MP, Sunderland PM, McDonald PR, Ganz E, et al. Brown-Roberts-Wells (BRW) stereotaxic frame modifications to accomplish magnetic resonant image (MRI) guidance in three planes: axial/coronal/sagittal. Poster session, Annual meeting AANS, April, 1985.
27. Kelly PJ, Daumas-Duport C. Definition of tumor boundaries. Presentation, Annual meeting AANS, April 1986.

12

Brain Tumor Radiobiology

*James D. Kolker, and
Ralph R. Weichselbaum*

Introduction

This chapter presents an overview of the principles of radiotherapy, the radiobiology of brain tumors, the effects of radiation on the central nervous system (CNS), and the implications for the use of radiotherapy to treat malignant tumors of the brain.

Types of Radiation

On the atomic scale, the term "radiation" includes electromagnetic radiation (photons or "x-rays"), nuclear elements (neutrons, protons, and electrons), heavy charged ions (nuclei of various elements including neon, carbon, etc.), and other particulate matter (including pi-mesons, which are negatively charged particles of mass 273 times that of an electron).[2] Radiobiology is the study of the interaction of these various forms of radiation with living biological material. This interaction involves the transfer of energy from the radiation to the atoms of the living matter. (The unit "rad" is a unit of absorbed dose, specifically 100 ergs/gram.) When energy is transferred, it is possible that the electrons in the biologic material may be either excited (raised to a higher energy state) or if enough energy is imparted it may be ionized (electrons ejected entirely from the

From: Kornblith PL, Walker MD (editors). Advances in Neuro-Oncology. Futura Publishing Company, Inc., Mount Kisco, NY, © 1988.

atom). Ionizing radiation has the ability to break chemical bonds and affect living tissue.[2]

The specific characteristic of interaction of radiation and biological material is dependent on both the type of radiation and the degree of potential energy that it carries. The type of radiation most commonly used in clinical radiotherapy is photon or x-ray radiation. This is high frequency (short wavelength) electromagnetic radiation, as opposed to visible light which has low frequency and long wavelength.[3] As the energy imparted to radiation increases, the wavelength decreases and its ability to penetrate increases. "Supervoltage" radiation refers to radiation produced with greater energy than 500 kV. Radiation from a cobalt-60 source produces energy in the 1.17 to 1.33 MeV range and linear accelerators from 4 to 20 MeV. Supervoltage radiation is the most clinically useful in the treatment of brain tumors. Its interaction with biological material is such that its maximum energy is deposited not at the surface, but at a specific depth depending upon the energy of the photon. For beams of higher energy, the dose at the surface becomes progressively less and the depth of maximum energy deposition also becomes deeper. The practical implication is that this radiation "spares" the skin and delivers the maximum dose to deeper structures. The depth of treatment is a function of beam energy.[3,4]

Electron radiation has different energy deposition characteristics compared to photons. Most of the electron energy is deposited near the surface; and while higher energy beams deliver more dose to deeper depths, the drop-off of this energy is more rapid than photons. "Skin sparing" is, therefore, lost, but the beam is much less penetrating within tissue. The depth of treatment is also a function of beam energy.[3,4]

Types of Interactions of Radiation with Matter

The previously enumerated types of radiation are all capable of causing ionizing events. They may be divided into the categories of charged or uncharged. The charged particles (including electrons, protons, or charged heavy ions) are capable of producing a direct ionizing event. Photons interact with orbital electrons and impart energy to eject the electron. These "secondary electrons" then produce an ionization. Uncharged neutrons interact with the nucleus of an atom, impart kinetic energy, and cause the recoil of charged particles such as protons or alpha particles (2 neutrons plus 2 protons) which then produce an ionizing event. These uncharged types of radiation are examples of indirectly ionizing radiation.[2-4]

Radiation may act upon a cell in a direct or indirect manner. The "critical structure" of a cell is DNA. If an ionization occurs in a molecule of DNA, a chemical bond may be broken or a chemical reaction may take place at that site. If this alteration is incompatible with the reproductive function of the cell, then it will die when it next undergoes mitosis. An event of this kind is a "direct action" of radiation. More likely, however, since most of the molecules of a cell are water, the radiation will react with water to produce an ion radical as follows:

$$H_2O \rightarrow H_2O^+ + e^-$$

H_2O^+ is both an ion, electrically changed because it has lost an electron, and a radical, because it has an unpaired electron in the outer shell. This highly reactive compound reacts within 10^{-10} seconds with another water molecule to produce another highly reactive molecule, the hydroxyl radical.

$$H_2O^+ + H_2O \rightarrow H_3O + OH\cdot$$

The hydroxyl radical has a lifespan in a biological system of 0.1 to 1 microsecond. During this time, this oxidizing agent can attack the DNA and produce molecular changes incompatible with current or future cell function. This chain of events is an example of indirect action, and it has been estimated that 75% of the damage to mammalian DNA is through the indirect action of photons to produce hydroxyl radicals.[2,3] After an indirect action of radiation, cellular lethality may occur.

Quality of Radiation

Linear energy transfer (LET) refers to the amount of energy transferred from the radiation to the biological material, but differs from "rad" (energy per unit mass of biological material) in that it describes the energy deposited as a function of unit length along the radiation track. The unit that is usually used is keV per micron of unit density material. Differences in LET account for the fact that although most radiation produces a qualitatively similar effect (ionization), there is a marked difference in the quantitative results of the various forms of radiation. Equal doses of radiation may translate into a very different biological result. This result is referred to as relative biological effectiveness (RBE). It is customary to compare other radiation forms and energies to the effect produced by 250 keV x-rays. The RBE can vary with the particular biologic system used as the measure. For many systems the RBE is related to LET, with RBE increasing with LET up to approximately 100 keV per micron then decreasing (see Fig. 1). Low LET radiation produces ionizations sparsely throughout biological material. More densely ionizing radiation, therefore, should have a greater biological effect. There reaches a point, however, where more than enough ionizations occur in a cell to inactivate it and the excess energy is wasted and RBE falls. Thus, there appears to be an optimal LET.[2,3,21,22]

Cell Cycle Effects

The lethal effects of ionizing radiation are cell cycle specific (see Figs. 2 and 3.) This effect can be demonstrated using synchronized populations of cells. A summary of the results of experiments on hamster and HeLa[12,13] cells is as follows:

1. Cells are relatively more sensitive at or near mitosis (M phase).
2. If G_1 is of significant length, resistance is seen early, followed by a more sensitive period as the S (synthetic) phase is approached.
3. Cells are more sensitive during early S but become progressively more resistant toward the end of the phase.
4. The G_2 (pre-mitotic) phase is usually as sensitive as the M phase. Several mechanisms have been suggested to integrate the experimental observations. If DNA is the major critical target affecting cell survival, then cell cycle effects might be explained on the basis of its number (haploid or diploid) and form (condensed or noncondensed). A very sensitive period also occurs as DNA condenses just prior to mitosis. Also, naturally occurring radiation protection agents such as sulfhydryl compounds vary with cell cycle and may exert an influence on survival.

Oxygen Effect

Cell survival is influenced by the oxic or hypoxic conditions under which they exist. Radiation damage is facilitated by oxygen. The ratio

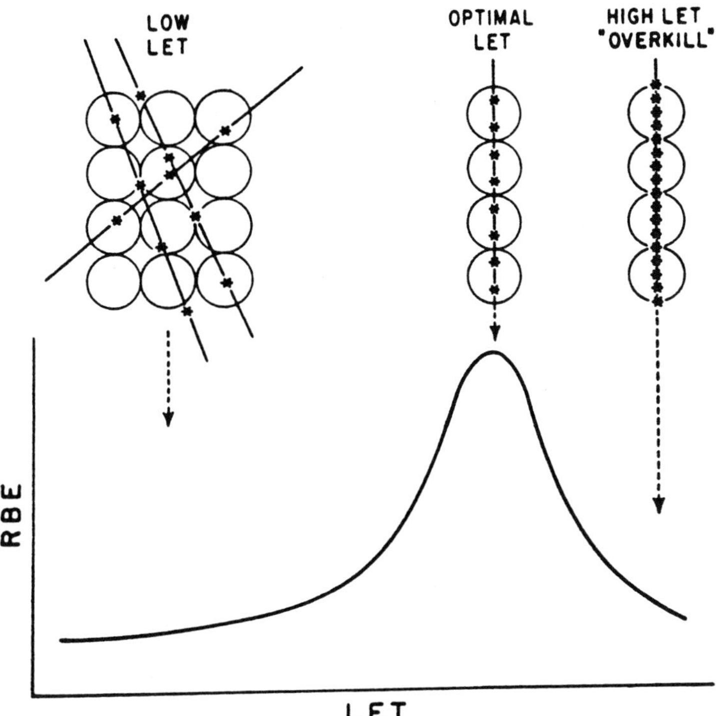

Figure 1. A diagrammatic representation of the relationship between LET and RBE is presented. For a cell to be killed, more than one ionizing event is necessary. At very low LET, energy is deposited sparsely along its track, thus ionizing events occur infrequently. More than one particle must pass through a cell in order to kill it. As LET increases, ionizing events occur more densely along its track and a single particle can produce enough damage to kill the cell, thus its efficiency or effectiveness is increased. As LET increases further, more energy is deposited than is minimally required to kill the cell, thus energy is wasted and efficiency is diminished. There is, therefore an optimal LET where just enough energy is deposited to kill the cell. (From Hall EJ. Radiation for the Radiobiologist, 2nd Edition, Philadelphia, Harper and Row Publishers, 1978.)

of the enhancement of cell kill in the presence of oxygen is called the oxygen enhancement ratio (OER) (Fig. 4) The magnitude of this effect varies with the type of radiation. For sparsely ionizing, low LET radiation such as x-ray photons, the OER is approximately 3. For moderately densely ionizing radiation, such as fast neutrons, the OER is

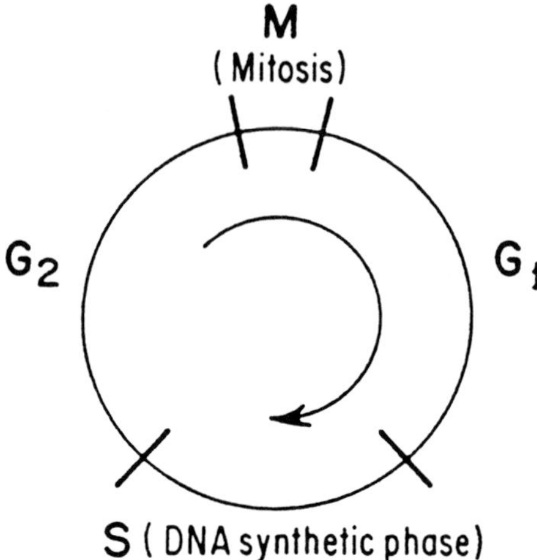

Figure 2. The stages of the mammalian cell cycle are schematically represented. There are intervals, (G_1 and G_2) between the mitotic phase (M) and the DNA synthetic phase (S) during which the cell appears to be inactive if judged by the uptake of radioactively labeled thymadine. There is a wide variation in the length of the G_1 phase among the mammalian cells, but relatively little between M, S, and G_2 phases. (From Hall EJ. Radiobiology for Radiobiologist, 2nd Edition, Philadelphia, Harper and Row Publishers, 1978.)

approximately 1.5. For densely ionizing radiation, such as alpha-particles, the OER is 1.0 (no enhancement). The precise mechanism of the oxygen effect is not known, but it is thought that oxygen participates in chemical reactions at the level of the free radicals. When the biological material is attached by the OH radical, it produces a free radical on the target, R·. If oxygen is present it can react to form RO_2 which is a permanent change in the structure. A chemical change is then fixed in the target tissue.[2]

Repair

After being exposed to ionizing radiation, one of four events is possible:

1. No damage may have occurred in the critical target and the cell is unaffected.
2. Lethal damage in which the critical target is irreversibly damaged.

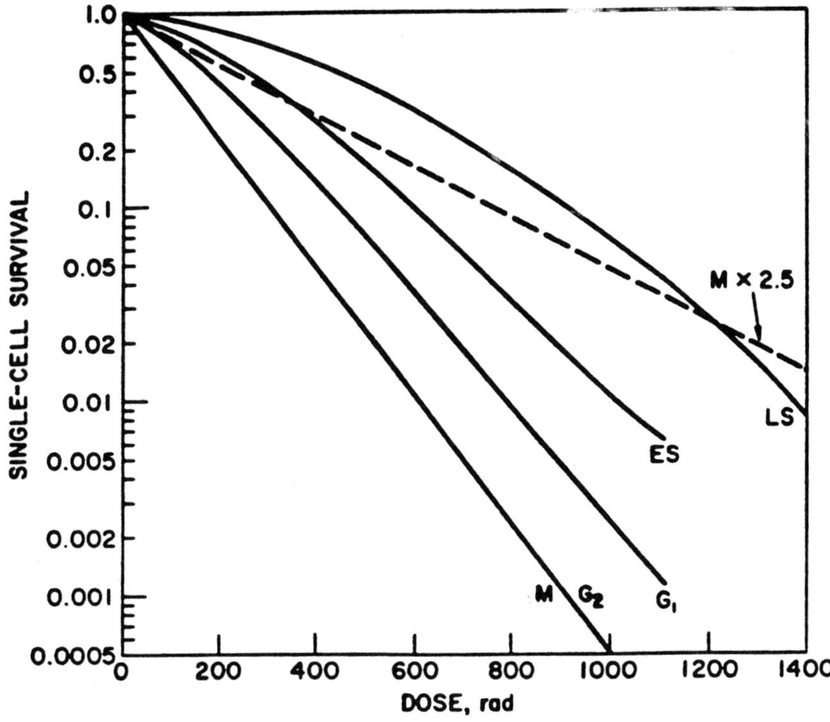

Figure 3. The cell survival curves from the Chinese hamster cells are illustrated. The dose of radiation required to kill cells varies with the phases of the cell cycle. Sensitivity is greatest for cells in late G and M phases and most resistant for late S (LS) phase. (From Hall EJ. Radiobiolgy for the Radiobiologist, 2nd Edition, Philadelphia, Harper and Row Publishers, 1978.)

3. Sublethal damage is damage to critical targets which can be repaired under a variety of experimental conditions. This is referred to as sublethal damage repair (SLDR).
4. Potentially lethal damage is operationally defined as damage which if unrepaired is lethal. This can be influenced by certain post-irradiation conditions and is referred to as potentially lethal damage repair (PLDR).[2,23,24]

Concepts of Radiosensitivity and Radiocurability

Cell kill can be measured with respect to the dose of radiation exposure. When plotted in a semi-logarithmic fashion, a cell survival

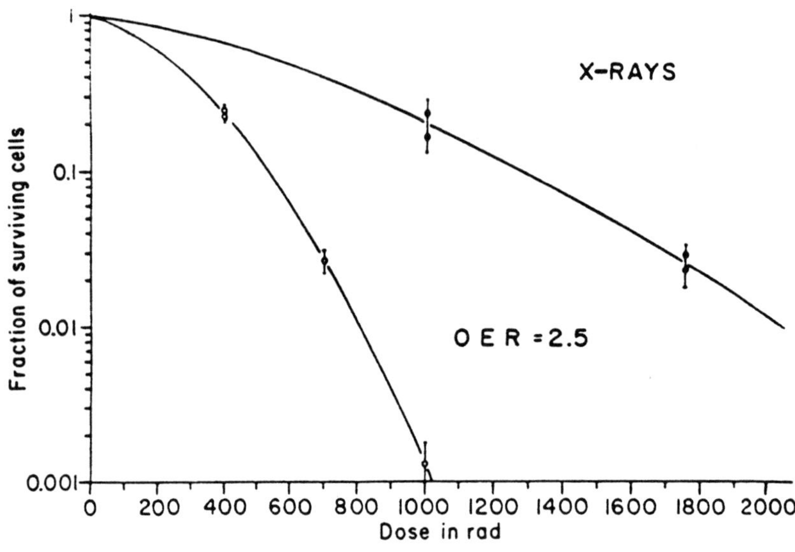

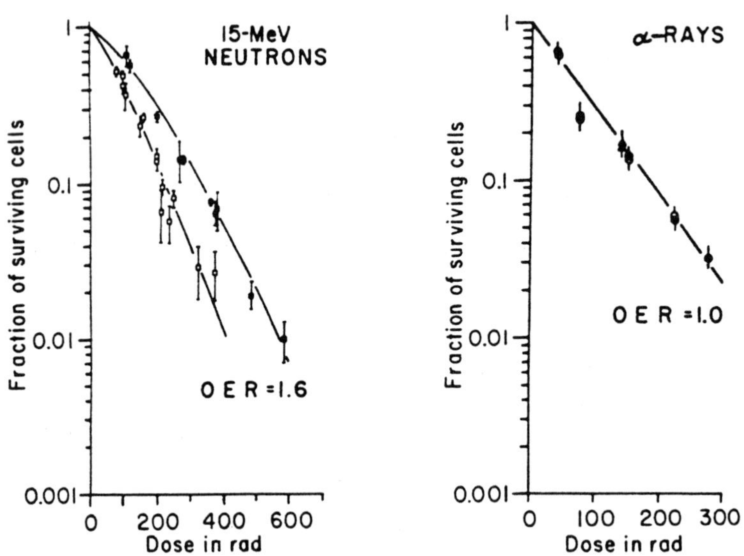

Figure 4. OER varies with the type of radiation. The greatest oxygen enhancement of cell kill occurs with low LET x-rays. As LET increases from neutron to alpha particles, for example, the advantage diminishes and the OER falls. (From Hall EJ. Radiobiology for the Radiobiologist, 2nd Edition, Philadelphia, Harper and Row Publishers, 1978.)

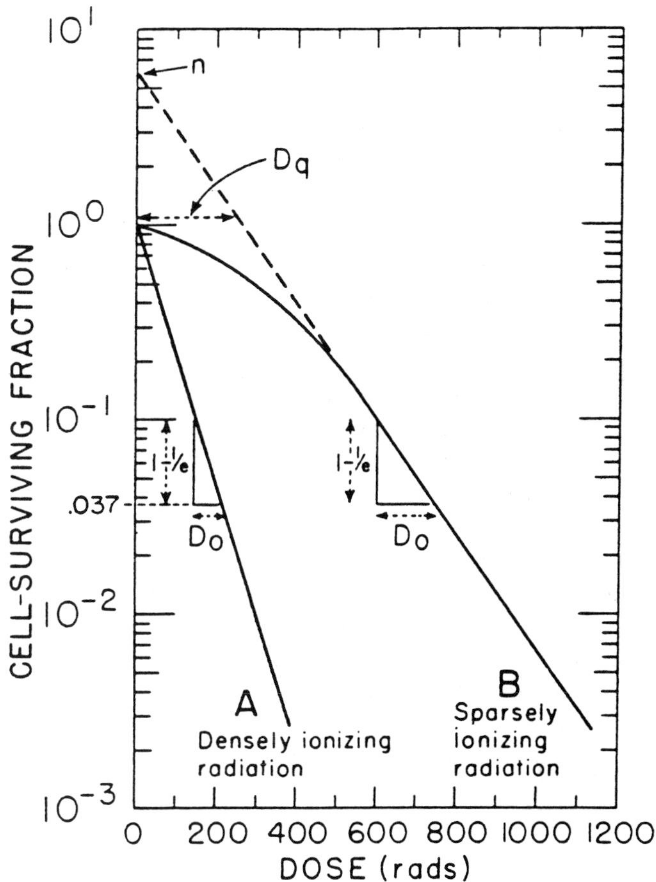

Figure 5. The typical survival curve for mammalian cells is illustrated. The initial portion is the shoulder of the curve and represents the ability of the cell to accumulate and repair sublethal damage. It is quantified by the extrapolation number, n, or by the quasi-threshold dose, D_q. The dose of radiation required in the straight line portion of the curve to reduce the clonogenic cell population to 37% of its original value is termed D_o. (From Hall EJ, Radiobiology for the Radiobiologist, 2nd Edition, Philadelphia, Harper and Row Publishers, 1978.)

curve is generated (Fig. 5). The inverse of the slope of the survival curve is a measure of radiosensitivity. In this exponential relationship, a constant proportion of cells (rather than a constant number of cells) is killed for a given dose increment. The dose of radiation required to reduce a cell population to 37% of its original number in the straight-line portion of the curve is referred to as D_o. This is the dose required to produce, on average, one lethal lesion per cell. The initial part of the curve is referred to as the shoulder and represents the ability of cells to accumulate and repair sublethal damage. The width of the shoulder can be quantified by extrapolating the straight portion of the curve back to the ordinate. This is the extrapolation number, n. The shoulder can also be expressed by the quasi-threshold dose, D_q, which is the dose measured from the projected linear portion of the curve back through unity of surviving fraction.[2,23]

Radiocurability is a clinical term that refers to whether a tumor is controlled locally by a dose of radiation. This dose is limited by the tolerance of normal surrounding tissue. *Radioresponsive* refers to the physical regression of measurable tumor after radiation, but not to whether the tumor is radiocurable. For example, carcinoma of the prostate is radiocurable,[46] but not radioresponsive. This tumor has a long cell doubling time. Cells that have sustained an inactivating lesion progress slowly through the cell cycle and express lethality at the subsequent mitosis. "Divisional death" explains why some radiocurable tumors do not appear radioresponsive. On the other hand, oat cell carcinoma of the lung is radioresponsive in that it regresses at relatively low doses of radiation, yet is not readily radiocurable, since it may often fail locally even with relatively high doses of radiation.[47]

Radiocurability and Dose

While the probability of tumor cure increases with dose, the dose that can be delivered is usually limited by radiation effects in the surrounding normal tissue. The relationship between the probability of tumor control or the probability of normal tissue complications with respect to dose is a sigmoid function (Fig. 6.) The separation between the tumor control and complication curves defines the therapeutic ratio.

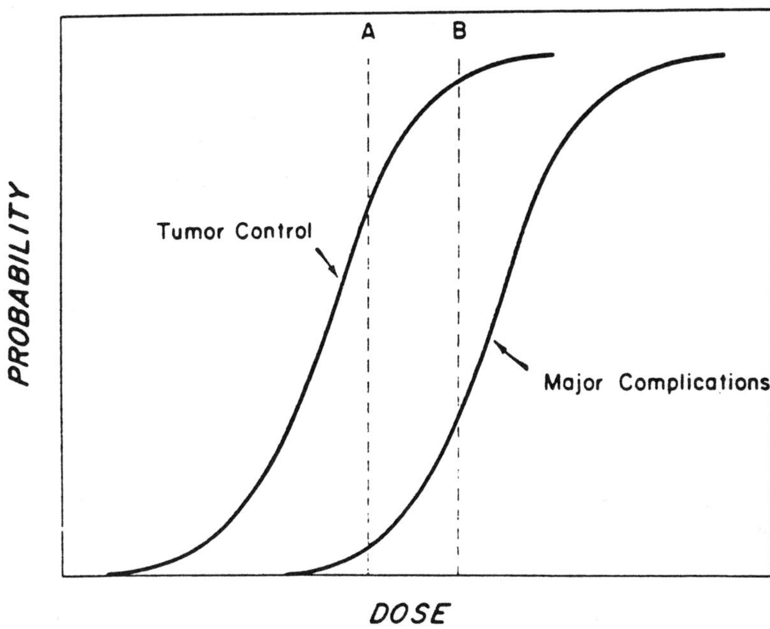

Figure 6. The relationship between tumor control and major complications to radiation dose is shown. The sigmoid curve on the left shows the relationship between local control and dose. For low doses no control is seen. However, as the dose is increased, an increased likelihood of local control is seen. Balanced against tumor control are complications observed in irradiated normal tissues. The sigmoid curve on the right traces the relationship between these complications and dose. The same sigmoid relationship is seen for both tumor control and complications. However, the complications curve is displaced to the right. If the curves are significantly separated, the likelihood of an uncomplicated curve is favorable. If they are in positions where they may be superimposed on one another, there is less chance for an uncomplicated cure. The choice of dose is dependent upon these factors. The optimal therapeutic ratio occurs when the complications curve is displaced as far to the right as possible. Note that both curves are extremely "steep" functions of the dose. (From Weichselbaum RR, Sherman D, Ervin TJ. Basic Principles of Radiotherapy. In: Oral Cancer, Shklar J, ed. Philadelphia, WB Saunders Company, 1984.)

Theories of Radiation Effects on Normal Brain

The exact mechanisms underlying the late effects of radiation on the CNS are not clearly understood, but it is fundamentally known that radiation affects cells capable of division.[5] With respect to division, the cells of the CNS may be divided into two groups: (1) the fixed post-mitotic neurons, and (2) the support glial elements and endothelial cells which undergo mitosis to a variable extent.[7-11] The former group is relatively insensitive to radiation effects, and therefore most theories of late effects center on this latter group of proliferating cells. If the loss of this collection of support cells exceeds the capacity of the brain to repair the damage, then those functions that depend on those cells also fails.[2,6] Since these cells serve different functions, the manifestation of radiation damage is heterogeneous.

Late effects can be grouped into two categories. The first is stem cell depletion. A stem cell population is a self-maintaining system whose function is to produce cells to repopulate a normal tissue. This reservoir of cells can be triggered to divide more rapidly if needed. If these cells have sustained lethal radiation damage, they will die during a subsequent mitosis and be unable to replete the population of functioning cells downstream. The mature functioning cells, on the other hand, will continue to perform their sustaining function for the duration of their natural life-span. The critical period for the organism occurs at a time approximately one "normal" mature cell life-span from the time of irradiation when there is inadequate replacement of mature cells. Proliferating stem cell populations in the CNS support the glial elements and capillary endothelial cells. The function that these mature cells serve may be compromised. The second category is late hyperproliferative vascular damage, perhaps in response to initial endothelial loss. This narrowing or obliteration of nutritive vessels results in diminished blood flow and possibly the death of the cell populations that they feed.[2,10,11] Hopewell[16-19] has proposed a theory of late effects based on the evidence that the type of damage produced is dose-related. Higher doses produced selective white matter necrosis while lower doses produced vascular changes in both grey and white matter, but after a much longer latent period. The white matter necrosis and vascular damage were separated in time, suggesting different target cells causing each lesion. The endothelial proliferation observed, presumably leading to vascular insufficiency, was suggested to be a growth response to initial cell loss. The earlier white matter necrosis could represent glial cell destruction. Van der Kogel[20] observes an analogous phenomenon in rat spinal cord.

The phenomenon known as the "blood-brain barrier" is the area that separates the lumen of the capillary and brain parenchyma. It is a complex structure, but the chief contributor to its qualities of exclusion and selective transport is thought to be the close approximation of endothelial cells in the form of tight junctions.[14] Caveness[6] has observed a late-delayed post-radiation syndrome in the brains of adult monkeys using fractionated and single dose supervoltage radiation. A delayed and rapidly progressive increase in CSF pressure has been noted. Edema was noted both in the irradiated volume and in remote areas of the brain. The hallmark lesion in the whole-brain irradiated monkeys was a minute focus of necrosis widely scattered throughout the forebrain white matter. Where there were acute lesions, there were breaks in the blood-brain barrier and brain swelling. Abnormal vascular channels making up patches of telangiectasias also contributed to brain damage and these lesions were progressively expressed over time. It should be noted that there was a great deal of variation in the latency and nature of the lesions with dose fraction size and age of animal. Even among monkeys of similar age and exposure, there was considerable variability in susceptibility to radiation damage. Remler[15] irradiated rat brains with 20 to 60 Gy single fractions and suggests that the dose-latency relationship produced suggests endothelial damage with breakdown of the blood-brain barrier as the primary mechanism causing the late radiation syndrome.

Radiobiology of Brain Tumors

Radiobiological parameters have been examined for a wide variety of human tumor cell lines in vitro.[24–32] Weichselbaum et al.[28] studied inherent radioresistance and repair of sublethal and potentially lethal damage of 29 human tumor cell lines. Nine tumor cell lines showed radioresistance which correlated with proficiency in the repair of potentially lethal damage. Some tumor cell lines exhibit a large ability to repair sublethal damage. Barranco et al.[25] studied three human melanoma lines which demonstrated a large ability to repair sublethal damage. Gerwick et al.[26] studied three human malignant glioma lines. Two of the three were resistant to the effects of ionizing radiation and one was within the range of normal fibroblasts.

Nilsson et al.[27] studied human glioblastoma lines and found them to be significantly more radioresistant than normal glial and/or human fibroblast lines. We conclude, therefore, although the number of human malignant glioma lines studied is limited, the data suggest that inherent radioresistance and/or ability to repair x-ray damage may be important in the clinical radiotherapy of human gliomas.

As a tumor grows, cells that have been well oxygenated by a feeding capillary get pushed farther away from their source of diffused oxygen by newly growing cells (Fig. 7). Oxygen concentration in diffusion falls with distance, thus cells farther away from the capillary are relatively hypoxic. This hypoxic fraction is relatively less radiosensitive. After a dose of radiation, the well-oxygenated cells die off more readily than the hypoxic cells, thus in the surviving tumor, there are proportionately more hypoxic cells. If the tumor reestablishes its normal structure, the previously hypoxic cells become reoxygenated and can be more readily killed in the next fraction of radiation.[2] Glioblastoma multiforme in humans containing areas of necrosis has been postulated to have areas of low oxygen tension.[34] The exact role of reoxygenation in human brain tumors is not clear. In an effort to sensitize hypoxic cells, chemical compounds have been developed to mimic the effects of oxygen. Because these compounds are only very slowly metabolized by cells, they can diffuse farther from the capillary and reach hypoxic cells. These electron affinic agents, most notably metronidazole and misonidazole, have been used in a number of clinical trials with high grade astrocytomas. Urtasun[1] reported the results of 36 patients, stratified by functional level then randomized to a control group of radiation alone versus radiation plus high-dose metronidazole. The group treated with radiation plus metronidazole had a significantly longer median survival (26 weeks) than the radiation alone group (15 weeks). The radiation scheme (3,000 rads in 9 fractions over 18 days), however, was suboptimal as evidenced by the poor median survival in the radiation alone group compared to other studies using higher doses of radiation.[12,13] The use of metronidazole compensated for the inadequate radiotherapy and produced a median survival almost comparable to studies using adequate radiation doses. There were no long-term survivors in either group. A subsequent study[41] by the same group compared standard dose conventional single daily fractionation (CF) with (adequate dose) multiple daily fraction radiation therapy (MDF) with and without misonidazole. They showed a significant advantage for the MDF scheme but no added advantage for misonidazole. In fact,

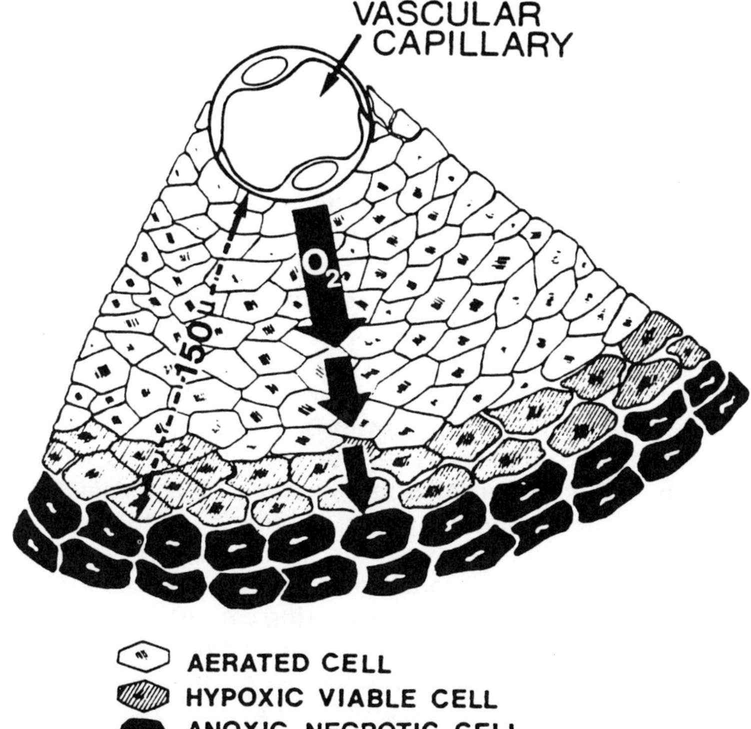

Figure 7. The diffusion of oxygen from capillary to surrounding tissue is illustrated. The distance that oxygen can diffuse from the capillary is limited by the initial partial pressure of oxygen and its metabolism by respiring cells through which it passes. Cells farther away from the capillary become progressively more hypoxic and, therefore, more radioresistant. (From Hall EJ. Radiobiology for the Radiobiologist, 2nd Edition, Philadelphia, Harper and Row Publishers, 1978.)

they have dropped the misonidazole arm of the study. Several other studies with these agents have also failed to demonstrate a significant clinical advantage.[35-37]

True radiosensitizers sensitize all cells that take up the agent. BUdR (5-bromodeoxyuridine) is formed by adding a bromide atom at the 5-position of a uridine molecule. It differs from thymidine which has a methyl group at that position. The van der Waals radius of the bromide and methyl groups are almost identical, however, and stereochemical similarities allow BUdR to be substituted for thymidine in DNA. For reasons that are not well understood, BUdR-substituted DNA is more radiosensitive. The increase in radiosensitivity of the cell is approximately a linear function with respect to thymidine replacement by BUdR.[48] Cells typically must move through several cycles to take up enough BUdR to be sensitized. To be clinically effective, the cell cycle time of the tumor cell should be shorter than that of the surrounding normal tissue, so that the tumor cell takes up more BUdR. Also, since BUdR is rapidly dehalogenated and catabolized in the liver, delivering adequate doses requires constant infusion.[49,50] Early uncontrolled trials with intra-arterial BUdR from Japan[51] suggested improved survival and local control in primary brain tumors without an increase in radiation damage to irradiated normal brain tissue. There was, however, significant morbidity from the indwelling arterial catheter in the internal carotid artery. The NCI has reported results from a phase I trial of intravenous infusion BUdR and radiotherapy for malignant glioma.[50] The median survival of 12 months for their 14 patients is not significantly better than recent historical studies for radiation alone.[12] Systemic toxicity has been significant. With improved indwelling catheter techniques now available, reconsideration is being given to intra-arterial infusion where higher BUdR doses can be delivered to the tumor.

Repopulation refers to the regrowth of cells after a killing event. In both normal and neoplastic tissues, the excessive loss of cells can trigger the proliferation of quiescent cells and shorten the cell cycle.[38,39] There are data to suggest that repopulation plays a role in clinical radioincurability of human tumors.

Split course radiotherapy is a technique where radiation is divided into two parts and separated by a rest pefiod. Parsons[40] has shown that this technique can lead to poorer tumor control than continuous course therapy. The inferior cure rates could be due to regrowth of tumor during the rest period. Conversely, if the radiation dose could be administered in a shorter period of time through smaller, more frequent fractions, then repopulation of tumor cells could be minimized. There is conflicting evidence for the clinical efficacy of hyperfractionation. Shin and Urtasun[41] demonstrated an advantage in median survival for a multiple daily fractionated regimen (39 weeks) compared to conventional single daily fractionation (27 weeks) in a prospective, randomized trial. No advantage in median survival could be demonstrated at the Princess Margaret Hospital[42] in a randomized trial comparing conventional daily fractionation with hyperfractionated therapy in which both groups received CCNU and hydroxyurea.

Redistribution refers to the change in proportion of surviving cells in various phases of cell cycle after radiation. A single dose of radiation changes this distribution by killing cells in the sensitive phases and causing a pre-mitotic block. The reassortment tends to synchronize cells within the cell cycle. Taking advantage of this synchrony is difficult in clinical practice. Adding to the difficulty is that only a small proportion of clonogenic cells are actively proliferating at any given time.[39]

Neutron radiation has several theoretical advantages over photon radiation. This high-LET radiation allows little or no repair of sublethal or potentially lethal damage. It has a lower OER (less dependent on the oxygen effect) than photons so it should kill hypoxic cells more efficiently. Also, there is less variation of cell sensitivity with phases of the cell cycle.[2] Thus far, however, this has not translated into a significantly better cure rate for high grade astrocytomas.[36,37,43] The dose of neutrons is limited by the late effects on normal brain. In studies where the dose of neutrons is high enough to usually sterilize tumor, the late effects on normal brain have compromised survival. Late effects have included a diffuse gliosis and white matter demyelination.[43,44]

Summary

There are many factors that contribute to a tumor's radiocurability. Not all types of brain tumors are radioincurable. Medulloblastoma, ependymoma, and dysgerminoma are malignant tumors that are both radioresponsive and relatively radiocurable.[45] High grade astrocytomas are mostly radioincurable. Factors contributing to the poor results may include the intrinsic properties of the tumor, the local envrionment, and the limitations of delivering adequate doses of radiation without causing excessive damage to normal surrounding brain tissue. There might be a small therapeutic window through which enough dose of low and/or high LET radiation (with or without chemotherapy or radiosensitizers) could be delivered to improve clinical results. As of yet, this has not been defined, but trials are ongoing.

REFERENCES

1. Urtasun R, Band P, Chapman JD, Feldstein ML, Mielke B, Fryer C. Radiation and high-dose metronidazole in supratentorial glioblastomas. N Engl J Med 1976; 294:1364.
2. Hall Eric J. Radiobiology for the radiobiologist, 2nd Ed. Philadelphia, PA, Harper and Row, 1978.
3. Johns HE, Cunningham, JR. The physics of radiobiology. Springfield, IL, Charles C Thomas, 1983.
4. Khan FM. The Physics of Radiation Therapy. Baltimore, Williams and Wilkins, 1984.
5. Zeman W. Disturbances of nucleic acid metabolism preceding delayed radionecrosis of nervous tissue. Proc Natl Acad Sci, USA 1968; 50:626.
6. Caveness WF, Experimental observations: delayed necrosis in normal monkey brain. In: Radiation Damage to the Nervous System, Gilbert HA, Kagan AR, eds. New York, Raven Press, 1980.
7. Jellinger K, Sturn KW. Delayed radiation myelopathy in man. J Neurol Sci 1971; 14:389–408.
8. Korr H, Schultze B, Maurer W. Autoradiographic investigations of glial proliferation in the brain of adult mice. II. Cycle time and mode of proliferation of neuroglia and endothelial cells. J Comp Neurol 1975; 160:477–490.
9. Korr H, Schultz B, Maurer W. Autoradiographic investigations of glial proliferation in the brain of adult mice. The DNA synthesis phase of neuroglia and endothelial cells. J Comp Neurol 1973; 150:169–176.
10. Casaret G. In: Cellular Basis and Aetiology of Late Somatic Effects of Ionizing Radiations. Harris, RJC, ed. New York, Academic Press, 1963.
11. Rubin R, Casaret GW. Clinical radiation pathology. Philadelphia, WB Saunders, 1969.
12. Walker MD, Strike TA, Sheline GE. An analysis of dose-effect relationship in the radiotherapy of malignant gliomas. Int J Radiat Oncol Biol Phys 1979; 5:1725.
13. Salazar OM, Rubin P, Feldstein ML, Pizzutiello R. High dose radiation in the treatment of malignant gliomas: Final report. Int J Radiat Oncol Biol Phys 1979; 5:1733.
14. Barr ML. The Human Nervous System, Hagerstown, MD, Harper and Row, 1974.
15. Remler MP, et al. The late effects of radiation on the blood brain barrier. Int J Radiat Oncol Biol Phys 1986; 12:1965–1969.
16. Hopewell JW, Young CMA. Changes in the microcirculation of normal tissues after irradiation. Int J Radiat Oncol Biol Phys 1978; 4:53–58.
17. Hopewell JW. Late radiation damage to the central nervous system: A radiobiological interpretation, Neuropathol Appl Neurobiol 1979; 5:329–343.
18. Reinhold HS, van Putten WLJ, Hopewell JW, van der Kogel AJ. The latent period in clinical radiation myleopathy. Int J Radiat Oncol Biol Phys 1984; 10:2385–2387.
19. Hopewell JW. Experimental studies of early and late responses in normal

tissues, In: The Biological Basis of Radiotherapy. Steel GG, Adams GE, Peckham MJ, eds. Amsterdam, Elsevier Science Publishers, 1983.

20. Van der Kogel AJ. Mechanisms of late radiation injury in the spinal cord. In: Radiation Biology in Cancer Research, Meyn RE, Withers HR, eds. New York, Raven Press, 1980.

21. Weichselbaum RR, Sherman D, Ervin TJ. Basic principles of radiotherapy. In: Oral Cancer. Shklar G, ed. Philadelphia, WB Saunders Co., 1984.

22. Skarsgard, LD. Survival, chromosome abnormalities and recovery in heavy-ion and x-irradiation mammalian cells. Radiat Res 1967; 7:208.

23. Elkind MM, Sutton H. Radiation responses of mammalian cells grown in culture. Repair of x-ray damage in surviving chinese hamster cells. Radiat Res 1960; 13:556.

24. Little JB, Hahn GM, Frindel F, et al. Repair of potential lethal radiation damage in vitro and in vivo. Radiology 1973; 106:689.

25. Barranco SC, Romdahl MM, Humphrey RM. The radiation response of human malignant melanoma cells grown in vitro. Cancer Res 1971; 31:830.

26. Gerwick LE, Kornblith PL. Radiation sensitivity of cultured human glioblastoma cells. Radiology 1977; 125:231.

27. Nilsson S, Carlson JB, Ponten J. Survival of irradiated glia and glioma cells studied with a new cloning technique. Int J Radiat Biol 1980; 37:267.

28. Weichselbaum RR, Dahlbert W, Little JB. Inherently radio-resistant cells exist in some human tumors. Proc Natl Acad Sci USA 1985; 82:4732.

29. Weichselbaum RR, Little JB. The differential response of human tumours to fractionated radiation may be due to a post-irradiation repair process. Br J Cancer 1982; 46:532.

30. Weichselbaum RR, Nove J, Little JB. X-ray sensitivity of human tumor cells in vitro. Int J Radiat Oncol Biol Phys 1980; 6:437.

31. Weichselbaum RR, Little JB. X-ray sensitivity of repair in human tumour cells. In: The Biological Basis of Radiotherapy. Steel GG, Adams GE, Peckham MJ, eds. New York, Elsevier Science Publishers BV, 1983.

32. Weichselbaum RR, Epstein J, Little JB. In vitro cellular radiosensitivity of human malignant tumors. Eur J Cancer 1976; 12:47.

33. Leith JT, Schilling WA, Wheeler KT. Cellular radiosensitivity of a rat brain tumor. Cancer 1975; 35:1545.

34. Nelson JS, Isukada Y, Schoenfeld D, Fulling K, Lamarche I, Peress N. Necrosis as a prognostic criterion in malignant supratentorial, astrocytic gliomas. Cancer 1983; 52:550.

35. EORTC brain tumor group: Misonidazole in radiotherapy of supratentorial malignant brain gliomas in adult patients. A randomized double-blind study. Eur J Cancer Clin Oncol 1983; 19:39.

36. Kapp DS, Wagner FC, Lawrence R. Glioblastoma multiforme: Treatment by large dose fraction irradiation and metronidazole. Int J Radiat Oncol Biol Phys 1982; 8:351.

37. Kurup PD, Pajak TF, et al. Fast neutrons and misonidazole for malignant astrocytomas. Int J Radiat Oncol Biol Phys 1985; 11:679.

38. Tubiana M. Cell kinetics and radiation oncology. Int J Radiat Oncol Biol Phys 1982; 8:1471.

39. Tubiana M. The causes of clinical radioresistance, In: The Biological

Basis of Radiotherapy, Steel GG Adams GE, Peckham MJ, eds. New York, Elsevier Science Publishers BV, 1983.

40. Parsons JT, Bova FTJ, Million RR. A re-evaluation of split course technique for squamous cell carcinoma of the head and neck. Int J Radiat Oncol Biol Phys 1982; 6:1645.

41. Shin KH, Urtasun RC, Fulton D, et al. Multiple daily fractionated radiation therapy and misonidazole in the management of malignant astrocytoma. A preliminary report. Cancer 1985; 56:758.

42. Payne DG, Simpson WJ, Keen C, Platts ME. Malignant astrocytoma: hyperfractionated and standard radiotherapy with chemotherapy in a randomized prospective clinical trial. Cancer 1982; 50:2301.

43. Catterall M, Bloom JG, et al. Fast neutrons compared with megavoltage x-rays in the treatment of patients with supratentorial glioblastoma: a controlled pilot study. Int J Radiat Oncol Biol Phys 1980; 6:261.

44. Laramore GE, Griffin TW, Gerdes AJ, Pancer RG. Fast neutron and mixed beam teletherapy for grade III and IV astrocytomas. Cancer 1978; 42:96.

45. Kornblith PL, Walker MD, Cassady JT. Neoplasms of the central nervous system. In: Cancer: Principles and Practice of Oncology. Devita VT, Hellman S, Rosenberg SA, eds. Philadelphia, Lippincott Co., 1985.

46. Bagshaw MA. Potential for radiotherapy alone in prostate cancer. Cancer 1985; 55:2079.

47. Cox JD, Holoye PV, Libnoch JA. The role of consolidation irradiation in combined modality therapy of small cell carcinoma of the lung. Int J Radiat Oncol Biol Phys 1982; 8:1271–1276.

48. Erickson RL, Szybalski W. Molecular radiobiology of human cell lines. V. Comparative radiosensitizing properties of 5–halodeoxycytidines and 5-halodeoxyuridines. Radiat Res 1963; 20:252.

49. Kriss JP, Revesez L. The distribution and fate of bromodeoxyuridine in the mouse and the rat. Cancer Res 1962; 22:254.

50. Kinsella TJ, Mitchell JB, Russo A, Morstyn G, Glatstein E. The use of halogenated thymidine analogs as clinical radiosensitizers: rationale, current status, and future prospects: Non-hypoxic cell sensitizers. Int J Radiat Oncol Biol Phys 1984; 10:1399.

51. Hoshino T, Sano K. Radiosensitization of malignant brain tumors with bromouridine (thymidine analogue). Acta Radiol 1969; 8:15.

13

External Beam Radiation Therapy of Gliomas

Judith L. Bader and Eli Glatstein

Introduction

Gliomas represent a major therapeutic challenge for surgical, radiation, and medical oncologists. Local control remains the predominant obstacle to cure. This chapter will review first the results of "standard" external beam photon radiation for gliomas, including the influence of prognostic factors and details of radiation delivery on outcome. Second, hypotheses regarding radiotherapeutic obstacles to cure will be analyzed. Finally, recent advances in technique and strategy for cure will be presented.

Results of "Standard" Postoperative Radiation Therapy for Gliomas

Low Grade Lesions

In 1975, Sheline published an excellent review of the radiation therapy of brain tumors.[1] For low grade lesions, he tabulated the eight series (all retrospective) which provided sufficient details about grade and clearly distinguished results for treatment by surgery alone versus surgery plus radiation therapy. He showed that 3- and 5-year

From: Kornblith PL, Walker MD (editors). Advances in Neuro-Oncology. Futura Publishing Company, Inc., Mount Kisco, NY, © 1988.

survival appeared improved by adding postoperative radiation therapy to surgery. With surgery alone, 3- and 5-year survival ranged from 52–64% and 13–65%, respectively. With postoperative radiation, 3- and 5-year survival ranged from 62–74% and 36–85%, respectively. Although based on nonrandomized trials, the case for postoperative radiation seemed clear.

Since that review, several additional large case series have appeared which distinguish patients by grade and treatment. Leibel, Sheline et al. confirmed the survival benefit of combining radiation with surgery in *incompletely* resected patients and indicated the prognostic significance of grade 1 vs. 2.[2] Fazekas made similar findings and commented that survival correlated with increasing radiation dose.[3] Rutten et al. could not confirm a dose-response effect, however.[4] Bloom, in an outstanding review of intracranial tumors, commented that about two-thirds of all patients with relatively low grade cerebral astrocytomas progressed to higher grade at the time of recurrence, due either to natural history or to prior treatment.[5] Garcia et al., using a slightly different grading system, also showed the benefit of postoperative radiation.[6] Data from Laws et al. at the Mayo Clinic suggested no benefit, but at doses not currently considered adequate and in a series extending over six decades.[7] In Table 1, the 3- and 5-year results of these reports are summarized. In papers which reported results at 10 years, the survival typically continued to diminish except in patients with completely excised lesions. Major problems exist, however, in comparing results from these series over many decades. The methods of radiologic diagnosis, availability of supportive care, and technical aspects of both surgery and radiation therapy have changed dramatically. In addition, no consensus existed among pathologists for criteria of grading tumors.

High Grade Lesions

The 1975 review by Sheline also presented survival data from 10 retrospective, nonrandomized series of patients with malignant gliomas (grades 3 and 4).[1] For patients receiving surgery alone, 1- and 2-year survival ranged from 0–32% and 3–6%, respectively. With postoperative radiation, 1- and 2-year survival ranged from 14–39% and 5–27%, respectively. Only grade 3 patients survived longer than 2 years. Subsequently published *retrospective* series which classify by grade and treatment report similar results.[4–6,8]

Table 1
Treatment of Low Grade Gliomas with Surgery and Radiation

Author, Years of Study, [Ref]	Grade	Radiation Dose	3-Year Survival (%)			5-Year Survival (%)		
			Complete Resection	Incomplete Resection Alone	Incomplete Resection Plus XRT	Complete Resection	Incomplete Resection Alone	Incomplete Resection Plus XRT
Leibel et al., 1942–1967 [2]	1	3500–5500	n.r.	n.r.	n.r.	100	25	58
	2	rads at 180	n.r.	n.r.	n.r.	100	0	25
	1 & 2	rads/d	100	27	59	100	19	46
Fazekas, 1958–1974 [3]	1 & 2	850–1450 ret*	n.r.	n.r.	57	90	13	41
Rutten et al., 1957–1978 [4]	2	4000–6500 rads at 200 rads/day	n.r.	n.r.	50	n.r.	n.r.	44
Bloom, 1952–1970 [5]	1	n.r.	n.r.	n.r.	n.r.	n.r.	n.r.	33
	2	n.r.	n.r.	n.r.	n.r.	n.r.	n.r.	21
Garcia et al., 1950–1979 [6]	"well differentiated"	5000–6100 rads at 180–200 rads/d	80	n.r.	100	80	n.r.	100
Laws et al., 1915–1975 [7]	1 & 2	none or <4000 rads	n.r.	n.r.	87	n.r.	n.r.	34
	1 & 2	>400 rads	n.r.	n.r.	65	n.r.	n.r.	49

n.r.: not reported
* ret: Using the Ellis formula, a measure of the nominal standard dose.

Two neuro-oncology groups have concluded randomized, *prospective* studies evaluating among other things the role of postoperative radiation in malignant gliomas. In Brain Tumor Study Group trial 69-01, patients who had received radiation therapy (5,000–6,000 rad) with or without carmustine chemotherapy had significantly improved survival at 1 year (24–36%) compared to patients receiving only supportive care (3%) or chemotherapy alone (12%).[9] In study 72-01, the three arms with radiation therapy with or without chemotherapy produced longer survival at 1 year (34–50%) than the fourth arm with postoperative chemotherapy alone (15%).[10] In addition, data combined from 69-01, 72-01, and 66-01 (surgery ± mithramycin chemotherapy) revealed not only a survival benefit for postoperative radiation but also an increasing dose-response relationship.[9–12]

In 1981, the Scandinavian Glioblastoma Study Group reported a trial comparing surgery alone to surgery plus radiation with or without bleomycin.[13] Despite receiving a relatively low dose (4,500 rad), radiated patients survived longer than patients who did not receive radiotherapy.

Although the evidence clearly points to survival benefit from radiation, the percent of patients cured with high grade lesions remains almost anecdotal, indicating the need for improvements over standard surgery plus radiation. Although grade 1 and 2 patients live longer than those with high grade, 5- and 10-year follow-up of low grade patients with incompletely resected lesions shows continuing relapse and death. Two- or three-year follow-up is usually sufficient to observe the natural history of treated high grade lesions.

Influence of Prognostic Factors on Survival

Although the glioma literature emphasizes the impact of treatment on outcome, the picture is more complex. Over the years, a number of prognostic variables have emerged from both retrospective and prospective clinical trials. The following variables have been reported as favorably influencing survival: good performance status, clinically "silent" tumor location, completeness of the surgical excision, young age, used of steroid medication, lower pathological grade (e.g., Kernohan grade, Nelson class, etc.), a variety of other pathological features, low glucose utilization by tumor on PET scan, absence of aneuploidy of tumor DNA, and the use of supportive care.[5,12,14-23] These factors may bias treatment outcome and determine survival at least as much as treatment parameters and must be considered when evaluating any report. In retrospective studies, these factors are seldom completely specified. In prospective studies, they may or may not be included as stratification variables.

Details of Radiation Therapy

Knowledge of treatment *details* is also crucial, particularly in radiation therapy. For example, the following factors can be *at least as important* as total dose in determining outcome and complications of therapy: dose per fraction, field size, method of imaging tumor and determining treatment volume, machine energy, method of prescribing dose (e.g., to a point, to an isodose line), method of setting up fields, and total time of treatment. Any primary report of radiation therapy should specify all of these parameters.

Obstacles to Cure by Radiation Therapy

Local Control

Distant metastases occur rarely with gliomas.[24,25] Local failure continues to be the overwhelming problem in achieving cure.[26] Partial surgical resection followed even by optimal radiation therapy fails to sterilize all remaining clonogenic cells, particularly in grade 4 lesions. Residual tumor eventually grows, causes increasing neurological and systemic problems leading to death. Rarely, high grade tumors may seed the spinal cord, an outcome which is treatable but usually associated with rapid demise.[27]

Tumor Localization for Radiation Targeting

In years past, tumor imaging was less precise with radionuclide brain scan, pneumoencephalogram, and arteriogram. In addition, for a variety of reasons, whole brain radiation therapy was not routine. "Marginal misses" or failure to include the entire tumor in the treated volume was thought to account for many local failures.[28] This notion led to the current common practice of initially treating the whole brain (particularly in high grade lesions) followed by a reduced volume (cone down field) to boost to higher dose only the area of known disease as determined on the best imaging studies and the operative report. The whole brain was also treated initially in order to encompass (1) areas of contiguous parenchymal microscopic spread, (2) normal routes of potential spread (e.g., periventricular), and (3) those areas possibly contaminated by the surgical procedure. New data correlating autopsy findings with previous CAT scans suggest that these modern imaging studies adequately delineate the limits of a brain tumor in most patients.[29] Therefore, treating only several centimeters around the visible abnormality on CAT scan, rather than whole brain, appears reasonable.

Sheline has recently recommended treating less than whole brain initially when good imaging studies are available and no adverse factors indicate risk for wider spread.[30] Additional refinements in imaging with MRI scans, particularly with contrast agents, may permit further reductions in the radiation target volume by distinguishing between edema and tumor. The hypothesis is that a smaller volume could be treated to a higher dose, resulting in improved local control without increase in normal tissue late effects.

Normal Tissue Tolerance

In theory, any tumor might be radiocurable if sufficient dose could be delivered without damaging normal tissue. The clinical problem is that, depending on prior surgery, radiation treatment volume, dose rate, techniques used, fraction size, and age of the patient, normal tissue brain tolerance may be reached at around 6,000 rad with conventional fractionation, whereas higher doses are apparently needed for cure. A variety of methods and formulae, including those of Ellis and others, have been proposed to compare effects of different fractionation schemes and establish safe doses for brain irradiation.[31–34] The development of brain necrosis can be fatal, even if tumor were controlled. If higher dose is needed for cure, new techniques will have to be developed for radiation delivery to increase the *therapeutic ratio* between the dose needed to kill tumor and the dose which produces necrosis. Several attempts in this direction will be discussed below.

Hypoxic Cells, Slowly Dividing Cells, Clonogenic Cells in Resting Phase, Ability of Cells to Accumulate Radiation Damage

Cell killing by conventional photon radiation is thought to be dependent on *oxygen*, among other factors. Radioresistance of gliomas has been hypothesized to relate to the presence of *hypoxic*, relatively radiation-resistant cells within tumors. A measure of this oxygen dependence in vitro is the *oxygen enhancement ratio*, the nearly 3-fold difference in dose needed to kill the same cells in the oxic versus anoxic state.[35] In addition, glioma cells cycle relatively slowly and have a low growth fraction. Such cells are probably less radiosensitive than cells from tumors with high growth rate and growth fraction. Finally, the finding of higher *extrapolation numbers* for human glioblastoma cell lines irradiated in culture than for normal glial cells lines suggests that, when radiated, glioma cells are able to accumulate considerable *sublethal damage* before being killed, another possible mechanism accounting for relative radioresistance.[35]

Several recent studies have correlated key parameters of survival curves from a variety of cell lines irradiated in vitro with clinical responsiveness of the same tumors in vivo.[36,37] These measures of intrinsic radiosensitivity of human cell lines appear to predict poor clinical tumor radioresponsiveness for glioma with conventionally fractionated photon irradiation.

Clinical Attempts to Improve Cure of Gliomas

Technical Advances

Imaging

In past years, the most common methods of imaging brain tumors included radionuclide brain scans, pneumoencephalogram, and arteriogram. The recent innovations, CAT and MRI scanning, provide far more precise delineation of tumor size, shape, margins, location, tissue density, and possibly content. This information is used in both setting up radiation treatment fields and computerized treatment planning. With improved localization and confidence about tumor margins, the *initial* radiation therapy fields may no longer need to include the whole brain (vide supra), just to avoid missing any portion of the original tumor volume.[30]

Computerized Dose Calculations and Display

Computers have automated radiation dose calculations so that dose distributions are rapidly obtainable at an infinite number of points in multiple planes. Using information about the outside contour or shape of the patient, the size (length by width) of the radiation beam, beam energy, and certain other physical and geometric factors, computers can make repetitive dose calculations inside and outside the field in any plane. Computerized dose calculations in a plane are displayed, by convention, according to "isodose" lines, points at which an equal dose is being delivered. The radiotherapist can then review and consider a variety of computer-simulated field sizes, shapes, field directions, beam weightings, and other parameters in order to select the optimal treatment plan for each individual patient, given the particular tumor size and location.[38] In addition, isodoses from moving rather than stationary beam treatments can also be easily calculated and displayed. Computer-calculated dosimetry replaces the extremely time-consuming and laborious single point hand calculations of the past, when usually only one or two points of interest within the treatment volume were calculated. Examples of several typical computerized isodose distributions for treating brain tumors are shown in Figures 1 and 2. Figure 1a shows the contour of a whole brain field, a tumor volume at the margin of the parietal lobe, and isodose lines for an initial treatment plan using bilateral opposed beams. Figure 1b shows one method, the wedged pair technique, of boosting the original tumor volume after completion of the whole brain field. Figure 1c shows the composite isodose curves from the whole brain and the cone down fields superimposed on the same contour.

Combining Newer Imaging Techniques and Computer Dose Displays: Computerized Treatment Planning

A second use of computers involves combining imaging techniques, (e.g., CAT or MRI scans) and computer-generated isodose dis-

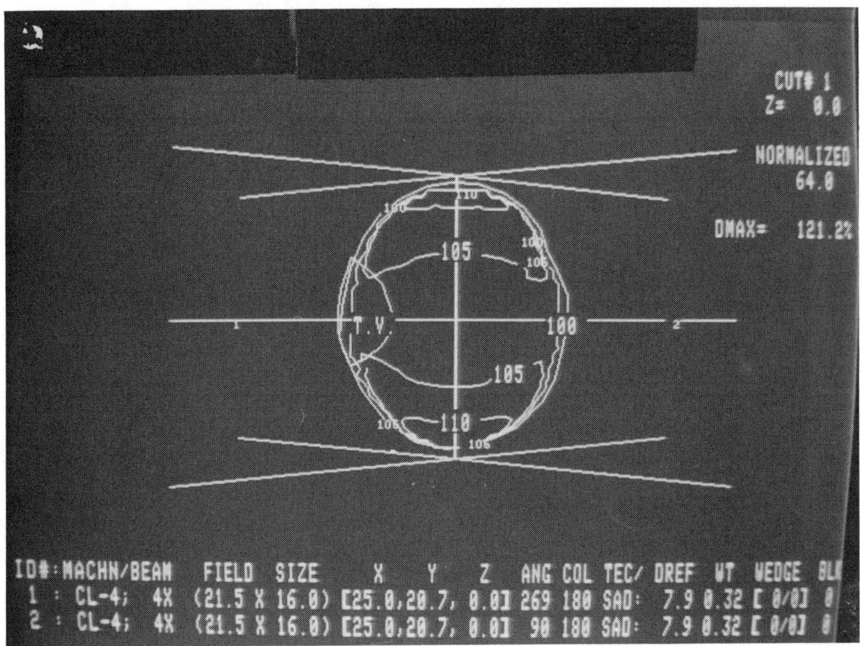

Figure 1a. Contour of whole brain, encircled tumor volume in parietal lobe (based on information from CAT scan), isodose lines for an initial treatment plan using bilateral opposed beams encompassing the whole brain.

plays.[39] The imaging provides a variety of features used in radiation therapy planning: (1) patient contour, (2) tumor location, size, shape, and borders, (3) relationship of the tumor to the surrounding normal structures, and (4) tissue density inside and outside the tumor volume. Multiple simulated treatment plans can be generated on the computer, superimposed on CAT scan image, and manipulated until an optimal plan in achieved. Figure 2a, a standard axial head CAT scan with the patient in the radiation therapy treatment position, shows the tumor volume for a low grade glioma with overlying isodose lines representing opposed lateral whole brain beams. Figure 2b represents the opposed lateral cone down beams, and Figure 2c represents the composite of the four beams together. By planning from a CAT scan, the radiation oncologist can optimize treatment of the tumor and sparing of the normal tissues. Elegant software has

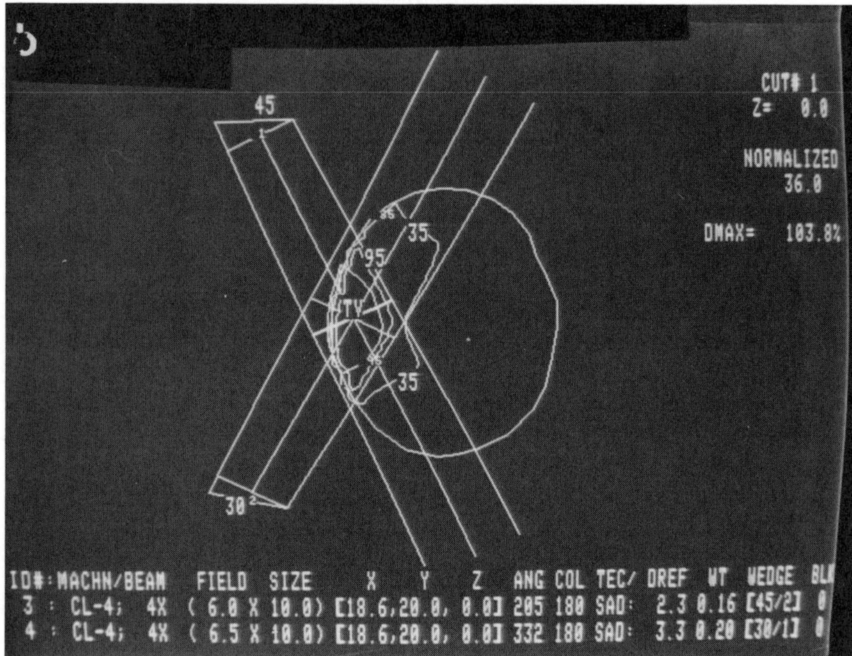

Figure 1b. Wedged pair technique used to boost the initial tumor volume after completion of the whole brain field.

been developed for manually outlining tumor shape in multiple planes on CAT scan (e.g., axial for brain tumors) and digitally reconstructing the tumor volume in the treatment plane (e.g., sagittal) to assist in the design of lateral treatment fields.[39]

Megavoltage Treatment Machines

Improvement in external beam therapy machines themselves has also been important in contemporary radiation therapy. The switch from ^{60}Co with an approximate energy of 1.25 million electron volts (MeV) to linear accelerators with typical energies from 4 to 20 MeV has allowed more homogeneous treatment of deeper tumors to higher dose with better sparing of more superficial normal structures. In addition, improvement in beam edge sharpness with linear accel-

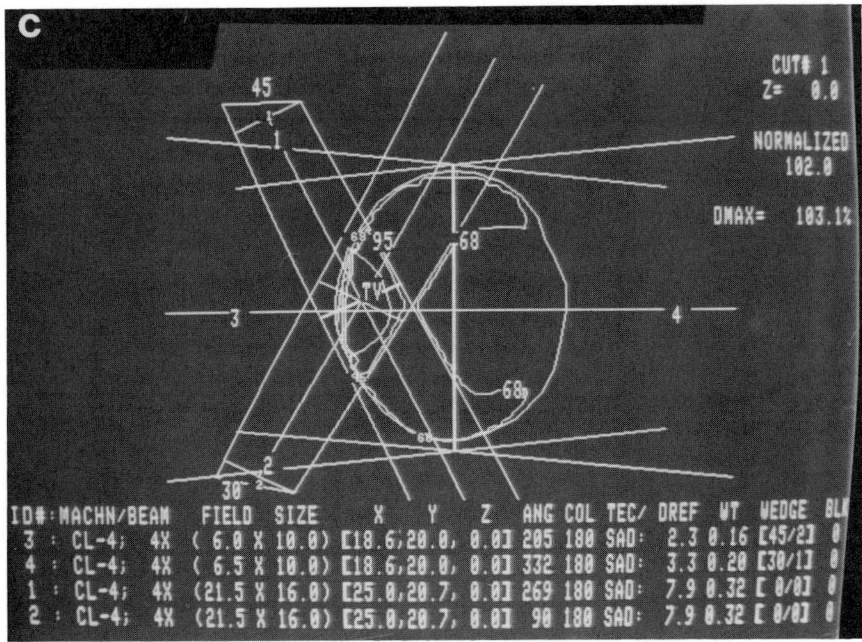

Figure 1c. Composite of isodoses from original and boost fields.

erators compared to ^{60}Co machines allows treatment closer to dose-sensitive structures, such as the lens of the eye.

Simulators

Another technical advance has been the development of a diagnostic x-ray machine which reproduces precisely the machine-to-patient geometry of high energy radiation therapy equipment. This "simulator" helps to set and record radiographically the boundaries of the treated fields with greater precision than ever before possible. Simulation and computerized treatment planning have contributed markedly to improved accuracy and sophistication of contemporary radiation therapy.

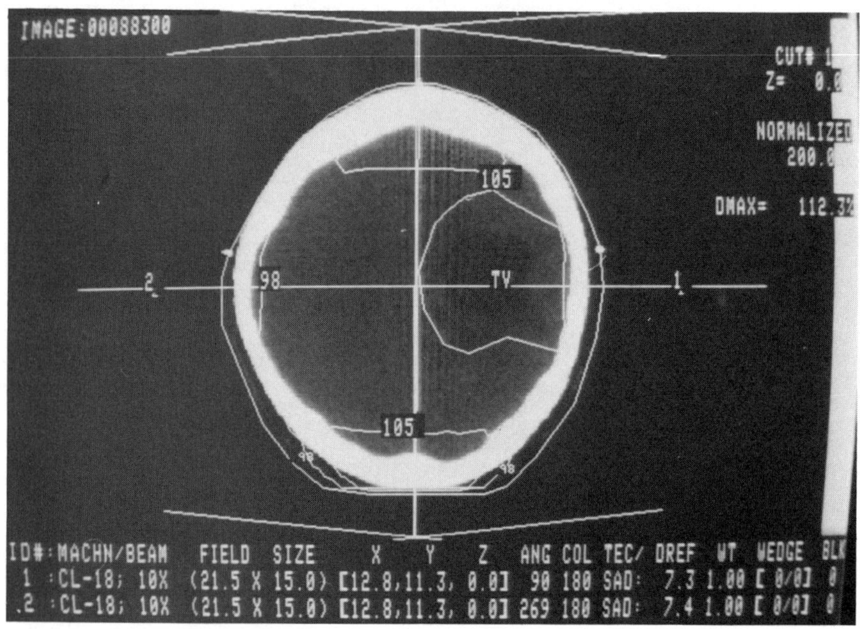

Figure 2a. Axial head CAT scan, taken with patient in the treatment position. Tumor volume for low grade glioma is outlined. Isodose lines for bilateral opposed whole brain fields are shown.

Attempts to Improve Cure Rate with Photons Alone

Pushing External Beam Photons to High Dose

A variety of studies using increasing dose with external beam radiation have been reported in recent years. Salazar et al. reviewed retrospectively patients with grades 3 and 4 gliomas treated post-operatively at their institution with final tumor minimum total doses of 5,000–5,500, 5,500–6,500, and 7,000–8,000 rad.[8] For grade 3 tumors, the data (based on relatively few patients) suggest that the highest dose range led to the longest median survival but the difference was no longer significant at about 4 years. For grade 4 patients, the same trend was apparent, with the survival difference disap-

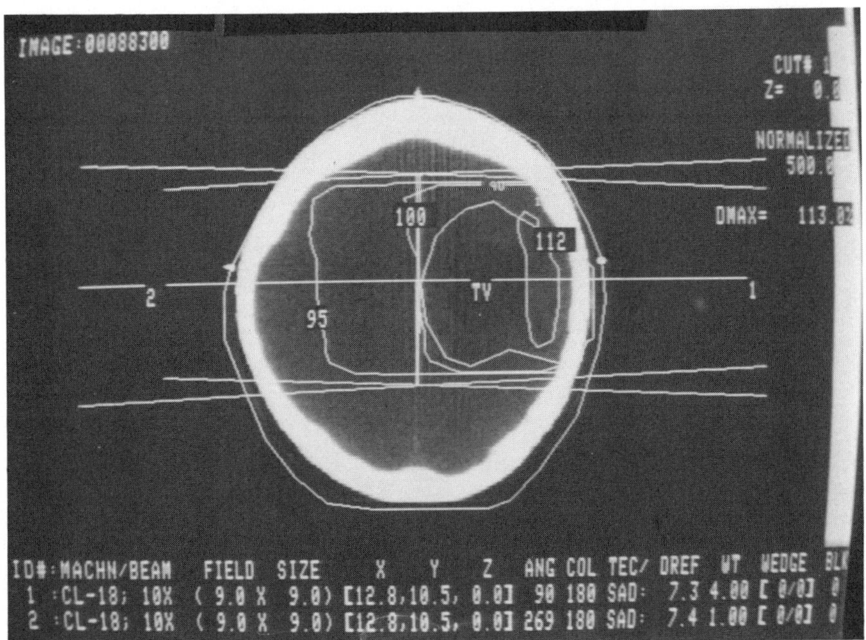

Figure 2b. Opposed lateral cone down field used to boost initial tumor volume after completion of the whole brain field.

pearing at 2 years. Local failure was the main problem in both grades 3 and 4, irrespective of dose, and areas suggestive of marked radiation effect or frank necrosis associated with tumor recurrence were commonly seen. The Brain Tumor Study Group retrospectively studied the relationship between dose and survival in 621 malignant glioma patients entered into three successive protocols (not specifically designed to evaluate dose-response) between 1966 and 1975.[12] Some patients also received chemotherapy. The data indicated an increasing median survival with increasing dose between 5,000, 5,500 and 6,000 rad. Unfortunately, however, ultimate survival was poor in all groups. Dose-response information from a joint RTOG-ECOG study suggested no survival difference between whole brain treatment to 6,000 rad and the same plus a 1,000 rad boost.[20]

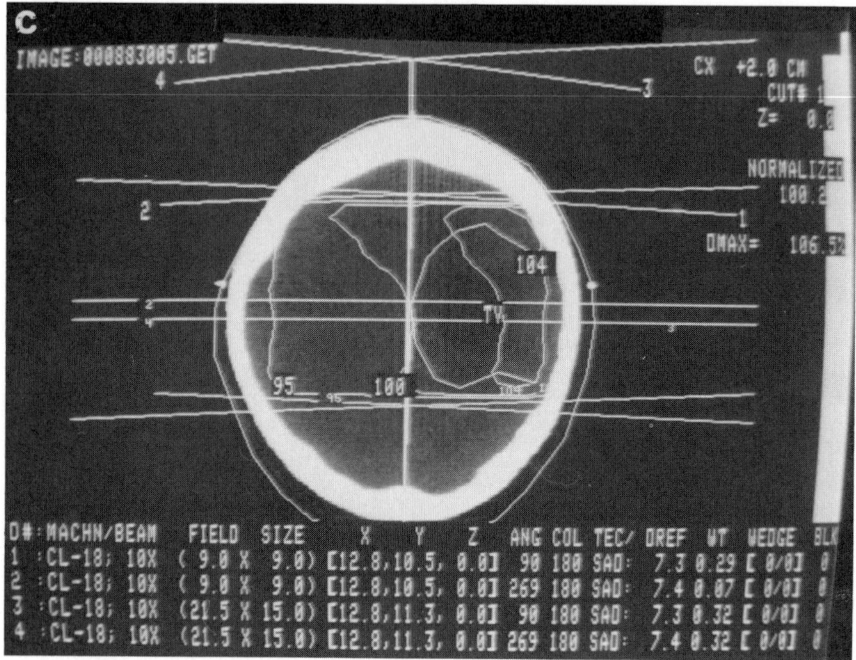

Figure 2c. Composite of isodoses from original and boost fields.

Use of Smaller Fields Pushed to Higher Dose

As mentioned above, improved imaging techniques may allow the use of smaller radiation field sizes. Because normal tissue tolerance in the brain is dependent upon dose, dose rate, and field size, it may be possible to increase the total tumor minimum dose slightly when smaller field sizes are used from the outset. The hope is that the tumor could receive a higher dose without exceeding the tolerance of surrounding normal tissues and possibly result in better local control and cure rate. Although a small volume cone down with external beam is one way to boost, brachytherapy (radioactive implant) to the original tumor volume is another.[40]

Alterations in Standard Fractionation

"Standard" technique for treating gliomas varies from one radiation department to another, but in general, a common practice is to

treat "curative" patients with 4,500–5,000 rad to the whole brain with *single* daily fractions of between 180 and 200 rad. Thereafter, a cone down or boost, targeted only to the area of original tumor, is give additional dose, bringing the tumor minimum dose to 6,000 rad. Higher doses are often used, particularly in patients with good performance status. This treatment is usually tolerated well and associated with clinical improvement, if not long-term cure. Most radiotherapists use dexamethasone during treatment if there is considerable brain edema, midline shift, large volume of tumor, or neurological problems reflecting mass effect.

Use of *more than one* daily radiation dose has been the subject of considerable research in recent years. Use of multiple *smaller than usual* daily fractions has been called *superfractionation* or *hyperfractionation*. Giving standard size fractions more than once a day is called *accelerated fractionation*. The overall number of days to completion of treatment is shortened with accelerated fractionation but similar to conventional treatment with superfractionation.

The rationale for superfractionation derives from several radiobiologic concepts.[41–44] (1) Giving smaller radiation fractions at more frequent intervals will permit greater total dose of radiation to be given without an increase in delayed toxicity because late reacting normal tissues (responsible for brain necrosis) show better tolerance with smaller doses per fraction. (2) Normal tissue repairs sublethal damage better than rapidly dividing tumor tissue. With an increased number of fractions, the therapeutic ratio can be exploited with each additional treatment. (3) With more fractions, there may be greater opportunity for redistribution of proliferating tumor cells into more sensitive phases of the cell cycle. (4) At lower dose per fraction, the oxygen effect is less important. (5) With more fractions, there may be greater chance for tumor reoxygenation after each dose. Although all these hypotheses have been proposed, only some may actually be clinically important in superfractionated radiation therapy of brain tumors as it has been delivered.[44]

Several major Canadian studies have investigated superfractionation in the treatment of gliomas. Between 1965 and 1968, the Princess Margaret Hospital studied nine different fractionation schedules in 134 patients with grades 3 and 4 glioma.[45] Total dose varied between 3,000 and 4,000 rad, dose per fraction ranged from 47 to 190 rad, time between fractions varied between 8 and 24 hours. In this relatively low dose, nonrandomized study, no clear benefit could be seen for any one of the treatment schedules. A second Princess Margaret Hospital study between 1977 and 1980 randomized 157 malignant glioma patients to *standard fractionation* (200 rad per fraction to 5,000 rad) or *superfractionation* (100 rad per fraction every 3 hours four times daily to 3,600–4,000 rad).[46] All patients received chemotherapy with CCNU and hydroxyurea. No significant survival or toxicity differences were seen between the two groups. Again, the total doses might be considered low, but when these clinical trials were initiated, concern was raised about how well multiple daily fractions would be tolerated and the tendency was to stop at a lower overall dose than would have been given by standard technique.

In another Canadian study, Shin et al. prospectively randomized 69 malignant glioma patients to *conventional fractionation* treatment (whole brain to 3,400 rad at 200 rad daily plus a 1,600 rad boost) or to superfractionation (4,000 rad whole brain at 89 rad three times a day plus 1,000 rad boost at 200 rad/fraction). All patients received CCNU. Although median survival was slightly longer in the superfractionation group, the difference was not significant.[47] In British Columbia in 1976, Douglas and Worth compared 30 consecutive malignant glioma patients treated with superfractionation (100 rad to the whole brain three times daily to 4,500, 5,400 or 6,000 rad, followed by a 1,000 rad boost) to 90 historical control patients treated with conventional daily radiation to doses between 4,000 and 5,000 rads.[48] Although a significant improvement for resected patients receiving superfractionated therapy is claimed, the survival rate for historical controls is below what might be expected and the groups are not strictly comparable for relevant prognostic factors.

Other studies using superfractionation with radiation sensitizers will be presented below in greater detail. This group of studies also shows no benefit for superfractionation, with two exceptions (see Table 2). Fulton et al. from Edmonton and Calgary, Canada, showed that survival was significantly prolonged in patients randomized to treatment with superfractionation (6,141 rad, 69 fractions, 89 rad/fraction t.i.d.) or the same plus misonidazole compared to conventional fractionation (5,800 rad, 30 fractions, 193 rad/fraction) with p = 0.002.[49] Shin et al. randomized 38 patients to conventional fractionation (CF) (5,800 rad/6 weeks/30 fractions), 43 patients to multiple daily fractions (MDF) (6,141 rad/4.5 weeks/69 fractions/89 rad every 3 hours/t.i.d.), and 43 to MDF plus misonidazole radiation sensitizer.[50] One year actuarial survival was 20% for CF, 41% for MDF, and 48% for the MDF plus sensitizer group; longer follow-up data were not available.

Table 2
Treatment of Malignant Gliomas with Radiation and Nitroimidazole Hypoxic Cell Sensitizers

Author/Group Name/ Year of Publication [Ref]	Years of Study	Randomized	Grades Studied	Sensitizer Used, Dose	Study Groups	No. Pts	Median Survival	% 1 Year Survival	Comments
Urtasun et. al., Edmonton, Alberta 1976, 1982 [66, 67]	74–?	Yes	4	Metro: 6 g/m sq 3×/wk, 4 hrs pre	Gp 1: 3000 rads, 9 fx, 333 rad/fx 3×/wk, 18 dys	13	15 wks	10	1. survival very poor in both groups 2. survival difference claimed significant but numbers very small 3. very low radiation dose 4. paper updating results shows curves crossing at 1 year
					Gp 2: same xrt + metro	16	26 wks	10	
Bleehan, Cambridge Glioma Group, 1981 [68]	?–78	Yes	3 &4	Miso: 3 g/m sq 4 hrs pre each rx	Gp 1: 5656 rads, 28 fx, 202 rads/fx 5.5 wks	20	251 dys	28	1. hard to detect differences in study with small numbers
					Gp 2: 4352 rads, 12 unequal fx, Mon & Wed: 294 rads, Fri: 500 rads	18	220 dys	26	
					Gp 3: same xrt as 2 + miso	17	270 dys	18	
Kapp et. al., Yale, 1982 [69]	79–81	No	4	Metro: 6 g/m sq 4 hrs pre	Gp 1: 4200 rads, 7 fx, 600 rads/fx, 1 fx/wk	19	9.4 mo	25	1. single fraction/week not optimal but not toxic either 2. no evidence of brain necrosis at autopsy
Carabell et al., Brain Tumor Study Group: 78-01, 1981 [70]	78–?	No	3 & 4	Miso: 2.5 g/m sq 4 hrs pre rx each Mon × 6	Gp 1: 6000 rads in 29 unequal fx: Mon: 400 rads per wk × 6, Tu, Th, Fri: 150 rads × 6 wks, boost of 180 x 5 d	49	39	30	1. a phase II trial, tolerance demonstrated, led to RTOG 79-18

continued

Table 2 (*continued*)

Treatment of Malignant Gliomas with Radiation and Nitroimidazole Hypoxic Cell Sensitizers

Author/Group Name/ Year of Publication [Ref]	Years of Study	Randomized	Grades Studied	Sensitizer Used, Dose	Study Groups	No. Pts	Median Survival	% 1 Year Survival	Comments
Cumberlin et al., BTSG: 77-02, 1983 [71]	78–80	Yes	3 & 4	Miso: 1.5 g/m sq each Mon & Thu × 6 wks	Gp 1: conventional fractionation (CF), 6000 rads/ 30–35 fx, 172–180 rads/ fx/day, 6–7 wks	N.R.	N.R.	N.R.	1. has been reported only in abstract form
					Gp 2: CF plus miso plus BCNU	N.R.	N.R.	N.R.	2. no significant difference in median survival or
					Gp 3: CF plus streptozotocin	N.R.	N.R.	N.R.	2-year actuarial survival between any of treatment
					Gp 4: multiple daily fractions: 6600 rads, 110 rads/fx, 2 fx/d, 60 fx, 6 wks	N.R.	N.R.	N.R.	arms
Ang et al., EORTC, 1982 [72]	79–81	No	3 & 4	Miso: 1.2 g/m sq 2 hrs pre 1st rx each day	Gp 1: 6000 rads, split course xrt, 200 rads/fx q 4 hrs 3 rx/d × 5d, 2 wk break, 200 rads/fx q 4 hrs 3 rx/d × 5d	34	N.R.	N.R.	1. multicenter pilot study 2. survival data not shown for +/− miso groups 3. multiple daily
					Gp 2: same xrt + miso	88	N.R.	N.R.	fractionation schedule well tolerated
Urtasun et al., Edmonton, Alberta 1982 [62]	76–?	Yes	3 & 4	Metro: 6 g/m sq 4 hrs pre each rx	Gp 1: 5800 rads, 30 fx, 193 rads/fx 5 dys/wk, 6 wks	19	26 wks	28	1. no statistical difference in survival between 3 treatment groups
				Miso: 1.25 g/m sq 4 hrs pre each rx	Gp 2: 3897 rads, 9 fx, 433 rads/fx 3 rx/wk, 3 wks, plus metro	17	19 wks	0	2. compared to previous metro trial (66, 67), results not improved for raising total radiation dose and dose per fraction
					Gp 3: same xrt as Gp 2 plus miso	23	27 wks	22	3. residual tumor present in all patients autopsied

Study	Yrs	Random	Grade	Drug	Radiation	n	Median survival	%	Comments
Nelson et al., RTOG: 79-18, 1983 [63]	79–82	Yes	3 & 4	Miso: 2.5 g/m sq 4 hrs pre rx each Monday	Gp 1: 6000 rads, 170–200 rads/fx, 5 dys/wk, 6–7 wks plus BCNU	114	54 wks	54	1. no statistcal difference in survival between the 2 groups
					Gp 2: 6000 rads, unequal fx: Mon: 400 rads/dy × 6 wks + miso. Tu, Th, Fri: 150 rads/dy × 6 wks, plus boost 180 rads/dy × 5 dys, plus BCNU	112	46 wks	46	2. multicenter study
Eortc Brain Tumor Group, 1983 [73]	78–80	Yes double blind	3 & 4 & oligo	Miso: 1.3 g/m sq 4 hrs pre rx for first 9 rx	Gp 1: 4950 rads, 15 unequal fx, 5 wks, qod rx, 350 rads/fx × 9 fx, then 300 rads/fx × 6 fx.	81	46.1 wks	38	1. no statistical difference in survival between the two groups
					Gp 2: same xrt plus miso for first 9 fx	82	44.5 wks	42	
MRC Working Party on Misonidazole in Gliomas, 1983 [74]	79–81	Yes double blind	3 & 4	Miso: 600 mg/m sq 4 hrs pre each rx	Gp 1: 4500 rads, 20 equal fx, 5 dys/wk, 4 wks, 225 rads/fx plus placebo pre each fx	196	8 mos	28	1. no statistical difference in survival between the 2 groups
					Gp 2: same xrt plus miso pre each rx	188	9 mos	25	2. low daily dose of miso may have been sufficient 3. relatively low total radiation dose
Fulton et al., Edmonton and Calgary 1984 [49]	81–82	Yes	3 & 4	Miso: 1.25 g/m sq 3×/wk for first 9 rx	Gp 1: conventional fractionation (CF): 5800 rads, 30 equal fx, 6 wks, 193 rads/fx/d	38	29 wks	23	1. survival significance prolonged in MDF or MDF + miso compared to CF
					Gp 2: multiple daily fractions (MDF): 6141 rads, 69 fx, 4.5wks, 89 rads/fx, 3 fx/d q 4 hrs	42	45 wks	45	2. no statistical difference between MDF and MDF + miso
					Gp 3: same as gp 2 plus miso	37	50 wks	43	
					Gp 4: high dose multiple daily fractions: 7120 rads, 80 fx, 5.5 wks, 89 rads/fx, 3 fx/d q 4 hrs	11	N.R.	N.R.	

continued

Table 2 *(continued)*
Treatment of Malignant Gliomas with Radiation and Nitroimidazole Hypoxic Cell Sensitizers

Author/Group Name/ Year of Publication [Ref]	Years of Study	Randomized	Grades Studied	Sensitizer Used, Dose	Study Groups	No. Pts	Median Survival	% 1 Year Survival	Comments
Stadler et al., Vienna, Austria 1984 [75]	77–?	Yes	3 & 4	Miso: 2.1 g/m sq 4 hrs pre each 400 rad fx	Gp 1: 6650 rads, 31 unequal fx, 7.5 wks, wk 1, 2, 8: 400 rads/fx/ dy Mon & Thu, 2 fx/wk wk 3–7: 170 rads/fx/dy, 5 fx/wk	Gp 1 + 2 45	9.8 mos	25	1. no statistical difference between 2 groups 2. survival curves cross at 24% at 24 months
					Gp 2: same xrt plus miso		13.8 mos	64	
Hatlevoll et al., Scandinavian Glioblastoma Study Group, 1985 [76]	79–82	Yes	3 & 4	Miso A: 1.2 g/m sq 4 hrs pre each rx	Gp 1: 4000 rads, 5 wks, 400 rads/fx twice wkly, 10 fx. ± Miso A, ± CCNU	119	10.5 mos	42	1. no significant difference between 2 or 5 fx/wk, ± miso, ± CCNU
				Miso B: 48 g/m sq 4 hrs pre each rx	Gp 2: 5000 rads, 5 wks, 200 rads/fx/dy × 5 fx/ wk, 25 fx, ± Miso B, ± CCNU	125	10.5 mos	42	
Shin et al., Alberta and Edmonton, Canada 1985 [50]	81–84	Yes	3 & 4	Miso: 1.25 g/m sq each Mon, Wed, Fri × 9 doses	Gp1: conventional fractionation (CF); 5800 rads/6 wks/30 fx/ 193 rad fx	38	27 wks	20	1. statistically significant difference between CF and MDF groups 2 and 3
					Gp 2: multiple daily fractions (MDF); 6141 rads/4.5 wks, 69 fx, 89 rads q 3 h t.i.d.	43	39 wks	41	2. no statistical difference between MDF and MDF plus miso
					Gp 3: MDF plus miso	43	49 wks	45	3. CF group had excess of grade 4 patients 4. CF dose could have been higher 5. follow-up trial is testing MDF 6141 vs MDF 7120

The rationale for *accelerated fractionation* is primarily to decrease the opportunity of clonogenic cells to proliferate between treatments by administering the radiation in a shorter overall time with a reduced inter-treatment interval.[51] Larger than standard single daily fractions have also been advocated for three reasons: (1) to overcome resistance in tumors with a wide shoulder on the radiation survival curve and large extrapolation number, (2) to sensitize with various compounds the maximum number of rad when clinical toxicity limited the number of sensitizer doses, and (3) to follow early sensitizer experimental suggestions that the drugs worked better with larger fraction doses.[50] It was found, however, that for equal total doses, large fractions increased late tissue injury over conventional fractionation and apparently resulted in poorer tumor control.[43,51] Large dose per fraction for glioma has usually been studied with sensitizers, as shown in Table 2, and with split course radiation.[52] No benefit was observed.

Use of Chemotherapy and Radiation Therapy

Several randomized neuro-oncology studies have prospectively investigated the role of chemotherapy in conjunction with postoperative radiation. Although there was early enthusiasm for this modality, most of the trials failed to show major clinical benefit for drug treatment. This topic is reviewed elsewhere in this book.

Radiation Sensitizers

Radiation sensitizers have been investigated in neuro-oncology in order to improve the unsatisfactory outcome seen with conventional treatment alone. The goal is to *differentially* increase the killing per rad or per fraction of radiation without producing a concomitant increase in the normal tissue toxicity. Thus, with the same overall dose, it might be possible to obtain better local control and hence cure. Several classes of radiosensitizing agents have received extensive laboratory investigation: oxygen, hypoxic cell sensitizers, pyrimidine analogs, thiol-depleting agents, and inhibitors of potentially lethal damage (PLD) repair.[53] Only the first three have been clinically tested against human gliomas.

Hypoxic Cells

Experimental work has shown that cells in rapidly growing tumors become hypoxic as they outgrow their blood supply, with 1–30% hypoxic cells in most solid rodent tumors. X-ray exposure is known to produce two to three times more efficient cell killing per rad in oxic versus anoxic cells, the so-called "oxygen enhancement ratio." Thus, if more oxygen could be made available to hypoxic cells in tumors, cure of tumors could improve—*if* failure to kill these hypoxic tumor cells represented the major determinant of local failure in radiation therapy. Because hypoxic cells are present in tumors but not in normal cells, sensitizers would provide a differential effect, especially if the soluble agent were *not* metabolized by the euoxic cells.[54]

Oxygen

Molecular oxygen itself (hyperbaric therapy) was the first hypoxic cell sensitizer investigated for human gliomas. Although its use was complicated under certain circumstances by decreased cortical blood flow, seizures, and lung toxicity, a clinical trial seemed warranted in view of the laboratory evidence suggesting possible radiation enhancement. In 1963, Chang and others at Columbia University began a study (not strictly randomized) of grades 3 and 4 supratentorial glioma patients.[55] With five different radiation schedules and doses ranging between 3,600–6,000 rads, 42 patients received postoperative cobalt radiation alone and 38 received radiation plus hyperbaric oxygen at 3 atmospheres of pressure. Actuarial analysis revealed median survival of 38 weeks in the oxygen group and 31 weeks for the controls, a difference not statistically significant. At 36 months, all controls had died and three others were living, although two subsequently died with tumor. Toxicities reported were seizures ($n = 2$), otitis media after myringotomy, acute skin desquamation, and autopsy evidence of extensive radiation necrosis adjacent to normal brain "attributable to oxygen effect." The main conclusion from the study was that hyperbaric oxygen treatment was feasible, although it failed to improve the outcome significantly. Although other hyperbaric oxygen trials did suggest some improvement for cervix and head and neck cancers, the expense, cumbersome technology, and potential physiological problems led investigators to search for other strategies.

Nitroimidazoles

A search ensued for chemicals that would mimic the oxygen effect. It was shown that radiation initially produced free radicals which caused lesions in DNA. These highly toxic moieties could either be repaired by receiving electrons from endogenous sulfhydryl groups or fixed through electron transfer to oxygen or other electron-affinic compounds. Thus, electron-affinic compounds were sought which would (1) diffuse deeply into poorly vascularized hypoxic areas, (2) unlike oxygen, resist metabolism by tumor cells through which they passed, and (3) achieve clinically significant sensitization at serum levels which were relatively nontoxic. The nitroimidazole compounds were the first hypoxic cell sensitizers to receive wide clinical testing, after being shown to be stable, relatively nontoxic and effective radiosensitizers in a wide spectrum of animal tumors.[56] The two compounds that have undergone widest testing, metronidazole and misonidazole, are shown in Figure 3.

MISONIDAZOLE

2-NITROIMIDAZOLE DERIVATIVE

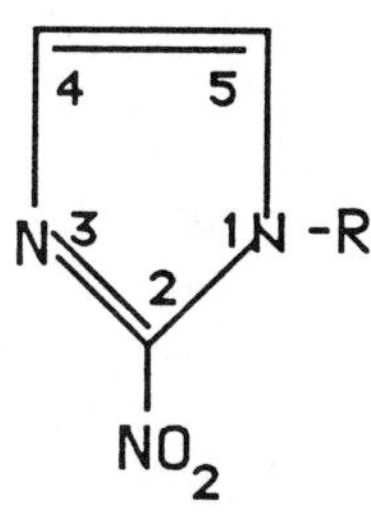

$R = CH_2CHOHCH_2OCH_3$

METRONIDAZOLE

5- NITROIMIDAZOLE DERIVATIVE

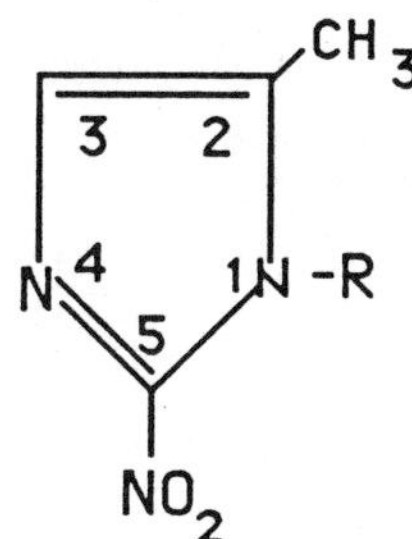

$R = CH_2CH_2OH$

Figure 3. Hypoxic cell sensitizers used in clinical treatment of gliomas.

Radiosensitization depends on the electron-affinity of a molecule. For nitroimidazoles, this property is determined by the ring structure. Penetration of drug into neural tissue (across the blood-brain barrier) depends on lipophilicity, which for the nitroimidazoles, is governed by the aliphatic side chain at the 1-position in the ring. The side chain also determines plasma half-life.[57]

The radiobiologic measure of the effectiveness of a sensitizer is called the (*sensitizer*) *enhancement ratio:* the ratio of doses in the absence and in the presence of the drug which produces the same biological effect. Enhancement ratios for nitroimidazoles, highly dependent on experimental conditions, have usually been reported in the range of 1.0–2.0.[58]

Nitroimidazole compounds have other properties that may also contribute to therapeutic efficacy. After prolonged incubation under experimental hypoxic conditions, they cause direct cytotoxicity to hypoxic cells and a reduction in the shoulder of the radiation survival curve. These effects could enhance cell killing during fractionated radiotherapy. In addition, there appears to be direct interaction between the drugs and cytotoxic agents, particularly alkylating agents.[53,57] Other actions have also been postulated.[57] In addition, some in vitro work recently published has suggested that nitroimidazole radiosensitizers may have oncogenic potential.[60]

Metronidazole was the first nitroimidazole tested widely in humans. It was quickly followed by misonidazole when the latter was shown to be a more efficient sensitizer mole for mole on hypoxic mammalian tumors.[61] Although other nitro compounds have been investigated in vitro and in vivo (e.g., desmethymisonidazole, SR-2508, SR-2555), only metro and misonidazole have been extensively tested and reported on for human gliomas.[57]

Toxicity for the nitro compounds is dose-dependent. Metronidazole has been associated with anorexia, nausea, vomiting, and CSN symptoms of encephalopathy (ataxia, shuffling gait, somnolence, and seizure activity). Misonidazole has produced nausea, vomiting, and a dose-limiting peripheral neuropathy, and occasional central neuropathy, ototoxicity, allergies, and skin problems.[61–64] Clinical evidence has accumulated that dexamethasone may diminish peripheral neuropathy, and phenytoin or phenobarbital may diminish CNS toxicity.[53,61–64] Laboratory evidence suggests that pyridoxine may decrease neurotoxicity as well.[65]

The major glioma clinical trials with nitroimidazole hypoxic cell sensitizers are summarized in Table 2.[49,50,62,63,66–76] Although some studies were prospectively randomized, stratification variables were not uniform and a wide variety of radiation and drug doses, schedules, and techniques were employed. Because drug dose was limited by neurototoxicity, sensitization of the maximum number of rad was attempted in many studies by the use of larger than conventional doses per fractionation. At the time these studies were designed, it was thought that larger doses would produce greater enhancement of sensitization and permit sensitization of more radiation before the onset of clinical toxicity from sensitizer. The median survival and 1-year survival data in the table are reported from the text of each paper, when it was given. For the others, percent survival was estimated from actuarial survival curves provided in the paper. In aggregate, the studies indicate that nitroimidazole sensitizers as administered failed to improve significantly the outlook for patients with high grade gliomas. Although subgroup analysis in certain papers indicates that greatest prolongation of survival was achieved in good prognosis patients given the highest doses of radiation and sensitizer,[50] a major impact on long-term survival probably will not be achieved with the regimens tried.

A variety of possible reasons have been given for the failure of nitroimidazole sensitizers to match clinically the promise suggested initially in the lab: (1) inadequate drug dose delivered to tumor (limited by clinical toxicity or schedule chosen), (2) adverse effect of drug on survival, (3) inadequate dose and/or suboptimal schedule of the radiation itself, (4) overestimation of enhancement expected due to misinterpretation of early in vitro results, (5) erroneous assumption that hypoxic cells in tumors limit cure by radiation, (6) selection of highly unfavorable cases, (7) greater adaptability of human than rodent tumor cells to negate the effects of these compounds by altered intrinsic intracellular levels of glutathione.[53,77,78] Whatever the reason, early enthusiasm for hypoxic cell sensitizers has certainly waned. Additional investigations continue, however, some with newer and potentially more efficient drugs.[57,77] Simultaneous use of sensitizers that work by other methods, e.g., depletion of competing glutathione, may also improve the clinical outcome.[53,57]

Pyrimidine Analogs

The search for other clinically important radiation enhancers has led to the resuscitation of thymidine analogs, a group of chemicals

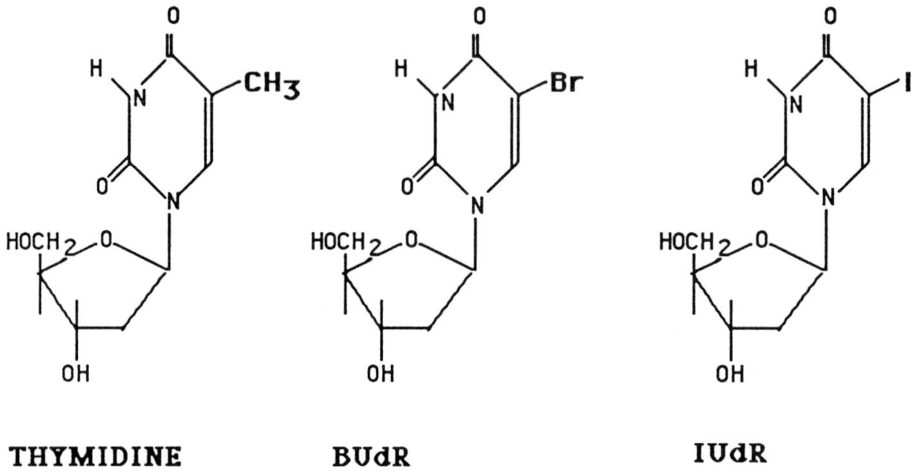

THYMIDINE   **BUdR**   **IUdR**

Figure 4. Chemical structure of thymidine and the two halogenated analogs (BUdR and IUdR) used as clinical sensitizers.

found in the 1950's to enhance mammalian cells to x-irradiation.[79] Those used in human clinical trials of gliomas to date include BUdR and IUdR (see Fig. 4).

Kinsella et al. have recently reviewed the history of the developmental work on thymidine analogs, mechanism of action, the early clinical trials, and the reintroduction of these drugs into clinical testing after a hiatus of about 15 years.[80] Cells need thymidine as a building block for incorporation into DNA. BUdR and IUdR can replace thymidine because of stereochemical similarities between the van der Waal's radius of the bromine or iodine atom and the methyl group at the 5-position of the uridine molecule. The analogs, like thymidine, must be phosphorylated prior to DNA incorporation. The drug is then *selectively* incorporated into dividing cells such as tumors undergoing DNA synthesis. With these substituted constituents, cells have a variety of altered properties in vitro: increased sensitivity to temperature and low pH, delay in cell cycle time, direct cytotoxicity, and increased radiosensitivity. The radiation sensitivity, which is dependent on dose, duration of exposure, and percent thymidine replacement, has been measured as an increase in the slope (D_o) of the cell survivial curve, an increase in the radiation sensitization factor (D_o control/D_o treated cells), and in some cases, a change in the shoulder (*n*) of the radiation survival curve.

The rationale for use of this group of drugs is the following: tumors, dividing more rapidly than surrounding noncycling normal cells (especially brain), should preferentially take up drug and thereby increase radiosensitivity. The precise mechanism of radiation sensitization remains unclear but appears to reflect both increase in DNA strand breaks and a marked inhibition of DNA repair. Clinical pharmacology has revealed that the drug is rapidly catabolized to a free base and subsequently dehalogenated, principally in the liver if the drug is infused as a bolus. The plasma half-life is short following bolus intravenous administration, and the intracellular metabolism is rapid. These factors initially led to the practice of administering the drug by continuous intra-arterial infusion via an indwelling catheter. Recent studies with prolonged intravenous infusions reveal nonlinear pharmacokinetics with gradual intra-arterial accumulation levels competitive with levels of thymidine (10^{-6}–10^{-5} m/l concentration). Safe and effective sensitization has been obtained by delivering relatively large drug doses via the less dangerous intravenous route with a portable infusion pump. Systemic toxicity in humans is dependent on dose, dose rate, and duration of exposure. Side effects have included neurotropenia, thrombocytopenia, skin rash, nail changes, alopecia, stomatitis, and cutaneous photosensitivity.

In the last 10 years, published clinical experience with BUdR and IUdR in gliomas has been limited to phase I and II studies performed at the National Cancer Institute, University of California at San Francisco (UCSF), and in Japan.[80–86] The NCI has investigated several drug escalation schemes and 12- or 24-hour continuous infusions of both drugs. Radiation fractionation was daily with BUdR and twice daily with IUdR. In all trials, 55 patients with high grade gliomas have been followed a minimum of 6 months. Median survival was 13.3 months and 1 year actuarial survival 57%.[86] Additional follow-up is needed to determine whether any subgroups of patients will have significantly benefited from radiosensitization. The studies have indicated that systemic toxicity limits BUdR delivery to about 700 mg/m^2/12 hours and IUdR to 1,200 mg/m^2/12 hours daily for 2–3 weeks. Photosensitivity is minimal with IUdR and drug levels two to three times higher than with BUdR.[84] The published UCSF phase I experience with BUdR for gliomas, as yet limited to 12 patients, reported tolerable toxicity with doses similar to those at the NCI.[85] The clinical pharmacology of pyrimidine analogs will no doubt continue to be studied in order to improve the therapeutic index and sensitization ratio.

Use of High LET Radiation and Proton Beam Therapy

Neutrons

Conventional external photon beam radiation is *sparsely ionizing, low linear energy transfer* (LET) radiation, meaning relatively low energy deposited per unit path length of the track of radiation. Radiation with neutrons or heavy charged particles is said to be high LET, i.e., more densely ionizing, with greater energy deposition per unit path length of radiation. With high LET, there is greater chance for energy deposition at multiple critical sites within a single cell leading to cell killing. Greatly simplified, the concept is that for a given dose of radiation, high LET yields greater cell killing (greater radiobiologic effect, RBE) than low LET. The RBE, however, is a complicated parameter and dependent on a variety of factors in addition to LET.[87]

High LET radiation is also less dependent on tissue oxygenation to produce its effect, a potentially important theoretical advantage in tumors with large hypoxic cores, and the major rationale for introduction of neutron therapy into experimental clinical practice. With neutrons, unlike photons, there is also little or no *repair* of sublethal radiation damage and less sensitivity to the variations of cell sensitivity with the phases of the mitotic cycle.[87]

Relatively few centers in the world provide clinical neutron radiation therapy.[88,89] Significant variations in equipment (machine energy, method of beam production, collimation, ability of beam to rotate, beam penumbra) and the beam quality (depth dose characteristics and especially RBE) of the radiation beam from each individual center make comparisons of clinical results from different centers very complicated.[89,90] Nevertheless, some literature has accumulated on the results of treating high grade gliomas with neutrons alone, mixed beams (photon plus neutron boost), and neutrons plus radiation sensitizers. This material is summarized in Table 3.[91–96] Two major conclusions emerge: (1) no significant improvement in quality of life or survival was observed, and (2) radiation pathology of autopsied patients often showed a consistent pattern of features: extensive coagulative necrosis of tumor, dense infiltration by collagenous connective tissue, phagocytic reaction, marked reduction to absence of viable tumor identified, abnormal astrocytic proliferation, and areas of gliosis and white matter degeneration in areas remote from the tumor site. In patients who received high dose neutron treatment, it was rare to find infiltrative tumor cells resembling those

Table 3
Results of Neutron Beam Treatment for Malignant Gliomas

Author, Group, [Ref]	Study Groups	No. Pts	Median Survival (mos)	1-Year Survival (%)
Griffin et al., Seattle, [91]	Neutrons alone	26	7	22
	Gp 1: 1550–1850 neutron rads, 150 rads/fx, twice weekly: Monday, Friday, whole brain	15		
	Gp 2: 1650–1850 neutron rads, 100 rads/fx/dy thrice weekly: Mon, Wed, Fri, whole brain	5		
	Gp 3: miscellaneous whole brain fractionated neutron doses	6		
	Mixed Beam	10	5	19
	Gp 4: neutrons: 600–6600 neutron rads whole brain, 60 rad/fx/day, twice weekly: Mon, Fri, then 120–180 neutron rad tumor boost @ 60 rads/fx photons: 2800–3200 photon rads whole brain, 180 rads/fx/day, thrice weekly (Tu, Wed, Th) plus 500–1000 rads local tumor boost	7		
	Gp 5: Mixed beam (treatment incomplete) whole brain without cone down	2		
	Photon 5000 rads (25 fx) then 450 neutron rads (5 fx)	1		
Griffin et al., RTOG: 76-11, 5 centers study [92]	Gp 1: 5000 photon rads whole brain, 180–200 rads/fx/d, 5 fx/wk, then 1500 rad photon boost @ same rate	80	9.8	40
	Gp 2: 5000 photon rads whole brain, 180–200 rads/fx/d, 5 fx/wk, then 1500 RBE adjusted neutron tumor boost @ same fx rate	78	8.6	40
Catterall et al., London [93]	Gp 1: 5000–5500 photon rads, one fx/day, 5 dys/wk	33	10	36.4
	Gp 2: 1300–1560 neutron rads, 12 fx, 26–33 days 3 rx/wk	30	10	30

Table 3 (*continued*)
Results of Neutron Beam Treatment for Malignant Gliomas

Author, Group, [Ref]	Study Groups	No. Pts	Median Survival (mos)	1-Year Survival (%)
Kurup et al., RTOG: 79-03, [79-03] [94]	1200 neutron rads whole brain: 300 neutron rads/fx @ one fx/wk × 4 weeks, then 600 neutron rads boost @ 300 rads/fx; also misonidazole 2.5 g/m sq given 4 hrs pre each rx.	25	12	50
Herskovic et al., Washington, D.C. [95]	Gp 1: neutrons alone; 1639–2200 neutron rads Gp 2: mixed beam: various schedules	17 13	n.r. n.r.	n.r. n.r.
Batterman, Amsterdam [96]	Gp 1: mixed beam: 3000 photon rads/3.5 wks, plus 1160 neutron rads boost	22	9	35

n.r.: not reported

seen prior to treatment, a finding common in autopsies of patients treated with photons.[93,97] In many neutron patients, death was thought to be due to the consequences of neutron effect on normal brain tissue rather than progressive tumor growth. These pathology findings, particularly the brain necrosis, led to a laboratory reinvestigation of neutron RBE for neural tissue specifically. Originally reported as 3, the RBE for neutrons in neural tissue is now considered between 5 and 6.[98] Lower doses per fraction and lower total neutron rad doses are now under investigation, whether for neutron only or neutron boost technique. Future studies will reveal whether adequate local tumor control without brain necrosis can be achieved with neutrons.

Heavy Charged Particle Radiation

Like neutrons, heavy charged particles provide the radiobiologic advantages of high LET radiation discussed above. In addition, they have greater deposition of energy per path length near the *end* of their path in the body, as the particle slows down (Bragg peak). This effect produces more effective destruction of tumor at the depth of the Bragg peak, potentially sparing the proximal and distal normal tissues in the particle's path.[90–100] By manipulating machine variables, the position of the Bragg peak can be made to correspond to the tumor volume inside the patient. Pioneering phase I and II work with heavy charged particle irradiation of malignant gliomas has recently been published by the University of California Lawrence Berkeley Laboratory in conjunction with the Northern California Oncology Group.[101] Thirty-three patients with high ($n = 23$) and low grade ($n = 10$) gliomas plus six with recurrent tumors were treated with helium, carbon, neon ions alone, or in combination with photon irradiation. A variety of doses and dose schedules were tried with very sophisticated treatment planning. The study was a phase I and II trial. The authors report no untoward toxicity; tumors persisted with the (relatively low) doses used, and brain necrosis was minimal. In addition, no improvement over conventional treatment was seen with this new technology. Additional studies are planned with different doses, dose schedules. chemotherapy, and sensitizers. Work defining the RBE for the various beams in different tissues is also needed.

Proton Beam Therapy

Proton beam therapy, with an RBE roughly equivalent to photons, is available at relatively few centers in the world.[102] Its importance in clinical medicine rests primarily on dose distribution properties, the Bragg peak, which is steep and can be very sharply focused.[100] Thus, tumors smaller than the typical glioma are most appropriate for treatment. The Harvard group has reported extensively on their successful treatment of choroidal melanomas, tumors abutting critical CNS structures, and arteriovenous malformations of the brain, as well as on radiobiology issues.[104–107] Groups from Japan and the USSR have also recently reported on proton therapy.[108,109]

Boron Neutron Capture

A clever use of low energy neutron radiation and immune targeting has been proposed for gliomas. Boron-loaded tumor-specific antiglioma antibodies could be administered to patients, with high affinity and highly specific localization of boron in the tumor. The high LET charged particles produced by the boron reaction would remain localized because the particles have ranges in tissue of less than 10 micrometers. With this technique, the hypothesis is that high doses of high RBE, high LET radiation might be exquisitely targeted at the tumor, sparing surrounding normal structures.[110] Major problems appear to be achieving a suitable concentration of boron within the tumor and an adequate flux of neutrons to activate the boron.

Other Treatments Used in Conjunction with External Beam Radiation

A variety of innovative approaches are currently under investigation to improve the effectiveness of glioma treatment, some to be used in conjunction with external beam radiation. Brachytherapy, the use of radioactive implants, is discussed in the following chapter. Others include hyperthermia, phototherapy, and tumor-specific monoclonal antibodies with radioactive tags.[111–115]

Conclusion

Despite considerable effort and investigation in the external beam treatment of human brain tumors, researchers have as yet produced few significant improvements in survival for patients with high grade malignant gliomas. Although modest advancement may result from more effective delivery of resources and techniques currently available, major leaps forward are likely to await the development of new biologic understanding of the development and growth characteristics of these very difficult tumors. Patients with gliomas, especially high grade lesions, should be considered for experimental protocols in an effort to improve the disappointing results from current conventional treatment.

REFERENCES

1. Sheline GE. Radiation therapy of primary tumors. Semin Oncol 1975; 2:29–42.
2. Leibel SA, Sheline GA, Wara WM, Boldrey EB, Neilsen SL. The role of

radiation therapy in the treatment of astrocytomas. Cancer 1975; 35:1551–1557.

3. Fazekas JT. Treatment of grades I and II brain astrocytomas. The role of radiotherapy. Int J Radiat Oncol Biol Phys 1977; 2:661–666.

4. Rutten EH, Kazem I, Slooff JL, Waler AH. Postoperative radiation therapy in the management of brain astrocytomata-retrospective study of 142 patients. Int J Radiat Oncol Biol Phys 7:191–195.

5. Bloom HJ. Intracranial tumors: Response and resistance to therapeutic endeavors, 1970–1980. Int J Radiat Oncol Biol Phys 8:1083–1113.

6. Garcia DM, Fulling KH, Marks JE. The value of radiation therapy in addition to surgery for astrocytomas of the adult cerebrum. Cancer 1985; 55:919–927.

7. Laws ER, Taylor WF, Clifton MB, Okazaki H. Neurosurgical management of low-grade astrocytoma of the cerebral hemispheres. J Neurosurg 1984; 61:665–673.

8. Salazar OM, Rubin P, Feldstein ML, Pizzutiello R. High dose radiation therapy in the treatment of malignant gliomas: Final report. Int J Radiat Oncol Biol Phys 1979; 5:1733–1740.

9. Walker MD, Alexander E, Hunt WE, MacCarty CS, Mahaley MS, Mealey J, Norrell HA, Owens G, Ransohoff J, Wilson CB, Gehan EA, Strike TA. J Neurosurg 1978; 49:333–343.

10. Walker MD, Green S, Byar DP, Alexander E, Batzdorf U, Brooks WH, Hunt W, MacCarty C, Mahaley MS, Mealey J, Owens G, Ransohoff J, Robertson JT, Shapiro W, Smith KR, Wilson CB, Strike TA. Randomized comparisons of radiotherapy and nitrosoureas for the treatment of malignant glioma after surgery. N Engl J Med 1980; 303:1323–1329.

11. Walker MD, Alexander E, Hunt WE, Leventhal CM, Mahaley MS, Mealey J, Norrell HA, Owens G, Ransohoff J, Wilson CB, Gehan EA. Evaluation of mithramycin in the treatment of anaplastic gliomas. J Neurosurg 1976; 44:655–667.

12. Walker MD, Strike T, Sheline GE. An analysis of dose-effect relationship in the radiotherapy of malignant gliomas. Int J Radiat Oncol Biol Phys 1979; 5:1725–1731.

13. Kristiansen K, Hagen S, Kollevold T, Torvik A, Holme I, Nesbakken R, Hatlevoll R, Lindgren M, Brun A, Lindgren S, Notter G, Andersen AP, Elgen K. Combined modality therapy of operated astrocytomas grade III and IV. Confirmation of the value of postoperative irradiation and lack of potentiation of bleomycin on survival time: A prospective multicenter trial of the Scandinavian Glioblastoma Study Group. Cancer 1981; 47:649–652.

14. Gilbert H, Kagan AR, Cassidy F, Wagner J, Fuchs K, Fox D, Macri I, Gilbert D, Rao A, Nussbaum H, Forsythe A, Eder D, Latino F, Youleles L, Chan P, Hints BL. Glioblastoma multiforme is not a uniform disease! Cancer Clin Trials 1981; 4:87–89.

15. Sheline GE. The importance of distinguishing tumor grade in malignant gliomas: treatment and prognosis. Int J Radiat Oncol Biol Phys 1976; 1:781–786.

16. Giangaspero F, Burger PC. Correlations between cytologic composition

and biologic behavior in the glioblastoma multiforme; a postmortem study of 50 cases. Cancer 1983; 52:2320–2333.

17. Fulling KH, Garcia DM. Anaplastic astrocytoma of the adult cerebrum, prognostic value of histologic features. Cancer 1985; 55:928–931.

18. Burger PC, Vogel FS, Green S, Strike TA. Glioblastoma multiforme and anaplastic astrocytoma, pathologic criteria and prognostic implications. Cancer 1985; 56:1106–1111.

19. Hirakawa K, Suzuki K, Ueda S, Nakagawa Y, Yoshino E, Ibayashi N, Hayashi K. Multivariate analysis of factors affecting postoperative survival in malignant astrocytoma. J Neuro-Oncol 1984; 2:331–340.

20. Chang CH, Horton J, Schoenfeld D, Salazar O, Perez-Tamayo R, Kramer S, Weinstein A, Nelson JS, Tsukada Y. Comparison of postoperative radiotherapy and combined postoperative radiotherapy and chemotherapy in the multidisciplinary management of malignant gliomas; a joint Radiation Therapy Oncology Group and Eastern Cooperative Oncology Group study. Cancer 1983; 52:997–1007.

21. Nelson DF, Nelson JS, Davis DR, Chand CH, Griffin TW, Pajak TF. Survival and prognosis of patients with astrocytoma with atypical or anaplastic features. J Neuro-Oncol 1985; 3:99–103.

22. Nelson JS, Tsukada Y, Schoenfeld D, Fulling K, Lamarche J, Peress N. Necrosis as a prognostic criterion in malignant supratentorial, astrocytic gliomas. Cancer 1983; 52:550–554.

23. Petronas NJ, Di Chiro GS, Kufta C, Bairamain D, Kornblith PL, Simon R, Larson SM. Prediction of survival in glioma patients by means of positron emission tomography. J Neurosurg 1985; 62:816–822.

24. Pasquier B, Pasquier D, N'Golet P, Panh MH, Couderc. Extraneural metastases of astrocytomas and glioblastomas, Clinicopathologic study of two cases and review of literature. Cancer 1980; 45:112–125.

25. Campbell AN, Chan HS, Becker LE, Daneman, Park TS, Hoffman. Extracranial metastases in childhood primary intracranial tumors. Cancer 1984; 53:974–981.

26. Salazar OM, Rubin P, McDonald JV, Feldstein ML. Patterns of failure in intracranial astrocytomas after irradiation: analysis of dose and field factors. Am J Roentgenol 1976; 126:279–292.

27. Erlich SS, Davis RL. Spinal subarachnoid metastasis from primary intracranial glioblastoma multiforme. Cancer 1978; 42:2854–2864.

28. Concannon JP, Kramer S, Berry R. The extent of intracranial gliomata at autopsy and its relationship to techniques used in radiation therapy of brain tumors. Am J Roentgenol 1960; 84:99–107.

29. Hochberg FH, Pruitt A. Assumptions in the radiotherapy of glioblastoma. Neurology 1980; 30:907–911.

30. Sheline GE. Radiotherapy of adult primary cerebral neoplasms. In: Walker M, ed. Cancer treatment and research series: Oncology and the Nervous System, The Hague, Holland, Martinus, 1982.

31. Sheline GE, Wara WM, Smith V. Therapeutic irradiation and brain injury. Int J Radiat Oncol Biol Phys 1980; 6:1215–1228.

32. Wigg DR, Koschel K, Hodgson GS. Tolerance of the mature human nervous system to photon irradiation. Br J Radiol 1981; 54:787–798.

33. Marks JE, Baglan RJ, Prassad SC, Blank WF. Cerebral radionecrosis:

Incidence and risk in relation to dose, time, fractionation and volume. Int J Radiat Oncol Biol Phys 1981; 7:243–252.

34. Pezner RD, Archambeau JO. Brain tolerance unit: A method to estimate risk of radiation brain injury for various dose schedules. Int J Radiat Oncol Biol Phys 1981; 7:397–402.

35. Russo A, Kinsella T, Morstyn G, Glatstein E. Determinants of radiosensitivity. Semin Oncol 1985; 12:332–349.

36. Fertil B, Malaise EP. Intrinsic radiosensitivity of human cell lines is correlated with radioresponsiveness of human tumors: Analysis of 101 published survival curves. Int J Radiat Oncol Biol Phys 1985; 11:1699–1707.

37. Matsuda K, Aramaki R, Takaki T, Wakisaka S. Possible explanation of radioresistance of glioblastoma in situ. Int J Radiat Oncol Biol Phys 1983; 9:255–258.

38. Glatstein E, Lichter A, Fraas B, Kelly B, van de Geign. The imaging revolution and radiation oncology: Use of CT, ultrasound, and NMR for localization, treatment planning and treatment delivery. Int J Radiat Oncol Biol Phys 1985; 11:299–314.

39. Griggin BR, Shuman W, Luk KH, Tong D. Locate: an application of computed tomography in radiation therapy treatment planning with emphasis on tumor localization. Int J Radiat Oncol Biol Phys 1984; 10:555–559.

40. Gutin PH, Phillips TL, Hosobuchi Y, Wara WM, Mackay AR, Weaver KA, Lamb S, Hurst S. Permanent and removable implants for the brachytherapy of brain tumors. Int J Radiat Oncol Biol Phys 1981; 7:1371–1381.

41. Zeman EM, Bedford JS. Changes in early and late effects with dose-per-fraction: alpha, beta, redistribution and repair. Int J Radiat Oncol Biol Phys 1984; 10:1039–1047.

42. Thames H, Withers HR, Peters LJ, Fletcher GH. Changes in early and late radiation responses with altered dose fractionation: implications for dose survival relationships. Int J Radiat Oncol Biol Phys 1982; 8:219–226.

43. Fowler JF. Non-standard fractionation in radiotherapy. Int J Radiat Oncol Biol Phys 1984; 10:755–759.

44. Withers HR. Biologic basis for alter fractionation schemes. Cancer 1985; 55:2086–2095.

45. Simpson WJ, Platts ME. Fractionation study in the treatment of glioblastoma multiforme. Int J Radiat Oncol Biol Phys 1976; 1:639–644.

46. Payne DG, Simpson WJ, Kee C, Platts ME. Malignant astrocytoma: Hyperfractionated and standard radiotherapy with chemotherapy in a randomized prospective clinical trial. Cancer 1982; 50:2301–2306.

47. Shin KY, Muller PJ, Geggie PH. Superfractionation radiation therapy in the treatment of malignant astrocytoma. Cancer 1983; 52:2040–2043.

48. Douglas BG, Worth AJ. Superfractionation in glioblastoma multiforme: Results of a phase II study. Int J Radiat Oncol Biol Phys 1982; 8:1787–1794.

49. Fulton DS, Urtasun RC, Shin KH, Geggie PH, Thomas H, Muller PJ, Moody J, Tanasichuk, Mielke B, Johnson E, Curry. Misonidazole com-

bined with hyperfractionation in the management of malignant glioma. Int J Radiat Oncol Biol Phys 1984; 10:1709–1712.

50. Shin KH, Urtasun RC, Fulton D, Geggie PH, Tanasichuk, Thomas H, Muller PJ, Curry B, Mielke B, Johnson E, Feldstein M. Multiple daily fractionated radiation therapy and misonidazole in the management of malignant astrocytoma. Cancer 1985; 56:758–760.

51. Thames HD, Peters LJ, Withers HR, Fletcher GH. Accelerated fractionation vs hyperfractionation: rationales for several treatments per day Int J Radiat Oncol Biol Phys 1983; 9:127–138.

52. Caldwell WL, Aristizabal SA. Treatment of glioblastoma multiforme. Acta Radiol [Ther] [Stockholm] 1975; 14:505–512.

53. Phillips TL, Wasserman TH. Promise of radiosensitizers and radioprotectors in the treatment of human cancer. Cancer Treat Rep 1984; 68:291–302.

54. Hall EJ. Radiobiology for the radiologist. 2nd ed. Philadelphia, Harper and Row, 1978; pp. 180–194.

55. Chang CH. Hyperbaric oxygen as a radiation sensitizer in the treatment of malignant gliomas. In: Chang CH, Housepian EM, eds. Tumors of the central nervous system: Modern radiotherapy in multidisciplinary management. New York, Masson Publishing, 1982; pp. 23–30.

56. Asquith JC, Watts ME, Patel K, Smithen CE, Adams GE. Electron affinic sensitization. V. Radiosensitization of hypoxic bacteria and mammalian cells in vitro by some nitroimidazoles and nitropyrazoles. Radiat Res 1974; 60:108–118.

57. Brown JM. Clinical perspectives for the use of new hypoxic cell sensitizers. Int J Radiat Oncol Biol Phys 1982; 8:1491–1497.

58. Adams GE. Hypoxia-mediated drugs for radiation and chemotherapy. Cancer 1981; 48:696–706.

59. Stratford IJ. Mechanisms of hypoxic cell radiosensitization and the development of new sensitizers. Int J Radiat Oncol Biol Phys 1982; 8:391–398.

60. Hei TK, Geard CR, Osmak RS, Hall EJ. In vitro assessment of the oncogenic potential of nitroimidazole radiosensitizers. Int J Radiat Oncol Biol Phys 1985; 11:1653–1658.

61. Urtasun RC, Feldstein ML, Partington JP. Hypoxic cell sensitizers and radiotherapy for malignant gliomas. In: Chang CH, Housepian EM, eds. Tumors of the Central Nervous System: Modern Radiotherapy in Multidisciplinary Management. New York, Masson Publishing, 1982; pp. 31–38.

62. Urtasun R, Feldstein ML, Partington J, Tanasichuk H, Miller JD, Russell DB, Agboola O, Meilke B. Radiation and nitroimidazoles in supratentorial high grade gliomas: A second clinical trial. Br J Cancer 1982; 46:101–108.

63. Nelson DF. A randomized comparison of misonidazole sensitized radiotherapy plus BCNU and radiotherapy plus BCNU for treatment of malignant glioma after surgery; preliminary results of an RTOG study. Int J Radiat Oncol Biol Phys 1983; 9:1143–1151.

64. Wasserman TH, Stetz J, Phillips TL. Radiation Therapy Oncology Group clinical trials with misonidazole. Cancer 1981; 47:2383–2390.

65. Eifel PJ, Brown DM, Lee W, Brown JM. Misonidazole neurotoxicity in mice decreased by administration with pyridoxine. Int J Radiat Oncol Biol Phys 1983; 9:1513–1519.
66. Urtasun R, Band P, Chapman JD, Feldstein ML, Mielke B, Fryer C. Radiation and high-dose metronidazole in supratentorial glioblastoma. N Engl J Med 1976; 294:1364–1367.
67. Urtasun R, Band P, Chapman JD, Feldstein ML. Radiation plus metronidazole for glioblastoma. N Engl J Med 1977; 296:757.
69. Bleehan NM. The Cambridge glioma trial of misonidazole and radiation therapy with associated pharmacokinetic studies. Cancer Clin Trials 1980; 3:267–273.
70. Carabell SC, Bruno L, Weinstein AS, Richter MP, Chang CH, Weiler CB, Goodman RL. Misonidazole and radiotherapy to treat malignant glioma: A phase II trial of the Radiation Therapy Oncology Group. Int J Radiat Oncol Biol Phys 1981; 7:71–79.
71. Cumberlin RL, Sheline GE, Strike TA. Treatment of malignant glioma: Results of BTSG 77-02. A J Clin Oncol (Cancer Clin Trials) 1983; 6:145 (abstract).
72. Ang KK, van der Schueren E, Notter G, Horiot C, Chenal C, Fauchon F, Raps J, van Perperzeel H, Goffin JC, Vessiere M, Van Glabbeke M. Split-course multiple daily fractionated radiotherapy schedule combined with misonidazole for the management of grade III and IV gliomas. Int J Radiat Oncol Biol Phys 1982; 8:1657–1664.
73. EORTC Brain Tumor Group. Misonidazole in radiotherapy of supratentorial malignant brain gliomas in adult patients: A randomized double-blind study. Eur J Cancer Clin Oncol 1983; 19:39–42.
74. MRC Working Party on Misonidazole in Gliomas. A study of the effect of misonidazole in conjunction with radiotherapy for the treatment of grades 3 and 4 astrocytomas. Br J Radiol 1983; 56:673–682.
75. Stadler B, Karcher KH, Kogelnik DH, Szepesi T. Misonidazole and irradiation in the treatment of high-grade astrocytomas: Further report of the Vienna Study Group. Int J Radiat Oncol Biol Phys 1984; 10:1713–1717.
76. Hatelvoll R et al. Combined modality treatment of operated astrocytomas grade 3 and 4: A prospective and randomized study of misonidazole and radiotherapy with two different radiation schedules and subsequent CCNU chemotherapy. Stage II of a prospective multicenter trial of the Scandinavian Glioblastoma Study Group. Cancer 1985; 56:41–47.
77. Brown JM. Clinical trials of radiosensitizers: What should we expect? Int J Radiat Oncol Biol Phys 1984; 10:425–429.
78. Dische S, Saunders MI, Anderson P, Stratford MR, Minchinton A. Clinical experience with nitroimidazoles as radiosensitizers. Int J Radiat Oncol Biol Phys 1982; 8:335–338.
79. Djordjevic B, Szbalski W. Genetics of human cell lines. III Incorporation of 5-bromo and 5-iododeoxyuridine into the deoxyribonucleic acid of human cells and its effect of radiation sensitivity. J Exp Med 1960; 112:509–531.
80. Kinsella TJ, Mitchell JB, Russo A, Morstyn G, Glatstein E. The use of

halogenated thymidine analogs as clinical radiosensitizers: Rationale, current status, and future prospects: non-hypoxic cell sensitizers. Int J Radiat Oncol Biol Phys 1984; 10:1399–1406.

81. Mitchell JB, Kinsella TJ, Russo A, McPherson S, Rowland J, Smith B, Kornblith PL, Glatstein E. Radiosensitization of hematopoietic precursor cells (CFUc) in glioblastoma patients receiving intermittent intravenous infusions of bromodeoxyuridine (BUdR). Int J Radiat Oncol Biol Phys 1983; 9:457–463.

82. Kinsella TJ, Russo A, Mitchell JB, Rowland J, Jenkins J, Schwade J, Myers C, Collins J, Speyer J, Kornblith P, Smith B, Kufta C, Glatstein E. A phase I study of intermittent intravenous bromodeoxyuridine (BUdR) with conventional fractionated irradiation. Int J Radiat Oncol Biol Phys 1984; 66–76.

83. Kinsella TJ, Mitchell JB, Russo A, Aiken M, Morstyn G, Hsu SM, Rowland J, Glatstein E. Continuous intravenous infusions of bromodeoxyuridine as a clinical radiosensitizer. J Clin Oncol 1984; 2:1144–1150.

84. Kinsella TJ, Russo A, Mitchell JB, Collins J, Rowland J, Wright D, Glatstein E. A phase I study of intravenous iododeoxyuridine as a clinical radiosensitizer. Int J Radiat Oncol Biol Phys 1985; 11:1941–1946.

85. Phuphanich S, Levin EM, Levin VA. Phase I study of intravenous bromodeoxyuridine used concomitantly with radiation therapy in patients with primary malignant brain tumors. Int J Radiat Oncol Biol Phys 1984; 10:1769–1772.

86. Jackson D, Kinsella TJ, Wright D, Katz D, Main D, Collins J, Rowland J, Kornblith P, Glatstein E. Halogenated pyrimidines as radiosensitizers in the treatment of high grade glioma. Am J Clin Oncol (Cancer Clin Trials) 1986 (in press, abstract).

87. Hall E. *op. cit.* pp. 95–110.

88. Hall E. *op. cit.* p. 302.

89. Hall EJ, Kellerer AM, Fried H. Dependence on neutron energy of the OER and RBE. Int J Radiat Oncol Biol Phys 1982; 8:1567–1572.

90. Catterall M. The assessment of the results of neutron therapy. Int J Radiat Oncol Biol Phys 1982; 8:1573–1580.

91. Griffin TW, Blasko JC, Laramore GE. Neutron teletherapy for grades III and IV astrocytomas. In: Chang CH, Housepian EM, eds. Tumors of the Central Nervous system: Modern Radiotherapy in Multidisciplinary Management. New York, Masson Publishing, 1982; pp. 39–46.

92. Griffin TW, Davis R, Laramore G, Hendrickson F, Rodrigues-Antunez A, Hussey D, Nelson J. Fast neutron radiation therapy for glioblastoma multiforme. Am J Clin Oncol (CCT) 1983; 6:661–667.

93. Catterall M, Bloom JG, Ash D, Walsh L. Richardson A, Uttley D, Gowing NF, Lewis P, Chaucer B. Fast neutrons compared with megavoltage x-rays in the treatment of patients with supratentorial glioblastoma: A controlled pilot study. Int J Radiat Oncol Biol Phys 1980; 6:261–266.

94. Kurup PD, Pajak T, Hendrickson FR, Nelson JS, Mansell J, Cohen L, Awschalom M, Rosenberg I, Ten Haken RK. Fast neurons and misonidazole for malignant astrocytomas. Int J Radiat Oncol Biol Phys 1985; 11:679–686.

95. Herskovic A, Ornitz RD, Shell M, Rogers CC. Treatment experience:

Glioblastoma multiforme treated with 15 MeV fast neutrons. Cancer 1982; 49:2463–2465.

96. Batterman JJ. Fast neutron therapy for advanced brain tumors. Int J Radiat Oncol Biol Phys 1980; 6:333–335.

97. Shaw C-M, Sumi SM, Alvord EC, Gerdes AJ, Spence A, Parker RG. Fast-neutron irradiation of glioblastoma multiforme. J Neurosurg 1978; 49:1–12.

98. Hornsey S, Morris CC, Myers R, White A. Relative biologic effectiveness for damage to the central nervous system by neutrons. Int J Radiat Oncol Biol Phys 1981; 7:185–189.

99. Hall E. Radiobiology for the radiologist. 2nd ed. Philadelphia, Harper and Row, 1978; pp. 22–29.

100. Hall EJ. New modalities in cancer treatment: heavy charged particles. Br J Radiol 1981; 54:773–781.

101. Castro JR, Saunders WM, Austin-Seymour MM, Woodruff KH, Gauger G, Chen GT, Collier JM, Phillips TL, Zink SR. A phase I–II trial of heavy charged particle irradiation of malignant glioma of the brain: A Northern California Oncology Group study. Int J Radiat Oncol Biol Phys 1985; 11:1795–1800.

102. Hall E. Radiobiology for the Radiologist. 2nd ed. Philadelphia, Harper and Row, 1978; pp. 310.

103. Saunders WM, Chen GT, Austin-Seymour M, Castro JR, Collier JM, Gauger G, Gutin P, Phillips TL, Pitluck S, Walton RE, Zink SR. Precision, high dose radiotherapy. II. Helium ion treatment of tumors adjacent to critical central nervous system structures. Int J Radiat Oncol Biol Phys 1985; 11:1339–1347.

104. Suit H, Goitein M, Munzenrider J, Verhey L, Blitzer P, Gragoudas E, Koehler AM, Urie M, Gentry R, Shipley W, Urano M, Duttenhaver J, Wagner M. Evaluation of the clinical applicability of proton beams in definitive fractionated radiation therapy. Int J Radiat Oncol Biol Phys 1982; 8:2199–2205.

105. Seddon JM, Gragoudas ES, Albert DM, Hsieh CC, Polivogianis L, Freidenberg GR. Comparison of survival rates for patients with uveal melanoma after treatment with proton beam irradiation or enucleation. Am J Ophthal 1985; 99:282–290.

106. Kjellberg RN, Hanamura T, Davis KR, Lyons SL, Adams RD. Bragg-peak proton beam therapy for arteriovenous malformations of the brain. N Engl J Med 1983; 309:269–274.

107. Urano M, Verhey L, Goitein M, Tepper JE, Suit HD, Mendiondo O, Gragoudas E, Koehler A. Relative biological effectiveness of modulated proton beams in various tissues. Int J Radiat Oncol Biol Phys 1984; 10:509–514.

108. Chuvilo IV et al. ITEP synchrotron proton beam in radiotherapy. Int J Radiat Oncol Biol Phys 1984; 10:185–195.

109. Akunuma A et al. Compensation techniques in NIRS proton beam radiotherapy. Int J Radiat Oncol Biol Phys 1982; 8:1629–1635.

110. Wellum GR, Zamenhof RG, Tolpin EI. Boron neutron capture radiation therapy of cerebral gliomas: an analysis of the possible use of boron-

loaded tumor-specific antibodies for the selective concentration of boron in gliomas. Int J Radiat Oncol Biol Phys 1982: 8:1339–1345.
111. Silberman AW, Morgan DF, Storm FK, Rand RW, Benz M, Drury B, Morton DL. Combination radiofrequency hyperthermia and chemotherapy (BCNU) for brain malignancy. J Neuro-Oncol 1984; 2:19–28.
112. Winter A, Laing J, Paglione R, Sterzer F. Microwave hyperthermia for brain tumors. Neurosurgery 1985; 17:387–399.
113. Boggan JE, Bolger C, Edwards MS. Effect of hematoporphyrin derivative photoradiation therapy on survival in the rat 9L gliosarcoma brain-tumor model. J Neurosurg 1985; 63:917–921.
114. Kostron H, Swartz MR, Miller DC, Martuza RL. The interaction of hematoporphyrin derivative, light, and ionizing radiation in a rat glioma model. Cancer 1986; 57:964–970.
115. Bullard DE, Bigner DD. Application of monoclonal antibodies in the diagnosis and treatment of primary brain tumors. J Neurosurg 1985; 63:2–16.

14

Interstitial Radiobrachytherapy of Malignant Cerebral Gliomas

Zbigniew Petrovich, Michael L.J. Apuzzo, Gary Luxton, Joanne H. Jepson, and Deirdre Cohen

Introduction

Malignant cerebral gliomas are the most common primary tumors of this site in adult patients. They represent approximately one-third of all brain tumors and one-half of all gliomas, or over 4,500 new cases a year.[1,2] The total number of primary central nervous system tumors in the United States has been estimated to be 13,800 in 1986.[2]

To date, no consistently effective therapy is available for malignant gliomas.[1,3–6] The median survival of patients treated with surgery alone in a large randomized trial was 18.0 weeks.[3] The addition of postoperative radiotherapy in the same study increased the median survival to over 40 weeks. There was an apparent increase in survival with increase in the radiation dose, up to 60 Gy. Although one study demonstrated a higher survival with a radiation dose of 7,500 cGy,[4] most investigators would limit the dose to 60 Gy. Radiation doses over 60 Gy, particularly when given to a large volume of tissue, are

From: Kornblith PL, Walker MD (editors). Advances in Neuro-Oncology. Futura Publishing Company, Inc., Mount Kisco, NY, © 1988.

expected to result in a relatively high incidence of serious complications such as cerebral necrosis.[1,7,8] The rationale behind the treatment of a large volume of brain in malignant gliomas was provided by a study reported by Concannon et al.[9] A more recent report, however, questioned this rationale, since 80% of the recurrent cases of malignant gliomas occur at or close to the original tumor.[10] Additionally, less than 5% of glioblastomas were found to be multicentric, and therefore more limited field radiotherapy for these tumors is warranted. Its use may result in a reduction of late toxicity of radiotherapy.

The use of fast neutron teletherapy has failed to significantly influence the survival of patients with grades III and IV astrocytomas.[11,12] Similarly, radiosensitizers did not improve survival of patients compared to radiotherapy alone.[13,14] Currently of greater interest is a concept of altered fractionation.[15–17] In a small study from Calgary, Canada, superfractionation radiotherapy patients experienced a better survival in comparison to the conventional fraction radiotherapy group.[17] Further work will be required to define the role of superfractionation in the treatment of malignant gliomas.

The addition of chemotherapy to the radiation treatment resulted in a modest increase in the median survival of patients, especially those between 40 and 60 years of age.[1,5] Toxicity of chemotherapy in the treatment of malignant gliomas is considerable; therefore, in our opinion, the routine use of this modality should not be contemplated.

One of the most significant new methodologies in the management of malignant gliomas came with the introduction of computerized tomography and associated guided stereotaxis.[18–21] This allowed for better tumor definition and more precise radiation treatment both in teletherapy and brachytherapy modes. Afterloading interstitial brachytherapy has rapidly evolved and at the present time it is being evaluated as a prospective standard therapy for recurrences, and together with teletherapy for selected primary, supratentorial malignant gliomas.[21–23]

Basic Radiation Physics and Biology

Radiation used in clinical radiotherapy can be conveniently grouped into electromagnetic and particle beams.

Electromagnetic Radiation

In electromagnetic radiation (EMR), energy is transferred through space, in the form of waves. This energy transfer is not continuous, but occurs in discrete packets, called quanta. Quanta or "bullets" of energy of visible light, x-rays, and gamma rays are called *photons*. All EMR is propagated in straight lines, at the same speed of approximately 3×10^8 m/sec in vacuum. This speed of EMR is commonly called the speed of light. EMR beams are characterized by wavelength, frequency, energy, and intensity. In the EMR spectrum, low frequency and long wavelength are represented by radio, TV, and radar waves. Intermediate frequency is represented by infrared, visible light, and ultraviolet. X-rays and gamma rays represent high frequency, short wavelength EMR. The basic difference between gamma rays and x-rays is their origin. Gamma rays are produced in processes taking place within the nucleus of an atom, while x-rays are produced through change in the state of orbital atomically bound electrons or through the slowing down process ("bremsstrahlung") of a fast-moving unbound electron.

A commonly used apparatus in clinical radiotherapy producing deep penetrating gamma rays is the cobalt-60 teletherapy unit. The cobalt-60 beam has a mean quantum energy of 1.25 meV (million electron volts), which is in a useful range for treatment of CNS malignancy. In recent years, cobalt-60 beams have lost much of their popularity in favor of linear accelerator (linac) generated x-ray beams. These x-ray beams are available at various energies from 4 to 25 MV. Besides having a selectable energy, the linac x-ray beams have more sharply defined geometrical edges, thereby allowing for additional treatment improvement when compared to the cobalt-60 beam. The higher the beam energy, the greater the penetration (greater depth dose), and the greater the sparing of more superficial tissues.

In the treatment of brain or spinal cord tumors, the lower energy (4–6 MV) x-ray beams are typically used while in treatment of centrally located lesions such as pituitary tumors, beams of energy greater than 15 MV are more desirable. Using a higher energy beam, one can effectively deliver the treatment to the tumor with a much lower incidence of radiation injury to cerebral cortex than with a lower energy x-ray beam.

Gamma rays are produced not only by man-made radioactive isotopes, such as cobalt-60 or iridium-192, but also by naturally occurring radioactive isotopes such as those in the series produced by the decay of radium-226.

Particle Radiation

A number of different particles, moving at a speed approaching the speed of light, are used in clinical radiotherapy. The most frequently used beams are accelerated subatomic particles such as electrons. Characteristics of these particles are shown in Table 1.

Electrons are negatively charged particles with a small mass about 1,840 times smaller than that of the proton. Accelerated electrons are used in radiotherapy in the form of beams of various energy. When produced by the decay of radioactive isotopes, electrons are referred to as beta rays. Tissue penetration of an electron beam depends on the energy. The higher the beam energy, the greater the penetration. The higher the beam intensity (number of electrons per second) the higher the dose rate. Clinically, electron beams are used for treatment of superficial tumors of up to several centimeters in depth.

The *neutron* is a particle with no charge and with a mass about 0.1% greater than that of the proton. A common source for a useful neutron beam is the cyclotron. Clinically useful neutrons can also be obtained from the radionuclide californium-252. The use of neutron beams in treatment of CNS malignancies has been increasing both in teletherapy and interstitial brachytherapy.[11,12,24]

Protons are positively charged subatomic particles which, when accelerated to high energy, form a useful beam, particularly for the treatment of pituitary lesions and primary melanoma of the eye.[25] Other lesions suitable for proton beam therapy include those in the

Table 1
Subatomic Particles Used in Radiotherapy

Particle	Symbol	Charge	Mass Units	Mass (gm) or (g)
Electron	e^-	-1	5.5×10^{-4}	9.1×10^{-28}
Proton	p	$+1$	1.0073	1.7×10^{-24}
Neutron	n	0	1.0087	1.7×10^{-24}
Pi Mesons	π	-1	.15	2.5×10^{-25}

proximity of the spinal cord such as chondrosarcoma or osteogenic sarcoma of the cervical spine. In this particular clinical situation, a proton beam is not only useful in treating the tumor but will also, with proper planning, greatly reduce the risk of radiation injury to the spinal cord compared to therapy with x-ray beams.

Pi mesons are subatomic particles, positively or negatively charged with a mass 273 times greater than that of the electron. Beams of negatively charged pi mesons, while biologically very promising, are utilized for therapy in only a few facilities in the world[26,27] because of their high cost and complexity.

In recent years, accelerated nuclei of several elements have been used in radiotherapy and biological research. These heavy particle beams are represented by the following: nuclei of helium, argon, boron, carbon, neon, and nitrogen. These beams are extremely useful, but similar limitations apply here as for pi meson beams.[28–30]

Basic Definitions

A discussion of the use of radiation in treatment of any neoplasm requires certain basic definitions.

A unit of absorbed dose of radiation is the *rad*. More recently, a new unit of absorbed dose has received international recognition. This unit, called the *Gray (Gy)*, is one joule of energy absorbed per kilogram in the form of ionizing radiation. Numerically, the Gray is equal to 100 rads. The locus of points of equal dose is called an *isodose curve*. Typically, in radiation oncology, a tumor dose is defined to a certain isodose level, which is a surface in three dimensions. In interstitial therapy of malignant gliomas, for example, we define the tumor dose to be 5,500 rads given at 40 to 55 rads per hour. This means that all points encompassed by the 5,500 rad isodose line in a particular plane will receive at least this dose.

To define a beam of radiation one should specify its nature, for example, whether electron or photon, its particle *energy* in MeV, or peak quantum energy in MV, kV, or kVp, and its quality. Beam quality gives information on beam attenuation through standard absorber materials. The thickness of an absorber that reduces the intensity of an incident beam by 50% is called the *half-value layer* or half-value thickness (HVL or HVT). HVL depends on beam energy and the type of absorber material. The HVL of x-ray beams from 10 kVp to 150 kVp ranges from less than one-tenth up to several millimeters of aluminum while for cobalt-60 and 4 MV x-ray beams it is greater than 10 mm of lead.[31]

Since radiation effect on tissue occurs through *ionization*, this term deserves an explanation. Ionization is the process of removal or addition of electrons. The charged atom is highly reactive chemically.

Radioactive isotopes decay at a statistically predictable rate. The time required for half of a given isotope to decay is called the *half-life*. There is a large variation in the half-life of commonly used radionuclides. It is more than 1,600 years for radium-226, 60 days for iodine-125, 8 days for iodine-131, and can be as short as a fraction of a second for some isotopes.[31] Isotope activity is defined by the number of nuclear disintegrations per second. The unit of radioactive isotope activity is the Curie (Ci). One curie = 3.70×10^{10} disintegration/sec.[32] In interstitial therapy, typically mCi quantitites of isotopes are used.

Radioactive Isotopes Used in Brachytherapy

In 1895, Wilhelm Roentgen discovered x-rays. This was followed a few weeks later by the discovery of natural radioactivity or gamma rays by Henri Becquerel. In 1898, Marie and Pierre Curie discovered radium and polonium.[33] Radium was immediately recognized as a powerful source of gamma rays and useful in the treatment of cancer. Radium-226 and its daughter product radon-222, remained unchallenged as the most important sources of radiation for cancer therapy for half a century. Following the development of nuclear reactors in the 1940s, numerous man-made isotopes became available to radiation oncologists as a source of radiation for brachytherapy. Radionuclides such as cesium-137 substituted for radium-226 in intracavitary therapy while iridium-192 and iodine-125 displaced radium-226 and radon-222 in interstitial therapy. The new radionuclides allowed for much better radiation protection, as well as providing a much wider technical scope for the optimization of interstitial radiotherapy. At this time, one can choose an isotope with appropriate characteristics to satisfy even the most complex clinical needs such as that of interstitial radiotherapy of tumors of the brain.

A number of radioactive isotopes have been used in interstitial radiotherapy of brain tumors. In a study of over 1,200 patients, from 1950 to 1980, Mundiger reported using several radionuclides for the

Table 2
Distribution of Patients by Radioactive
Isotope Used in Therapy

Isotope	No. of patients	%
Iridium-192	737	60
Cobalt-60	179	15
Gold-198	128	10
Iodine-125	109	9
Yttrium-90	44	4
Tantalum-182	21	2
Phosphorus-32	6	<1
Total	1,224	100

treatment of such tumors.[23] Table 2 shows the distribution of patients by radionuclide used in their therapy. Although seven different isotopes were used in this study, two clearly dominated. Iridium-192 was used in 737 patients (60%), and iodine-125 in 179 (15%). Further discussion on radioactive isotopes will be limited to either those used at the University of Southern California Medical Center Hospitals or felt by the authors to be interesting for potential utilization in interstitial radiotherapy of brain tumors. Table 3 shows important characteristics of such radionuclides and also gives a comparison with radioactive isotopes not used in treatment of CNS malignancy at this time. Iridium-192 is the radionuclide used by us. Its accessibility, low cost, and the ability to obtain a desired activity on short notice are the key factors. Iridium-192 is used like other isotopes in brachytherapy, encapsulated in the form of sealed seeds. It is the most widely used isotope in brachytherapy.[21,23,34] Iridium-192 has a half-life of 74 days and an average quantum energy of about 370 KeV, giving it an HVL in tissue of 6 cm.

Iodine-125 is a very useful radionuclide, particularly in interstitial therapy of supratentorial tumors. Its half-life is 60 days with an average photon energy of 28 keV. This relatively low energy of iodine-125 is clinically important. A collimated beam has an HVL in tissue of only 2 cm, compared to 6 cm for iridium-192 and 8 cm for cesium-137. The rapid dose fall-off of iodine-125 allows for better protection of critical structure during the treatment of brain or eye tumors. This isotope has been used in removable and permanent radioactive implants. The latter is commonly utilized for the treatment of adeno-

Table 3
Physical Characteristics of Brachytherapy Isotopes

Isotope	Half-Life	Energy of Radiation	Nominal 50% Attenuation Length in Tissue*
^{226}Ra	1,600 yrs.	184 KeV – 2.4 MeV weighted average: 830 KeV	10 cm
^{137}Cs	30.0 yrs.	662 KeV	8 cm
^{60}Co	5.26 yrs.	1.17, 1.33 MeV	11 cm
^{192}Ir	74.2 days	110 KeV – 1.38 MeV weighted average: 370 KeV	6 cm
^{125}I	60 days	27 KeV – 35 KeV weighted average: 28.5 KeV	2 cm
^{90}Sr/^{90}Y	27.7 yrs.	beta spectrum average: 1.1 MeV	1.5 mm

*Attenuation length excludes effects of scatter.

carcinoma of the prostate and tumors of the lung, head, and neck.[35] Brain tumors are commonly treated with removable iodine-125 implants.[22,23] Some centers, however, prefer the use of permanent iodine-125 implants.[36] An additional benefit of using Iodine-125 is its higher relative biological effectiveness (RBE), when compared with iridium-192 or cesium-137.[35,37,38] This higher RBE will be discussed later.

Californium-252 is a radionuclide used as a source of neutrons in brachytherapy of CNS, pelvic, and head and neck tumors.[24,39,40] It offers a low dose rate neutron radiation of high RBE. This radiation is of proven effectiveness in controlling selected tumors. Due to the problems with radiation safety in handling of californium-252, its use in the United States is limited.[39,40]

An interesting radioactive isotope with a potential usefulness for the treatment of CNS tumors is ruthenium-106. This radionuclide delivers a high dose of beta radiation to a small volume of tissue.[41,42] Ruthenium-106 decays, through rhodium-106 to a stable palladium-106, emitting several bands of high energy beta radiation. The useful energy band has a maximum energy of 3.5 MeV. This beta spectrum gives a superior tissue penetration compared to strontium-90/yttrium-90 beta rays. A large number of patients with ocular melanoma has been treated with ruthenium-106, resulting in a gratifying outcome.[42] The use of this radionuclide may also be considered in patients with smaller brain tumors, particularly those in the proximity of critical structures such as the midbrain or the optic chiasm. A wide clinical use of ruthenium-106 in the United States is not expected, due to practical difficulties of obtaining the isotope.

Biological Consideration

Ionizing radiation, including EMR and particle beams used by radiation oncologists for treatment of tumors, produces its cancerocidal effect through a release of ionizing energy in tissue. The degree of energy absorption within a limited distance from the particle track is extremely variable. Some particles, such as alpha particles or heavy nuclei, produce dense ionization in their path. This is called a high *linear energy transfer* (LET) radiation. Additionally, there is an increase in the energy deposition per unit track length at the end of their path. This dose enhancement is called the *Bragg peak*. By choosing an appropriate particle beam energy, one can utilize this phenomenon as well in treatment of tumors, with increased relative sparing of the normal tissue. Photon beams and electron beams are low LET radiation. Energy is gradually released by secondary electrons along their tracks, without Bragg peak effect.

It is thought that the most important target in the cell is the DNA molecule. It can be damaged directly by the passage through it of a beam particle, the usual means of damage from heavy charged particle beams, or indirectly by secondary electrons as occurs from cell exposure to photon beams. Ionization or excitation produced by radiation can result in damage to the DNA molecule. Frequently, this is accomplished through active radicals, which are extremely short-lived. The active radical credited with the greatest potential for causing biological damage is the hydroxyl radical.

The most critical target in the cell is the DNA, although there are other important targets, such as the cell membrane where radiation damage can lead to cell death. The cell, however, has a very efficient repair system. The results of cellular damage and repair are predictable only statistically. Thus some cells exposed to a single dose of radiation will die while others will repair sublethal injury and fully recover. To overcome this problem of repair from sublethal injury, while limiting the damage to nearby normal tissues, tumors are treated with multiple fraction radiotherapy.

Most tumors seen clinically have a significant proportion of cells in a state of hypoxia. Since the effect of ionizing radiation is strongly enhanced by the presence of oxygen, hypoxic cells are expected to more successfully survive exposure to ionizing radiation than fully oxic cells. Therefore, the dose of radiation required to achieve the same biologic effect for hypoxic cells will be greater than for fully oxygenated cells. The ratio of these doses of radiation is called the *oxygen enhancement ratio* (OER). For low LET radiation such as EMR, OER at the dose rate typically employed in external beam radiotherapy approaches 3. On the other hand, a high LET radiation such as alpha particles or heavy nuclei will have an OER close to 1. The neutron beam OER has an intermediate value.[43] OER also depends on dose rate, with lower values being obtained for the low dose rate continuous irradiation typical of interstitial brachytherapy.[35]

Equal doses of different radiation beams do not result in the same degree of biological damage. In order to compare the effect of various beams of radiation, 250 kVp x-ray beam is used as the standard. The ratio of a dose of 250 kVp radiation producing certain biologic effect to the dose of a radiation beam being tested is called the *relative biologic effectiveness* (RBE). RBE for commonly used x-ray beams is close to 1, while it may be two to ten times higher for fast neutron beams depending upon the biological end-point measured. RBE depends on multiple factors including the following given by Eric Hall: radiation quality, radiation dose, number of dose fractions, dose rate, and biological system or end-point.[43] Among radionuclides used in brachytherapy of the brain, iodine-125 is considered as having an RBE slightly greater than 1.[37,38]

Interstitial Brachytherapy

As discussed in the introduction, treatment results for malignant gliomas are disappointing.[1-6] In spite of the use of high doses of external beam radiotherapy, almost all recurrences occur in the area of the original lesion.[10] This factor, in addition to a low incidence of multicentricity and metastatic disease in malignant gliomas, makes the use of interstitial brachytherapy very appealing. With the use of brachytherapy, one can preferentially deliver much higher doses of radiation to the tumor and minimize unncessary radiation exposure to uninvolved brain tissue. This need for the protection of the normal brain tissue is greatest in patients who present with a recurrent tumor following a full course of teletherapy.

Although interstitial brachytherapy of brain tumors was used more than 50 years ago,[44] more precise treatment had to wait for the development of computer tomographic guidance stereotaxis.[18-23] A CT scan allowed for precise tumor localization and appropriate volume measurements. Stereotactic devices allowed precise placement of radiation sources at desired locations within the tumor. More recent developments in brain imaging with the use of magnetic resonance imaging have further increased our ability to define the tumor volume. In most reported studies, removable iodine-125 or iridium-192 radioactive implants are used. One recent report describes the use of iodine-125 seeds imbedded in Gelfoam strips as a permanent implant.[36] This method of implantation is utilized in patients following gross tumor removal. In view of this fact, as well as the fact that there is a considerable problem with radiation dosimetry, this method has limited applicability.

The largest series of patients treated with interstitial radiotherapy has been reported by Mundiger.[23] From 1950 to 1980, a total of 1,224 patients were treated with seven different radioactive isotopes. Most of them (75%) were treated with iodine-125 or iridium-192. In the past several years, there has been a very low complication rate. The treatment results are difficult to evaluate in this study. They appear good for low grade tumors. It is not immediately apparent what the treatment results were for malignant gliomas.

In a University of California (San Francisco) study, high intensity (greater than 25 mCi) iodine-125 sources were used in removable implants and a high dose of radiation was given. In a group of 41 patients with recurrent malignant astrocytomas, more than half had a good clinical response. In an additional six patients, there was no tumor progression, while in 14 (34%) the tumor continued to grow.[22] A disturbing problem in the UCSF study is a high incidence of serious complications.[22,44]

In a study reported by a group from Washington University, small recurrent tumors were treated.[45] Due to the limited number of patients and the short period of follow-up, treatment results are difficult to assess.

An interesting study has been reported by Maruyama et al.[24,39] The authors used californium-252 as a source of fast neutrons. Due to a small number of patients, the treatment outcome is difficult to evaluate in this study.

The Department of Neurological Surgery of the University of Southern California has had intense interest in the use of the stereotactic techniques,[20,21] and the technique of radioactive implantation under stereotactic guidance has evolved to a level of precision where these procedures can be performed with negligible acute and chronic toxicity.

Surgical Techniques

Within the University of Southern California Medical Center Hospitals, multiple point source interstitial brachytherapy is undertaken with the assistance of a Brown-Roberts-Wells Stereotactic Guidance System.[46] This instrumentation is operatively used in conjunction with imaging data derived from the use of CT imaging devices including General Electric 9800, Phillips 310 Tomoscan, and Picker 1200 units (Table 4).

Table 4
Surgical Steps in Catheter Placement

1. Anesthesia attends for local standby procedure.
2. Application of base ring (BRW stereotactic system).
3. Placement of localizer, contrast-enhanced CT.
4. Determine catheter target points with radiation therapist (one or more planes).
5. In operating room, select entry site for initial catheter placement.
6. Derive target coordinates and stereotactic arc settings for catheter array in parallel distribution.
7. Individual catheter placement.
    a. Set arc coordinates.
    b. Set target check on phantom base.
    c. Check depth arc angle settings to target.
    d. Following $\frac{1}{4}$ inch scalp incision $\frac{1}{4}$ twist drill calvarial perforation.
    e. Suture silastic cuff to scalp at incision.
    f. Introduce catheter through silastic cuff to target point.
    g. Apply aron alfa acrylic seal (catheter to cuff).
    h. Apply steri-strip marker to catheter cuff margin.
8. Following completion of afterloading with dummy and active ribbon with radiographic monitor, fix ribbon position with large vascular clip at cuff margin.
9. Apply sterile dressing.

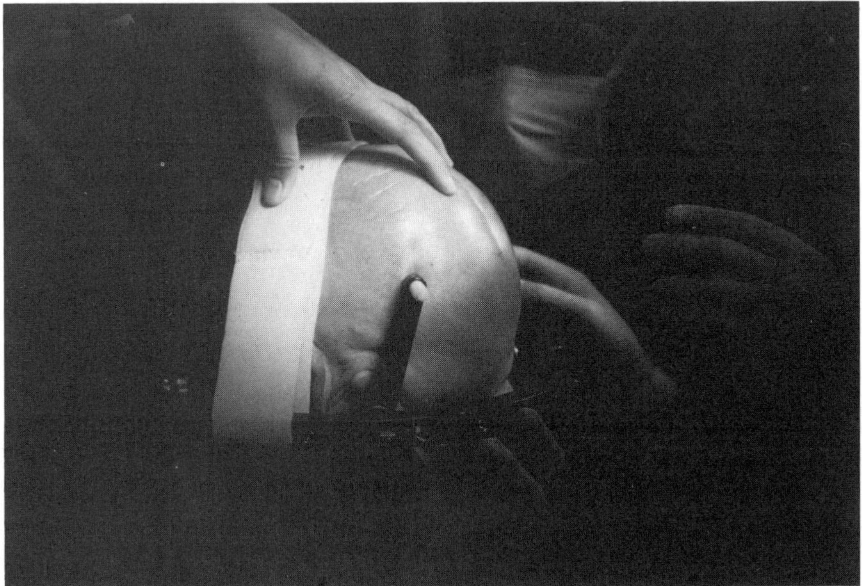

Figure 1. Base ring of stereotactic guidance system is applied with care regarding previous craniotomy flap. Carbon fiber rod in center of field with nylon set screw reduces artifact during scanning process.

Patients undergo application of the unit's base ring in an operating room area (Fig. 1) and are then moved to the scanner unit (Fig. 2) where multiple slice tomography is undertaken with reference to a previously derived data base of three-dimensional computed tomography, magnetic resonance, and digital subtraction venous angiographic imaging. Targets for transcutaneous catheter placement are derived at the scanner console by representatives of neurosurgical, radiation therapy, and radiation physics facilities, and the patient is transferred to the operating room for the remainder of the procedure.[20,21]

Employing x and y plane pixel coordinates of intralesional target points, as well as entry coordinates, three-dimensional trajectory transits are derived for placement of a parallel catheter array on an Epson HX-20 programmable computer.

Appropriate settings are entered into the stereotactic system's arc and each trajectory and target are individually checked extracranially on a phantom base unit (Fig. 3).

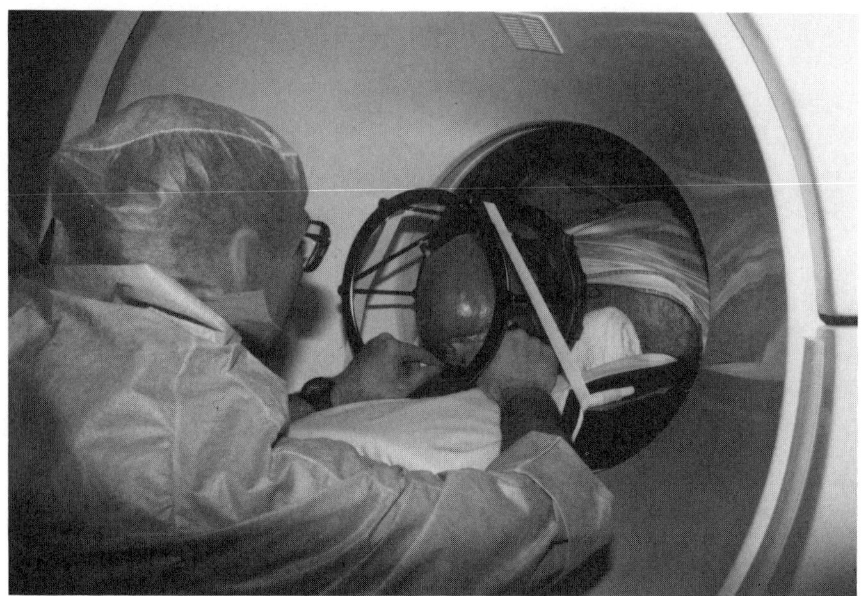

Figure 2. Patient in scanner gantry with localizer unit fixed to base ring for scanning process. Surgeon affixes marker to scalp as an aid in entry point selection in respect to tumor target volume.

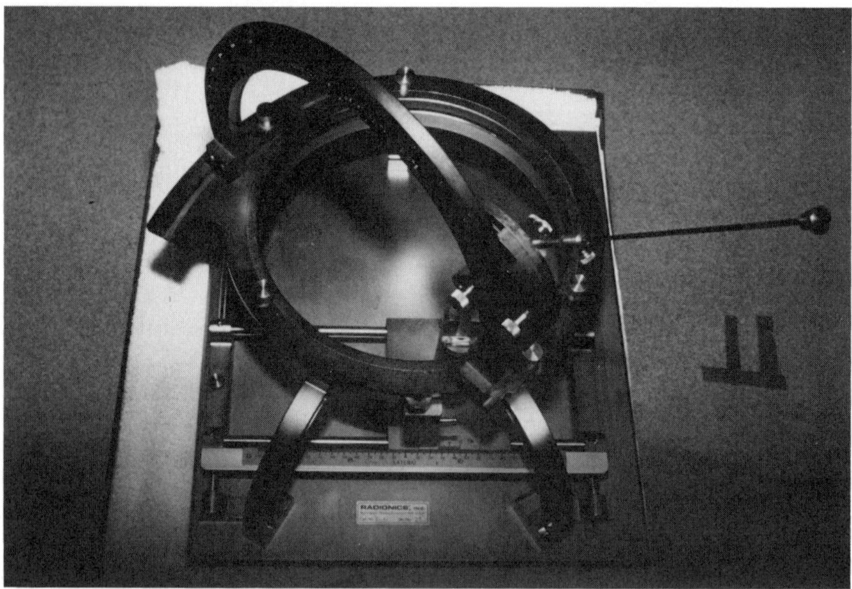

Figure 3. Stereotactic arc guidance system placed on phantom base unit. Phantom extracranially reproduces intracranial target points and allows for check of arc system settings for each catheter placement.

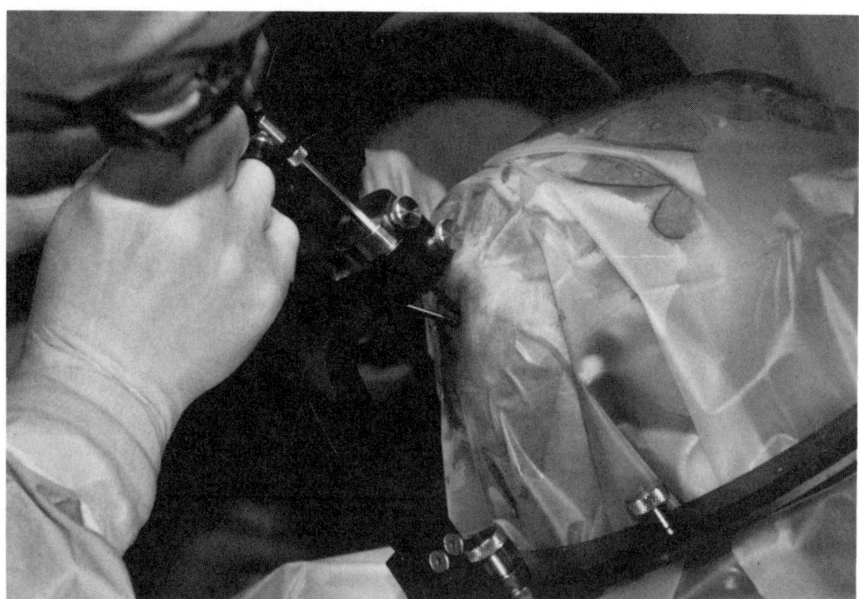

Figure 4. Twist drill calvarial perforation prior to passing catheter to target volume in transcutaneous technique. Note that drill is set in a rigid bushing in direct line of transist to target.

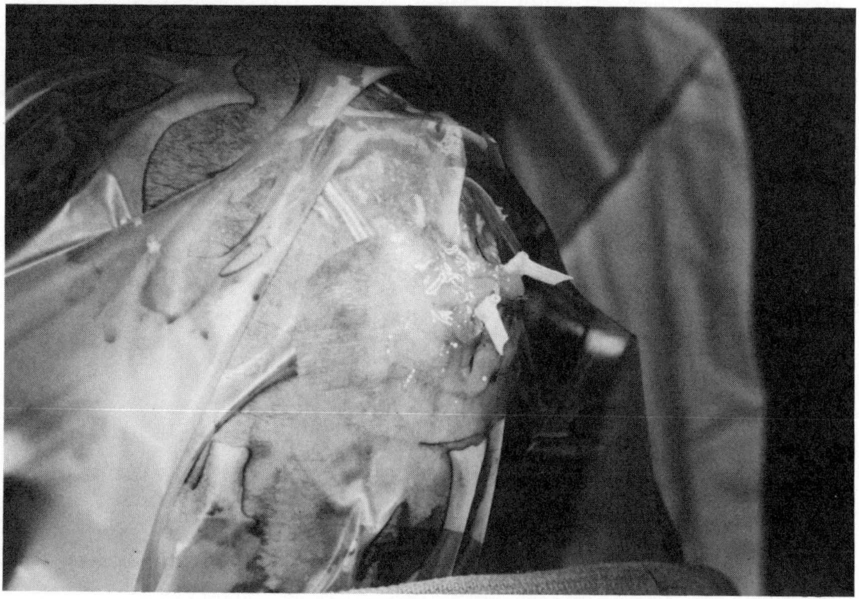

Figure 5. Two catheter arrays completed with silastic cuff sutured to scalp for stability. Catheter structures are covered by layer of antibiotic ointment.

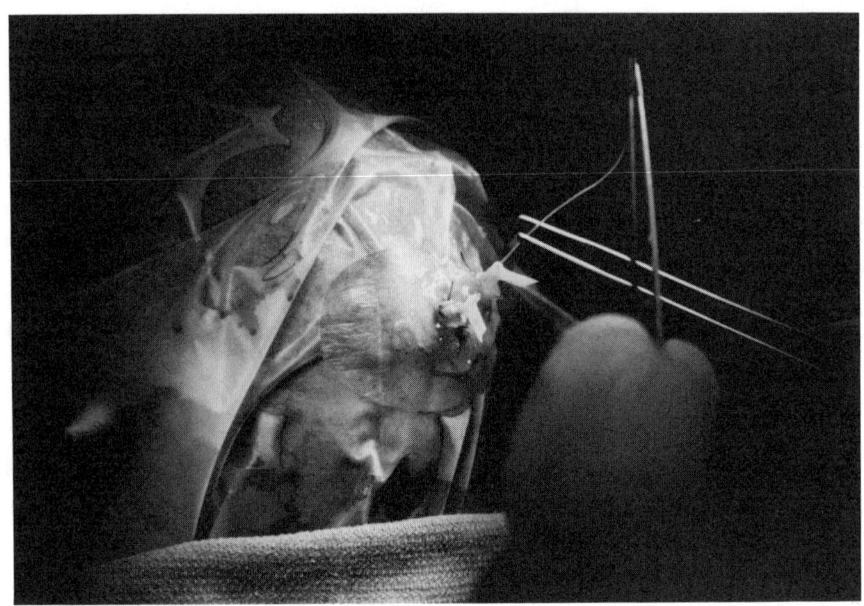

Figure 6. Catheters are afterloaded with ribbons of radionuclide.

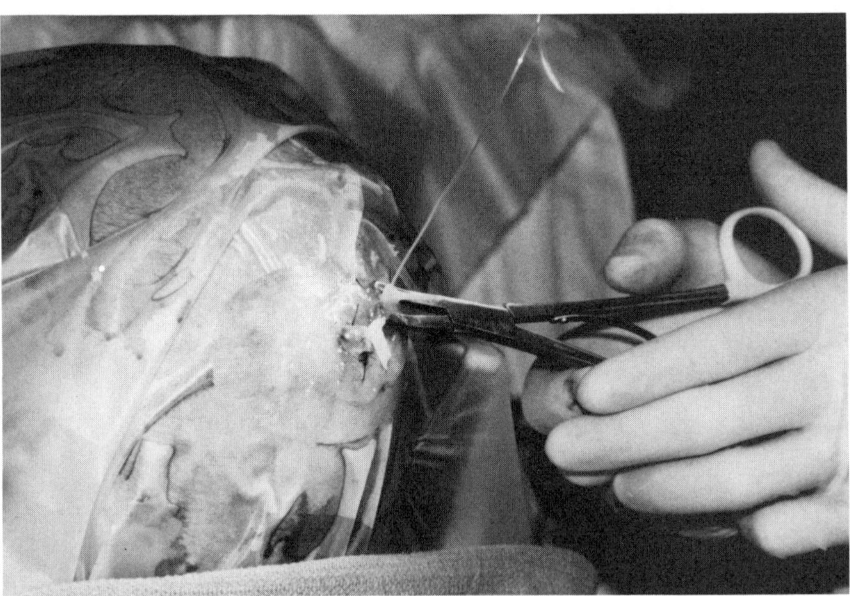

Figure 7. Cuff, catheter, ribbon complex is fixed securely as a single unit with a large vascular clip.

Silastic catheters specially designed for afterloading with iridium-192 sources are transcutaneously introduced through $\frac{1}{4}$ inch twist drill perforations made along trajectory lines in the arc system's rigid bushing holder (Fig. 4). Depending on the requirements of the procedure, one to seven catheters have been introduced under local standby anesthesia with the patient's full cooperation and response. Following placement of the multiple catheter array, afterloading is completed in the operating room and the catheter source ribbon complex is secured with a vascular clip prior to dressing and radiographic assessment of source placement (Figs. 5–10).

At dose schedules of 40–55 rads per hour, patients are required to be hospitalized 4 to 6 days for the completion of the individual therapeutic regimen. Catheters and sources are removed at the bedside with single sutures placed at each scalp incision site.

General Methodology

The patients are jointly evaluated for interstitial radiotherapy by a team consisting of: a neurosurgeon, radiation oncologist(s), a

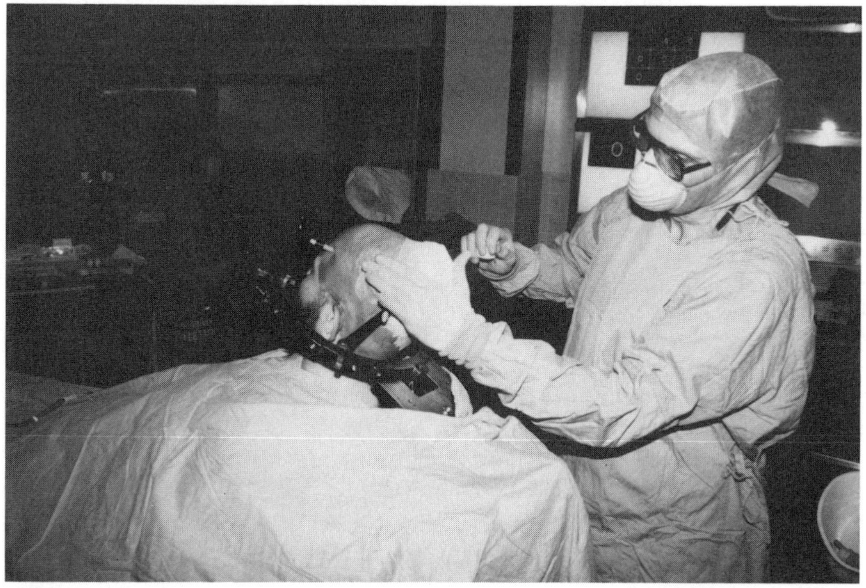

Figure 8. After ribbon and catheters are trimmed, a sterile dressing of fluff is applied that will not be changed until the bedside catheter removal.

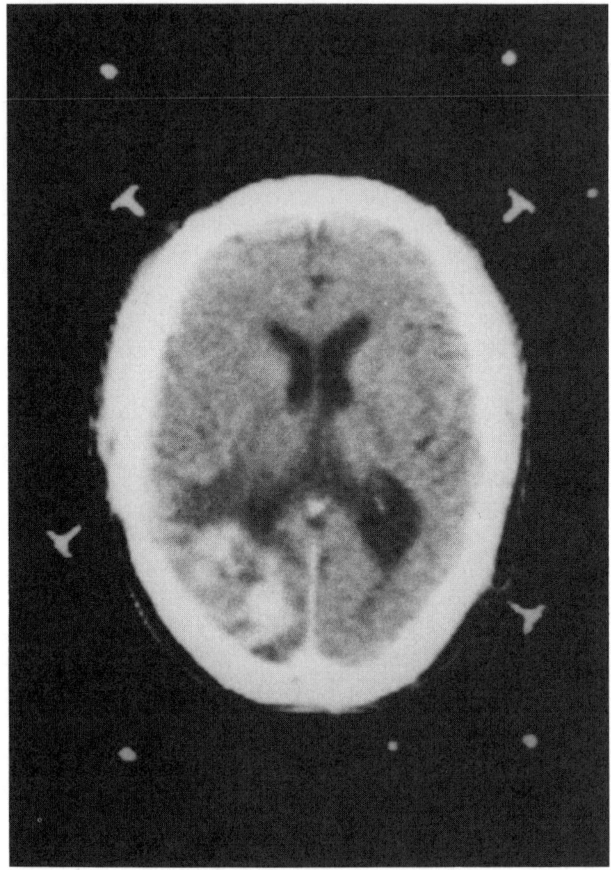

Figure 9. Preoperative CAT scan. Stereotactic base ring in place. Area of increased uptake of contast is target volume.

physicist, and a nurse (Table 5). All patients with recurrent and/or persistent gliomas are considered for this therapy. For those patients seen at USC from the beginning of their treatment, the total dose of external beam radiotherapy was 4,500 cGy given in five fractions per week at a daily dose of 180 cGy with the 4 MV x-ray beam. The volume of interest in the treatment of malignant gliomas prior to 1984 was the whole brain. Due to a lack of tumor recurrence outside of the primary site, and because of concern for neural injury in long surviving patients, much more conservative treatment fields have been

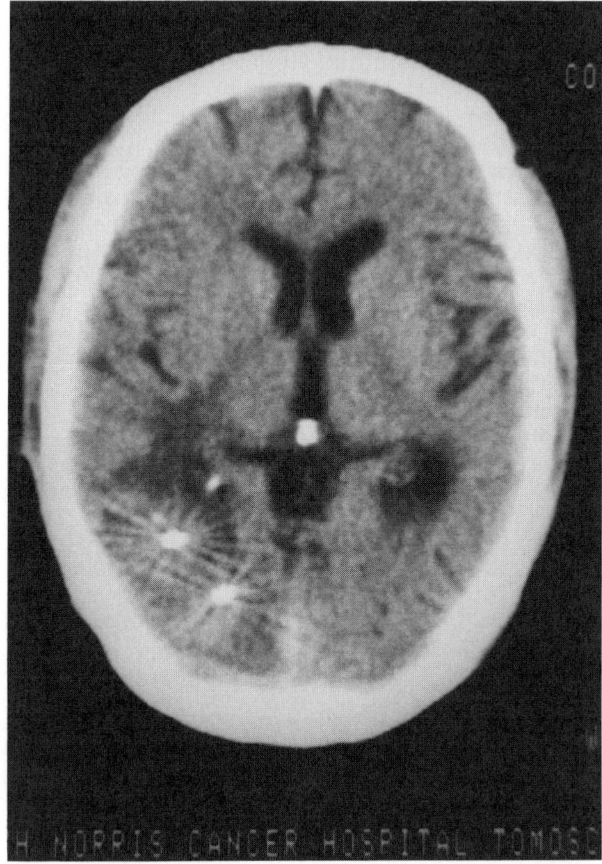

Figure 10. Same patient as Figure 1. Postoperative CAT scan showing right parieto-occipital location of plastic catheters afterloaded with iridium-192.

used. A boost dose was then given to the tumor site to bring the total tumor dose to 5,500 cGy (rads). For those patients with recurrent and/ or persistent gliomas, removable implants of iridium-192 have been used. Total doses given depended on previous radiation received, site of the implant, and the radiation tolerance of surrounding structures. Brachytherapy doses did not exceed 5,500 cGy (rads). No attempt was made to treat suspected tumor extensions which were not demonstrable on imaging studies. The dose rate was 40 to 55 cGy/hr. The reason for this low dose rate was an attempt to minimize the

Table 5

Steps in Interstitial Radiobrachytherapy

1. Obtain three-dimensional computerized tomography, magnetic resonance.
2. Radiation physics simulates by calculation a program for different catheter arrays and patterns in relation to source geometry and intensity.
3. Planning conference to determine appropriate catheter array, neurosurgery, radiation therapy, radiation physics.
4. Admit patient for procedure.
5. Determine target sites in CT scanner.
6. Place silastic catheters.
7. Afterload active source ribbons and radiographically localize.
8. Computerized tomography for final localization.
9. Determine actual isodose curves.
10. Finalize treatment plan.
11. Complete treatment period.
12. Remove catheters and sources.

toxicity of radiotherapy. There is strong laboratory evidence that high dose radiotherapy may result in a greater incidence of serious late complications when compared with a lower dose rate radiotherapy.[47-49] The clinical experience seems to support the laboratory data.[3,8,50,51] It is our belief, in view of the available data on radiation toxicity, that one is required to use meticulous techniques both in brachytherapy and teletherapy to limit the volume of tissue treated. In teletherapy, a daily dose of 180 cGy is preferable and in no clinical situation should it be substantially exceeded unless a long-term survival is not expected. Similarly, we have tried not to exceed in interstitial brachytherapy a dose rate of 55 cGy/hour. In order to promote dose homogeneity through the treated volume, at least two catheters are used for masses greater than 2.5 cm in diameter. In larger tumors, five or more catheters may be required. Due to irregular shape of many lesions, five or more catheters do not give a totally satisfactory dose distribution. Figures 13 and 14 demonstrate these problems. Typical dose distributions in our radioactive implant of the brain are shown in Figures 11, 12, and 14.

In recent years in our clinics, with increasing frequency, we are seeing larger recurrent or persistent malignant gliomas. It is felt that an increase in the dose of radiation is not the answer. The incidence of complications would not be acceptable. We have elected to study

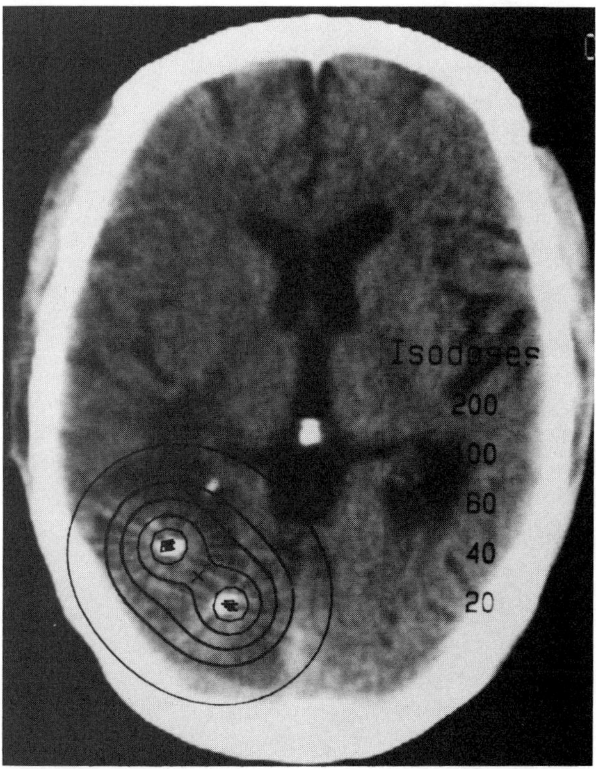

Figure 11. Same patient. Superimposed isodose curves show dose distribution from 20 rads/hr to 200 rads/hr. The 40 rad/hr line was selected as covering the tumor volume.

interstitial microwave hyperthermia in combination with iridium-192 radiation. It is hoped that the hyperthermia and radiotherapy combination can address the problem of control of larger tumors better than interstitial radiotherapy alone. There is strong clinical and laboratory evidence that this can be accomplished.[52,53] Phase I–II clinical pilot study is in a preparatory stage.

Although available data does not permit a statistically valid statement regarding the impact of this form of therapy on malignant gliomas, our current experience indicates a response rate of approximately 70%. Acute complications are rare. Late complications such as radionecrosis are also uncommon. Our data suggest that the tech-

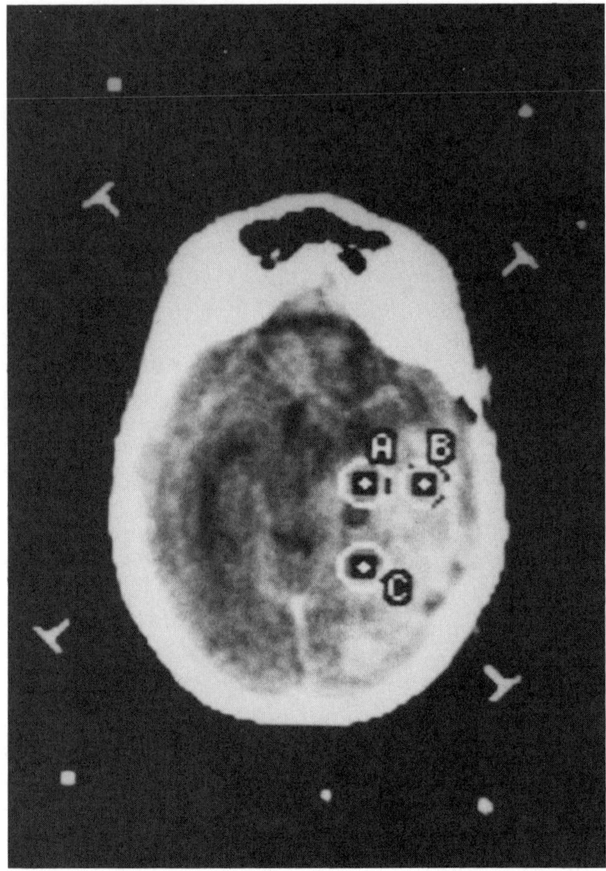

Figure 12. Recurrent glioma of left parietal region. Stereotactic base ring in place. A, B, and C are target sites selected for catheter placement.

nique should be considered in individuals who have the following characteristics.

1. Histology: malignant astrocytoma, or highly selected patients with solitary metastatic disease.

2. Age: less than 55 years.

3. Lesion Size: less than 5 cm maximal linear dimension.

4. Lesion: CT definable.

5. No midline involvement.

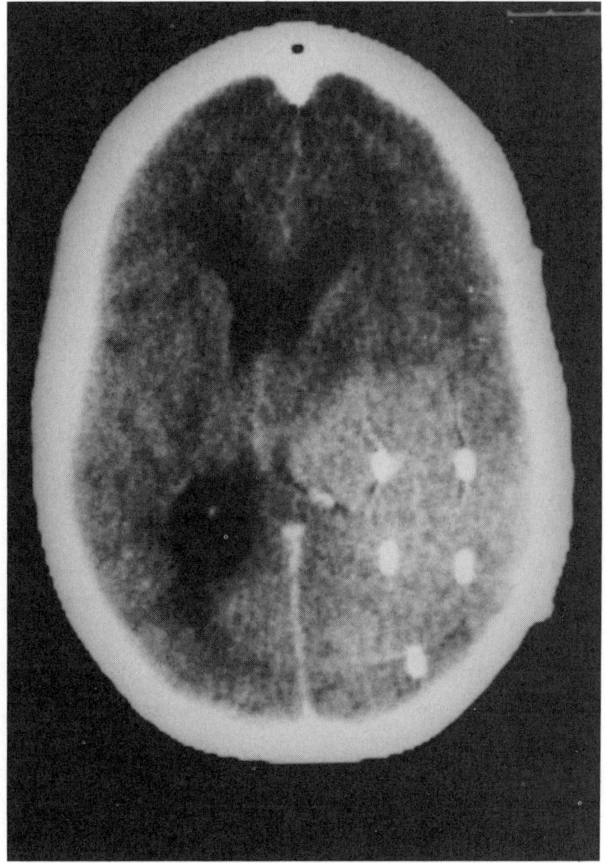

Figure 13. Postoperative CAT scan on same patient as Figure 4 showing all five catheters in position. These have already been afterloaded with iridium-192.

6. Initial performance status greater than 70 on the Karnofsky scale.

In our view, no data base is currently available to predict or define the value of optimal technique in applying this methodology in malignant invasive central nervous system tumors. Until such data are available, the applications of the technique should be confined to major medical centers. Such centers are expected to have appro-

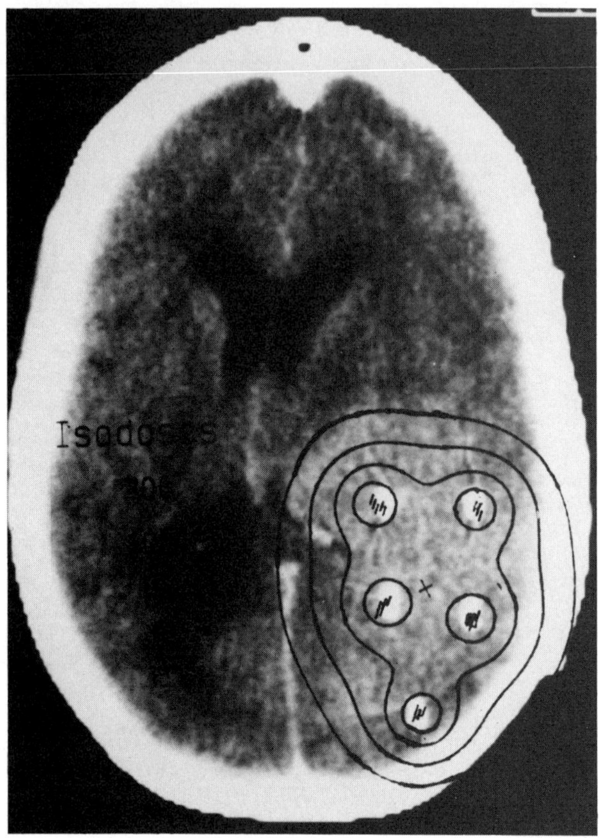

Figure 14. The computer-generated isodose curves are superimposed on the CAT scan. The outermost isodose curve of 40 rads/hr covers most of the tumor volume. There is a poor margin at the antero-medial border. Isodose curves of 60, 80, 100, and 200 rads/hr are also shown.

priate expertise to allow application of this complex technique in a multidisciplinary fashion.

REFERENCES

1. Chang Ch, Horton MB, Schoenfeld D. Comparison of postoperative radiotherapy and combined postoperative radiotherapy and chemotherapy

in the multidisciplinary management of malignant gliomas. A joint Radiation Therapy Oncology Group and Eastern Cooperative Oncology Group study. Cancer 1983; 52:997–1007.
2. American Cancer Society. Cancer statistics. Cancer 1986; 36:16–17.
3. Walker MD, Strike TA, Sheline GE. An analysis of dose-effect relationship in the radiotherapy of malignant gliomas. Int J Radiat Oncol 1979; 5:1725–1731.
4. Salazar OM, Rubin P, Feldstein ML. High dose radiation therapy in the treatment of malignant gliomas. Final report. Int J Radiat Oncol 1979; 5:1733–1740.
5. Walker MD, Alexander E, Hunt WE. Evaluation of BCNU and/or radiotherapy in the treatment of anaplastic gliomas. J Neurosurg 1978; 49:333–343.
6. Salcman M. Survival in glioblastoma. Historical perspective. Neurosurgery 1980; 7:435–439.
7. Lindgren M. On tolerance of brain tissue and sensitivity of brain tumors to irradiation. Acta Radiol 1958; 170:1–73.
8. Marks JE, Baglan RJ, Prassad SC. Cerebral necrosis: Incidence and risk in relation to dose, time, fractionation and volume. Int J Radiat Oncol 1981; 7:243–252.
9. Concannon JP, Kramer S, Berry R. The extent of intracranial gliomata at autopsy and its relationship to technique used in radiation therapy of brain tumors. Am J Roentgenol 1960; 84:99–107.
10. Hochberg FH, Pruitt A. Assumptions in the radiotherapy of glioblastoma. Neurology 1980; 30:907–911.
11. Laramore GE, Griffin TW, Gerdes TW. Fast neutron and mixed (neutron, photon) beam teletherapy for grades III and IV astrocytomas. Cancer 1978; 42:96–103.
12. Catteral M, Bloom HJ, Ash DV. Fast neutrons compared with megavoltage x-rays in the treatment of patients with supratentorial glioblastoma. A controlled pilot study. Int J Radiat Oncol 1980; 6:261–266.
13. Urtasun R, Band P, Chapman JD. Radiation and high dose metronidazole in supratentorial glioblastoma. N Engl J Med 1976; 294:1364–1367.
14. Bleehen, NM, Wiltshire CR, Plowman PN. A randomized study of misonidazole and radiotherapy for grade III and IV cerebral astrocytoma. Br J Cancer 1981; 43:436–442.
15. Simpson WJ, Platt ME. Fractionation study in the treatment of glioblastoma multiforme. Int J Radiat Oncol 1976; 1:639–644.
16. Douglas BG. Superfractionation: Its rationale and anticipated benefits. Int J Radiat Oncol 1982; 8:1143–1153.
17. Shin KH, Muller PJ, George PHS. Superfractionation radiation therapy in the treatment of malignant astrocytoma. Cancer 1983; 52:2040–2043.
18. Scarabin JM, Pecker J, Brucker JM. Stereotaxic exploration in 200 supratentorial brain tumors. Neuroradiology 1978; 16:591–593.
19. Lewander R, Bergstrom M, Boethius J. Stereotaxic computer tomography for biopsy of gliomas. Acta Radiol 1978; 19:867–888.
20. Apuzzo MLJ, Sabshin JK. Computed tomographic guidance stereotaxis in the management of intracranial mass lesions. Neurosurgery 1983; 12:277–285.

21. Apuzzo MLJ, Jepson JH, Luxton G, Little FM. Ionizing and nonionizing radiation treatment of malignant cerebral gliomas; specialized approaches. Clin Neurosurg 1984; 31:470–496.
22. Gutin PH, Phillips TL, Wara WM. Brachytherapy of recurrent malignant brain tumors with removable high activity iodine–125 sources. J Neurosurg 1984; 60:61–68.
23. Mundiger F. Die stereotaktische interstitielle therapie nicht reserzierbarer intrakranieller tumoren mit iridium–192 and jod-125. Strahlentherapie 1981; 76:90–112.
24. Maruyama Y, Chin HW, Young BA. Implantation of brain tumors with CJ–252. Radiology 1984; 152:177–181.
25. Gragoudas ES, Goitein L, Verhey J. Proton beam irradiation. An alternative to enucleatin for intraocular melanomas. Ophthalmology 1980; 87:581.
26. Bush SE, Smith AR, Zink S. Pion radiotherapy at Lampf. Int J Radiat Oncol 1982; 8:2181–2186.
27. Goodman GB, Douglas BG, Jackson SM. Pions, Vancouver. Int J Radiat Oncol 1982; 8:2187–2190.
28. Char DH, Castro JR, Anivey JM. Helium ion charged particle therapy for choroidal melanoma. Ophthalmology 1980; 87:565–570.
29. Castro JR, Quivey JM. Clinical experience and expectation with helium and heavy ion irradiation. Int J Radiat Oncol 1977; 3:127–131.
30. Wheeler KT, Deen DF, Leith JT. Cellular response of rat brain to a therapeutic carbon ion beam. Radiology 1979; 133:755–760.
31. Quimby EH, Goodwin PN, Morgan RH. Natural and artificial radioactivity. In: Physical Foundations of Radiology, New York, Harper and Row 1970; 4:218–240.
32. Johns HE, Cunningham JR. The Physics of Radiology. 4*th* Edition. Springfield, IL, Charles C Thomas, 1983; 456 p.
33. del Regato JA, Currie Sklodowska M. Int J Radiat Oncol 1976; 1:345–353.
34. Paine CH. A modified afterloading technique for small implants using iridium–192 wires for interstitial therapy. Clin Radiol 1977; 28:295–297.
35. Marchese MJ, Hall EJ, Hilaris BS. Clinical, physical and radiobiological aspects of encapsulated iodine–125 in radiation oncology. Endocurie Hypertherm Oncol 1985; 1:67–82.
36. Marchese MJ, Nori D, Anderson LL. A versatile permanent planner implant technique utilizing iodine–125 seeds imbedded in gelfoam. Int J Radiat Oncol 1984; 10:747–751.
37. Hall EJ. Radiation dose-rate. A factor of importance in radiobiology and radiotherapy. Br J Radiol 1972;45:81–97.
38. Zeitz L, Kim SH, Kim JH. Determination of relative biological effectiveness (RBE) of soft x-rays. Radiat Res 1977; 70:552–563.
39. Maruyama Y, Feda JM, Beach LJ. A tumor/normal tissue advantage for low dose rate neutron brachytherapy. Int J Radiat Oncol 1983; 9:1715–1721.
40. Maruyama Y. Work in progress: californium–252 brachytherapy plus fractionated irradiation for advanced tonsillar carcinoma. Radiology 1983; 148:247–251.

41. Lommatzsch PK. Treatment of choroidal melanomas with ru-106/rh-106 beta ray applicators. Surv Ophthalmol 1974; 19:85–100.
42. Lommatzsch PK. Radiotherapie der intraokularen tumoren, insbesandere bei arderhautmelanom. Klin Mbl Augenheilkd 1979; 174:948–958.
43. Hall EJ. Radiobiology for the Radiologists, New York, Harper and Row, 1978.
44. Leibel SA, Gutin PH, Phillips TL. Interstitial implantation of high-activity iodine–125 sources for treatment of recurrent malignant brain tumors. Int J Radiat Oncol 1984; 10:144.
45. Rao DV, Simpson JR, Marchosky JA. Afterloading interstitial irradiation for CNS tumors. Int J Radiat Oncol 1984; 10:144.
46. Heilbrun MP, Roberts TS, Apuzzo MLJ, Wells TH, Sabshin JK. Preliminary experience with Brown-Roberts-Wells computerized tomographic stereotaxic guidance system. J Neurosurg 1983; 59:217–222.
47. Withers RH. Biologic basis for altered fractionation schemes. Cancer 1985; 55:2086–2095.
48. Van der Vogel AJ. Radiation tolerance of the rat spinal cord. Time dose relationship. Radiology 1977; 122:505–509.
49. Leith JT, DeWyngaert JK, Glicksman AS. Radiation myelopathy in the rat. An interpretation of dose-effect relationship. (In press)
50. Sheline GE. Radiation therapy of brain tumor. Cancer 1977; 39:873–881.
51. Hindo WA, DeTrana FA, Lee MS. Large dose increment irradiation in treatment of cerebral metastasis. Cancer 1970; 26:138–141.
52. Winter A, Laing J, Pagliane R. Microwave hyperthermia for brain tumors. Neurosurgery 1985; 17:387–399.
53. Salcman M, Samaras GM. Hyperthermia for brain tumors: biophysical rationale. Neurosurgery 1981; 9:327–335.

15

Clinical Factors Affecting Brain Tumor Chemotherapy

Patrick A. LaSala

Introduction

The discussion of chemotherapy for brain tumors will be restricted to malignant gliomas—anaplastic astrocytoma and glioblastoma multiforme. Their combined incidence is approximately 3/100,000 persons per year or 6,600 new cases in the United States.[1-3] Standard therapy includes an operative resection to reduce tumor burden followed by external beam radiation with 5,500 to 6,000 rads delivered in 30 to 35 fractions, with five treatments given per week. Chemotherapy is usually employed either as an adjuvant therapy along with or following radiation therapy. Alternatively, chemotherapy is used in an attempt to control tumor recurrence. The drug is administered when there is clinical evidence of tumor regrowth and usually after previous tumor surgery, radiotherapy and possibly chemotherapy. Malignant gliomas usually recur 8 to 11 months after the initial treatment[4-7] with a median survival from the time of recurrence of approximately 35 weeks.[8-10]

A comprehensive review of chemotherapy for brain tumors was carried out in 1980 by Edwards[11] and more recently by Kornblith.[29] In the intervening time, several single drug trials for recurrent tumor have been carried out. Additionally, there have been a series of multidrug treatment studies published, which will be reviewed. Over this time frame, there has not been a major chemotherapeutic break-

From: Kornblith PL, Walker MD (editors). Advances in Neuro-Oncology. Futura Publishing Company, Inc., Mount Kisco, NY, © 1988.

through with more efficacious drugs or a curative regimen. There has been, however, an increase in the understanding of the variables that effect brain tumors. The studies reviewed pay careful attention to such factors as age and neurological status at diagnosis and stage of disease evaluated by computed tomography. In recent years, in vitro chemosensitivity techniques, initially designed to study drug resistance, are now taking on a greater role in drug screening. In vitro assays potentially predict the clinical response to specific drugs and this may be a valuable tool in drug selection and individualized therapy.

Clinical Factors Affecting Brain Tumor Chemotherapy

Many variables, other than drug efficacy, effect the outcome of patients receiving chemotherapy for brain tumors. The first group includes age, neurologic status and extent of disease at diagnosis.[12] A poorer prognosis exists in the elderly and there is less of a response to chemotherapy. Neurological status and disease stage are particularly important determinants prior to chemotherapy. Advanced neurologic signs such as obtundation are not associated with a good response to chemotherapy. Large tumors such as bilateral tumors are difficult to debulk and provide little time for chemotherapeutic agents to show an effect. These factors are now considered before entry into clincal trials.

Chemotherapeutic response rates are relatively low for the patient population with brain tumors. If a single agent shows a small response, synergistic agents are likely to be necessary to achieve an adequate response rate for inclusion in a phase III trial. Preselection of patients who are likely to be responsive to a particular drug would achieve the same goal of increasing the response rate in a trial group. This concept is being tested at the cellular level with in vitro chemosensitivity techniques.[13–15] These techniques and their implications will be described in more detail below and in the chapter by Darling and Thomas.

In addition to clinical factors effecting chemotherapeutic efficacy, important biologic variables are active. Among them are the blood-brain barrier, the tumoral microenvironment, cell-cycle kinetics, cellular heterogeneity and the development of drug resistence. The blood-brain barrier is located in the endothelium of the majority of cerebral capillaries. There is pentalaminar fusion of adjacent cell membranes which form a relatively continuous zone obstructing the passage of substances having a molecular weight greater than 200 daltons. Drugs which are nonionized or have readily reversible ionization equations pass through the blood-brain barrier. High lipid-solubility of a drug will also result in passage across the blood-brain barrier. Capillary endothelial cells within tumor tissue have been shown to have abnormal or discontinous tight junctions. Enhanced computerized tomographic scans depend upon BBB breakdown for entry of large protein molecules to differentiate tumor tissue from the surrounding normal brain. While this suggests chemical or drug access to the tumor tissue, there is evidence reported of at least partial preservation of a blood-tumor barrier in the proliferating zones of the tumor.[16] This has resulted in methods to modify the BBB (BTB) with modification agents such as mannitol to increase the availability of agents to the tumor.[17]

Histological preparations of glioblastoma multiforme often show areas of necrosis in the center portion of the tumor with an active proliferating edge of tumor which is well vascularized. This is adjacent to an outer zone which interfaces with the surrounding brain. Each of these areas is considered to have a distinct pharmocologic environment with tumor cells in very different proportions and with different kinetic parameters. Overall, the environment differs in that there is no lymphatic system and, therefore, drugs and their metabolites are handled differently in the extracellular space than in other regions. Normal glia do not replicate in adults and older children. Supporting structures along with the cerebral vasculature turnover at a relatively slow rate. Malignant brain tumor cells by their nature replicate. High-grade gliomas have a small portion of the cells actively replicating. Cell kinetics have been investigated and a wide distribution of kinetic parameters identified.[18-24] Labeling indexes on the order of 0% to 15% have been reported. Low grade and intermediate gliomas have lower labeling indices while glioblastoma has LI's in the higher range.[20] The growth fraction has been calculated to be 0.30 and variable. The cell cycle time is estimated to be 70 to 80 hours with a computed cell loss of 85%. Clinical doubling time is therefore approximately 6 to 8 weeks. Cell kinetics have obvious important implications for chemotherapeutic planning.[18] Heterogeneity of cells within a tumor and between tumors[25,26] represents a difficult problem for treatment with chemotherapeutic agent. Shapiro[25,27] has demonstrated that chromosome numbers vary in cloned tumor cells from near diploid to hyperdiploid. They demonstrated that in general, cell populations with near diploid karyotypes are drug resistant while the hyperdiploid karyotypes are sensitive.[28,73]

Specific Chemotherapy Agents

Nitrosoureas

Of the cytotoxic agents, the chloroethyl nitrosoureas are the most commonly used chemotherapeutic agents for brain tumors. As a group, the nitrosoureas are considered highly lipid-soluble and essentially nonionized and readily cross the blood-brain barrier. They degrade in the bloodstream into two compounds, one with carbamylation activity and the other into an alkylating agent. The basic nitrosourea moiety can be modified to alter the solubility properties, the amount of carbamylation or alkylating activity and toxicity. Kornblith[29] reviewed clinical series utilizing carmustine (BCNU) in a controlled setting. In these series, BCNU was employed following surgery and radiation therapy (see Table 1).[30–34] Median survival time improved to between 51 and 73 weeks when compared to control patients receiving irradiation alone (median survival time approximately 35 weeks). Other studies found BCNU to have only an equivocal effect or no effect at all.[33]

Attempts have been made to improve the therapeutic index of BCNU. Ultra-high doses of BCNU with total bone marrow destruction and autologous bone marrow rescue have been used.[35] The bone marrow is the dose-limiting organ for delivery of BCNU and therefore bone marrow rescue will allow increased drug concentrations to be achieved. Hochberg et al.[36] treated 11 patients with recurrent malignant glioma. A single high dose BCNU regimen was used with doses ranging from 600 to 1,400 mg/sg m. The median survival time for this group was 7 months. The authors demonstrated that single high dose BCNU with autologous bone marrow transplantation could be safely performed. Enhanced therapeutic efficacy over standard intravenous therapy could not be determined. Intra-arterial administration of BCNU and other chemotherapeutic agents represents another method of delivery, providing higher concentration of the drugs, to the tumor area. While indeed a higher concentration of drug is achievable, there is great concern regarding toxicity. Retinal damage is commonly observed when BCNU is given below the level of the ophthalmic artery. Several authors[37,38] have reported neurotoxicity with superselective injections which were devised to overcome the retinal problems. Overall the method has several advantages and a series of cooperative studies are underway to assess the value of the currently available agents delivered by this route.

BCNU remains the most effective single agent. Its efficacy is limited by cumulative myelosuppression, hepatic dysfunction, and increasing incidence of pulmonary fibrosis when a total cumulative dose of more than 1,450 mg is administered.

The question of timing the administration of BCNU is not yet resolved. In most cases, radiotherapy follows immediately after surgery and chemotherapy is withheld until radiotherapy is completed. An argument can be made for instituting chemotherapy earlier. The loss of 6 weeks in a condition with short survival times may reduce the drug's overall effect. Vascular changes associated with radiation therapy may reduce penetration of the drug, rendering it less effective. Factors mitigating for later use are the observation that BCNU seems to be more effective against recurrent tumor and therefore may be better reserved for recurrences than traditional surgery and radiotherapy as the first arms of the treatment plan. Currently, the most common approach is to use irradiation and BCNU as a combined modality following surgery. Further information is needed to resolve the issue of timing BCNU therapy.

Other Nitrosoureas

Lomustine (CCNU) has been compared to several different agents including others in the nitrosourea group.[31,33,39–43] CCNU has been found to be relatively ineffective when used alone or in combination with other drugs or when compared to radiotherapy alone. With radiotherapy, CCNU is approximately as effective as BCNU and radiotherapy, albeit in smaller series. The radiosensitizer misonidazole was used as a potentiator for CCNU with little effect.[44] Pompili et al.[45] undertook a retrospective analysis of seven patients, four with basal ganglia tumors and three with brainstem tumors. Tumor diagnosis was made radiographically and the only therapy given was CCNU at a dosage of 130 mg/sq m every 6 weeks. There was no increase in survival when compared to patients with similar lesions receiving methylprednisolone alone. The dose-limiting side effect of CCNU is myelosuppression with thrombocytopenia representing the greatest hazard. Nephrotoxicity has been reported.[46] When compared to BCNU, CCNU has less favorable pharmacokinetics and absorption characteristics. Its oral administration, however, makes out-patient therapy feasible which actually increases compliance in some cases. In terms of fully established efficacy, only BCNU has withstood the scrutiny of a phase III trial.

1-(2-Chloroethyl)-3-(2,6-dioxo-3-piperidyl)-1-nitrosourea (PCNU) is considered active against brain tumors. It shares similar toxicity characteristics with other nitrosoureas, mainly cumulative delayed myelosuppression. PCNU has been compared to azinidinylbenzoquinone (AZQ) in a controlled study[47] and found to be significantly better than AZQ. To date, it has not been shown to be either more effective or less toxic than BCNU.

Semustine (MeCCNU) is an oral agent with extreme lipid-solubility. It was included in a large cooperative study[48] where MeCCNU was used following surgery with and without radiation therapy and was compared to radiation therapy alone, and radiation therapy and BCNU. MeCCNU was not effective alone and did not enhance the effects of radiation. There is no improvement in the therapeutic index with this agent, and it is not actively used.

(1-4-Amino-2-methyl-5-pyrimidinyl)-methyl-3-(2-chloroethyl)-3-nitrosourea (ACNU) has been used in high dose with bone marrow rescue.[49] Additionally, it has been used in a combination study with fluorouracil.[50] It has been shown to be active and warrants further study. BCNU remains the most effective nitrosourea against brain tumors. The other nitrosoureas have not proven to be more effective or less toxic. Therefore, attention is now being directed towards optimizing delivery of BCNU. Efforts include changes in dosage schedule and direct delivery of BCNU to the tumor bed.

Procarbazine

Procarbazine (Matulan or Natulan) is an alkylating agent which requires hepatic metabolic activation. It has been studied as a single agent[51] and in combination with other drugs.[52,53] In the single-agent trial,[51] the mean survival time of patients following radiation therapy was 47 weeks. This compares favorably with the 50-week mean survival for the reference group treated with BCNU. Procarbazine has been utilized in combination with CCNU and vincristine[52,53] and no advantage was achieved. Toxicity includes nausea and vomiting.

Cis-platin

Cis-platin (CDDP, Platinol) is a heavy metal compound that inhibits DNA synthesis. It has been evaluated in recurrent brain tumors and found to be active, suggesting further studies of this agent are needed.[54,64] Side effects from administration of cis-platin include gastrointestinal disturbance with vomiting and ototoxicity. Its role in the treatment of brain tumors in the pediatric age group is still being defined.

Aziridinylbenzoquinone

AZQ, an alkylating agent, has been evaluated in phase I and II trials.[47-55] This agent appears to be effective in at least some patients with malignant glioma and, therefore, requires more study. AZQ therapy results in a partial response rate of 20% and may be useful in a selected patient population. In the above studies, AZQ is well tolerated. The major toxicity is delayed progressive thrombocytopenia.

Chemical Modifiers of Radiation

Radiosensitizers

While not chemotherapeutic agents per se, radiosensitizers modify the effects of radiation therapy. Two general groups of drugs have been used as radiosensitizers, the halogenated pyrimidines and nitroimidazole.

Pyrimidines

Bromodeoxyuridine (BUdR) and iododeoxyuridine (IUdR) are pyrimidines that are incorporated into DNA in place of thymidine making the cells substantially more sensitive to radiation in vitro.[65] BUdR and IUdR are taken up nonselectivity by dividing cells. The rationale for their use in brain tumors is based on cell populations within glioblastomas dividing more rapidly than surrounding cells. Kinsella et al.[66] have demonstrated nuclear uptake of the halogenated pyrimidines in tumor tissue with an anti-BUdR monoclonal antibody technique. Nuclear uptake ranges from 50–70%. Systemic toxicity with this form of therapy includes dose-limiting thrombocytopenia and dry desquamation of the palms and soles. Local toxicity includes moist desquamation of skin in the radiated area. Clinical trials are thus far limited to phase I and II studies and therefore definitive assessment of efficacy is not yet possible. The concept and approach remains promising.

Nitroimidazole

Misonidazole is a synthetic nitroimidazole with radiosensitizing properties. It has been evaluated in extensive controlled trials.[67–71] Various radiotherapeutic treatment fractions have been coordinated with peak plasma levels of misonidazole. No therapeutic gain over radiation therapy alone was demonstrated and survival is not increased. No increase in survival was demonstrated when misonidazole was added to 6,000 rads of radiotherapy followed by BCNU.[72]

In Vitro Chemosensitivity Testing

In addition to the work presented by Darling and Thomas in their chapter, we felt it worthwhile to provide some additional information on the potentially valuable technique of in vitro chemosensitivity testing. In vitro chemosensitivity testing was designed initially to study drug resistance, which remains a difficult problem.[73,74] In vitro assay techniques are currently being tested to predict clinical response to a given chemotherapeutic agent and to aid in selecting specific regimines. In vitro testing is based first on being able to explant glioma tissue and facilitate the tissues growth in culture. Permanent cell lines can be obtained in some cases.

An important consideration in tissue culture technique and chemosensitivity testing is the selection of nutrient medium. A variety of formulas are available for use. The author's laboratory uses Ham's F12 medium mixed with Dulbecco's modified essential medium. In general, this media requires supplementation with fetal calf serum to insure adequate growth of tumor cells. The addition of serum, however, adds variables to in vitro study design which can possibly be avoided or reduced by use of a chemically defined medium. Morrison[75] reported the use of a chemically defined medium to facilitate the growth of purified astrocytes. The above medium is supplemented with a combination of hormones and growth factors which promote attachment and growth of cells. Our chemically defined medium includes hydrocortisone, insulin, biotin, and sodium selinite.

In Vitro Assay

In vitro drug assays can be used to select prospective therapy and to screen new agents as they become available. In vitro systems are useful for assessing the effectiveness of combination therapy and in determining appropriate drug concentrations. There are several inherent difficulties in applying the results of tissue culture chemosensitivity. First, there are several techniques, including colony forming assay, microcytotoxicity assay, organ culture[76,77] and MTS assay,[78–80] sister chromatid exchange assay (SCE), and radiolabeled precursor inhibition assay. These techniques measure different parameters and end-points and therefore internal comparison is not possible. Second, the pharmokokinetics of drug treatment are complex and cannot be completely duplicated in an in vitro model. Most chemotherapeutic regimens include a short infusion of the drug with peak plasma levels occurring for less than 1 hour. Most in vitro assays use a 1 hour drug exposure. Plasma or serum concentration may not reflect tumor tissue concentration adding another variable to drug concentration in vitro. As a result, a dose-response curve is generated by testing dosages around the expected dose used clinically.

In vitro assay systems do not take into account such factors as the blood-brain barrier, microcirculation, and microenvironment of tumors. These factors raise questions about drug penetrance and exposure. The in vitro model allows for a uniform exposure of drug to tumor cells. In vitro pharmokokinetics are dependent upon factors such as drug concentration, temperature, pH, serum binding, and binding to plastic.

Microcytotoxicity Assay

For this assay, tumor cells are plated in small wells after exposure to a test drug.[81,82] Drug exposure is usually 1 hour. After an interval, usually 24 hours, the cells are stained and counted. This method then provides a dose-cell survival curve. The method's main advantages is short processing time. The method does not allow differentiation between cell kill and inhibition of cell growth.

Colony-Forming Assay

In this assay developed by Rosenblum,[83,84] single cells are disaggregated from a tumor biopsy. Cells are exposed to various drug concentrations for a defined interval, usually 1 to 2 hours, and then the cells are plated at a known concentration either into soft agar or as a monolayer for 2 to 4 weeks. At that point, the number of cells forming colonies can be counted providing a colony-forming efficiency (CFE). The number and size of colonies can be compared to untreated cells. Results are expressed as the concentration of drug that reduces colony formation by 50%. There are technical pitfalls with this technique.[85,86] The process of disaggregation may result in cell clumps as well as single cells. Cell clumps form colonies more readily than single cells which would directly effect the colony-forming efficiency. When growing colonies from a malignant glioma, colonies can form from normal astrocytes which may be obtained from the leading edge of the tumor. Morphological features alone will not differentiate the two cell types.[87] Growth of clones in nude mice may help to make the distinction. Other problems include a low CFE for brain tumors ranging from 0.001% to 2%.[84] This can be improved substantially by allowing a few passages in culture before drug testing.[88,89] Culture conditions must be optimal for adequate growth in monolayer or agar. The media used is not well standardized and often contains serum, which as discussed above, makes analysis complex. The use of a chemically defined medium may obviate some of these problems. Despite these problems, the technique is reproducible and directly measures cell survival and proliferation.

Radioisotope Based Inhibition Assay

This method measures the inhibition of radiolabeled precursors of DNA, RNA, or protein synthesis. The technique is dependent on cell synthesis. Cells with long cycling times may not be suitable for this assay. A cell suspension is exposed to a drug for a set time. Recovery is allowed to occur, up to 10 days and then the cells are exposed to the precursor and the radioactivity is counted. The assay is straightforward and less time-consuming than other techniques. However, the assay measures only inhibition of cell synthesis and therefore discloses no information about cell death. Cellular inhibition may be temporary, and depending on recovery time, the test may yield false-positive results.[90] False-negative results are possible if cell division proceeds for a time before cell death. The technique may not be useful for each class of chemotherapeutic agent due to differences in mechanism of drug action. Several investigations have demonstrated a reasonable correlation of this technique with the colony formation assay.[91–93]

The DNA alkaline elution assay[94] and the sister chromatid exchange assay[95] are more recently developed assay systems. Their role in chemosensitivity testing is not yet fully established.

Clinical Chemosensitivity

Several reports are available comparing clinical response to a specific drug and in vitro chemosensitivity using one of the methods outlined above. Kornblith et al.[81,96] studied 58 patients with malignant gliomas, using the microcytotoxicity assay and testing BCNU. Study criteria required patients to have had at least two doses of nitrosourea and to have had two or more CT scan examinations. Fourteen patients met these criteria. Tumor size increased in all five patients whose tumor did not respond to BCNU in the microcytotoxity assay. Six of the nine patients whose tumor in culture showed significant sensitivity to BCNU showed a clear decrease in tumor size over periods ranging from 17 to 48 months. In this study based on the microcytotoxicity assay, resistance to BCNU was correctly predicted in each case and there was a 67% correct prediction of sensitivity.

Rosenblum and Gerosa[97] reported on 71 patients with malignant gliomas. They utilized the colony-forming assay and tested BCNU. Ninety percent of the patients were tested and 48% were sensitive to BCNU. Twenty-four patients were evaluated for clinical response. Five of 11 patients sensitive to BCNU in culture showed a clinical response. Thirteen tumors resistant in vitro showed no clinical response.

Summary

In summary, there are at present a limited number of options in chemotherapy of human brain tumors. Only BCNU has passed successfully through phase III trials with consistent success. Other secondary useful agents are primarily in the nitrosourea group and include procarbazine, CCNU, and PCNU. Cis-platin and AZQ have a relatively low response rate, but may be useful in some patients.

Our understanding of the variables and limitations of chemotherapy as it applies to the therapy of malignant gliomas has clearly advanced rapidly. What is essential now is to develop therapeutic programs custom designed to fit the special requirement of efficacy. The heterogeneity, resistance and access issues certainly complicate the successful treatment strategies.

Among the most promising avenues of study which now appears ready to produce useful data for improving clinical chemotherapy is the approach of in vitro chemosensitivity testing. This modality described by David Thomas in detail in his chapter in this book and reviewed above offers the potential of guiding us in the use of currently available agents and helping in the development of new agents.

Alternate routes of delivery such as intraarterial therapy have the critical advantages but have so far lacked a sufficient therapeutic index to play a major role.

Clearly we need better agents to make chemotherapy a more valuable part of the therapeutic armamentarium. Through our greater understanding of basic mechanisms and with the use of in vitro assays, we may be able to proceed more rapidly in this quest.

REFERENCES

1. Harch GR, Levin VA, Gutin PH, et al. Reoperation for recurrent glioblastoma and anaplastic astrocytoma. Neurosurgery 1987; 5:615–620.
2. Cobb CA, Youmans JR. Glial and neuronal tumors of the brain in adults. In: Youmans JR (ed). Neurological Surgery, Philadelphia, WB Saunders, 1982; p 2762.
3. Liebermann AN, Ransohoff J. Treatment of primary brain tumors. Med Clin North Am 1979; 63:835–848.
4. Levin VA, Wilson CB, Davis R, Wara WM, Pischer TL, Irwin L. A phase III comparison of BCNU, hydroxyurea, and radiation therapy for treatment of primary malignant gliomas. J Neurosurg 1979; 51:526–532.
5. Gerosa MA, DiStefano E, Olivi A. VM–26 monochemotherapy trail in the treatment of recurrent supratentorial gliomas: Preliminary report. Surg Neurol 1981; 15:128–134.
6. European Organization for Research on Treatment of Cancer (EORTC) Brain Tumor Group. Evaluation of CCNU, VM–26 plus CCNU, and procarbazine in supratentorial brain gliomas: Final evaluation of a randomized study. J Neurosurg 1981; 55:27–31.

7. Eagan RT, Creagan ET, Biseal HF, Layton DD, Grover RV, et al. RC. Phase II study of dianhydrogalactitol based combination chemotherapy for recurrent brain tumors. Oncology 1981; 38:4–6.

8. Eagan RT, Dinapoli RP, Herman RC, Groover RV, Layton DD, et al. Combination carmustine (BCNU) and dianhydrogalactitol in the treatment of primary brain tumor recurring after irradiation. Cancer Treat Rep 1982; 66:1647–1649.

9. Eagan RT, Scott M. Evaluation of prognostic factors in chemotherapy of recurrent brain tumors. J Clin Oncol 1983; 1:38–44.

10. Haid M, Khandekar JD, Christ M, Johnson CM, Miller SJ, et al. Oxyridinylbenzoquinone in recurrent, progressive gliomas of the central nervous system: A phase II study by the Illinois Cancer Council, Cancer 1985; 56:1311–1315.

11. Edwards MS, Levin VA, Wilson CB. Brain tumor chemotherapy: an evaluation of agents in current use for phase II and III trials. Cancer Treat Rep 1980; 64:1179–1205.

12. Gethan EA, Walker MD. Prognostic factors for patients with brain tumors. Natl Cancer Inst Monogr 1977; 46:189–195.

13. Thomas DGT, Darling JL, Paul EA, et al. Assay of anticancer drugs in tissue culture: relationship of relapse free interval (RFI) and in vitro chemosensitivity in patients with malignant cerebral glioma. Br J Cancer 1985; 51:525–532.

14. Rosenblum ML, Gerosa MA, Wilson CB, et al. Stem-cell studies of human malignant brain tumors. Part 1: Development of the stem-cell assay and its potential. J Neurosurg 1983; 58:170–176.

15. Kornblith PL, Smith BH, Leonard LA. Response of cultured human brain tumors to nitrosoureas: correlation with clinical data. Cancer 1981; 47:255–265.

16. Front D, Israel O, Kohn S, Nir I. The blood-tissue barrier of human brain tumors. Correlation of scintigraphic and ultrastructural findings. J Nucl Med 1984; 25:461.

17. Heimberger K, Samec P, Binder H, et al. Blood brain barrier disruption interventional neuroradiology in brain tumor therapy. Ann Radiol (Paris) 1986; 29(2):230–232.

18. Hoshino T. Therapeutic implications of brain tumor cell kinetics. Natl Cancer Inst Monogr 1977; 46:29–35.

19. Hoshino T. A commentary on biology and growth kinetics of low-grade and high-grade gliomas. J Neurosurg 1984; 61:895–900.

20. Hoshino T. Barker M, Wilson CB, et al. Cell kinetics of human gliomas. J Neurosurg 1972; 37:15–26.

21. Hoshino T. Townsend JJ, Muraoka I, et al. An autoradiographic study of human gliomas: growth kinetics of anaplastic astrocytoma and glioblastoma multiforme. Brain 1980; 103:967–984.

22. Hoshino T. Wilson CB. Cell kinetic analyses of human malignant brain tumors (gliomas). Cancer 1979; 44:956–962.

23. Hoshino T, Wilson CB. Review of basic concepts of cell kinetics as applied to brain tumors. J Neurosurg 1975; 42:123–131.

24. Hoshino T, Wilson CB, Rosenblum ML, et al. Chemotherapeutic impli-

cations of growth fraction and cell cycle time in glioblastomas. J Neurosurg 1975; 43:127–135.

25. Shapiro JR, Shapiro WR. Clonal tumor cell heterogeneity. Prog Exp Tumor Res 1984; 27:49–66.

26. Shapiro JR, Shapior WR. The subpopulations and isolated cell types of freshly resected high grade gliomas: their influence on the tumor's evolution in vivo and behavior and therapy in vitro. Cancer Metastasis Rev 1985; 4:107–124.

27. Shapiro JR, Yung WKA, Shapiro WR: Isolation, karyotype and clonal growth of heterogeneous subpopulations of human malignant gliomas. Cancer Res 1981; 41:2349–2359.

28. Shapiro JR, Pu PY, Shapiro WR. Resistant cell types in human gliomas. In: Salmon SE, Trent JM (eds). Human Tumor Cloning. Orlando, Grune & Stratton, 1984; pp 113–142.

29. Kornblith PL, Walker M. Chemotherapy for malignant gliomas. J Neurosurg 1988; 68:1–17.

30. Chang CH, Horton J, Schoenfeld D, et al. Comparison of postoperative radiotherapy and combined postoperative radiotheray and chemotherapy in the multidisciplinary management of malignanat gliomas. A joint Radiation Therapy Oncology Group and Eastern Cooperative Oncology Group study. Cancer 1983; 52:997–1107.

31. Levin VS, Wilson CB, Rubenstein L, et al. Adjuvant chemotherapy with BCNU or the combination of CCNU, procarbazine, and vincristine following irradiation and hydroxyurea for glioblastoma multiforme. Proc Ann Meet Am Assoc Cancer Res 1980; 21:474 (Abstract).

32. Nelson DF, Schoenfeld D, Weinstein AS, et al. A randomized comparison of misonidazole sensitized radiotherapy plus BCNU for treatment of malignant glioma after surgery; preliminary results of an RTOG study. Int J Radiat Oncol Biol Phys 1983; 9:1143–1151.

33. Solero CL, Monfardini S, Brambilla C, et al. Controlled study with BCNU vs. CCNU as adjuvant chemotherapy following surgery plus radiotherapy for glioblastoma multiforme: Cancer Clin Trials 1979; 2:43–48.

34. Walker MD, Alexander E Jr, Hunt WE, et al. Evaluation of BCNU and/or radiotherapy in the treatment of anaplastic gliomas. A cooperative clinical trial. J Neurosurg 1978; 49:333–343.

35. Mortimer JE, Hewlett JS, Bay J, et al. High dose BCNU with autologous bone marrow rescue in the treatment of recurrent malignant gliomas. J Neuro-Oncol 1983; 1:269–273.

36. Hochberg FH, Parker LM, Takvorian T, et al. High-dose BCNU with autologous bone marrow rescue for recurrent glioblastoma multiforme. J Neurosurg 1981; 54:455–460.

37. Foo SH, Ransohoff J, Berenstein A, et al. Intra-arterial BCNU chemotherapy for malignant gliomas. J Neurosurg 1985; 62:458–459 (Letter).

38. Greenberg HS, Ensminger WD, Chandler WF. Intra-arterial BCNU chemotherapy for treatment of malignant gliomas of the central nervous system. J Neurosurg 1984; 61:423–429.

39. Cianfriglia F, Pomili A, Riccio A, et al. CCNU-chemotherapy of hemispheric supratentorial glioblastoma multiforme. Cancer 1980; 45:1289–1299.

40. Garrett MJ, Hughes HJ, Freedman LS. A comparison of radiotherapy alone with radiotherapy and CCNU in cerebral glioma. Clin Oncol 1978; 4:71–76.
41. Payne DG, Simpson WJ, Keen C, et al. Malignant astrocytoma. Hyperfractionated and standard radiotherapy with chemotherapy in a randomized prospective clincial trial. Cancer 1982; 50:2301–2306.
42. Seiler RW, Zimmerman A, Markwalder H. Adjuvant chemotherapy with VM 26 and CCNU after operation and radiotherapy of high-grade supratentorial astrocytomas. Surg Neurol 1980; 13:65–68.
43. Eyre HJ, Qualgliana JM, Eltringham JR, et al. Randomized comparisons of radiotherapy and CCNU versus radiotherapy, CCNU plus procarbazine for the treatment of malignant gliomas following surgery. A Southwest Oncology Group Report. J Neuro-Oncol 1983; 1:171–177.
44. Fulton DS, Urtasun RC, Shin KH, et al. Multiple daily radiation and misonidazole in the management of malignant glioma. Proc Annu Meet Am Soc Clin Oncol 1983; 2:C–885 (Abstract).
45. Pompili A, Riccio A, Jandolo B, et al. CCNU chemotherapy in adult patients with tumors of the basal ganglia and brain stem. J Neurosurg 1980; 53:361–363.
46. Ellis ME, Weiss RB, Kuperminc M. Nephrotoxicity of lomustine. A case report and literature review. Cancer Chemother Pharmacol 1985; 15:174–175.
47. Green SB, Byar DP, Strike TA, et al. Randomized comparisons of BCNU, streptozotocin, radiosensitizer, and fractionation of radiotherapy in the postoperative treatment of malignant glioma (Study 7702). Proc Annu Meet Am Soc Clin Oncol 1984; 3:C–1018 (Abstract).
48. Walker MD, Alexander E Jr, Hunt WE, et al. Evaluation of BCNU and/or radiotherapy in the treatment of anaplastic gliomas. A cooperative clinical trial. J Neurosurg 1978; 49:333–343.
49. Hara T, Miyazaki S, Ishii E, et al. High-dose 1-(4-amino 2-methyl-5-pyrimidinyl)-methyl-3-(2-chloroethyl)-3-nitrosourea hydrochloride (ACNU) with autologous bone marrow rescue for patients with brain stem tumors. Child's Brain 1984; 11:369–374.
50. Mori T, Mineura K, Katakura R. Chemotherapy of malignant brain tumor by a water soluble anti-tumor nitrosourea, ACNU. Neurol Med Chir 1979; 19:1157–1171.
51. Green SB, Byar DP, Walker MD, et al. Comparisons of carmustine, procarbazine, and high-dose methylprednisolone as additions to surgery and radiotherapy for the treatment of malignant glioma. Cancer Treat Rep 1983; 67:121–132.
52. Eyre HJ, Quagliana JM, Eltringham JR, et al. Randomized comparisons of radiotherapy and CCNU versus radiotherapy, CCNU plus procarbazine for the treatment of malignant gliomas following surgery. A Southwest Oncology Group Report. J Neuro-Oncol 1983; 1:171–177.
53. Levin VA, Wilson CB, Rubenstein L, et al. Adjuvant chemotherapy with BCNU or the combination of CCNU, procarbazine, and vincristine following irradiation and hydroxyurea for glioblastoma multiforme. Proc Annu Meet Am Assoc Cancer Res 1980; 21:474 (Abstract).
54. Stewart DJ, O'Bryan RM, Al-Sarraf M, et al. Phase II study of cisplatin

in recurrent astrocytomas in adults: a Southwest Oncology Group Study. J Neuro-Oncol 1983; 1:145–147.

55. Feun LG, Stewart DJ, Maor M, et al. A pilot study of cisdiaminedichloroplatinum and radiation therapy in patients with high grade astrocytomas. J Neuro-Oncol 1983; 1:109–113.

56. Bjornsson TD, Schold SC, Friedman HS, et al. Pharmacokinetics of diaziquone after three different dosage regimens. Cancer Treat Rep 1985; 69:1383–1385.

57. Curt GA, Kelley JA, Kufta CV, et al. Phase II and pharmacokinetic study of aziridinylbenzoquinone (2,5-diaziridinyl 3,6-bis(carboethoxyamino)–1,4-benzoquinone, Diaziquone, NSC 182986) in high-grade gliomas. Cancer Res 1983; 43:6102–6105.

58. Decker DA, Al-Sarraf M, Kresge C, et al. Phase II study of aziridinylbenzoquinone (AZQ: NSC–182986) in the treatment of malignant gliomas recurrent after radiation. Preliminary report. J Neuro-Oncol 1985; 3:19–21.

59. Greenberg HS, Ensminger WD, Layton PB, et al. Phase I-II evaluation of intra-arterial diaziquone for recurrent malignant astrocytomas. Cancer Treat Rep 1986; 70:353–357.

60. Madajewicz S, Spaulding M, Bhimani S, et al. Phase I-II diaziquone chemotherapy in brain tumors. Cancer Treat Rep 1984; 68:913–914.

61. Maral J, Poisson M, Pertuiset BF, et al. Phase II evaluation of diaziquone (CI–904, AZQ) in the treatment of human malignant glioma. J Neuro-Oncol 1985; 3:245–249.

62. Taylor SA, McCracken JD, Eyre HJ, et al. Phase II study of aziridinylbenzoquinone (AZQ) in patients with central nervous system malignancies: a Southwest Oncology Group Study. J Neuro-Oncol 1985; 3:131–135.

63. Feun LG, Yung WK, Leavens ME, et al. A phase II trial of 2,5-diaziridinyl 3,6-bis(carboethoxy amino) 1,4-benzoquinone (AZQ, NSC 182986) in recurrent primary brain tumors. J Neuro-Oncol 1984; 2:13–17.

64. EORTC Brain Tumour Group. Effect of AZQ (1,4-cyclohexadiene-1,4-diacarbamic acid-2,5-bis(1-aziridinyl)-3,6-dioxodiethylester) in recurring supratentorial malignant brain gliomas-a phase II study. Eur J Cancer Clin Oncol 1985; 21:143–146 (Letter).

65. Djordjevic B, Szybalski W. Genetics of human cell lines. III. Incorporation of 5-bromo- and 5-iododeoxyuridine into the deoxyribonucleic acid of human cells and its effect on radiation sensitivity. J Exp Med 1960; 112:509–531.

66. Kinsella TJ, Mitchell JB, Russo A, et al. Continuous intravenous infusions of bromodeoxyrinidine as a clinical radiosensitizer. J Clin Oncol 1986; 2(10):1144–1150.

67. MRC Working Party on Misonidazole in Gliomas. A study of the effect of misonidazile in conjunction with radiotherapy for the treatment of grades 3 and 4 astrocytomas. Br J Radiol 1983; 56:673–682.

68. Nelson DF, Schoenfeld D, Weinstein AS, et al. A randomized comparison of misonidazole sensitized radiotherapy plus BCNU for treatment of malignant glioma after surgery; preliminary results of an RTOG study. Int J Radiat Oncol Biol Phys 1983; 9:1143–1151.

69. EORTC Tumor Group. Misonidazole in radiotherapy of supratentorial malignanat brain gliomas in adult patients: randomized double-blind study. Eur J Cancer Clin Oncol 1983; 19:39–42.

70. Fulton DS, Urtasun RC, Shin KH, et al. Misonidazole combined with hyperfractionation in the management of malignanat glioma. Int J Radiat Oncol Biol Phys 1984; 10:1709–1712.

71. Stadler B, Karcher KH, Kogelnik HD, et al. Misonidazole and irradiation in the treatment of high-grade astrocytomas: further report of the Vienna Study Group. Int J Radiat Oncol Phys 1984; 10:1713–1717.

72. Walker MD, Green SB, Byar DP, et al. Randomized comparisons of radiotherapy and nitrosoureas for maligant glioma after surgery. N Engl J Med 1980; 303:1323–1329.

73. Kimmel DW, Shapiro JR, Shapiro WR. In vitro drug sensitivity testing in human gliomas. J Neurosurg 1987; 66:161–171.

74. Shapiro WR. Treatment of neuroectodermal brain tumors. Ann Neurol 1982; 12:231–237.

75. Morrison RS, de Vellis J. Growth of purified astrocytes in a chemically defined medium. Proc Natl Acad Sci 1981; 78:7205–7209.

76. Rubinstein LJ, Herman MM, Foley VL. In vitro characteristics of human glioblastomas maintained in organ culture systems. Light microscopy observations. Am J Pathol 1973; 71:61–80.

77. Saez RJ, Campbell RJ, Laws ER Jr. Chemotherapeutic trials on human malignant astrocytomas in organ culture. J Neurosurg 1977; 46:320–327.

78. Darling JL, Oktar N, Thomas DGT. Multicellular tumor spheroids derived from human brain tumors. Cell Biol Int Rep 1983; 7:23–30.
    79 Tofilon PJ, Buckley N, Deen DF. Effect of cell-cell interactions on drug sensitivity and growth of drug-sensitive and resistant tumor cells in spheroids. Science 1984; 226:862–864.

80. Nedermann T. Growth of tumor cells as multicellular spheroids and anti-tumor drug evaluation. In: Dendy PP, Hill BT (eds): Human Tumour Drug Sensitivity Testing In Vitro: Techniques and Clinical Applications. London, Academic Press, pp 147–162.

81. Kornblith PL, Smith BH, Leonard LA. Response of cultured human brain tumors to nitrosoureas: correlations with clinical data. Cancer 1981; 47:255–265.

82. Kornblith PL, Szypko PE. Variations in response of human brain tumors to BCNU in vitro. J Neurosurg 1978; 48:580–586.

83. Rosenblum ML, Knebel KD, Vasquez DA, Wilson CB. Brain tumor therapy, quantitative analysis using a model system. J Neurosurg 1977; 46:145–154.

84. Rosenblum, ML, Vasquez DA, Hashino T, Wilson CB. Development of a clonogenic cell assay for human brain tumors. Cancer 1978; 41:2305–2314.

85. Rosenblum MR, Dougherty DV, Reese C. Potentials and possible pitfalls of human stem cell analysis. Cancer Chemother Pharmacol 1981; 6:227–235.

86. Selby P, Buick RN, Tannock I. A critical appraisal of the "human tumor stem-cell assasy." N Engl J Med 1983; 308:129–134.

87. Rosenblum ML, Dougherty DA, Brown JM, Barker M, Hoshino T, Deen

DF. Improved methods of disaggregating single cells from solid tumors. Cell Tissue Kinet 1980; 13:667.

88. Rosenblum ML. Chemosensitivity testing for human brain tumors. In: Salmon SE (ed). Cloning of Human Tumor Stem Cells. New York, Alan R. Liss, 1980; pp 259–276.

89. Rosenblum ML, Gerosa MA, Wilson CB. Stem cell studies of human malignant brain tumors. Part 1: Development of the stem cell assay and its potential. J Neurosurg 1983; 58:170–176.

90. Freshney RI, Paul J, Kane IM. Assay of anti-cancer drugs in tissue culture; conditions affecting their ability to incorporate ^{3}H-lencine after drug treatment. Br J Cancer 1980; 41:857–866.

91. Kaufmann M. Biochemical short-term predictive assay: results of correlative trials in comparison to other assays. Recent Results Cancer Res 1984; 94:151–160.

92. Volm M, Kaufmann M, Mattern J. Results obtained using a short-term radionucleotide assay and clinical observation. In: Dendy PP, Hill BT (eds). Human Tumour Drug Sensitivity Testing In Vitro: Techniques and Clinical Applications. London, Academic Press, pp 251–258.

93. Silvestrini R, Sanfilippo O, Daidone MG. An attempt to use incorporation of radioactive nucleic acid precursors to preduct clinical response.In: Dendy PP, Hill BT (eds): Human Tumour Drug Sensitivity Testing In Vitro: Techniques and Clinical Applications. London, Academic Press, pp 281–290.

94. Sariban E, Kohn KW, Zlotogorski C. DNA cross-linking responses of human malignant glioma cell strains to chloroethylnitrosoureas, cis-platin and diaziquone. Cancer Res 1987; 47:3988–3994.

95. Tofilon PJ, Williams ME, Barcellos MH, et al. Comparison of the sister chromatid exchange and cell survival assays as a measure of tumor sensitivity in vitro to cis-diaminedichloroplatinum (II). Cancer Res 1983; 43:3511–3513.

96. Kornblith PL, Szypko PE. Variations in response of human brain tumors to BCNU in vitro. J Neurosurg 1978; 48:580–586.

97. Rosenblum ML, Gerosa MA. Stem cell sensitivity. Prog Exp Tumor Res 1984; 28:1–17.

16

Chemosensitivity of Human Glioma: Current Results and Future Prospects

*John L. Darling and
David G.T. Thomas*

Introduction

Tumors of the central nervous system are not rare and the prognosis of patients with malignant glioma, which perhaps constitutes 50% of all primary brain tumors, is uniformly poor. In addition to surgery and radiotherapy, both of which have established roles to play, chemotherapy as an adjunctive treatment is now becoming more widespread. Its general adoption is hampered by a number of biological problems, perhaps more theoretical than practical. There is the question of tumor heterogeneity and this is manifest in two ways. First, intertumor variation produces the clinical observation that not all patients with histologically similar tumors respond identically to a particular drug. Second, there is the question of heterogenity of cells within a single neoplasm. Additionally, chemotherapy is not without toxicity, which with certain agents may be severe. There is also little doubt that while agents such as the nitrosoureas and procarbazine are effective in an adjuvant situation, their effect is only modest and there is a clear need for more effective drugs.

From: Kornblith PL, Walker MD (editors). Advances in Neuro-Oncology. Futura Publishing Company, Inc., Mount Kisco, NY, © 1988.

Acknowledgment: Work in the authors' laboratory is supported by the Brain Research Trust and the Cancer Research Campaign.

The response of a tumor to cytotoxic drugs is determined by a large number of factors. Some of these are concerned with the tumor itself, while others are concerned with the host or the interaction between the host and tumor. It is difficult or perhaps impossible to determine the exact importance of each of these factors or to determine if one is more important than another. However, the rationale for chemosensitivity testing either in vitro or in vivo relies heavily on the assumption that intrinisic cellular sensitivity is the major and overriding factor determining chemotherapeutic response. In recent years, considerable effort has been invested in the examination of drug sensitivity of isolated human tumor cells, taken either from the tumor or in the form of long- or short-term cell cultured lines. In this chapter, we intend to describe how these tests have been or can be applied to human brain tumors to answer questions about heterogeneity, toxicity, in vitro/clinical correlations, and the the search for new drugs.

However the end-point is determined, the basic design of an in vitro chemosensitivity assay is the same. Tumor biopsies are prepared, either as disaggregated cells for clonogenic, dye exclusion, or short-term radioisotopic assay, or for culture as monolayer, explants, or organ cultures. In the former case, the identification of malignant cells is less important than in the latter as it is said that the clonogenic assay selects only for malignant cells and the short-term drug exposures used in the dye exclusion assay and Volm-type assays are not long enough for significant overgrowth of normal cell contaminants to occur. In the latter case, overgrowth by stromal cells remains a problem with some types of tumor, for example, breast carcinoma, where it is usual for fibroblasts to overgrow most primary cultures. However, with malignant glioma, fibroblast overgrowth is extremely rare. Nevertheless, it is important to be able to identify the malignant cells within cultures and ensure that they are representative of the original tumor biopsy.

The next stage of a chemosensitivity assay involves exposing tumor cells to drugs. This may be for a short (1–2 hours) or a protracted period (1–3 days. Drug exposure must take into account a number of considerations such as relevance to in vivo exposure levels, in vivo activation, and drug stability in vitro. The proliferative state of the cells must also be considered. Will all the cells have passed through one or more cell cycles during drug exposure? Is the apparent in vitro sensitivity stable after a short exposure?

After drug exposure, a period of recovery is often allowed before residual viability is determined. This can be short (1–4 hours) enabling only the equilibration of acid-soluble pools and the efflux of unbound drugs from the cell surface, or quite long (2–3 days or 1–3 cell population doublings) allowing the cells to recover from sublethal damage and reversible metabolic effects. The seven population doublings (14–21 days) needed for a single cell to produce a colony of over 100 cells in the clonogenic assay should be considered an extreme form of recovery period.

Review of Chemosensitivity Assays for Human Brain Tumors

Morphological Assays

These tests rely on the subjective and semiquantitative inspection of cells either by phase contrast microscopy or by the examination of fixed and stained monolayers to assess the degree of cell damage. These tests have been extensively used by a number of workers who have produced evidence of a correlation between the in vitro assay results and clinical response.[1,2] Using this type of assay on short-term cultures of brain tumors has made it possible to demonstrate a considerable variation in the response between cultures.[3–6] These tests have only been applied to small numbers of cultures and no in vitro/clinical correlations have been reported for brain tumors. With regard to the technical nature of the assay, it is difficult to automate the visual examination of cultured material and produce results in a reproducible manner. It is likely that there is considerable variation between operators in determining the degree of damage, and the relationship between morphological changes and cytotoxicity is difficult to assess.

Cell Counting Assays

As an attempt to develop a quantitative assay, several workers have used cell counting techniques based on intact monolayers, fixed and stained monolayers, or by counting cell suspensions produced from drug-treated monolayers using either electronic cell counting or hemocytometry. By growing cells on glass coverslips in culture tubes[7] and estimating the number of cells per unit area with a calibrated eyepiece graticule, it was possible to screen 12 glioma cultures against a range of chemotherapeutic agents and to demonstrate a considerable range of ID_{50} values.[8]

This approach, again in small numbers of patients, appears to have some clinical utility, as there is some relationship between drug-induced diminution of cell numbers and clinical response,[9,10] although other authors have reported that there was no correlation between in vitro sensitivity and clinical response.[11]

By determining the number of cells remaining adherent after drug treatment in microtitration plate wells, two groups have been able to demonstrate considerable variation in the response of cultures derived from malignant glioma to BCNU[12–14] and radiation.[12]

Kornblith et al.[14] compared the chemosensitivities of cultures derived from 14 patients with malignant glioma with the clinical response of the patients to BCNU. In the assay, cells were exposed to BCNU for 1 hour and allowed to recover for 20–24 hours after which they were fixed, stained, and counted under a microscope.[13] All patients had histologically confirmed malignant astrocytomas, and all had undergone postoperative radiotherapy (4,500–5,000 cGy), at least two courses of BCNU or CCNU, and had two or more CT scans during chemotherapy. In reality, only one of the 14 patients had ever been treated with BCNU, and had received only a single course of BCNU followed by eight courses of CCNU. Of the others, 11 had been treated with CCNU, one had been given CCNU, vincristine, and procarbazine, and one had CCNU and methotrexate. The in vitro response was defined as a 25% or greater cell kill at a clinically achievable dose of BCNU and there was a correct prediction in 10/13 patients (five true positives, five true negatives). There were three false positives (cases where the in vitro test suggested sensitivity, but where there was no clinical response), but there were no false negatives. Using a similar microtitration assay, Yung et al.[15] have found considerable heterogeneity in sensitivity to BCNU and *cis*-diamine-dichloroplatinum (CDDP) between six karyotypically distinct clonal cell lines isolated from two malignant gliomas.

Intermediate Duration Assays Using Radioisotope Uptake

In situations where it is possible to produce monolayer cell cultures which retain features of the tumors of origin, it is possible to use radioisotope-uptake assays of relatively long duration (e.g., 3–10 days). Assays of this type have a number of distinct advantages. They often use microtitration plates which make it easier to handle a large number of replicate cultures. This permits the testing of multiple drug concentrations and drug combinations in vitro, and as radioactive isotopes are used automation can be employed. With an assay of this kind it is possible to produce sensitivity readings after a drug exposure of 24, 48, 72 hours or longer, to measure the rate at which drug sensitivity develops over the exposure period, and to determine the maximum sensitivity expressed, which may be a stable figure if a plateau is reached. If a recovery period is allowed after drug exposure, the reversibility of drug action can also be estimated.

Using Radiolabeled Amino Acids

One of the first assays of this kind was developed using ^{3}H-leucine incorporation as a measure of residual protein synthesis.[16] The assay was validated using HeLa cells in order to determine the optimal time for drug exposure, recovery and isotopic labeling and it was found that short drug exposures, less than one cell cycle, gave misleading sensitivities. Indeed, prolonged drug exposures and recovery were required for reproducible, stable ID$_{50}$'s.

When the assay was allowed to proceed, after drug exposure, until just before density-dependent inhibition of growth was apparent, the microtitration assay was found to correlate closely with a monolayer cloning assay.[17] The end-point was determined by extracting the acid insoluble residue in sodium hydroxide solution and measuring ^{3}H-leucine uptake by scintillation spectrometry. This approach was rather laborious and attempts were made to simplify the assay.[18,19] If a higher energy β-emitting amino acid was substituted for ^{3}H-leucine, such as ^{35}S-methionine, it is possible to treat radioisotopically labeled cells in situ with a fluorescent material—organic solvent-based scintillation fluid;[20] or salicylic acid;[21] and carry out scintillation autofluorography (Fig. 1). Fluorography of this kind is used extensively for the detection of labeled proteins or nucleic acids on polyacrylamide gels and thin-layer chromatograms. Gels are equiliberated with fluors such as PPO dissolved in DMSO, dried, and exposed to x-ray film at −70°C. The β-particles, instead of interacting directly with the photographic emulsion as in conventional autoradiography, induce the fluor to produce multiple photons of visible light which can be detected on blue-sensitive x-ray film. In the chemosensitivity assay, x-ray film is placed against the underside of the

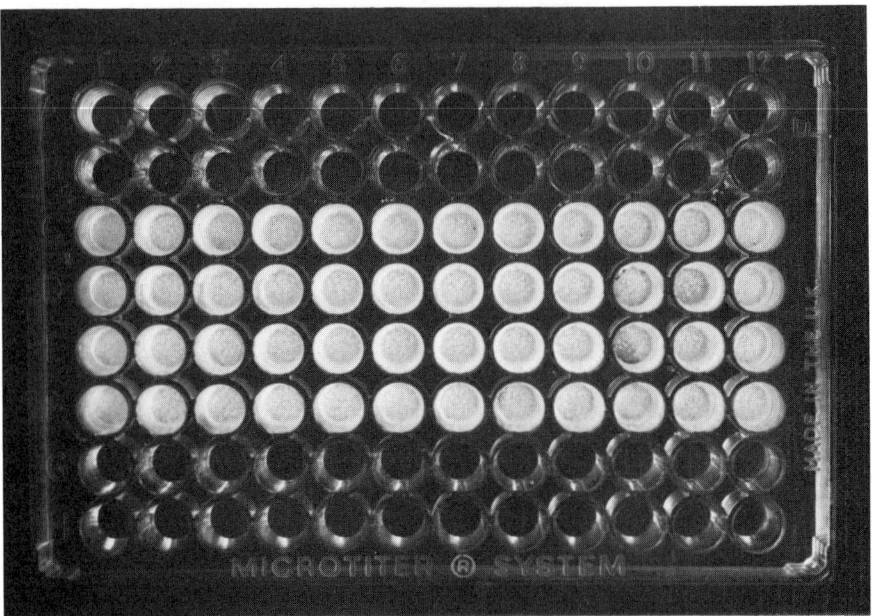

Figure 1. An example of a microtitration plate on which rows C–F have been seeded with U251 MG human glioma cells which have subsequently been labeled with ^{35}S-methionine. An aliquot of a saturated solution of sodium salicylate in methanol was added to each well and dried by centrifugation at 20°C.

microtitration plate and held tightly against the well bases with a polythene sponge and aluminum pressure plate. The x-ray film negative which is produced can be developed with a high-contrast black and white developer, fixed and scanned with a conventional scanning densitometer. An advantage with this type of end-point determination, is that a permanent record of each experiment is produced. This is illustrated in Figure 2 which shows fluorograms produced from microtitration plates which have been seeded with cells from an established human glioma cell line, U251MG. The cells have been pulsed with 2 μCi/ml of ^{35}S-methionine for 4 hours, washed and fixed in situ on the plates with methanol. Unincorporated label was extracted with two washes in ice-cold trichloroacetic acid. The wells on plate A were filled with 50 μl of toluene-based scintillation fluid and the wells on plate B with 100 μl of a saturated solution of sodium

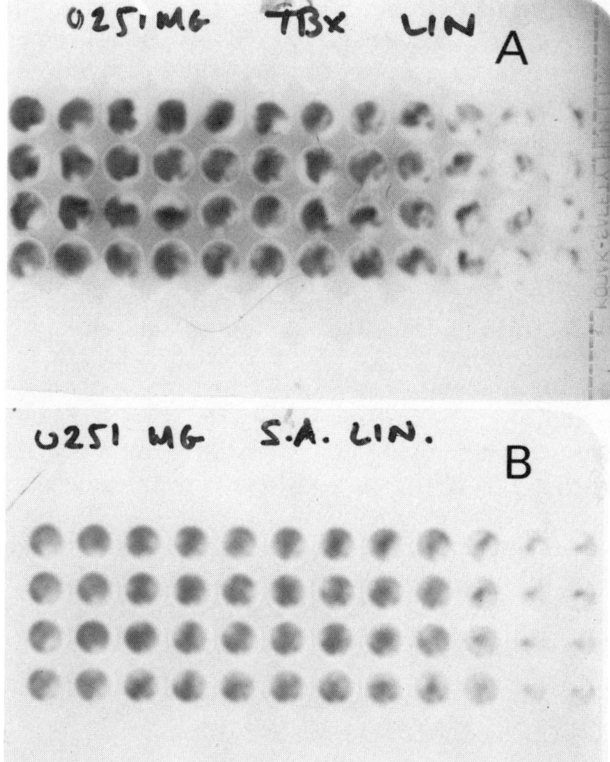

Figure 2. An example of an autofluorograph taken from a plate similar to that shown in Figure 1. Details of the preparation of this are given in the text.

salicylate in methanol. The plates were dried by centrifugation at 250 × g and a piece of x-ray film placed against the base of each microtitration plate. After exposure at −70° the films were developed in D-19 developer, fixed and washed. This procedure will work if ^{3}H-leucine is used as the isotope, although the image takes 3–5 times as long to be produced.[18]

A major advantage of a microtitration plate method involving relatively long-term exposure to cytotoxic drugs is that changes in chemosensitivity over time can be investigated. Using ^{3}H-leucine incorporation, we have investigated the changes in sensitivity of short-term glioma cell cultures against four drugs. It was clear that in many cases and particularly with 5-FU that a plateau level was reached after 3 days of drug treatment and a prolonged recovery period. Our reason for long drug exposures is that a 3-day exposure period allows most proliferating cells to pass through the cell cycle at least once in the presence of drug. The doubling time of many short-term human glioma cultures is relatively long in comparison to many established cell lines, and as cell cycle times vary, both within a population of cells derived from one tumor and between cell lines, it is possible that unless prolonged drug exposure times are used, some cells will not have completed a full cycle in the presence of drug. The development of cytotoxicity in three cell lines derived from a spontaneous murine astrocytoma[22,23] is shown for two drugs, AZQ and VP16-213 (Fig. 3). There is rapid change in cytotoxicity over the initial stages of drug exposure and only after 48–72 hours' exposure is the maximum cytotoxicity reached. It follows that attempts to use short-term drug exposures would result in a situation where the ID_{50} was determined from a part of the curve where rapid changes in sensitivity were taking place (for example, over the first 24 hours of exposure to drug) and consequently the exact sensitivity measurement would depend on the time at which it was made. Small differences in when the determination was carried out would result in large differences in apparent sensitivity.

Using Radiolabeled Nucleic Acid Precursors

As inhibition of cell proliferation is the ideal goal of predictive chemosensitivity testing, it has been suggested that radiolabeled nucleotides provide a better end-point than labeled amino acids as inhibition of nucleotide uptake should be a realistic indicator of inhibition of cell proliferation. However, there are a number of significant problems associated with their use. Drugs can influence the transport of labeled nucleosides across the cell membrane[24] and a variety of anti-neoplastic drugs have been shown to interfere with the size of intracellular nucleotide pools. Another potential pitfall is the increased estimate of DNA synthesis that can occur as a result of increased salvage synthesis caused by drugs that inhibit the de novo pathway. It is also apparent that tritiated thymidine is toxic to proliferating cells in culture[25] including cultures of human glioma.[26] In recent studies, Pertuiset et al.[26] were able to demonstrate a correlation between cellular sensitivity to tritium-induced DNA damage

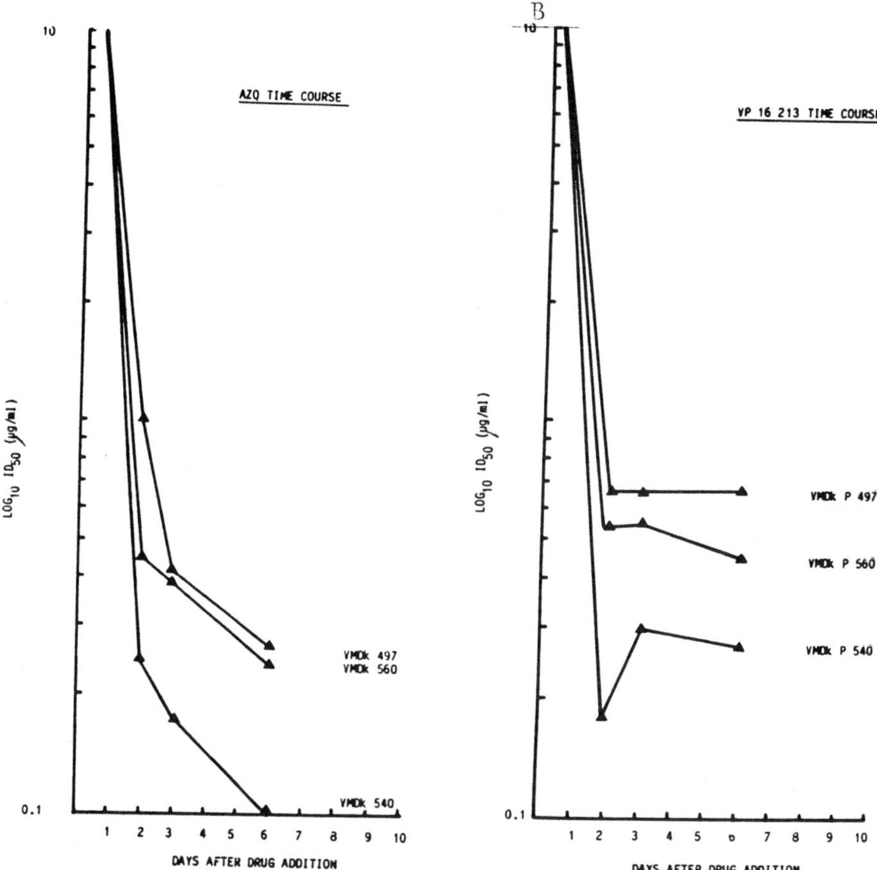

Figure 3. Development of a plateau level of apparent ID_{50} in cultures of three established cell lines (P497, 540, and 560) derived from a spontaneous murine astrocytoma. Replicate cultures were treated for either 2 or 3 days with either (A) AZQ or (B) VPI6-213 and the ID_{50} determined either at these time points or after 3 days of recovery in fresh medium.

in vitro and response to external-beam irradiation in patients who underwent radiation therapy and who had cultures prepared from their tumor. However, from within this sample of patients, radiation therapy was not the only treatment used; in fact, all but three had chemotherapy with a variety of agents including alkylating agents.

Clonogenic Assays

As cell proliferation is the critical factor determining tumor growth, the ability to measure the effect of cytotoxic drugs on cell proliferation in vitro is of considerable experimental importance.

In essence, chemosensitivity assays based on colony formation are simple. Single cell suspensions from tumors are treated with drugs and then suspended in a soft agar overlayer in a petri dish or tube. As each viable cell is theoretically capable of division to form a macroscopic colony, the number of colonies produced can be compared to that produced in control cultures and a surviving fraction determined.

In experimentally produced animal tumors, it is thought that the cells which give rise to colonies in in vitro or in vivo assays represent the stem-cell component of the tumor (see ref. 27, for review). In human tumors, the evidence that all cells forming colonies in soft agar are stem-cells is less convincing.[28] In normal self-renewing tissues such as intestine, testis, or the hematopoetic system, stem-cells are responsible for repopulation. These stem-cells are undifferentiated, but during clonal expansion, they give rise to transitional cells which begin to acquire differentiated characteristics, while gradually losing their ability to proliferate. The increasing differentiation of transitional cells results in terminally differentiated end cells which have acquired the differentiated feature of the tissue but have lost their ability to proliferate. There is some evidence that a similar cellular hierachy exists within tumors,[27,28] although the relationship between stem-cells and cells capable of forming colonies in soft agar remains obscure.

As early as 1955, Puck and Marcus[29] produced colonies from HeLa cells and noted that almost all the HeLa cells were clonogenic. They incorporated a feeder layer of X-irradiated HeLa cells to supply conditioning factors and using this colony forming assay determined the x-ray sensitivity of HeLa cells in vitro.[30]

Cells transformed by oncogenic viruses can be assayed by colony formation on glass or plastic surfaces,[31] although this system does not distinguish completely between normal and malignant cells as there is tendency for some normal cells to form colonies.[32,33] In an attempt to produce an assay that suppressed the growth of normal cells, without impairing colony formation by transformed cells, cultures were prepared in soft (0.3%) agar in petri dishes, base coated with 0.5% agar.[32]

Mouse myeloma cells were found to form colonies in soft agar and could be assayed for colony-forming efficiency as there was a linear relationship between the number of tumor cell colonies formed and the number of cells plated.[34] This method has also been used to assay mouse myeloma cells for their in vitro sensitivity to melphalan.[35] Such an assay system, however, proved unsuitable for the growth of human myeloma cell colonies[36] and, in consequence, a considerable amount of effort has been expended in developing clonogenic assays for human tumor cells.

Two main methodologies have been proposed for the assay of clonogenic cells from human tumors. The first is the Hamburger-Salmon assay[36–38] where tumor cells are plated in an enriched semi-solid medium in petri dishes, over a base layer of agar incorporating a complex range of growth factors including media conditioned by adherent spleen cells from BALB/C mice. Subsequent work has shown that for some tumor types the medium can be simplified and that conditioned medium is only essential for human myeloma cells.[38] Colonies form within 14–21 days of incubation. It has been possible to characterize the cells that form colonies and this has confirmed their tumor cell origin.[36–39]

The second assay system was originally developed for the in vitro assay of clonogenic cells from animal tumors such as Lewis lung tumor and B–16 melanoma.[40] For human tumor cells, the assay has been modified and is carried out in tubes with a replenishable liquid phase[41–43] and the cells suspended in a soft agar plug at the bottom of the tube. Additions to the agar include red blood cells (RBC) from August rats which undergo lysis during the assay, releasing growth factors which seem to be important in tumor cell growth. Another feature of this assay is the use of gassing mixtures which contain low levels of oxygen (less than 5%). The addition of RBC and use of reduced oxygen tensions has been found to increase the colony formation of mouse marrow cells in vitro.[44] In comparative studies, the colony forming efficiency (CFE) of cells taken directly from melanomas, ovarian carcinomas, and gliomas is higher in the Courtenay assay than in the Hamburger-Salmon assay.[45]

A major problem with all colony-forming assays is the relatively poor CFE of cells from solid tumors. Even using the Courtenay assay, plating efficiencies of neuroblastomas, squamous cell carcinomas of the head and neck, and colorectal carcinomas are often less than 1%, and in the majority of cases no colonies formed at all.[46] Other authors consider that up to 60% of solid tumors can be assayed in the Hamburger-Salmon assay[47,48] with ovarian carcinomas, bladder carcinomas, and melanomas giving the highest colony forming efficiencies.[48] Cells from malignant effusions form colonies in 80–90% of cases.[47]

A second major problem has been in efficiently producing single cell suspensions from human tumors and ensuring that clumps of cells are not plated. Some authors consider that a majority of "colonies" which develop in clonogenic assays arise from pre-existing clumps of cells.[49]

Clonogenic Assays for Brain Tumors

Monolayer cloning assays have been developed for animal[50] and human[51] brain tumors. In these assays, tumor biopsies are disaggregated with proteolytic enzymes,[52] treated with drugs, and plated together with heavily X-irradiated 9L gliosarcoma feeder cells. The resultant colonies have glial- and malignancy-related characteristics.[52,53] However, claims that colonies can be produced from 95% of surgical specimens[52] are inconsistent with the low colony-forming efficiencies observed in these tumors.[53,54]

Initial studies indicate that there is a relationship between in vitro resistance and clinical resistance.[54] In a series of six patients, only one tumor showed a cell kill greater than 50% against BCNU and this patient responded clinically to the drug. The remaining five patients had maximum cell kills in the range 0–42% and none responded clinically.[54] In larger series it is apparent that the clonogenic assay tends to overpredict clinical sensitivity.[52] Another interesting feature of this assay is the apparent relationship between patient age and in vitro cell kill[55] with younger glioma patients tending to have more sensitive tumors in vitro. Monolayer cloning assays have also been used to determine the in vitro radiosensitivity of human gliomas.[56–59]

Recently, preliminary results have been published by two groups which indicate that cells from human malignant gliomas grow well in soft agar culture and between 60% and 80% of samples can successfully be assessed for drug sensitivity.[60,61]

There are, however, in addition to the disadvantages which are common to all clonogenic assays, a number which are unique to human brain tumors. In monolayer cloning, cells derived from normal brain have similar cloning efficienies to cells derived from malignant glioma.[62] In these studies, the normal brain was derived from a series of brains used in a head injury study and not from around a malignant tumor. Tumor astrocytes are highly motile and it has been reported[63] that these cells wander away from monolayer colonies before they have achieved the 25–50 cells needed to constitute a colony in vitro.

The relationship between clonogenicity in liquid overlay (monolayer cloning) and clonogenicity in suspension culture in semi-solid medium has not been examined in any major study and this relationship needs to be accurately defined. In particular, the identity of cells which produce colonies under these different sets of experimental circumstances and the relationship of these to the stem-cell population of the original tumor has not been established.

A further consideration must be the question of the applicability of end-points such as clonogenic cell survival to the clinical situation with malignant glioma. With the drugs that are presently available, it is unrealistic to suggest that these will ever be curative although they provide a worthwhile remission, with a modest increase in relapse-free interval. It is, therefore, a matter of debate as to whether an assay which measures the effect of drugs on the stem-cell population, which must only constitute a relatively small proportion of the bulk of a tumor, is of any importance in determining the transient responses observed clinically in cases of malignant glioma. It is difficult to believe that changes in the number of stem-cells can determine significant short-term changes in tumor bulk. It may be of course, that these "stem-cell" assays do not measure the effect of drugs on stem-cells alone, but also on the larger cell population which still retains limited potential for proliferation. In that case, the use of such assays must be weighed against the very considerable difficulties which they pose technically, when compared to intermediate duration assays using short-term cultures which may provide all the information necessary to predict short- to medium-term clinical response.

When drugs do become available which provide the reasonable liklihood of cure, the clonogenic assays will assume a new importance as in this case control of the stem-cell population will be critical. Indeed, the very development of such new drugs may depend on our understanding of the biology of brain tumor stem-cells. Consequently, the identity of cells which constitute colonies in both the monolayer and suspension culture clonogenic assay will have to be critically evaluated in order to be assured that they truly represent the stem-cell population of the tumor.

Organ Culture

Organ culture systems, where explants of tumors are grown on gelfoam matrices, or rafts in liquid medium, have a number of advantages over disaggregated cells. Cellular interrelationships are maintained and the function of the tissue is to some extent intact, indicating that repair mechanisms and metabolic cooperation between cells might still operate.

Human brain tumors have been grown and extensively characterized in organ culture and appear to retain many characteristics of the tumor of origin.[64,65] Human brain tumor fragments grown on gelfoam rafts[66] will infiltrate the matrix in a manner similar to their in situ infiltration of normal brain.[67] This substrate has been used for the growth of malignant astrocytomas and using microfluorometric estimates of NADH as a quantitative index, the effectiveness of a range of drugs has been determined.[68] It has been possible to use [125]IUdR uptake[69] to quantitate the effects of PCB, CCNU, vincristine, and 5-FU on organ cultures of malignant astrocytomas.

Multicellular Tumor Spheroids (MTS)

MTS are tumor cells growing in a three-dimensional structure, simulating the growth and micro-environmental conditions of tumors. Their preparation was first described by Sutherland, McCredie, and Inch[70] who noted that V79 Chinese hamster lung carcinoma cells removed from monolayer culture and inoculated into spinner flasks initially underwent a rapid phase of aggregation to form clumps of cells. These clumps then continued to grow by cell proliferation. An alternative method of MTS production has been to plate dissociated cells into plastic cell-culture flasks that have been base-coated with agar. As the cells cannot attach to the agar, they tend to form aggregates which continue to proliferate.[71] Once a critical diameter has been reached, a central area of hypoxia begins to develop surrounded by a rim of viable cells. This viable rim is a constant width irrespective of the size of the spheroid and represents the maximum distance through which oxygen will diffuse into the spheroid from the tissue-culture medium.

MTS provide several advantages over monolayer or suspension cell cultures. Not only are the oxygenation characteristics of human tumors modeled, but also the intimate contacts between cells and cell-cycle heterogeneity (i.e., within some areas of a single spheroid, cells divide at rates comparable to cells in monolayer culture and in other areas they become arrested in G_0 phase). It has also been noted that there is a correlation between tumor growth rate in vivo and spheroid growth rate, which is not apparent in monolayer cell culture.[71] A unique advantage of MTS is the ability to sequentially "strip off" layers of cells from the surface in order to determine the chemosensitivity of cells in different positions of the spheroid. In this way it will be possible to study the effect of three-dimensional structure on chemotherapeutic response.

Established human glioma cell lines (U215MG, U118MG) have also been grown as MTS,[72] but the general histological and ultrastructural pattern of a thin rim encompassing a large volume of nonproliferating cells was not observed. In addition, these spheroids did not show central degeneration, although readily reaching diameters in excess of 600 μm.[73] Conversely, MTS produced from early passage cultures of human gliomas, by plating cells onto agarose-coated petri dishes[52,74] did have a thin outer rim and a large area of central necrosis. The 9L gliosarcoma cell line underwent MTS formation[75,76] when grown in suspension culture and the cell-cycle characteristics and growth fraction of cells within the spheroid closely resembled those of the intracerebral tumor.

The chemotherapeutic responsiveness of MTS can be measured in a number of ways. The most widely used is where the growth of individual spheroids are monitored by microscopy after drug treatment. There is usually a dose-dependent lag period before the growth rate of drug-treated MTS resumes that of the untreated controls.[77] The second method employed measures cell survival. Drug-treated spheroids are pooled, disaggregated with trypsin, and plated onto plastic petri dishes at low cell density and the number of colonies produced are scored,[78,79] The third method involves the determination of the dose of drug or irradiation which will "sterilize" (i.e., render incapable of growth) 50% of treated spheroids.[80] Recently, the chemotherapeutic sensitivity of cells within a spheroid have been measured using a sister chromatid exchange assay which has proved useful for determining the responsiveness of spheroids composed of mixed populations of drug resistant and sensitive cells.[81]

Future Prospects for Chemosensitivity Testing of Human Brain Tumors

Identity of Cells Used in Chemosensitivity Assays of Human Brain Tumors

It is fortunate that a considerable amount is known about the biology of cells within the CNS. This is due, in part, to the considerable numbers of cell-type specific markers which have been identified. Use of these in vitro markers has not been fully exploited in determining the relationship between cells grown from brain tumor biopsies and their normal counterparts in the adult CNS, although it seems reasonable that in the very near future information on the lineages of many cell types and the interrelationships between cell types will soon become apparent.

The observation that cultures derived from grade III and grade IV astrocytomas do not appear to have radically different chemosensitivities may overlook the subdivisions that these tumors may be put into on the basis of monoclonal antibody testing. It is clear that some glioma cell cultures, whether derived from grade III or IV tumors, respond particularly well to drugs and equally a number of tumors do not. Whether this represents a continuous spectrum of responsiveness within a heterogeneous population or whether these sensitive or resistant cultures are representative of subgroups of gliomas which are inherently sensitive or insensitive to cytotoxic drugs remains to be seen.

Development of Established Cell Lines from Human Brain Tumors

Although cell lines seem reasonably easy to establish from a high proportion of human malignant gliomas, with figures as high as 25–30% quoted[82] in some tumor types the development of such lines has been very difficult. For example, medulloblastomas appear to be refractory to establishment in vitro as do lines from cerebral lymphomas and ependymomas. There is a clear need for established cell lines from both immediate clinical reasons: e.g., for determining therapy and for long-term biological studies. Long-term lines would be useful from meningiomas for studies on hormonal regulation of growth and from craniopharyngiomas for studies on the mechanisms of radiation sensitivity. One approach which has been reported recently for the successful establishment of long-term lines from human sarcomas[83] relies on a period of 3–5 alternate monolayer/multicellular spheroid passage. This may be due to limiting the diffusion of growth factors in the inital stages of culture establishment and would seem particularly applicable to tumors such as medulloblastoma where there is often a tendency to spontaneously form spheroid-like structures in monolayer culture.

New Assay Methods for Human Brain Tumors

Because of the relative insensitivity of clonogenic assays for determining drug response in vitro, Tofilon et al.[84] have investigated the use of an assay which measures the induction of sister chromatid exchanges (SCE) in 9L cells treated with cytotoxic drugs. This has the advantage that cytotoxicity is measured not at the cellular level, but at the chromosome level. In a comparative study, there was a good correlation between SCE induction and cell kill for a panel of nitrosoureas with alkylating activity. There was also evidence that the SCE assay could detect evidence of drug-induced damage at an earlier stage than a colony-forming assay. One nitrosourea, BHCNU which has carbomoylating activity but no alkylating activity did not produce SCE at levels which were toxic to more than 90% of the cells. This would indicate that a considerable amount of caution should be exercised in using the SCE assay without an adequate control in the form of some kind of alternative assay running in parallel when drugs of unknown modes of action are being assayed. However, this assay method does not seem to be limited to conventional alkylating agents as a number of cytotoxic drugs with very different modes of action are known to induce SCEs including 5-FU, VCR, cis-PLAT and hydroxyurea.[84] This assay has been used, with similar results, for human glioma cell lines.[85] A particular advantage to this method is that as it is based on an analysis of single cells; it can be used to distinguish between drug-resistant and drug-sensitive cells in mixed cultures.[81]

There are clearly improvements that can be made in the existing clonogenic assays available for human brain tumors. There have been only sparse reports of the use of the Courtenay clonogenic assay,[45] and no reports of the use of the combined cloning and ^{3}H-thymidine update assay.[86]

Design of Clinical Trials for Testing In Vitro Hypotheses

There is a pressing need for large scale clinical trials for chemosensitivity testing with malignant brain tumors. Although there are indications from the present authors' work that sensitivity to at least two drugs is linked with improved relapse-free interval, this needs to be confirmed in larger retrospective studies which are carefully controlled for the effects of other known prognostic factors. In our series, 107 patients with grade III or IV gliomas were treated with adjuvant chemotherapy using procarbazine, CCNU, and vincristine following whole-head irradiation. Cell cultures were prepared from 40 of these patients and their sensitivity to each drug assessed using our ^{35}S-methionine uptake assay. Twenty-two patients (40%) responded to PCB and/or CCNU in vitro and sensitivity to these drugs was linked with increased relapse-free interval (RFI), while sensitivity to VCR was not. The RFI of patients who had responded to PCB or CCNU in vitro was significantly longer than the RFI of patients whose tumors failed to respond in vitro or patients who had not been tested. There was no difference in sex ratio, extent of operation, radiation treatment, and degree of steroid cover between responders, nonresponders, and untested groups. Further statistical analysis taking prognostic factors such as age and grade into account indicated that there was an association between chemosensitivity in vitro and RFI.[87] There have been indications from work done with other types of cancer that clinical outcome and drug sensitivity in vitro are linked.[88] It seems that chemosensitivity testing is only likely to be helpful if there is a clear link between in vitro drug sensitivity and a favorably increased relapse-free interval or survival. It has been argued that in trials where there is a correlation between improved clinical outcome and in vitro chemosensitivity, this relationship may also be true in groups of patients who have not recieved chemotherapy. That is to say, in vitro chemosensitivity testing is simply measuring a "cellular prognostic factor" which is unrelated to intrinsic chemosensitivity. It has been suggested, albeit without any experimental evidence, that this might be related to expression of particular oncogenes or oncogene products, for example, growth factors. Although it is difficult to believe that cellular chemosensitivity could be an indirect measure of oncogene expression or growth factor production in untreated patients, it is quite possible that in treated patients, if drug resistance is associated with the amplification of particular oncogenes, this could be detected with the assay. Naturally, we shall be in a better position to answer this question when we know more about the expression of oncogenes in untreated and treated gliomas. In any event, we are currently reanalyzing our results in patients who have not received chemotherapy but whose tumors where assayed in vitro. There may be problems associated with this approach because of the bias introduced by considering patients who where thought unsuitable for chemotherapy on medical grounds because of their poorer intrinsic prognosis.

The validity of chemosensitivity testing must also be tested in prospective clinical trials, although the exact design of these is not clear. It is certain that in order to answer such questions, multicenter trials will be necessary as few single centers see sufficient patients with malignant gliomas.

Drug Resistance In Vitro

Radiation and drug treatment is only palliative for patients with malignant glioma, and these tumors eventually recur. It is thought that this is due to the development of resistance, although there is little evidence for this using human material in vitro. It is unclear if drug resistant cells are present in tumors all the time but only in small numbers or if drug-resistant cells develop during treatment. The molecular mechanisms of glioma cell drug resistance are only now beginning to be investigated. Preliminary results with drug-resistant 9L cells indicate that the mechanism of resistance of these cells to the chloroethyl nitrosoureas is highly specific indicating that glioma cells resistant to these agents need not be cross-resistant to other agents which cross-link DNA.[89] In BCNU-resistant human glioma cells, resistance may be linked with the ability of these cells to repair 0^6-alkylguanine DNA adducts.[90] It is clear that considerable work needs to be done in relation to drug resistance in human glioma using clinical material. It is by no means certain that the mechanisms by which cells in the laboratory become resistant to cytotoxic drugs is relevant to clinical drug resistance. It is probably only by examining pre-therapy and post-therapy samples in the same patient, perhaps taken by stereotactic methods, that it will be possible to answer important questions about clinical drug resistance.

Conclusions

There is little doubt that in vitro methods for determining radio- and chemosensitivity are of considerable importance in neuro-oncology. The demonstration by a number of authors that clinical progress and in vitro chemosensitivity are linked is interesting, but futher, long-term trials must be carried out to validate these observations. Such studies may also throw some light on the molecular mechanisms of radio- and chemosensitivity. It is important to bear in mind that many in vitro techniques are only applicable when it is possible to produce representative cell cultures from tumors. Human adult glioma is one of the few tumor types that does produce such cultures and although the development of such cultures for many pediatric brain tumors has currently lagged behind, this is likely to change in the future. These factors provide an impetus to apply molecular biological techniques to the important question of the therapeutic sensitivity of human brain tumors.

REFERENCES

1. Limburg H, Heckmann U. Chemotherapy in the treatment of pelvic malignant diseases with special reference to ovarian cancer. J Obstet Gynaec Br 1968; 75:1246–1255.
2. Wheeler TK, Dendy PP, Dawson A. Assessment of an in vitro screening test of cytotoxic agents in the treatment of advanced malignant disease. Oncology 1974; 362–376.
3. Wilson CB, Barker M. Sensitivity of cell cultures of neural tumors to vinblastine sulfate (NSC-49842). Cancer Chemo Rep 1965; 44:9–13.
4. Wilson CB, Barker M. Relative cytotoxicity of mithramycin and vinblastine sulfate in cell cultures of human neural tumors. J Natl Cancer Inst 1967; 38:458–467.
5. Gazo LR, Afra D. Study on the effect of actinomycins in tissue cultures from human brain tumors. Acta Neurochir 1969; 21:139–152.
6. Bogdahn U. Chemosensitivity of malignant human brain tumors: Preliminary results. J Neuro-Oncol 1983; 1:149–166.
7. Ambrose EJ, Andrews RD, Easty DM, et al. Drug assays on cultures of human tumour biopsies. Lancet 1962; i:24–25.

8. Easty DM, Wylie JAH. Screening of 12 gliomata against chemotherapeutic agents in vitro. Br Med J 1963; ii:1589–1592.
9. Holmes HL, Little JM. Tissue culture microtest for predicting response of human cancer to chemotherapy. Lancet 1974; ii:985–987.
10. Lickiss JN, Cane KA, Baikie AG. In vitro drug selection in antineoplastic chemotherapy. Eur J Cancer 1974; 10:809–814.
11. Berry RJ, Laing AH, Wells J. Fresh explant culture of human tumours in vitro and the assessment of sensitivity to cytotoxic chemotherapy. Br J Cancer 1975; 31:218–227.
12. Mealey J Jr, Chen TT, Shupe R. Response of cultured human glioblastomas to radiation and BCNU chemotherapy. J Neurosurg 1979; 41:339–349.
13. Kornblith PL, Szypko PE. Variations in response of human brain tumors to BCNU in vitro. J Neurosurg 1978; 48:580–586.
14. Kornblith PL, Smith BH, Leonard LA. Response of cultured human brain tumors to nitrosoureas: Correlation with clinical data. Cancer 1981; 47:255–265.
15. Yung WKA, Shapiro JR, Shapiro WR. Heterogeneous chemosensitivities of subpopulations of human glioma cells in culture. Cancer Res 1982; 42:992–998.
16. Freshney RI, Paul J, Kane IM. Assay of anti-cancer drugs in tissue culture: Conditions affecting their ability to incorporate ^{3}H-leucine after drug treatment. Br J Cancer 1975; 31:89–99.
17. Morgan D, Freshney RI, Darling JL, et al. Assay of anticancer drugs in tissue culture: Cell cultures of biopsies from human astrocytoma. Br J Cancer 1983; 47:205–214.
18. Freshney RI, Morgan D. Radioisotopic quantitation in microtitration plates by an autofluorographic method. Cell Biol Int Rep 1978; 2:375–380.
19. Thomas DGT, Darling JL, Freshney RI, et al. In vitro chemosensitivity assay of human glioma by scintillation autofluorography. In: Multidisciplinary Aspects of Brain Tumor Therapy, Paoletti P, Walker MD, Butti G, Knerich R, eds. Amsterdam, Elsevier North Holland Biomedical Press, 1979; pp. 19–35.
20. Carlsson J, Lundqvist H, Ponten J. The measurement of spatial precursor distributions in cell culture. In Vitro 1976; 12:571–579.
21. Chamberlain JP. Fluorographic detection of radioactivity in polyacrylamide gels with the water soluble fluor, sodium salicylate. Anal Biochem 1979; 98:132–135.
22. Pilkington GJ, Darling JL, Lantos PL, et al. Cell lines (VmDk) from a spontaneous murine astrocytoma: Morphological and immunocytochemical characterization. J Neurol Sci 1983; 62:115–139.
23. Pilkington GJ, Darling JL, Lantos PL, et al. Tumorigenicity of cell lines (VmDk) derived from a spontaneous murine astrocytoma: Histology, fine structure and immunocytochemistry of tumors. J Neurol Sci 1985; 71:145–164.
24. Nakata YS, Bader JP. The uptake of nucleosides by cells in culture:II inhibition by 2-mercapto-1-(β-4-pyridethyl) benzimidazole. Biochim Biophys Acta 1969; 190:250–256.

454 • ADVANCES IN NEURO-ONCOLOGY

25. Ehmann UK, Wheeler KT. Cinemicrographic determination of cell progression and division abnormalities after treatment with 1,3 bis (2-chloroethyl)-1-nitrosourea. Eur J Cancer 1979; 15:461–473.
26. Pertuiset B, Dougherty D, Cromyer C, et al. Stem cell studies of human malignant brain tumors. Part 2: Proliferation kinetics of brain tumor cells in vitro in early passage cultures. J Neurosurg 1985; 63:426–432.
27. Steel GG. Growth kinetics of tumours: Cell population kinetics in relation to the growth and treatment of cancer. Oxford, UK, Clarendon Press, 1977.
28. Selby P, Buick RN, Tannock I. A critical appraisal of the "human tumor stem-cell" assay. N Engl J Med 1983; 308:129–134.
29. Puck TT, Marcus PI. A rapid method for viable cell titration and clone production with HeLa cells in tissue culture: The use of x-irradiated cells to supply conditioning factors. PNAS (USA) 1955; 41:432–437.
30. Puck TT, Marcus PI. Action of x-rays on mammalian cells. J Exp Med 1956; 103:653–666.
31. Stoker M, MacPherson I. Studies on transformation of hamster cells by polyoma viruses in vitro. Virology 1961; 14:359–370.
32. MacPherson I, Montagnier L. Agar suspension culture for the selective assay of cells transformed by polyoma virus. Virology 1964; 23:291–294.
33. MacPherson I. Soft agar techniques. In: Tissue Culture: Methods and Applications, Kruse PF, Patterson MK, eds. New York/London, Academic Press, 1973; pp. 276–280.
34. Park CH, Bergsagel DE, McCulloch EA. Mouse myeloma tumor stem cells: A primary cell culture assay. J Natl Cancer Inst 1971; 46:411–422.
35. Ogawa M, Bergsagel DE, McCulloch EA. Chemotherapy of mouse myeloma: Quantitative cell culture predictive of response in vivo. Blood 1973; 41:7–15.
36. Hamburger A, Salmon SE. Primary bioassay of human myeloma stem cells. J Clin Invest 1977; 60:846–854.
37. Hamburger AW, Salmon SE. Primary bioassay of human tumor stem cells. Science 1977; 197:461–463.
38. Hamburger AW. The Salmon-Hamburger "stem" cell assay. In: Human Tumour Drug Sensitivity Testing In Vitro: Techniques and Clinical Application, Dendy PP, Hill BT, eds. London, Academic Press, 1983; pp 113–119.
39. Salmon SE. Cloning of Human Tumor Stem Cells. New York, Alan R. Liss, 1980.
40. Courtenay VD. A soft agar colony assay for Lewis lung tumor and B16 melanoma taken directly from the mouse. Br J Cancer 1976; 34:39–45.
41. Courtenay VD, Mills J. An in vitro colony forming assay for human tumours grown in immune-suppressed mice and treated in vivo with cytotoxic agents. Br J Cancer 1978; 37:261–268.
42. Courtenay VD, Selby PJ, Smith IE, et al. Growth of human tumour cell colonies from biopsies using two soft agar techniques. Br J Cancer 1978; 38:77–81.
43. Courtenay D. The Courtenay clonogenic assay. In: Human Tumour Drug Sensitivity Testing In Vitro: Techniques and Clinical Application, Dendy PP, Hill BT, eds. London, Academic Press, 1983; pp 103–111.

44. Bradley TR, Telfer PA, Fry P. The effect of erythrocytes on mouse bone marrow colony development in vitro. Blood 1971; 38:353–359.
45. Tveit KM. Evaluation of the Courtenay assay for drug sensitivity prediction in vivo. In: Human Tumour Drug Sensitivity Testing In Vitro: Techniques and Clinical Application, Dendy PP, Hill BT, eds. London, Academic Press, 1983; pp 305–316.
46. Rupniak HT, Hill BT. The poor cloning ability in agar of human tumour cells from biopsies of primary tumours. Cell Biol Int Rep 1980; 4:479–486.
47. Salmon SE, von Hoff DD. In vitro evaluation of anticancer drugs with the human tumor stem cell assay. Semin Oncol 1981; 8:377–385.
48. Cowan JD, von Hoff DD. The human tumor cloning assay: An in vitro assay for antitumor activity in solid tumors. In: Cancer Chemotherapy 1, Cancer Treatment and Research, Vol 7, Muggia FM, ed. The Hague, Martinus Nijhoff, 1983; pp. 103–121.
49. Agrez MV, Kovach JS, Lieber MM. Cell aggregates in the soft agar human tumour stem-cell assay. Br J Cancer 1982; 46:880–887.
50. Rosenblum ML, Knebel KD, Wheeler KT, et al. Development of an in vitro colony formation assay for the evaluation of in vivo chemotherapy of a rat brain tumor. In Vitro 1975; 44:264–273.
51. Rosenblum ML, Vasquez DA, Hoshino T, et al. Development of a clonogenic cell assay for human brain tumors. Cancer 1978; 41:2305–2314.
52. Rosenblum ML, Gerosa MA, Wilson CB, et al. Stem cell studies of human malignant brain tumors. Part 1: Development of the stem cell assay and its potential. J Neurosurg 1983; 58:170–176.
53. Rosenblum ML. Chemosensitivity testing for human brain tumors. In: Cloning of Human Tumor Stem Cells, Salmon SE. New York, Alan R. Liss, 1980; pp 259–276.
54. Rosenblum ML, Dougherty DA, Deen DF, et al. Analysis of clonogenic human brain tumour cells: Preliminary results of tumour sensitivity testing with BCNU. Br J Cancer 1980; 41(Suppl IV):181–185.
55. Rosenblum ML, Gerosa M, Dougherty DV, et al. Age-related chemosensitivity of stem cells from human malignant brain tumours. Lancet 1982; i:885–887.
56. Weichselbaum RR, Epstein J, Little JB, et al. Inherent cellular radiosensitivity of human tumors of varying clinical curability. Am J Roentgenol 1976; 127:1027–1032.
57. Weichselbaum RR, Epstein J, Little, JB, et al. In vitro cellular radiosensitivity of human malignant tumors. Eur J Cancer 1976; 12:47–51.
58. Weichselbaum RR, Liszczak TM, Phillips JP, et al. Characterization and radiobiologic parameters of medulloblastomas in vitro. Cancer 1977; 40:1087–1096.
59. Gerweck LE, Kornblith PL, Burlett P, et al. Radiation sensitivity of cultured human glioblastoma cells. Radiology 1977; 125:231–234.
60. Georges PM, Sanders C, Rombaut C, et al. Drug screening for brain tumor chemotherapy: Results of 102 stem cell assays. J Neuro-Oncol 1984; 2:287.
61. Mulne AF, Salgaller ML, Yates AJ, et al. Growth of brain tumors in the

human tumor stem cell assay. Proc Am Assoc Cancer Res 1984; 25 (Abstract 113).

62. Freshney RI, Hart E. Clonogenicity of human glia in suspension. Br J Cancer 1982; 46:459.

63. Shapiro JR, Shapiro WR. The subpolulations and isolated cell types of freshly resected high grade human gliomas: Their influence on the tumor's evolution in vivo and behavior and therapy in vitro. Cancer Metastasis Rev 1985; 4:107–124.

64. Holmstrom T, Saksela E. Growth of human brain tumor explants in matrix cultures in different human sera. Acta Pathol Microbiol Scand 1971; (A)79:399–406.

65. Rubinstein LJ, Herman MM, Foley VL. In vitro characteristics of human glioblastomas maintained in organ culture systems: Light microscopy observations. Am J Pathol 1973; 71:61–80.

66. Raafat M, El-Bolkainy N, Rifaat M, Sorour O. A new technique for growing intracranial tumors in vitro. Med J Cairo University 1972; 11:1–13.

67. Sorour O, Raafat M, El-Bolkainy N, Rifaat M. Infiltrative potential of brain tumors in organ culture. J Neurosurg 1975; 43:742–747.

68. Saez RJ, Campbell RJ, Laws ER. Chemotherapeutic trials on human malignant astrocytomas in organ culture. J Neurosurg 1977; 46:320–327.

69. Masters JRW, Krishnaswamy A, Rigby CC, et al. Quantitative organ culture: an approach to predictive tumor response. Br J Cancer 1980; 41(Suppl IV):199–202.

70. Sutherland RM, McCredie JA, Inch WR. Growth of multicell spheroids as a model of nodular carcinomas. J Natl Cancer Inst 1971; 46:113–120.

71. Yuhas JM, Li AP, Martinez AO, et al. A simplified method for production and growth of multicellular tumor spheroids. Cancer Res 1977; 37:3639–3643.

72. Haji-Karim M, Carlsson J. Proliferation and viability in cellular spheroids of human origin. Cancer Res 1977; 38:1457–1464.

73. Carlsson J, Brunk U. The fine structure of three-dimensional colonies of human glioma cells in agarose culture. Acta Pathol Microbiol Scand (A) 1977; 85:183–192.

74. Pertuiset BF, Rosenblum ML, Poisson M, et al. Cinetique de spheroides multicellularies developpes a partir d'un glioblastome humain et action de la 1,3 bis (2-chloroethyl)-1-nitrosouree. Sem Hop Paris 1983; 59:468–472.

75. Deen DF, Hoshino T, Williams ME, et al. Development of a 9L rat brain tumor cell multicellular spheroid system and its response to 1,3 bis(2-chloroethyl)-1-nitrosourea and radiation. J Natl Cancer Inst 1980; 64:1373–1381.

76. Sano Y, Deen DF, Hoshino T. Factors that influence initiation and growth of 9L rat brain gliosarcoma multicellular spheroids. Cancer Res 1982; 42:1223–1226.

77. Yuhas JM, Tarleton AE, Hartman JG. In vitro analysis of the response of multicellular tumor spheroids exposed to chemotherapeutic agents in vitro or in vivo. Cancer Res 1978; 38:3595–3598.

78. Twentyman PR. Experimental chemotherapy studies: Intercomparison of assays. Br J Cancer 1980; 41(Suppl IV):279–287.

79. Twentyman PR. Response to chemotherapy of EMT6 spheroids as measured by growth delay and cell survival. Br J Cancer 1980; 42:297–304.
80. Porreau-Schneider N, Malaise EP. Relationship between surviving fractions using the colony method, the LD_{50} and the growth delay after irradiation of human melanoma cells grown as multicellular spheroids. Radiat Res 1981; 85:321–332.
81. Tofilon PJ, Buckley N, Deen DF. Effect of cell-to-cell interactions on drug sensitivity and growth of drug-sensitive and -resistant tumor cells in spheroids. Science 1984; 226:862–864.
82. Westermark B, Ponten J, Hugosson R. Determinants for the establishment of permanent tissue culture lines from human gliomas. Acta Path Microbiol Scand (A) 1973; 81:791–805.
83. Bruland O, Fodstad O, Pihl A. The use of multicellular spheroids in establishing human sarcoma cell lines in vitro. Int J Cancer 1985; 35:793–798.
84. Tofilon PJ, Williams ME, Deen DF. Nitrosourea-induced sister chromatid exchanges and correlation to cell survival in 9L rat brain tumor cells. Cancer Res 1983; 43:473–475.
85. Deen DF, Kendall LE, Marton LJ, Tofilon PJ. Prediction of human tumor cell chemosensitivity using the sister chromatid exchange assay. Cancer Res 1986; 46:1599–1602.
86. Friedman HM, Glaubiger DL. Assessment of in vitro drug sensitivity of human tumor cells using ^{3}H-thymidine incorporation in a modified human tumor stem cell assay. Cancer Res 1982; 4683–4689.
87. Thomas DGT, Darling JL, Paul EA, et al. Assay of anticancer drugs in tissue culture: Relationship of relapse free interval (RFI) and in vitro chemosensitivity in patients with malignant cerebral glioma. Br J Cancer 1985; 51:525–532.
88. Dendy PP, Hill BT. Human Tumour Drug Sensitivity Testing In Vitro: Techniques and Clinical Application. London, Academic Press, 1983.
89. Bodell WJ, Gerosa M, Aida T, et al. Investigation of resistance to DNA cross-linking agents in 9L cells with different sensitivities to chloroethylnitrosoureas. Cancer Res 1985; 45:3460–3464.
90. Bodell WJ, Aida T, Berger MS, et al. Increased repair of O^6-alkylguanine DNA adducts in glioma-derived human cells resistant to the cytotoxic and cytogenetic effects of 1,3-bis(2-chloroethyl)-1-nitrosourea. Carcinogenesis 1986; 7:879–883.

17

Non-Nuclear Targets of DNA Cross-Linking Agents in Glioma-Derived Cell Lines: Implications for In Vitro Assay Systems for the Prediction of Clinical Sensitivity and Resistance

B.H. Smith, M.A. Oberc-Greenwood,
C.J. Cummins, J. Ellis, C. Gibson,
P.E. McKeever, and P.L. Kornblith

Introduction

The possibility that in vitro assays can be used to predict the clinical response of patients with gliomas to available, or new, chemotherapeutic agents is an attractive one. Recent evidence indicates that such predictive systems are achievable[1,2] (see also Thomas et al., this volume). A number of issues remain unsettled.[3] An important issue is whether one or more in vitro assays are required for an optimal predictive system.

From: Kornblith PL, Walker MD (editors). Advances in Neuro-Oncology. Futura Publishing Company, Inc., Mount Kisco, NY, © 1988.

Stimulated by differences between microcytoxicity data[1,4] and the results of DNA alkaline elution assays[5,6] on the sensitivity of human glioma-derived cell lines to BCNU (1,3-bis (2-chloroethyl)-1-nitrosourea), as well as direct observation of BCNU-induced cell death at times too early to be accounted for by DNA alkylation and/or cross-linking,[4,7] we have attempted to begin to answer the question of what might constitute an optimal in vitro system. Knowing that BCNU, AZQ (aziridinylbenzoquinone, 2,5 diaziridiayl-3,6-bis-(carboethoxyamino)-1,4-benzoquinone), and cis-platinum (cis-dichloroamine-platinum (II)) have all been considered to achieve their cytotoxic effects by damaging DNA,[5,6,8–11] we asked whether cytoplasmic toxicity is also a significant component of the antitumor actions of these drugs; whether the agents differ in the patterns of cytoplasmic toxicity they induce; and whether these changes would be better evaluated by single- or multiple-assay systems.

Materials and Methods

The details of the methodology used have already been provided.[1,4,7,12,13] Only a relevant summary is provided here.

The cell lines utilized in these experiments were derived from malignant gliomas obtained at operation and grown from explants as stationary monolayers in Ham's F-10 nutrient medium (GIBCO, Grand Island, New York) with 10% fetal calf serum (FCS, GIBCO) at 37°C. Lines were routinely subcultured, using 1.0 ml trypsin-EDTA solution (0.05% trypsin and 0.02% EDTA solution) in a 10-minute incubation. To be certain of stable cell line properties, all experiments were done within the same passage, which in some cases required the use of cryopreserved cells. Lines were also screened routinely for mycoplasma by the flourochrome technique. None were positive.

Drug dilutions were prepared as previously described.[1,4,7,12,13] Taking into account the rapid decomposition of BCNU in medium, concentrations delivered to the cells were 80, 15, 5.0, 3.0, 2.0, and 1.0 µg/ml. Controls utilized the diluent, ethanol.

AZQ was delivered to the cells either in aqueous solution at 25-50 µg/ml or by surface plating of AZQ (by evaporation from an ethanol solution of AZQ. AZQ concentrations of 3.1 or 6.2 µg/ml were chosen based on microtiter assays showing that these concentrations plated on the culture surface by evaporation produced 50% or greater cell killing. Solubilization for the aqueous-phase testing of AZQ required dimethylacetamide (0.5%) in the nutrient medium. Since DMA, used in the aqueous assay, modifies the cell physiology (for example, it causes irreversible binding of hexokinase to the mitochondrial membrane), the surface plating assay provided a useful control. The surface-plating and aqueous delivery techniques, in fact, yielded similar cytotoxicity and ultrastructural data.

Cis-platinum was dissolved in the nutrient medium to achieve concentrations of 25, 50 and 100 μg/ml.

Cells were exposed to the drugs for periods of from 5 minutes to 72 hours. For BCNU, the short-exposure times were critical and both light (microcinematographic and histological) and electron microscopic methods were utilized to follow the cells. For the details of the microcinematography, see reference 6. Some changes occurred within minutes, and cell death was maximal by 18–24 hours. AZQ induced ultrastructural changes in the cells within the first few hours, but none in less than 1 hour. Maximal changes occurred by 48 hours. For cis-platinum, nonspecific cell rounding was seen as early as 4 hours, but the ultrastructural changes in the cytoplasm were not maximal until 72 hours, at which time the cell damage indicated by the microcytotoxicity assay was also high.

For preparation for electron microscopic examination, the cells were fixed in prewarmed (37°C) Karnovsky's fixative (pH 7.4) for 1 hour. They were then washed three times (10 minutes each) in 0.1 M cacodylate buffer, also at pH 7.4. Osmication used 1% osmium tetroxide in cacodylate buffer for 1 hour at 25°C. After graded cold (4°C) methanol dehydration, cells were embedded in Poly-Bed 812.

After polymerization the plastic disks were removed from the Costar tray wells and thick (1 μm) and thin (60–70 nm) sections were cut on an LKB-IV microtome. In the case of the thick sections for light microscopy, toluidine blue-0 staining was used. For the thin sections, saturated uranyl acetate and 0.5% lead citrate counterstaining was employed. Thin sections were examined with a JEOL 1OOCX electron microscope, with a minimum of 50 cells per experimental condition being utilized to define any changes.

Results

BCNU

BCNU-sensitive cells (with "sensitivity" defined in the microcytoxicity assay by 40% or greater cell death of up to 60 μg/ml) showed membrane blebbing and retraction within minutes of exposure to BCNU. Neither BCNU-resistant nor control cells showed these changes. The results with microcinematography, light microscope histology, and electron microcopy were all consistent.

In the sensitive cells, response was dependent on BCNU concentration. At 15 µg/ml, 69% of cells had blebs by 30 minutes, 87% by 90 minutes, and 100% by 4 hours. Lower concentrations produced lesser changes, with little or no change being seen at 2.0 and 1.0 µg/ml. On microcinematography,[7] some cells became quiescent after vigorous blebbing activity, but by 24 hours, almost universal cell death was evident.

On detailed ultrastructural examination, the blebs were filled with an homogenous, granular cytoplasm, generally stained more lightly than nonbleb cytoplasm and devoid of cytoplasmic organelles. Extensive cytoplasmic rearrangements could be seen. Four to 6 nm microfilaments stretched across the base of the blebs, with contraction or pinching-off evident. Consistent with this, membrane-bound cytoplamsic packets appeared to be shed by the cells. A perinuclear ring of 8–9 nm filaments was also evident in BCNU-treated cells, but not in controls.

AZQ

The pattern of change in the AZQ-treated cells was quite different.[12] There was no early bleb formation. Instead, within the first few hours of AZQ exposure, the formation of intracytoplasmic membranous whorls was a prominent but transient feature, more marked in the aqueous-treated cells. Mitochondrial changes, initially mitochondrial swelling and the appearance of diffuse, amorphous material in the spaces between cristae, were first seen 4 hours after AZQ exposure at the highest drug concentrations delivered by surface plating. These changes were progressive both in severity and in the number of cells affected. At 4 hours only 3–4% of cells showed such changes. At 8 hours, 45% of cells in one line and 12% in a second line had evidence of damaged mitochondria.

AZQ-induced mitochondrial changes became even more striking after 12 hours of exposure to both surface and aqueous deliveries at concentrations of 6.2 µg/mm² and 50 µg/ml, respectively. Approximately 50% of cells were involved in both lines with surface delivery. Light microscopy showed extensive vacuolization of the cells, which, on electron microscopy, could be seen to consist of mitochondria in varying stages of destruction. Remnants of cristae and electron-dense material were found within the mitochondria, the outer membranes of which were still intact.

By 24 hours, similar effects of the lower doses could also be seen. At 48 hours, the mitochondrial damage was observed in virtually 100% of cells at all doses. Some cell sections were devoid of any mitochondria, indicating severe disruption and actual breakdown.

Other changes induced by AZQ involved the nucleus and the endoplasmic reticulum. These included condensation of chromatin along the nuclear membrane and marked dilation of the endoplasmic reticulum, both beginning at 12 hours and increasing progressively to 48 hours, with the effects again dose-dependent.

Cis-Platinum

The pattern of cytotoxicity was different again for cis-platinum. Four changes were consistent: cell rounding and reduced nuclear-cytoplasmic ratio, nuclear chromatin clumping, vesiculation, and swelling of the Golgi apparatus, and dilation of the smooth endoplasmic reticulum, especially in the subplasmalemmal region. No mitochondrial changes or blebbing were seen.

Changes were detectable in all three structures as early as 4 hours; and although there were differences between lines in the appearance or degree of changes at a particular time, by 72 hours, virtually all of the cells showed nuclear and Golgi changes, and approximately 80% showed dilation of the endoplasmic reticulum.[13]

Discussion

The findings reported here make clear that distinct patterns of cytoplasmic toxicity in glioma-derived cells are associated with the DNA cross-linking agents, BCNU, AZQ, and cis-platinum. In addition, these cytoplasmic effects are relevant to the in vitro cell-death patterns observed, especially with BCNU and AZQ, in in vitro microcytotoxicity assays.

These investigations began with the question as to what might constitute an optimal in vitro assay system for the prediction of clinical response of patients with gliomas to available, or new, chemotherapy agents. Clearly, different effects of the agents being screened will be seen, depending on the particular assay used. With BCNU, for example, the microcytotoxicity assay used in our laboratory indicates, at least in part, early membrane damage, while the alkaline elution assay measures DNA alkylation and cross-linking.[1,4-6] The two assays do not contradict one another. They simply don't show the same types of cell injury. However, if both nuclear and non-nuclear targets are important in glioma cell death and a single assay is relied upon exclusively, some of the conclusions about sensitivity and/or resistance are likely to be misleading. At the least, potentially useful information will be lost.

Based on these findings, it would appear that multiple assays to screen for both nuclear and cytoplasmic effects may be required, if a reliable, predictive in vitro sensitivity-resistance system is to be developed. Useful assays include DNA assays, microcytotoxicity determinations of various types, colony-forming assays, immunological (humoral and/or cell-mediated) cytotoxicity assays, electron microscopy, and specific biochemical measurements, as they are suggested by the particular biology of the cell type or therapeutic agent in question. Given some, even preliminary, insights as to a given agent's range of cellular effects, a set of assays especially suited for that drug, yet practical and simple enough to provide useful, predictive information within a clinically relevant time could be defined. Beyond this, one would hope that the system of in vitro assays would provide a means to look at better drug combinations and metabolic, differentiation, and surface membrane manipulations designed to enhance chemotherapeutic agent effectiveness without increasing toxicity to patients. While in vitro systems can never duplicate in vivo host complexity, they have an important role to play in more accurately defining probabilities of effectiveness, enhancement of antitumor action, and avoidance of unnecessary patient toxicity.

Several questions remain to be answered about the findings reviewed here. First, the relationship of the cytoplasmic changes to the in vitro patterns of cell death needs to be established in much more quantitative detail. Secondly, can the cytoplasmic effects of BCNU, AZQ, and cis-platinum, as well as other agents, be manipulated in vitro to increase tumor cell death, especially at lower, less patient-toxic doses of chemotherapy agents? Are there opportunities for therapeutic synergy? Turning the issue around, are these non-nuclear cytotoxic effects important in the often therapy-limiting, normal-cell toxicity from chemotherapeutic agents? Could normal cells be protected at least in vitro? It seems very likely that normal bone marrow cells or lymphocytes, for example, should be included as part of an "optimal" in vitro chemotherapy agent screening program.

A crucial question is whether the non-nuclear changes seen in these experiments are clinically relevant? We cannot give a clear answer to that question as yet. Ultimately one would need tumor regression data, and relapse-free interval and survival data under conditions in which these effects were maximized to draw any firm conclusion. However, because we can correlate cell death patterns with these effects in vitro in the case of at least two of the three chemotherapy agents we have examined, it seems very likely that the effects are relevant and might be used to therapeutic advantage.

How could some of these effects be manipulated to therapeutic advantage? A specific example can be given for BCNU.

BCNU-induced glioma-cell membrane damage correlates with suppression of the glutathione-dependent peroxide detoxification system (Sanchez, Cummins, and Smith, unpublished observations). BCNU's carbamylating action apparently results in the covalent inactivation of glutathione reductase and thus the peroxidase system.[14,15] Nathan et al. have shown that pretreatment of murine tumors with BCNU in vitro increases macrophage-generated and exogenous peroxide-radical, induced cell killing, suggesting the possibility of using BCNU plus a peroxide-generating system to enhance the destruction of glial tumor tissue in vivo.[16] In addition, Nathan and Cohn have shown complete experimental tumor regression in mice treated with a combination of BCNU and a peroxide-generating system, with BCNU and peroxide by themselves being ineffective.[17] Taken together, the evidence at hand indicates that BCNU's antitumor actions should be thought of not only in relation to alkylation and cross-linking of DNA, but also inhibition of peroxide-detoxification mechanisms. Combination therapy based on this or parallel concepts not only offers the possibility of enhanced tumor-cell kill in tumors without alkylation repair capability, but also the possibility of using BCNU to treat tumors that have such repair capability and are thus "BCNU-resistant in relation to DNA alkylation."

Similarly, a broader concept of the potential antitumor effects of AZQ and cis-platinum might open new therapeutic approaches. Increasing response rate to a given agent, or even just enhancing the degree of antitumor effect in those who are responsive, are valuable goals. For example, could small doses of AZQ or other quinone derivatives, by impairing mitochondrial function, enhance the DNA-damaging effects of another chemotherapy agent, while minimizing bone marrow toxicity? Microsomal reduction of AZQ and other quinones has led to the suggestion that the free-radical intermediate, and perhaps subsequent superoxide production, may be necessary to the cytotoxic activity of AZQ. Could superoxide production be enhanced?[18,19]

The dramatic effects of cis-platinum on the endoplasmic reticulum, especially in the subplasmalemmal zone, and reports indicating that it alters the surface properties of tumor cells, and thereby their susceptibility to immune destruction,[20-25] suggest still another approach: the combination of cytotoxic chemotherapy with immunotherapy. This takes on particular significance for glial tumors because some glioma cell populations secrete an extracellular mucopolysaccharide "halo" or coat that can inhibit the approach of cytotoxic lymphocytes.[26,27] If cis-platinum can both damage tumor cell DNA and reduce the effectiveness of the extracellular "coat" as a shield against cytotoxic lymphocytes, then we may have an important new anti-glioma therapy. In other words, thinking of cis-platinum as a membrane-active as well as a DNA cross-linking agent opens up new therapeutic possibilities.

If the use of multiple-assay systems brings out such new therapeutic possibilities, while increasing the accuracy of in vitro prediction of clinical sensitivity and resistance, the promise of such systems will have more than been fulfilled.

Summary

The use of in vitro assays to predict clinical response to chemotherapy for glioma patients is attractive and, current evidence indicates, achievable. A critical question is what constitutes an optimal in vitro system. Should it consist of a single assay or multiple assays of different types? If DNA is the primary target of a drug, is an assay that evaluates changes in DNA sufficient?

Alkylation and/or cross-linking of DNA have been considered to be the critical antitumor actions of BCNU (1,3-bis (2-chloroethyl)-1-nitrosourea), AZQ (aziridinylbenzoquinone, 2,5-diaziridinyl-3, 6-bis-(carboethoxyamino)-1,4-benzoquinone), and cis-platinum (cis-dichloroammineplatinum [II]). However, each of the three agents also causes a specific pattern of cytoplasmic injury.

BCNU produces striking blebbing of the membrane of the tumor cells within minutes, and this effect correlates with the early cell death (18–24 hours) seen in one microcytotoxicity assay, but not in DNA assays. With AZQ, mitochondrial toxicity is prominent and consistent with multifactorial cytotoxicity indicated by a variety of assays. Cis-platinum causes dilated subendoplasmic reticulum, and swelling and vesiculation of the perinuclear golgi apparatus. However, cell-death time patterns are consistent with DNA damage.

The data suggest that the non-nuclear targets can be important in determining tumor cell cytotoxicity for DNA cross-linking agents and that a panel of in vitro assays may be required to reliably predict in vivo clinical sensitivity or resistance. In addition, understanding the non-nuclear damage, even if it is not the primary factor in tumor cell death, may suggest ways to enhance chemotherapeutic agent effectiveness.

REFERENCES

1. Kornblith PL, Smith BH, Leonard LA. Response of cultured human brain tumors to nitrosoureas: correlation with clinical data. Cancer 1981; 47:255–265.
2. Thomas DGT, Darling JA, Paul EA, Mott TJ, Godlee JN, Tobias JS, Capra LG, Collins CD, Mooney C, Bozek T, Finn GP, Arigbabu SO, Bullard DE, Shannon N, Freshney RI. Assay of anticancer drugs in tissue culture: Relationship of relapse-free interval (RFI) and in vitro chemosensitivity in patients with malignant cerebral glioma. Br J Cancer 1985; 51:525–532.
3. Kimmel D, Shapiro JR, Shapiro WR. In vitro drug sensitivity testing in human gliomas. J Neurosurg 1987; 66:161–171.
4. Kornblith PL, Szypko PE. Variations in response of human brain tumors to BCNU in vitro. J Neurosurg 1978; 48:580–586.
5. Erickson LC, Laurent G, Sharkey NA, Kohn KW. DNA Cross-linking and monoadduct repair in nitrosourea-treated human tumor cells. Nature 1980; 288:727–729.
6. Sariban E, Kohn KW, Zlotogorski C, Laurent G, D'Incalci M, Day RS III, Smith BH, Kornblith PL, Erickson LC. DNA cross-linking response in human malignant glioma cell strains to chloroethylnitrosoureas, cisplatin, and diaziquone. Cancer Res 1987; 47:3988–3994.
7. Smith BH, Vaughn M, Greenwood MA, Kornblith PL, Robinson A, Shitara N, McKeever PE. Membrane and cytoplasmic changes in 1,3-bis(2-chloroethyl)-1-nitrosourea (BCNU)-sensitive and -resistant human malignant glioma-derived cell lines. J Neuro-Oncol 1983; 1:237–248.
8. Kohn KW. Mechanistic approaches to new nitrosourea development. Rec Res Cancer Res 1981; 76:141–152.
9. Zwelling LA, Kohn KW. Mechanism of action of cis-dichloro-diammineplatinum (II). Cancer Treat Rep 1979; 63:1439–1443.

10. Akhtar MH, Begleiter A, Johnson D, Lown JW, McLaughlin L, Sim SK. Studies related to antitumor antibiotics. Part IV. Correlation of covalent cross-linking of DNA by bifunctional aziridinoquinones with their neoplastic activities. Can J Chem 1975; 53:2891–2905.

11. Rosenberg B. Possible mechanism for the antitumor activity of platinum coordination complexes. Cancer Chemother Rep 1975; 59: 589–598.

12. Oberc-Greenwood MA, Smith BH, Cooke C, Ellis JR, Kornblith PL, McKeever PE. Mitochondrial toxicity of 2,5-diaziridinyl-3,6-bis-(carboethoxyamino)-1, 4-benzoquinone. JNCI 1983; 71:723–733.

13. Oberc-Greenwood MA, Smith BH, Cooke C, Pepin C, Kornblith PL. Selective cytoplasmic and membrane changes induced by cis-platinum. J Neuro-Oncol, in press, 1988.

14. Babson JR, Reed DJ. Inactivation of glutathione reductase by 2-chloroethylnitrosourea-derived isocyanates. Biochem Biophys Res Comm 1978; 83:754–762.

15. Frischer H, Ahmad T. Severe generalized glutathione reductase deficiency after antitumor chemotherapy with BCNU (1,3-bis(chloroethyl)-1-nitrosourea). J Lab Clin Med 1977; 89:1080-1091.

16. Nathan CF, Arrick BA, Murray HW, DeSantis NM, Cohn ZA. Tumor cell antioxidant defenses. Inhibition of the glutathione redox cycle enhances macrophage-mediated cytolysis. J Exp Med 1981; 153:766–782.

17. Nathan CF, Cohn ZA. Antitumor effects of hydrogen peroxide in vivo. J Exp Med 1981; 153:766–782.

18. Bachur NR, Gordon SL, Gee MV, Kon H. NADPH cytochrome P-450 reductase activation of quinone anticancer agents to free radicals. Proc Natl Acad Sci USA 1979; 76:954–957.

19. Gutierrez PL, Friedman RD, Bachur NR. Biochemical activation of AZQ [3,6-diaziridinyl-2,5-bis(carboethoxyamino) 1,4-benzoquinone] to its free radical species. Cancer Treat Rep 1982; 66:339–342.

20. Juckett DA, Rosenberg B. Actions of cis-platinum on cell surface nucleic acids in cancer cells as determined by cell electrophoresis. Cancer Res 1982; 42:3565–3573.

21. Kleinerman ES, Howser D, Young RC, Bull J, Zwelling LA, Barlock A, Decker JM, Muchmore AV. Defective monocyte killing in patients with malignancies and restoration of function during chemotherapy. Lancet 1980; Nov:1102–1105.

22. Aggarawal SK, Sodhi A. Cytotoxic effects of cis-dichlorodiammineplatinum (II) on mammalian cells in vitro: A fine ultrastructural study. Cytobiologie 1973; 7:366–374.

23. Aggarawal SK, Niroomand-rad I. Effect of cisplatin on the plasma membrane phosphatase activities in ascites sarcoma-180 cells. A cytochemical study. J Histochem Cytochem 1983; 31:307-317.

24. Sodhi A. Ultrastructural observations on the effect of cis-dichlorodiammineplatinum (II) on the cells of ascites fibrosarcoma in mice: Part I. Interaction of macrophages with fibrosarcoma cells. Ind J Exp Biol 1979; 17:623–627.

25. Sodhi A, Bali Prasad S. Ultrastructural and fluorescence microscopical observations on the effect of cis-dichloro diammineplatinum (II) on the surface of normal and tumor cells. Ind J Exp Biol 1981; 19:328–332.

26. Dick SJ, Macchi B, Papazoglou S, Oldfield EH, Kornblith PL, Smith BH, Gately M. The production of mucopolysaccharide coats by human glioma cells: a mechanism by which tumors may escape cell-mediated immune attack. Science 1983; 13:739–742.
27. Oberc-Greenwood MA, Muul LM, Gately MK, Kornblith PL, Smith BH. Ultrastructural features of the lymphocyte-stimulated halos produced by human glioma-derived cells in vitro. J Neuro-Oncol 1986; 3:387–396.

18

Preclinical Models for Differentiation Therapy

Daniel L. Dexter and Janet L. Gross

Introduction

The concept that naturally produced substances or synthetic compounds can induce a more differentiated phenotype in tumor cells is not novel. Markert, in 1968 in a seminal paper dealing with the subject, defined cancer as "a disease of differentiation."[1] Van Potter's biochemical theory of cancer 20 years ago referred to the disease as a case of "oncogeny is blocked ontogeny,"[2,3] another way to state Markert's hypothesis. The spontaneous differentiation observed in murine teratocarcinomas in the laboratories of Pierce, Stevens, and others two to three decades ago[4,5] led Pierce to postulate that directed maturation of cancer cells could serve as an alternative to cytotoxic chemotherapy.[6] He postulated that differentiation might be induced in cancer cells by naturally produced "physiological" inducers or by chemical agents.[6] Indeed, Landau and Sachs in the 1960s identified a substance produced by normal embryo cells that differentiated mouse myeloid leukemia cells to macrophages and granulocytes.[7] The factor, designated MGI, was later shown to be a specific colony stimulating factor (CSF) involved in hematopoietic stem cell differentiation.[8] In 1967, Dyke and Mulkey interpreted several cases of spontaneous regressions of neuroblastomas in children as being due to the maturation of malignant neuroblastoma to benign gan-

From: Kornblith PL, Walker MD (editors). Advances in Neuro-Oncology. Futura Publishing Company, Inc., Mount Kisco, NY, © 1988.

glioneuroma.[9] Their report, based on histological evidence, explained a phenomenon that had been observed occasionally with pediatric neuroblastomas since the early part of this century.[10,11] These observations[9-11] with neuroblastoma were important because they extended the thinking on cancer differentiation from murine tumors to human solid tumors in a clinical setting.

Thus the conceptual basis for considering differentiation therapy as an alternative, or adjunct, to conventional cancer treatment protocols, was advanced decades ago by several investigators, and was supported by data obtained with animal tumors and at least one type of human cancer. These findings were largely ignored during the advent of cancer chemotherapy in the 1960s and 1970s. Killing tumor cells with combinations of cytotoxic drugs, or drugs and ionizing radiation, following surgery, became the objective of clinicians facing an aggressive disease. Initial successes with childhood leukemia, lymphoma, choriocarcinoma, and more recently with testicular cancer offered hope that treatment with cytotoxic modalities might lead to significant reduction in cancer deaths.[12,13] Unfortunately, our armamentarium of drugs, radiation, and other modalities has not had significant impact on deaths due to solid tumors especially those of the lung, prostate and G.I. tract.[14] Accordingly, the utilization of naturally produced or synthetic chemical inducers of differentiation in maturational therapy protocols has become an attractive alternative approach in preclinical and clinical cancer research.

Work with Leukemia Cells

During the past 20 years when aggressive treatment with cytotoxic modalities was being developed through more sophisticated clinical trials,[15] there were continued laboratory investigations in cancer differentiation. This new interest was sparked primarily from the findings by Friend and co-workers that dimethylsulfoxide (DMSO), a polar solvent, could induce the maturation of a murine erythroleukemia cell line (MEL cells) to terminally differentiated, post-mitotic cells which produced hemoglobin.[16] Subsequent studies then showed that a variety of chemicals could induce erythroid differentiation in MEL cells[17-21]; the erythroid differentiation has since been elegantly characterized to the molecular level.[22-24]

These studies critically demonstrated for the first time that simple chemical agents could stimulate the differentiation of tumor cells.

However, the implication for therapy was not fully appreciated since the MEL cell model was a murine culture system which had been originally transformed by a virus. Also, there was no evidence for in vivo differentiation and finally, the relevance of the model could be questioned since erythroleukemia in man was not a significant clinical problem.

In 1977, the HL-60 cell line was described by Collins et al.[25,26] The HL-60 line was derived from leukemic cells from a patient with myeloid leukemia; these cells have proven responsive to a variety of differentiating agents from several distinct chemical classes.[27] In an important study, Fontana et al. demonstrated that HL-60 cells have a bidirectional differentiation potential; DMSO and retinoic acid induce the granulocyte phenotype whereas the phorbol diesters cause the maturation of HL-60 cells to a macrophage phenotype.[28] HL-60 cells have also been utilized to investigate the relationships among oncogene expression, proliferation, and differentiation. Various groups have reported modulation of oncogene expression including *c-myc*, *c-fms*, and *c-amv* following exposure of HL-60 cells to differentiating agents.[29-34] Thus, the HL-60 cell line has provided a relevant model for the study of the differentiation of human cancer cells at the morphological, biochemical, and genetic levels. This myeloid leukemia system has provided a great impetus for work with differentiating agents.

Studies with Solid Tumor Cells

Investigations have been conducted on the effects of differentiating agents on solid tumor cells as well as on leukemia cells. Mouse rhabdomyosarcoma cells treated with dimethylformamide (DMF) had a significantly reduced tumorigenicity compared to untreated cells. Creatine kinase activity (a biochemical marker of muscle differentiation) in these same cells was significantly increased when the rhabdomyosarcoma cells were cultured in the presence of sodium butyrate.[35] Murine neuroblastoma cells have shown a change in membrane potential following exposure to DMSO.[36] Teratocarcinoma cells treated with retinoic acid have also demonstrated a more benign phenotype.[37] Importantly, Speers has shown in vivo induction of differentiation in murine teratomas following administration of retinoic acid to mice bearing these tumors.[38,39] This was an important finding because it indicated that solid tumors may be susceptible to differentiation agents, and thus the induction process is not limited to cultured cancer cells.

Experiments in vitro have also been conducted using human solid tumor cells as targets for differentiating agents. DMSO treatment of human lung cancer cells has induced increased cilia formation, a marker of lung tissue.[40] Human melanoma cells exposed to the active phorbol diester 12-O-tetradecanoyl phorbol–13-acetate (TPA) or to DMSO have been converted to post-mitotic cells containing increased melanin.[41] Other groups have also studied the ability of retinoids to differentiate human melanoma cells.[42,43] We have recently reported that human glioma cells treated with butyrate have an altered malignant phenotype including marked reductions in the activity of the serine protease, plasminogen activator (PA), and in the clonogenicity of the glioma cells in soft agar.[44]

Maturational agents have also been used to induce a more benign phenotype in cultured human colon cancer cells. Exposure of human colon carcinoma cells to DMF caused a striking loss of malignant characteristics, including complete loss of clonogenicity in agar and a marked decrease in tumorigenicity in nude mice.[45] Differentiation markers have also been modulated in human colon cancer cells treated with maturational agents. Several cell lines (HCT–15, DLD–1, and two clones of DLD–1) have shown increased expression of membrane-associated carcinoembryonic antigen (CEA) following exposure to DMF.[46] Tsao et al. have demonstrated increased secretion of CEA following treatment of cultured HCT–18 rectal carcinoma cells with butyrate.[47] Normal colonic mucin antigen has been increased in HCT–15 and DLD–1 cells, and tumor colonic mucin antigen has been decreased, when these cells were cultured in the presence of DMF.[46] Expression of surface lipoproteins on colorectal tumor cells has been modulated by butyrate.[48] Glycogen levels in HCT–15 cells have increased following butyrate treatment,[49] and levels of purine metabolizing enzymes have been modulated by both butyrate and DMF in HCT–15, clone A and clone D colon cancer cells.[50] Thus, several biochemical markers of differentiation have been expressed following the exposure of human colon tumor cells to various differentiating agents.

Differentiating agents have also had significant effects on the growth of human solid tumors in vivo. Treatment with the polar solvents DMF or N-methylformamide (NMF) has been shown to inhibit the growth of two human colon tumors (DLD–2 and HCT–15) implanted s.c. in athymic mice. Intraperitoneal administration of 300 mg/kg NMF for 21 days to mice bearing subcutaneous implants of DLD–2 colon carcinoma produced a 75% inhibition in the growth of the solid tumor.[51] Similar results against human xenograft tumors were achieved when NMF and DMF were tested in the NCI Therapeutic Development Program.[52] Because of these results, NMF has been introduced into Phase 1/2 clinical trials.[52-54] However, it has not been established whether polar solvents inhibit the growth of human colon cancers in nude mice because of a differentiating mechanism or due to tumoricidal action.[55] The experiments described above do, however, establish that polar solvents that differentiate leukemia and solid tumor cells in tissue culture (at nontoxic concentrations) can also have an antitumor effect in vivo.

Classes of Differentiating Agents

Studies on leukemia cell differentiation have led to the important finding that many structurally unrelated classes of compounds can induce cancer cell maturation. The list of chemical inducers include polar solvents, retinoids, vitamin D analogs, certain phorbol disters, short chain fatty acids, and a number of (but not all) conventional anticancer drugs.[27,55-58] Cytotoxic agents that can induce the maturation of cultured murine and human leukemia cells at nontoxic concentrations include cytosine arabinoside (ara C) and adriamycin. The existence of distinct classes of maturational agents implies the operation of different mechanisms of differentiation induction, which will be agent-dependent. This has been demonstrated for leukemia cells wlth butyrate, polar solvents, and phorbol diesters, among others,[18,28,55,59,60] through the use of variant clones, although the specific mechanisms have not been elucidated.

The responses of various types of tumor cells to distinct classes of agents can also be quite diverse. Three examples will be presented here. Vitamin A has been associated with normal epithelial cell differentiation and has been identified as a potential inhibitor of carcinogenesis since the 1920s.[61,62] Retinoic acid, a vitamin A metabolite, is a good inducer of differentiation for cultured human melanoma cells.[41-43] In contrast, retinoic acid actually increases the proliferation of certain malignant cells[63] including the growth of colon cancer cells in soft agar.[64] The growth of tumor cells in soft agar is considered a property or marker of the malignant phenotype, and conversely, a loss of clonogenicity in agar indicates a cell with a benign phenotype.

Thus retinoids may be useful for the differentiation therapy of melanomas, but could be detrimental for the treatment of colon carcinomas. By comparison, agents such as DMF and NMF abrogate the clonogenicity of colon and other tumor cells in semi-solid medium,[45,65] and may be useful in the treatment of intestinal tumors. The phorbol diester TPA is a potent inducer of the macrophage phenotype in human HL-60 leukemia cells,[28] yet it antagonizes differentiation induction by polar solvents in MEL cells.[59] Again, the same agent can have distinct, even opposite effects on differentiation depending on the target tumor cell. The finding that TPA is a tumor promoter in vivo for normal cells,[66] whereas it is an inducer of differentiation for some cultured leukemia cell lines presents another paradox. Once again the biological effect of a chemical stimulus (TPA) will depend on the cell target.

Vitamin D analogs, like TPA, are potent inducers of macrophage differentiation in HL-60 cells; $1\alpha,25$-dihydroxy vitamin D_3 induces HL-60 maturation in the nanomolar range.[67,68] Moreover, like TPA, the dihydroxy vitamin D_3 analog enhances chemically induced transformation of 3T3 mouse fibroblasts to malignant cells and antagonizes the DMSO-induced differentiation of MEL cells.[69,70] However, differences in biological activity between TPA and dihydroxy vitamin D_3 have also been demonstrated. For example, Sasaki et al. recently reported that whereas TPA and dihydroxy vitamin D_3 enhanced the chemical transformation of mouse 3T3 fibroblasts, only TPA also induced ornithine decarboxylase during the transformation process.[71]

The above examples illustrate that the response of a cancer cell to a differentiation inducer will be agent-specific and will also depend on the type of cancer cell exposed to the agent. Moreover, when a given tumor cell differentiates to the same phenotypic end-point when treated with distinct differentiating chemicals, the mechanism of differentiation in each case may also be unique, The studies discussed above indicate that it will be important to match differentiating agents with tumor types if one wishes to successfully use differentiating agents in preclinical or clinical investigations.

The Development of Preclinical Models for the Differentiation Therapy of Solid Tumors

Although conventional and maturational therapies for the treatment of solid tumors have the same goal, i.e., the reduction and ul-

---

Table 1
Suggested Markers for Differentiation
of Solid Tumors

- General Markers for Solid Tumor Cells
    - Loss of clonogenicity in soft agar
    - Depression of plasminogen activator activity
    - Loss of proliferative capacity
    - Loss of tumorigenicity
    - Morphological changes
    - Alteration of oncogene expression
- Markers Specific for Distinct Tumor Tissue Types
    - Mucin and CEA antigens for colon cancer
    - Melanin and tyrosinase levels for melanomas
    - Estrogen receptor levels for breast cancer
    - Peptide markers for small cell lung cancer
    - Expression of glial fibrillary acidic protein (GFAP)
        and S100 protein for gliomas
    - Keratin for squamous cell carcinomas

---

timate eradication of tumor burden, the mechanism of action of maturational agents is expected to be different from that of cytotoxic drugs. Therefore, guidelines must be devised to administer compounds that act in the differentiation mode and to assess their efficacy from the standpoint of their effects on cellular differentiation as well as on tumor progression. A rational approach to evaluate compounds preclinically must be initiated first in vitro, and then in vivo with appropriate animal models, if maturational therapy is to have any chance of success in the clinic.

Several concepts are implicit in the use of maturational agents both preclinically and clinically. First, differentiation agents should arrest the growth of tumor cells at nontoxic doses. Second, these agents should induce the differentiation of cells as assessed by morphologic, biochemical, antigenic, or functional criteria; examples of both general and specific markers for differentiation of solid tumor cells are shown in Table 1. The general markers include characteristics common to all malignancies such as clonogenicity in agar and tumorigenicity in the appropriate host. A specific marker would be a molecule characteristic of the (differentiated) normal tissue from which the neoplasm developed. The markers listed in Table 1 have been discussed for the most part earlier in this review. Third, mat-

Table 2
Development of Maturational Agents

Cell Culture (In Vitro)	Animal Model (In Vivo)	Clinical
Loss of malignant properties 　growth arrest in monolayers 　loss of clonogenicity in soft agar 　loss of tumorigenicity of cultured cancer cells in appropriate animal host	Cessation of tumor growth or reduction in tumor burden at nontoxic doses	Cessation of tumor growth or reduction in tumor burden at nontoxic doses
Assessment of functional differentiation 　morphological 　biochemical 　antigenic	Assessment of functional differentiation 　histological 　bichemical 　antigenic *and* Toxicology Bio-availability Scheduling protocols Combination protocols	Assessment of functional differentiation 　histological　access to pre- 　biochemical　and post- 　antigenic　treatment tissues *and* Clinical Pharmacology Drug Metabolism
Specificity 　tumor type 　class of maturational agent	Specificity	Specificity

urational compounds should be tumor tissue-specific, that is each solid tumor type will have a characteristic pattern of response to each mechanistic or structural class of agent.

A schematic diagram of the development of maturational agents from preclinical to clinical protocols is shown in Table 2. Predictive in vitro and in vivo cancer models for each tumor tissue type will be essential for the identification of clinically efficacious maturational agents. In selecting a cancer cell line as representatlve of a given tumor type, the following factors should be considered. First, the line should be well characterized. Second, the line should be capable of differentiation in culture when exposed to known maturational agents. In order to assess this differentiation, the line should have known general or specific markers which can be modulated by maturational compounds. Third, the cells should be capable of expanded growth in vitro if cell injection into animals or large numbers of cells for biochemical analysis are required. Fourth, the line should produce tumors in animal hosts that develop with a reasonable and reproducible latency period and frequency. Ideally, the line should be capable of growth in an animal model at anatomical locations similar to those seen clinically. For instance, a human glioma line should be able to proliferate intracranially in a nude mouse model.

Once an animal model is established, such factors as scheduling protocols, reversibility of drug action, and pharmocokinetics can be evaluated for a given class of maturational agent. Maturational agents in animal models should cause at the minimum a cessation of tumor growth at nontoxic doses and should cause neoplastic tissue differentiation as assessed by histology or biochemical parameters. Toxicology studies should also be done with animals. Factors to be considered in toxicity tests would include conventional parameters and also effects on normal stem cell populations (i.e., those in the bone marrow, gut, and skin). When the animal model work is completed, the agent could be tested in phase 1/phase 2 protocols against the tumor type(s) for which the drug candidate has shown specificity in its preclinical evaluation. Factors which need to be addressed in cancer patients would be toxicity, drug metabolism, and pharmacokinetics, as well as efficacy and the induction of differentiation in the tumor.

In an effort to establish a preclinical model for the differentiation of human brain neoplasms, we examined the ability of two human glioma lines to propagate in vitro and in vivo in nude mice.[72] As general markers for solid tumor cell differentiation, two properties of each line in vitro were assessed: first, anchorage independence as measured by the ability of cancer cells to grow in soft agar,[65,73] and second, the activity of plasminogen activator (PA), a well-characterized serine protease. Elevated PA activity has been shown to correlate with tumorgenicity,[74] metastatic capacity,[74] and to be influenced by the differentiation state of the cell.[75] Our hypothesis, therefore, was (1) a highly tumorigenic and perhaps less-differentiated glioma would be clonogenic in soft agar and exhibit relatively high PA activity, and (2) maturational agents could modulate both these properties.

The activity of PA, as measured by the ^{125}I-fibrin plate assay,[76] was examined in detergent extracts from two human glioma lines as a function of growth in vitro. Although there were no significant dif-

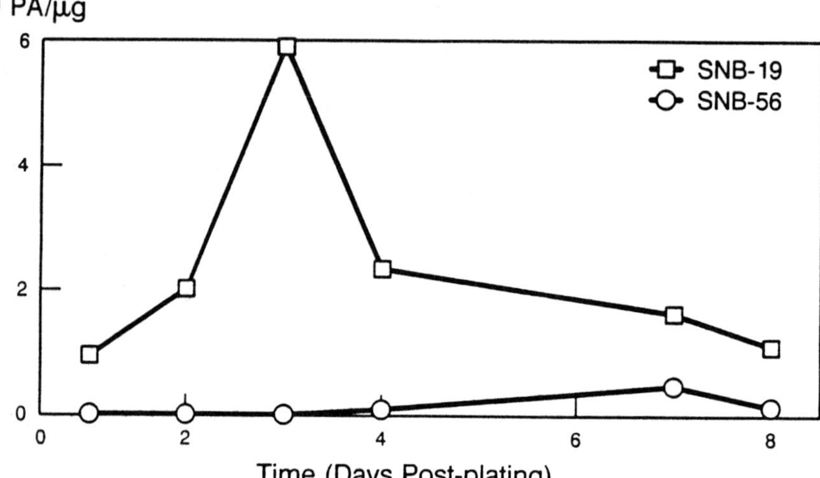

Figure 1. Kinetics of human glioma PA activity. Human glioma cells were plated on day 0. On various days post-plating, cells from triplicate cultures were extracted in Triton X–100 and 1 μg samples of the extracts were assayed for PA activity, as previously described.[76] (Adapted from Gross et al.[72])

Table 3
Correlation of PA Activity with Malignant Parameters

Glioma Line	PA Activity (mU/μg)	Clonogenicity Soft Agar (%)	Tumorgenicity Nude Mice
SNB-19	3.20	41.5	+ + + +
SNB-56	0.05	1.2	−

Glioma cells were plated on day 0 and fed daily with growth medium. On day three, triplicate cultures were extracted with detergent. Detergent extracts were assayed for PA activity. The ^{125}I-fibrin plate assay[76] data represents the average of three separate experiments and are expressed as mU PA activity per μg protein.

Clonogenicity in soft agar was assessed by counting colony formation from 90,000 cells/60 mm dish after a 4-week period.[72]

Tumorigenicity in nude mice was determined by measuring tumor growth during a 90-day period after injecting 10^7 cells of each line s.c. (10 mice/line).

Adapted from Gross et al.[72]

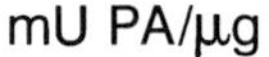

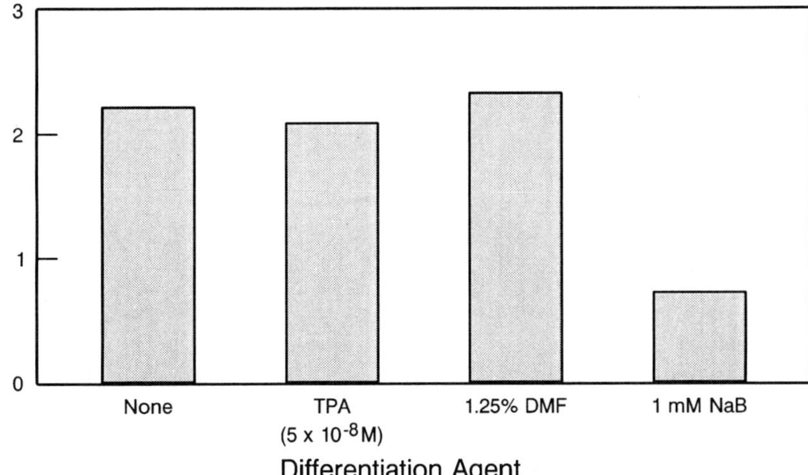

Figure 2. Effect of known differentiating agents on SNB-19 PA activity. SNB-19 cells were plated on day 0 and fed daily with fresh growth medium. Three days post-plating, varying concentrations of known differentiation agents were added. After 30 hours, cells from triplicate cultures were harvested, pelleted, and extracted with Triton X–100. Cell associated PA activity was assayed using 1 µg samples of cell protein.[76] (Modified from Gross et al.[72])

ferences in growth kinetics between the lines (data not shown), the kinetics of PA activity differed markedly, as shown in Figure 1. One line, SNB-19, exhibited maximal PA activity as cultures approached confluence; SNB-19 had very high PA activity which peaked 3–4 days post-plating. In contrast, another line, SNB-56 exhibited no significant PA activity at any time in culture.[72]

The relative PA activities of the two glioma lines correlated with other malignant parameters including anchorage independence and tumorigenicity in nude mice. As shown in Table 3, SNB-19, which had the highest intracellular PA activity, was the most clonogenic in soft agar and the most tumorigenic in nude mice when injected subcutaneously. SNB–56, which had no intracellular PA activity, was neither clonogenic in soft agar nor tumorigenic in nude mice (Table 3), in agreement with its low PA activity.[72]

Since PA activity has been modulated by differentiation agents in other solid tumor lines in vitro, the effects of knowm maturational agents on SNB-19 peak PA activity was examined. Three agents,

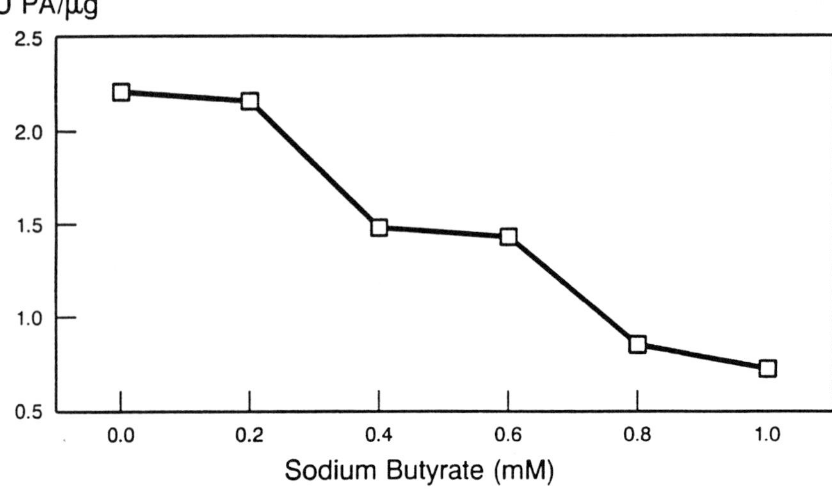

Figure 3. Effect of sodium butyrate on SNB-19 PA activity. SNB-19 cells were plated on day 0 and fed daily with fresh growth medium. Three days post-plating, varying concentrations of sodium butyrate were added to cells. Cells from triplicate cultures were harvested 30 hours later and extracted with Triton X-100. Cell extracts (1 μg) were assayed for PA activity.[76] (Adapted from Gross et al.[72])

known to affect differentiation in several solid tumor and leukemia lines,[55,77] were each added to day 3 SNB-19 cultures. Thirty hours after the addition of either the phorbol diester TPA (5×10^{-8}M), the polar solvent DMF (1.0% v/v), or sodium butyrate (NaB, 1 mH) at nontoxic concentrations, cell-associated PA activity was measured. As demonstrated in Figure 2, 1 mM NaB significantly reduced measurable PA activity, whereas the other agents had no effect on the activity of this protease.[72]

The effects of NaB on peak SNB-19 PA activity were both dose- and time-dependent. The dose-response for the NaB-induced reduction in SNB-19 PA activity is shown in Figure 3. The concentration required for a 50% reduction in peak SNB-19 PA activity was approximately 0.75 mM, which is below the concentration required to inhibit by 50% the growth of the cells (IC_{50} = 1.4 mM). Furthermore, the treated cells were 95% viable as measured by trypan blue dye exclusion. The kinetics of reduction of SNB-19 peak PA activity by NaB is depicted in Figure 4. Maximum reduction (84%) in PA activity was observed 48 hours after the addition of 0.75 mM NaB. NaB (0.5

mU PA/μg

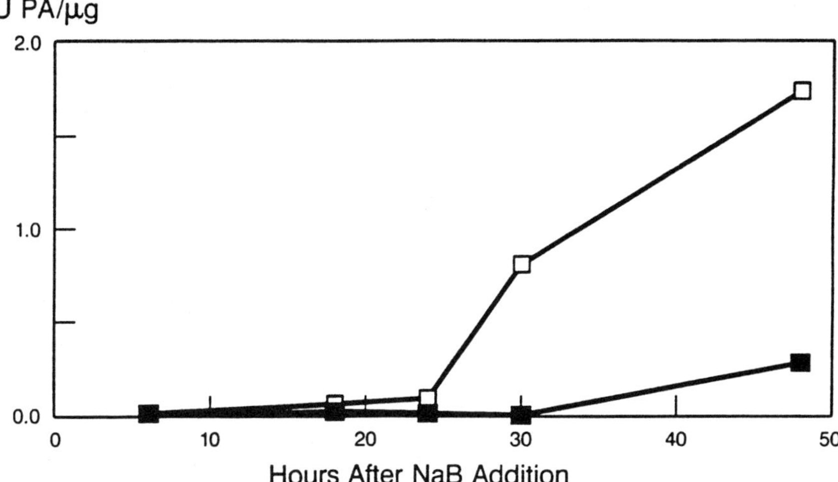

Figure 4. Kinetics of SNB-19 activity with sodium butyrate. SNB-19 cells were plated on day 0 and fed daily with fresh growth medium. Three days post-plating, growth medium with (■) or without (□) 0.75 mM sodium butyrate was added to the cultures. At various times after sodium butyrate addition, cells from triplicate cultures were harvested, pelleted, and detergent-extracted. Cell-associated PA activity was measured using 1 μg cell protein.

mM) also reduced SNB-19 clonogenicity in soft agar by 98% (data not shown).[76]

The results thus far suggest that the SNB-19 human glioma line may be a useful preclinical model for maturational agents both in vitro and in vivo. The cells have general biochemical markers of malignancy in vitro (PA and anchorage independence) which can be modulated by at least one differentiating agent, NaB. Specific glial/glioma markers such as glial fibrillary acid protein (GFAP), high affinity glutamic acid and α-amino butyric acid uptake, and glutamine synthetase activity[78] are potential targets for modulation by maturational agents and have not yet been examined. Our initial data indicate that the SNB-19 line might provide an appropriate in vivo preclinical model for maturational agents, since the cells grow easily in culture, the tumor incidence with 10^7 cells/inoculum is excellent (100%), and tumor growth occurs within a reasonable length of time. However, the induction of differentiation in SNB-19 gliomas growing in nude mice treated with maturational agents remains to be demonstrated. Ideally, the intracranial growth of SNB-19 cells would be most analogous to the clinical situation and the development of the intracranial model for differentiation therapy should be pursued.[79] In conclusion, our data indicate that glioma lines such as SNB-19 may be useful in the identification of differentiating agents that would be effective in the treatment of this neoplasm.

Summary

There has been significant progress in recent years in the development of differentiating agents for the treatment of cancer. This constitutes a novel approach to cancer therapy by which tumor progression may be controlled and the disease arrested through the maturation of cancer cells to benign cells. The concept of maturational therapy grew out of phenomenological observations made decades ago. However, this idea was not immediately accepted because of the prevailing view that "once a cancer cell always a cancer cell," necessitating the destruction of all the tumor cells in a patient in order to cure the individual. Therefore, emphasis was placed on aggressive therapy with combinations of cytotoxic drugs and radiation. Since several decades of cytotoxic therapy have not significantly affected 5-year survival rates for many of the solid tumors, alternative approaches, such as differentiation therapy, have recently generated considerable interest.

While clinicians were pursuing aggressive cytotoxic therapies, basic scientists began to make advances in the use of chemicals to induce the differentiation of cultured cancer cells, especially leukemia cells. From 1970, there has been steady progress in research directed at causing the differentiation of murine and human leukemia and solid tumor cells with maturational agents. More recently, efforts have been made in the laboratory to treat tumor-bearing mice with these agents in order to achieve a tumor response based on the triggering of differentiation events in the neoplasm. Thus, it is now possible to develop a preclinical approach to identify agents capable of differentiating tumor cells in vitro and in vivo, and to match the appropriate agent and tumor type for optimal efficacy. Each pairing of agent and tumor could be extended to the appropriate patient population in phase 1/phase 2 clinical trials.

It is most encouraging that clinical trials with differentiating agents have already been initiated. A number of trials have been conducted using low-dose ara C for the differentiation therapy of myelodysplastic syndrome and frank leukemia,[80-82] and many other trials are ongoing. Hexamethylene bisacetamide (HMBA), a polar planar molecule, has recently been introduced into the clinic as a differentiating agent.[83,84] Thus preclinical and clinical research efforts with maturational agents are converging, and coordinated investigations between basic researchers and medical and radiation oncologists are quite feasible and should lead to exciting new findings.

REFERENCES

1. Markert CL. Neoplasia, a disease of differentiation. Cancer Res 1968; 28:1908–1914.
2. Potter VR. Recent trends in cancer biochemistry: the importance of studies on fetal tissues. Can Cancer Conf 1968; 8:9–14.
3. Potter VR. Phenotypic diversity in experimental hepatomas: the concept of partially blocked ontogeny. Br J Cancer 1978; 38:1–22.
4. Pierce BG, Dixon FJ, Verney DL. Teratogenic and tissue forming potentials of cell types comprising neoplastic embryoid bodies. Lab Invest 1960; 9:583–602.
5. Stevens LC. Experimental production of testicular teratomas in mice. Proc Natl Acad Sci USA 1964; 52: 254–261.
6. Pierce GB. The benign cells of malignant tumors. In: Developmental Aspects of Carcinogenesis and Immunity, TJ King, ed. New York, Academic Press, 1974; pp. 3–22.
7. Landau T, Sachs L. Characterization of the inducer required for the development of macrophage and granulocyte colonies. Proc Natl Acad Sci USA 1971; 68:2540–2544.
8. Metcalf D. The granulocyte-macrophage colony-stimulating factors. Science 1985; 229:16–22.
9. Dyke PC, Mulkey D. Maturation of ganglioneuroblastoma to ganglioneuroma. Cancer 1967; 20:1343–1349.
10. Cushing H, Wolbach SB. The transformation of a malignant paravertebral sympathicoblastoma into a benign ganglioneuroma. Am J Pathol 1927; 3:203–230.
11. Fox F, Davidson J, Tumas LB. Maturation of a sympathicoblastoma into ganglioneuroma. Cancer 1959; 127:108–116.
12. Decade of Discovery: Advances in Cancer Research 1971–1981. JP Van Nevel, ed. NIH Publication No. 81–2323, Bethesda, 1981.
13. Einhorn LH, Williams SD. The role of cis-platinum in solid-tumor therapy. N Engl J Med 1979; 300: 289–291.
14. American Cancer Society, 1985 Cancer Facts and Figures Booklet. American Cancer Society, New York, 1988.
15. Carter SK, Schein PS. Clinical evaluation of new anticancer agents. In: Medical Oncology: Basic Principles and Clinical Management of Cancer, P Calabresi, PS Schein, SA Rosenberg, eds. New York, Macmillan, 1985; pp. 392–405.
16. Friend C, Scher W, Holland JG, Sato T. Hemoglobin synthesis in murine

virus-induced leukemic cells in vitro: stimulation of erythroid differentiation by dimethylsulfoxide. Proc Natl Acad Sci USA 1971; 68:378–382.

17. Tanaka M, Levy J, Terada M, Breslow R, Rifkind RA, et al. Induction of erythroid differentiation in murine virus infected erythroleukemia cells by highly polar compounds. Proc Natl Acad Sci USA 1975; 72:1003–1006.

18. Leder A, Leder P. Butyric acid, a potent inducer of erythroid differentiation in cultured erythroleukemic cells. Cell 1975; 5:319–322.

19. Reuben RC, Wife RL, Breslow R, Rifkind RA, et al. A new group of potent inducers of differentiation in cultured erythroleukemla cells. Proc Natl Acad Sci USA 1976; 73:862–866.

20. Bernstein A, Hunt DM, Crickley V, Mak TW. Induction by ouabain of hemoglobin synthesis in cultured Friend erythroleukemic cells. Cell 1976; 9:375–381.

21. Terada M, Epner E, Nudel V, Salmon J, Fibach E, et al. Induction of murine erythroleukemia differentiation by actinomycin D. Proc Natl Acad Sci USA 1978; 75:2795–2799.

22. Tapiero H, Fourcade A, Billard C. Membrane dynamics of Friend leukaemic cells. II. Changes associated with cell differentiation. Cell Differ 1980; 9:211–218.

23. McClintock PR, Papacomstantinou J. Regulation of hemoglobin synthesis in a murine erythroblastic leukemic cell: the requirement for replication to induce hemoglobin synthesis. Proc Natl Acad Sci USA 1974; 71:4551–4555.

24. Scher W, Friend C. Breakage of DNA and alteration in folded genomes by inducers of differentiation in Friend erythroleukemia cells. Cancer Res 1978; 38:841–849.

25. Collins SJ, Gallo RC, Gallagher RE. Continuous growth and differentiation of human myeloid leukemic cells in suspension culture. Nature 1977; 270:347–349.

26. Collins SJ, Ruscetti FW, Gallagher RE, Gallo RC. Terminal differentiation of human promyelocytic leukemia cells induced by dimethyl sulfoxide and other polar compounds. Proc Natl Acad Sci USA 1978: 75:2458–2462.

27. Collins SJ, Bodner A, Tinge R, Gallo RC. Induction of morphological and functional differentiation of human promyelocytic leukemia cells (HL–60) by compounds which induce differentiation of murine leukemia cells. Int J Cancer 1980; 25:213–218.

28. Fontana JA, Colbert DA, Deisseroth AB. Identification of a population of bipotent stem cells in the HL–60 human promyelocytic leukemia cell line. Proc Natl Acad Sci USA 1981; 78; 1386.

29. Westin EH, Wong-Staal F, Gelmann EP, Fawera RD, Papas TS, et al. Expression of cellular homologues of retroviral onc genes in human hematopoietic cells. Proc Natl Acad Sci USA 1982; 79:2490–2494.

30. Westin EH, Gallo RC, Arya SK, Eva A, Sonza LM, et al. Differential expression of the amv gene in human hematopoietic cells. Proc Natl Acad Sci USA 1982; 791; 2194–2198.

31. Reitsma PH, Rothberg PG, Astrin SM, Trial J, Bar-Shavit Z, et al. Regulation of myc gene expression in HL–60 cells by a vitamin D metabolite. Nature 1983; 306:492–494.

32. Grosso LE, Pitot HC. Transcriptional regulation of c-myc during chemically induced differentiation of HL–60 cultures. Cancer Res 1981; 45:847–850.
33. Sariban E, Mitchell T, Kufe D. Expression of c-fms proto-oncogene during human monocytic differentiation. Nature 1985; 316:64–66.
34. Matsui T, Takahashl R, Mihara K. Cooperative regulation of c-myc expression in differentiation of human promyelocytic leukemia induced by recombinant g-interferon and 1,25–dihydroxyvitamin D_3 Cancer Res 1985; 45: 4366–4371.
35. Dexter DL, Konieczny SF, Lawrence JB, Shaffer M, Mitchell P, et al. Induction by butyrate of differentiated properties in cloned murine rhabdomyosarcoma cells. Differentiation 1981; 18:115–122.
36. Kimhi Y, Palfrey C, Spector I, Barak Y, Littaner UZ. Maturation of neuroblastoma cells in the presence of dimethylsulfoxide. Proc Natl Acad Sci USA 1976; 73:462–466.
37. Strickland S, Mahdavi V. The induction of differentiation in teratocarcinoma stem cells by retinoic acid. Cell 1978: 15:393–403.
38. Speers WC. Conversion of malignant murine embryonal carcinomas to benign teratomas by chemical induction of differentiation in vivo. Cancer Res 1982; 42:1843–1849. 9. Speers WC, Altmann M. Chemically induced differentiation of murine embryonal carcinoma in vivo: Transplantation of differentiated tumors. Cancer Res 1984; 44:2129–2135.
40. Tralka TS, Rabson AS. Cilia formation in cultures of human lung cancer cells treated with dimethylsulfoxide. J Natl Cancer Inst 1976; 57:1383–1388.
41. Huberman E, Heckman C, Langenbach R. Stimulation of differentiated functions in human melanoma cells by tumor promoting agents and dimethylsulfoxide. Cancer Res 1979; 39:2618–2624.
42. Lotan R, Lotan D. Stimulation of melanogenesis in a human melanoma cell line by retinoids. Cancer Res 1980; 40:3345–3350.
43. Meyskens FL Jr, Fuller BB. Characterization of the effects of different retinoids on the growth and differentiation of a human melanoma cell line and selected subclones. Cancer Res 1980; 40:2194–2196.
44. Gross JL, Behrens DL, Kornblith PL, Dexter DL. Plasminogen activator and inhibitor activities in human glioma cells: modulation by sodium butyrate. Proc Am Assoc Cancer Res 1986; 27:157.
45. Dexter, DL, Barbosa JA, Calabresi P. N,N-Dimethylformamide-induced alteration of cell culture characteristics and loss of tumorigenicity in cultured human colon carcinoma cells. Cancer Res 1979; 39:1020–1025.
46. Hager JC, Gold DV, Barbosa JA, Fligiel Z, Miller F, Dexter DL. N,N-Dimethylformamide-induced modulation of organ- and tumor-associated markers in cultured human colon carcinoma cells. J Natl Cancer Inst 1980; 64:439–446.
47. Tsao D, Morita A, Bella A Jr, Luu P, Kim YS. Differential effects of sodium butyrate, dimethylsulfoxide, and retinoic acid on membrane-associated antigens, enzymes and glycoproteins of human rectal adenocarcinoma cells. Cancer Res 1982; 42;1052–1058.
48. Kim YE, Tsao D, Siddigui B, Whitehead JS, Arnstein P, et al. Effects of

sodium butyrate and dimethylsulfoxide on biochemical properties of human colon cancer cells. Cancer 1980; 45:1185–1192.

49. Dexter DL, Lev R, McKendall GR, Mitchell P, Calabresi P. Sodium butyrate-induced alteration of growth properties and glycogen levels in cultured human colon carcinoma cells. Histochem J 1984; 16:137–149.

50. Dexter DL, Crabtree GW, Stoeckler JD, Savarese TM, Ghoda LY, et al. N,N-Dimethylformamide and sodium butyrate modulation of the activities of purine-metabolizing enzymes in cultured human colon carcinoma cells. Cancer Res 1981; 41:808–812.

51. Dexter DL, Spremulli EN, Matook GM, Diamond I, Calabresi P. Inhibition of the growth of human colon cancer xenografts by polar solvents. Cancer Res 1982; 42:5018–5022.

52. National Cancer Institute Clinical Brochure: N-Methylformamide (NMF). NSC 3051. Bethesda, MD, National Cancer Institute, 1982.

53. Ettinger DS, Orr DW, Rice DP, Donehower RC. Phase 1 study of N-methylformamide in patients with advanced cancer. Cancer Treat Rep 1985; 69:489–493.

54. O'Dwyer PJ, Donehower M, Sigman LM, Fortner CL, Aisner J, et al. Phase 1 trial of N-methylformamide (NMF, NSC 3051). J Clin Oncol 1985; 3:853–857.

55. Spremulli EN, Dexter DL. Polar solvents: A novel class of antineoplastic agents. J Clin Oncol 1984; 2:227–241.

56. Gusella JF, Housman D. Induction of erythroid differentiation in vitro by purines and purine analogues. Cell 1976; 8:263–269.

57. Michalewicz R, Lotem J, Sachs L. Cell differentiation and therapeutic effect of low doses of cytosine arabinoside in human myelold leukemia. Leuk Res 1984; 8:783–790.

58. Schwartz EL, Sartorelli AC. Structure-activity relationships for the induction of differentiation of HL–60 human and acute promyelocytic leukemia cells by anthracyclines. Cancer Res 1982; 42:2651–2655.

59. Fibach E, Gambari R, Shaw PA, Naniatis G, Reuben RC, et al. Tumor promoter-mediated inhibition of cell differentiation: suppression of the expression of erythroid functions in murine erythroleukemia cells. Proc Natl Acad Sci USA 1979; 76:1906–1910.

60. Rovera G, Bonaiuto J, The phenotypes of variant clones of Friend mouse erythroleukemic cells resistant to dimethyl sulfoxide. Cancer Res 1976; 36:4057–4061.

61. Wolbach SB, Howe PR. Tissue changes following deprivation of fat-soluble A vitamin. J Exp Med 1925; 42:753–778.

62. Fujimaki Y. Formation of carcinoma in albino rats fed on deficient diets. J Cancer Res 1926; 10:469–477.

63. Lotan R. Effects of vitamin A and its analogs (retinoids) on normal and neoplastic cells. Biochim Biophys Acta 1980; 605:33–91.

64. Gross JL, Dexter DL. Unpublished findings.

65. Dexter DL. N,N-Dimethylformamide-induced morphological differentiation and reduction of tumorigenicity in cultured mouse rhabdomyosarcoma cells. Cancer Res 1977; 37:3136–3140.

66. Hecker E. Phorbol esters from crotin oil-chemical nature and biological activities. Naturwissenschaften 1967; 54:617–623.

67. Tanaka H, Abe E, Miyaura C, Kuribayashi T, Konno K, et al. I-25 Dihydroxycholecalciferol and a human myeloid leukemia cell line (HL–60). The presence of a cytosol receptor and induction and differentiation. Biochem J 1982; 204:713–719.
68. Murao S, Gemmeli MA, Callaham MF, Anderson HL, Huberman E. Control of macrophage cell differentiation in human promyelocytic HL–60 leukemia cells by 1,25 dihydroxy vitamin D_3 and phorbol–12–myristate–13-acetate. Cancer Res 1981; 43:4989–4996.
69. Kuruki T, Sasaki K, Chida K, Abe E, Suda T. 1α,25-Dihydroxy vitamin D_3 markedly enhances chemically-induced transformation in BALB 3T3 cells. Gann 1983; 74:611–614.
70. Suda S, Enomoto S, Abe E, Suda T. Inhibition by 1α,25–dihydroxy vitamin D_3 of dimethyl sulfoxide-induced differentiation of Friend erythroleukemia cells. Biochem Biophys Res Com 1984; 119:807–813.
71. Sasaki K, Chida K, Hashiba H, Kamata N, Abe E, Suda T, et al. Enhancement by 1α,25-dihydroxy-vitamin D_3 of chemically induced transformation of BALB 3T3 cells without induction of ornithine decarboxylase or activation of protein kinase C. Cancer Res 1986; 46:604–610.
72. Gross JL, Behrens DL, Kornblith PL, Mullins DE, Dexter DL. Plasminogen activator and inhibitor activity in human glioma cells: modulation by sodium butyrate. Cancer Res 1988; 48:291–296.
73. Shin S, Freedman, VH, Risser R, Pollack R. Tumorigenicity of virus-transformed cells in nude mice is correlated specifically with anchorage independent growth in vitro. Proc Natl Acad Sci USA 1975; 72:4435–4439.
74. Mullins DE, Rohrlich ST. The role of proteinases in cellular invasiveness. Biochim Biophys Acta 1983; 695:177–214.
75. Ossowski L, Belin D. Effect of dimethyl sulfoxide on human carcinoma cells, inhibition of plasminogen activator synthesis, change in cell morphology, and alteration of response to cholera toxin. Mol Cell Biol 1985; 5:3552–3559.
76. Gross JL, Moscatelli D, Jaffe EA, Rifkin DB. Plasminogen activator and collagenase production by cultured capillary endothelial cells. J Cell Biol 1982; 95:974–981.
77. Freshney RI. Induction of differentiation in neoplastic cells. Anticancer Res 1985; 5:111–130.
78. Frame MC, Freshney RI, Vaughan PFT, Graham DI, Shaw R. Interrelationship between differentiation and malignacy-associated properties in glioma. Br J Cancer 1984; 49:269–280.
79. Kaye AH, Morstyn G, Gardner I, Pyke K. Development of a xenograft glioma model in mouse brain, Cancer Res 1986; 46:1367–1373.
80. Winter JN, Variakojis D, Gaynor ER. Low dose cytosine arabinoside (ara-C) therapy in the myelodysplastic syndromes and acute leukemia. Cancer 1985; 56:443–449.
81. Jensen MK, Ahlbom G. Low dose cytosine arabinoside in the treatment of acute nonlymphocytic leukemia. Br J Haematol 1985; 34:261–263.
82. Griffin JD, Spriggs D, Wisch JS, Kufe, DW. Treatment of preleukemic syndromes with continuous intravenous infusing of low-dose cytosine arabinoside. J Clin Oncol 1985; 3:982–991.

83. Rowinski, EK, Ettinger DS, Donehower RC, Grochow LB, et al. Phase I
and pharmacokinetic study of hexamethylene bisacetamide (HMBA).
Proc Am Soc Clin Oncol 1986; 5:131.
84. Sigman LM, Van Echo DA, Egorin MJ, Whitacre MY, Aisner J. Phase 1
trial of 5-day continuous infusion hexamethylene bisacetamide (HMBA,
NSC 95580). Proc Am Soc Clin Oncol 1986; 5:34.

19

Prospects for Improved Chloroethylnitrosoureas and Related Haloethylating Agents

Kurt W. Kohn

The difficulty of drug delivery to tumors in the central nervous system has limited the range of compounds that could be developed for a potentially effective therapy. Since many of the chloroethylnitrosoureas have high lipid solubility which allows them to diffuse readily through membrane barriers and to penetrate into the cerebrospinal fluid, these compounds have been and continue to be among the most extensively used drugs for the treatment of brain tumors and for clinical trials of new protocols. Chloroethylnitrosoureas are often used together with other drugs in efforts to find more effective combination therapies.

The mechanism of action of chloroethylnitrosoureas has been studied extensively, and a great deal is now known about their chemical reactions and biochemical effects.[45-48,51,54,55] However, this basic knowledge has to a large extent not been utilized in the clinical development of these drugs. This has been due in part to pessimism

From: Kornblith PL, Walker MD (editors). Advances in Neuro-Oncology. Futura Publishing Company, Inc., Mount Kisco, NY, © 1988.

Abbreviations used in this chapter: BCNU = 1,3-bis(2-chloroethyl)-1-nitrosourea (carmustine); CCNU = 1-(2-chloroethyl)-1-nitroso-3-cyclohexylurea (lomustine); MeCCNU = 1-(2-chloroethyl)-1-nitroso-3-(4'*trans*-methylcyclohexylurea; PCNU = 1-(2-chloroethyl)-1-nitroso-3-(2,6-dioxo-1-piperidyl)urea; ACNU = 1-(2-chloroethyl)-1-nitroso-3-(4-amino-2-methyl-5-pyrimidinyl)methylurea.

generated by the limited effectiveness and severe toxicity encountered in the clinical use of chloroethylnitrosoureas and to a perception of these compounds as essentially nonspecific alkylating agents, not worthy of extensive new drug development efforts. Nevertheless, the chloroethylnitrosoureas remain among the most prominent drugs used in clinical investigations of the chemotherapy of brain tumors. Despite the variety of apparently nonspecific chemical reactions of these drugs with nucleic acids and proteins, extensive preclinical antitumor testing has shown the chloroethylnitrosoureas to have extraordinary activity against a broad spectrum of experimental tumors (screening data, Developmental Therapeutics Program, NCI).[60] Most of these chemical reactions probably are irrelevant to the antitumor activity and it may be that only one type of reaction—possibly a minor one—is crucial. If the crucial type of reaction could be identified, and if compounds could be designed to produce mainly this type of reaction, antitumor effectiveness might be greatly improved. This chapter considers how knowledge of chemical and biochemical mechanisms may be utilized in the clinical development of improved chloroethylnitrosoureas and related haloethylating agents.

The Problem of the Multiplicity of Chemical Reactions of Chloroethylnitrosoureas with Biological Target Molecules

Current evidence indicates that the major cytotoxic reaction of chloroethylnitrosoureas involves the production of crosslinking adducts at DNA guanine-O6 positions,[15,16,30,31,44,53,55,56,80] and that this reaction is responsible for the antitumor activity.[3,4,16,78] However, these drugs also produce extensive reactions of other kinds that do not contribute to the antitumor action and that may prevent the therapeutic potential from being fully realized. Before considering the specific reactions that may be responsible for the antitumor action, the chemical side reactions will be reviewed, since an appropriate direction for drug development would be to aim for compounds that have a minimum of unnecessary or potentially harmful chemical side reactions.

The chemical reactions of the chloroethylnitrosoureas are diverse and complicated, and only the essential aspects will be considered. The compounds are highly unstable and decompose in aqueous so-

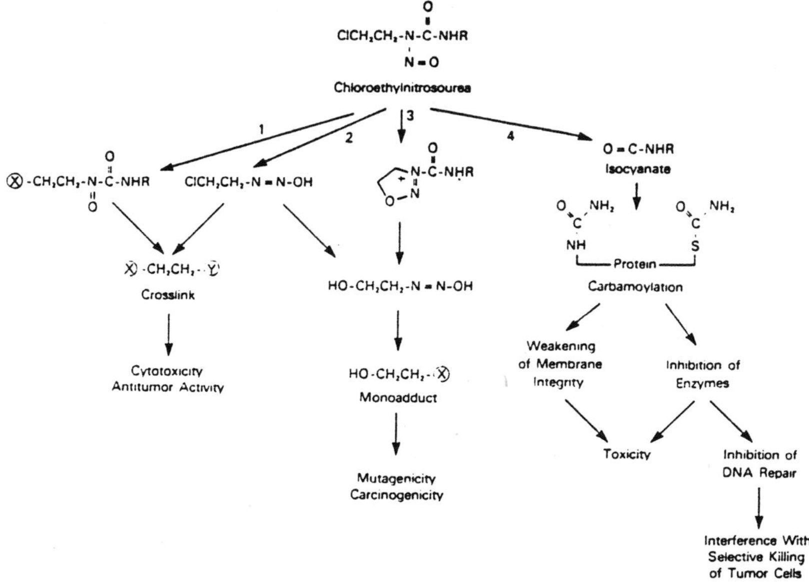

Figure 1. Outline of chemical reactions of chloroethylnitrosoureas and biological consequences, as suggested by current evidence. X and Y are sites on DNA which are alkylated by the drug. One molecule of isocyanate is generated (arrow 4) for each alkylating species, which may be generated by reaction path 1, 2, or 3. (Not all of the possible reaction paths are shown.)

lution with half-times at 37°C, ranging typically from a few minutes to approximately an hour. When a molecule of a chloroethylnitrosourea decomposes, two types of reactive intermediates are generally produced in approximately equal quantities: (1) alkylating diazo products and related cyclic intermediates, and (2) isocyanates (Fig. 1). The alkylating products are of two general types, one type capable of bifunctional reaction leading to the crosslinking of DNA (Fig. 2) or other biological macromolecules, and the other type capable only of the formation of monoadducts. The product that does the crosslinking may be either 2-chloroethyldiazohydroxide or a product generated by the initial loss of chloride.[36,51,52,62,63] Biochemical and structure-activity data implicate crosslinks as the source of the major cytotoxic and antitumor actions.[16,28,87] The products capable only of monofunctional reactions, which are detected as 2-hydroxyethyl adducts, are 2-hydroxyethyldiazohydroxide and certain cyclic intermediates.[50,79] Compounds that have only monofunctional reactivity,

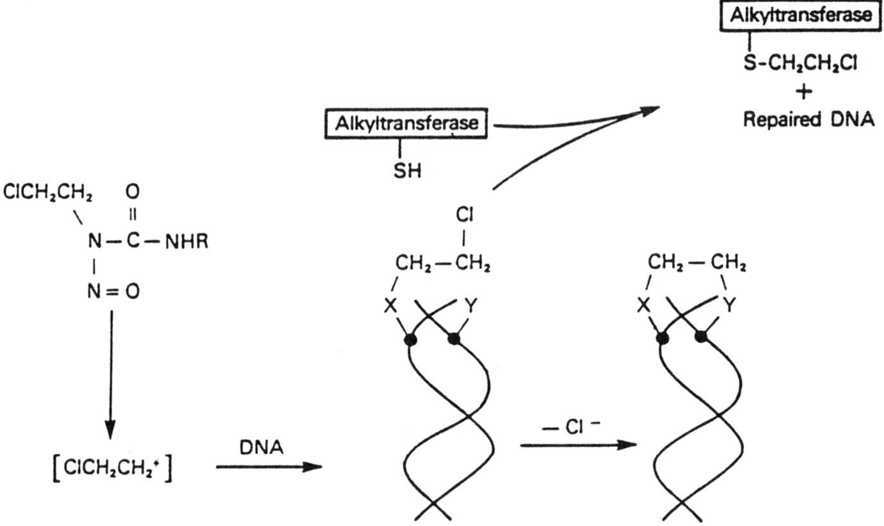

Figure 2. The formation of DNA interstrand crosslinks by a chloroethylating agent, and the prevention of crosslinking by guanine-O6-alkyltransferase. After the formation of a chloroethyl adduct at a DNA guanine-O6 site (labeled X), a second reaction occurs slowly with site Y to generate a crosslink. The alkyltransferase can rapidly remove the chloroethyl adduct before it reacts further to form a crosslink; the repaired DNA then is chemically normal. The alkyltransferase molecule which has accepted the alkyl group is permanently inactivated.

possess little or no antitumor activity but may be highly mutagenic and carcinogenic.

Compounds have been prepared that produce isocyanates exclusively.[41,42] Other compounds have been prepared that produce reactive monofunctional and bifunctional alkylating products, as well as isocyanates of a particular kind which rapidly self-inactivate by intramolecular reaction (Fig. 3) Preclinical studies of compounds generating only reactive alkylating products or only reactive isocyanate products have shown that the antitumor effects are entirely attributable to the alkylating products, and that the production of isocyanates neither confers nor contributes to antitumor activity (screening data, Developmental Therapeutics Program, NCI).

The chloroethylnitrosoureas most often employed clinically, BCNU, CCNU, and MeCCNU, generate isocyanates that do not self-inactivate. Thus the current clinical use of these drugs unnecessarily

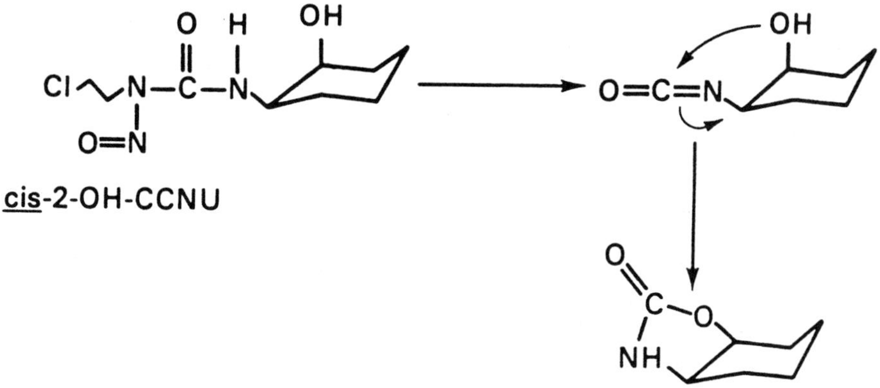

Figure 3. Example of a chloroethylnitrosourea that forms a self-inactivating isocyanate product. An OH group has been substituted onto the 2 position of the cyclohexyl ring of CCNU. From this position, it will be able to react with the isocyanate group to yield a stable molecule that does not react further.

subjects patients to isocyanates. Since alternative forms of the drug are available that do not produce reactive isocyanates and that have at least equal preclinical antitumor activity, the question must be addressed whether the isocyanate production, aside from being unnecessary, may in fact contribute significant toxicity or actually interfere with the potential antitumor action of the drug or of another drug in a combination.

Effects of Isocyanates

A large body of data has accumulated indicating that the isocyanate production can have a variety of effects that complicate the interpretation of clinical and preclinical studies employing BCNU, CCNU, or MeCCNU; the possibility cannot be excluded that significant potential advances in chemotherapy are being obscured by these effects. The known biologically relevant effects of isocyanates will be summarized. Isocyanates derived from BCNU, CCNU, or MeCCNU do not react with DNA or RNA, but do react with accessible amino and sulfhydryl groups of various proteins to generate carbamoyl derivatives of these protein sites (Fig. 1). Such carbamoylation reactions can inhibit the functions of a variety of enzymes and proteins.[8] For example, the polymerization of tubulin is inhibited by BCNU, CCNU, MeCCNU or trans-4-hydroxy-CCNU, all of which produce isocyanates that do not self-inactivate; on the other hand, chlorozotocin and cis-2-hydroxy-CCNU, which produce self-inactivating isocyanates, did not inhibit significantly.[19]

A particularly sensitive enzyme is glutathione reductase. It is carbamoylated by the isocyanate decomposition products of BCNU and CCNU.[7] This enzyme, as well as the related enzyme, lipoamide dehydrogenase, are carbamoylated at the reduced cysteine residues located within the oxidoreduction active site.[2] Glutathione reductase activity is consistently reduced in erythrocytes, leukocytes, and platelets in patients receiving chemotherapy in which BCNU is included;[33] other alkylating agents, including cyclophosphamide and procarbazine, did not have this effect. The onset of inhibition was rapid and there was a pattern of decreasing recovery with increasing number of doses. In the mouse, BCNU inhibited glutathione reductase activity in all tissues tested. Human platelets exposed in vitro to BCNU rapidly develop severe inhibition of glutathione reductase and become incapable of aggregating in response to various effectors.[58] The inhibition of glutathione reductase in lung tissue may enhance pulmonary oxygen toxicity by diminishing the lung's antioxidant capacity.[43,74] Glutathione reductase may protect against oxidative toxicity produced by drugs such as doxorubicin; BCNU when used together with doxorubicin may augment this toxicity.[6]

Of special concern is the inhibition of the ligase step of DNA repair. The isocyanates generated by BCNU or CCNU have been found to inhibit the rejoining of DNA strand breaks generated by ionizing radiation or that form in the course of nucleotide excision repair of DNA damage.[29,32,39,41,42] Nucleotide excision repair mechanisms act on a wide variety of DNA lesions, including alkylation damage, and there is evidence that isocyanate production by BCNU and CCNU inhibits the excision repair of general alkylation damage. The isocyanate production thus may interfere with the potential effectiveness of these drugs by blocking repair mechanisms that must remain intact to allow critical normal cells to recover.

Treatment of cells with BCNU or CCNU causes an accumulation of DNA strand breaks. This does not occur with equitoxic doses of derivatives, such as *cis*-2-hydroxy-CCNU, which do not generate active isocyanates.[67] The accumulation of strand breaks may be due to the inhibition of strand rejoining (DNA ligase reaction) in the course

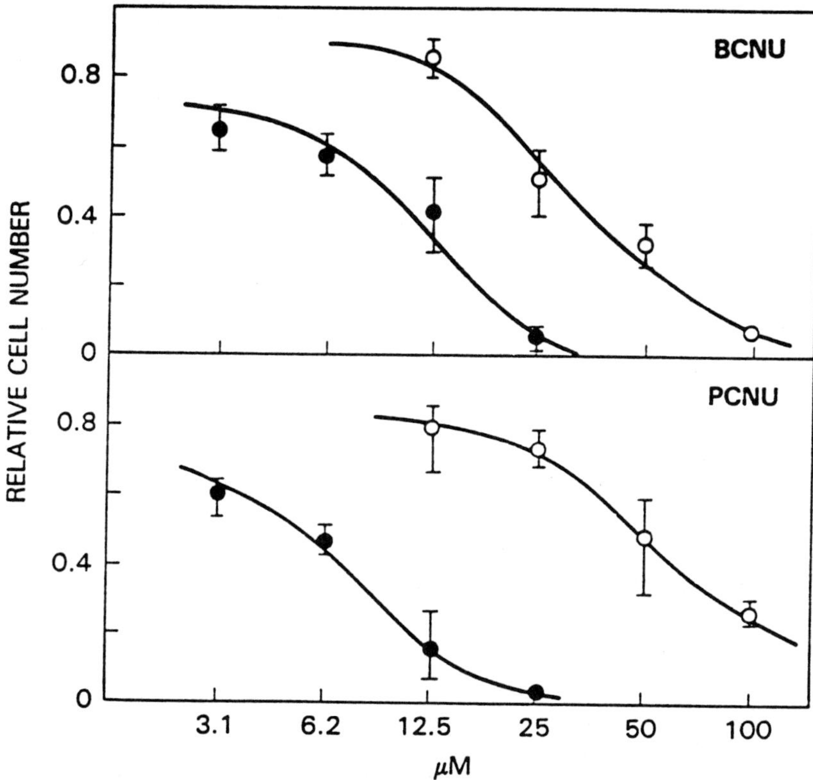

Figure 4. Isocyanate production reduces the selective toxicity of chloroe-thylnitrosoureas against Mer⁻ tumor cells. A Mer⁻ strain of human malignant glioma cells was compared with a Mer⁺ strain. The cells were treated for 2 hours with various concentrations of BCNU (a strong carbamoylator) or PCNU (a weak carbamylator). Cell number was determined 24 hours later; the cells were in exponential growth phase at the time of treatment. (From Sariban et al 1987.)

of DNA excision repair of the extraneous alkylation damage caused by the drugs. As will be discussed below, current evidence indicates that the antitumor action of the chloroethylnitrosoureas depends on guanine-O6 alkylations that can be repaired by a specific mechanism not involving excision repair, strand breaks or ligase. When BCNU, CCNU, or MeCCNU are combined with drugs such as cyclophospha-mide, melphalan, and cis-platin, the repair of alkylation damage pro-duced by these drugs would be inhibited. Since DNA repair may be essential to allow critical normal cells to recover, its inhibition may prevent the full expression of the therapeutic potential of such combinations.

There is evidence that the isocyanate production reduces the differential cytotoxicity of chloroethylnitrosoureas to potentially sensitive human tumor cells. The selectivity of killing of tumor cells that are defective in guanine-O6-alkyltransferase (Mer⁻ phenotype) is reduced in the case of BCNU or CCNU, compared to their noncarbamoylating or weakly carbamoylating congeners (Fig. 4). Moreover, the strongly carbamoylating drugs, including BCNU, CCNU, and MeCCNU, are more cytotoxic to normal human cells than are their weakly carbamoylating congeners.[67]

Isocyanate production by BCNU, CCNU, or MeCCNU also has been reported to cause cell membrane retraction and blebbing,[75-77] inhibition of calmodulin,[37] inhibition of RNA processing,[1,3,9] and may contribute to myelosuppression.[5]

Non-Carbamoylating Chloroethylnitrosoureas

The carbamoylating actions are reduced or eliminated if the isocyanate product has a hydroxyl or amino group positioned so as to react efficiently with the isocyanate group in the same molecule. This is easily accomplished, for example, by adding a hydroxyl group to the 2-position of the cyclohexyl ring of CCNU (Fig. 3). *Cis*-2-hydroxy-CCNU has been found to produce substantially less carbamoylation than CCNU,[83] to be at least as effective as CCNU against several murine tumors, including several intracranial tumors (J Plowman, Developmental Therapeutics Program, NCI, personal communication), and to produce a greater differential cytotoxicity than CCNU against Mer⁻, relative to Mer⁺, human tumor cells (LC Erickson, NW Gibson, and KW Kohn, unpublished data). Since CCNU is metabolized in the liver to various hydroxylated products (most of which do not have the hydroxyl group in the proper position to inactivate the isocyanate), it would be a straightforward matter to develop this compound as a replacement for CCNU.

Several chloroethylnitrosoureas with low carbamoylating activities have been used in clinical trials, including most prominently chlorozotocin and PCNU. Chlorozotocin has poor lipid solubility, does not penetrate into the cerebrospinal fluid and is ineffective against murine intracranial tumors. There has been considerable use of PCNU in clinical trials against brain tumors, and the compound seems to give results similar to BCNU. Even without demonstrated superiority, it would seem prudent to use the low-carbamoylating PCNU rather than BCNU, CCNU, or MeCCNU in clinical trials. To a lesser extent ACNU, another low-carbamoylator, has been used. The chemical structures of PCNU and ACNU are more complicated than that of CCNU, and these compounds may be suboptimal for extraneous reasons. A possibly better choice among compounds that have already been used clinically would be 2-chloroethyl-2-hydroxyethyl-nitrosourea, which has excellent activity against murine tumors and has a simple chemical structure that should self-inactivate the isocyanate product.[27]

The Key Role of Crosslinks Involving the Guanine-O6 Position

Alkylnitrosoureas in general can alkylate DNA to some extent at any nitrogen or oxygen atom.[72] In the case of chloroethylnitrosoureas, the 2-hydroxyethyl and 2-chloroethyl adducts at guanine-N7 and guanine-O6 of DNA have been identified as major monoalkylation products.[55,62,63,79,81] In addition, several products have been identified that are implicated in the formation of crosslinks between guanines on the same DNA strand and between guanine and cytosine on opposite strands.[55,81] These include (1) a diadduct in which two guanines are linked via an ethyl bridge between the two N7 positions, (2) a diadduct in which guanine is linked to cytosine via an ethyl bridge, and (3) a cyclic monoadduct—thought to be an intermediate in the formation of guanine-cytosine interstrand crosslinks—in which an ethyl group bridges between the O6 and N1 positions of the same guanine residue. The 2-hydroxyethyl products—which cannot form crosslinks—are produced to a considerably greater extent than are crosslinking adducts. The evidence which will be summarized next indicates that the cytotoxicity and antitumor activity are attributable to a minor adduct at guanine-O6 that produces interstrand crosslinks, and therefore that extraneous alkylations predominate over those that may give rise to the antitumor-effective crosslinks.

In order for chloroethylnitrosoureas to crosslink DNA, they must first form monoadducts on one of the DNA strands, and these monoadducts must then react with sites on the opposite strand. The second step of this sequence occurs slowly over a period of a few hours, both in purified DNA[44,53] and in cells.[28,31,45,47,48] Most human cells contain a DNA guanine-O6-alkyltransferase that can rapidly remove an alkyl group from the guanine-O6 position and transfer it to a sulfhydryl position on the enzyme.[64,69,87] The enzyme can remove guanine-O6 monoalkylations rapidly enough to prevent the formation of interstrand crosslinks (Fig. 2).[15,16,54,55] The activity of this enzyme in various human cell lines, and its ability to prevent interstrand crosslink formation, correlate with cell survival after treatment with chloroethylnitrosoureas.[4,11-14,23,25,26,28,30,61,70,85] A similar correlation with antitumor activity has been demonstrated in xenografts of human rhabdomyosarcomas having different alkyltransferase contents.[17] The level of interstrand crosslinking by chloroethylnitrosoureas in bone marrow has been found to parallel the extent of myelosuppression in mice.[9,10]

Approximately 25% of human tumor cell strains have abnormally low alkyltransferase activities.[20,88-90] Such strains—designated as possessing the Mer$^-$ phenotype[20,22]—respond to chloroethylnitrosoureas by the formation of relatively large numbers of interstrand crosslinks and by exhibiting greater cytotoxicity than do Mer$^+$ strains which have normal or high alkyltransferase activities.[28,30] Brent et al.[17] have demonstrated that xenografts of human rhabdomyosarcomas having low alkyltransferase activities exhibit greater reductions in size and longer growth delays of the solid tumors than do other strains of the same histologic type of tumor that have normal or high levels of the alkyltransferase. Thus there is considerable support for a relationship between reduced alkyltransferase activity, increased DNA interstrand crosslinking, and good antitumor responses.

Analog Development Efforts

Several directions have been explored under the NCI Drug Development Program aiming for compounds with reduced extraneous chemical reactivities, but retaining preclinical antitumor activities as good or better than those of the parent chloroethylnitrosoureas.

Hydroxy-CCNU Derivatives

CCNU derivatives were synthesized in which a hydroxyl group was added to the cyclohexyl 2 position, or both to the 2 and 6 positions, in the *cis* orientation relative to the nitrosourea moiety. These compounds were found to have much lower carbamoylating activities than the parent CCNU, but retained curative antitumor activity, similar to CCNU, against several murine intracranial tumors (J. Plowman, NCI Drug Development Program, personal communication). The compounds exhibited greater differential cytotoxicity than did CCNU against Mer⁻ human tumor cells in culture relative to Mer⁺ cells (L.C. Erickson and K.W. Kohn, unpublished data). Cis-hydroxy-CCNU, with its low carbamoylating activity, would be an appropriate replacement drug for CCNU, from which it does not differ in any other significant way (except for slightly better water solubility).

Fluoroethylnitrosoureas

Replacement of the 2-chloroethyl with a 2-fluoroethyl group would be expected to alter the alkylating properties of the drug, especially in bifunctional reactions. The fluoro analog of CCNU (FCNU, NSC-7974) produces 2-hydroxyethyl and 2-fluoroethyl adducts of DNA guanine-N7 and 2-hydroxyethyl adducts of guanine-O6.[81,82] Although a 2-fluoroethyl adduct of guanine-O6 was not identified, its possibly transient formation is not excluded. Since fluoride is a weaker leaving group than chloride, the further reaction of the fluoroethyl adducts to form crosslinks should be slower and less extensive than in the case of chloroethylnitrosoureas.[44] In accord with this expectation, interstrand crosslinking by FCNU in Mer⁻ cells was very slight, and appeared only after 24–48 hours, compared with 6–12 hours in the case of chloroethylnitrosoureas (L.C. Erickson and K.W. Kohn, unpublished data). Nevertheless, there was selective cytotoxicity to Mer⁻ cells relative to Mer⁺ cells, implicating a toxic reaction at guanine-O6 in alkyltransferase-deficient cells. Although the mechanistic picture is not entirely clear, the evidence shows that the reactions of FCNU with DNA are significantly different from those of CCNU.

Despite its lower efficiency of DNA interstrand crosslinking, the preclinical antitumor activity of FCNU in several systems was found to be as good as, or better than, CCNU. Cures were obtained in several intracranial tumor systems, including Zimmerman ependymoblastoma, glioma 26, glioma 261, B16 melanoma and, to a lesser degree, colon 26 (J. Plowman, NCI Developmental Therapeutics Program, personal communication). In the case of intracranially implanted

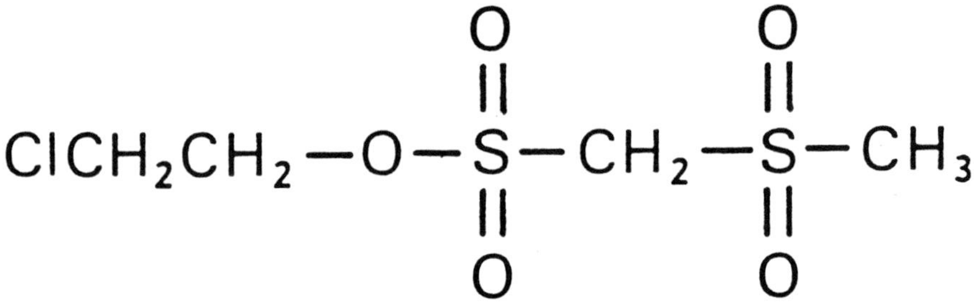

$$CICH_2CH_2-O-\underset{\underset{O}{\overset{\overset{O}{\|}}{\|}}}{S}-CH_2-\underset{\underset{O}{\overset{\overset{O}{\|}}{\|}}}{S}-CH_3$$

Figure 5. Structure of 2-chloroethyl(methanesulfonyl)methanesulfonate (clomesone, NSC338947).

Lewis lung carcinoma, the drug increased survival time significantly but did not produce long-term survivors.

Contrary to the chloroethylnitrosoureas, FCNU was found to induce convulsions in mice (reports to the NCI Developmental Therapeutics Program by J.A. Montgomery and by R.K. Johnson). This toxicity was attributable to the stoichiometric production of 2-fluoroethanol, which is metabolized to fluoroacetate and then to the Krebs cycle inhibitor, fluorocitrate. Some degree of protection was afforded by co-administration of sodium acetate. By using small daily doses of FCNU, instead of a large single dose, it was possible to obtain full activity against B16 melanoma well below neurotoxic doses. Thus it should be possible to avoid neurotoxicity by means of an appropriate divided dose schedule, and, if necessary, by monitoring serum levels of fluoroethanol and fluoroacetate.

Clinical trial of FCNU, although unfortunately not as yet planned, would determine whether or not the differences in the nature and kinetics of the reaction with DNA would allow the extraordinary preclinical antitumor activity of the 2-haloethylnitrosoureas to be more fully expressed in man.

Clomesone

Clomesone (Fig. 5) represents a new class of chloroethylating agents that lack several of the unnecessary chemical reactivities of the nitrosoureas. This new drug was developed by Shealy et al.[71] who synthesized a series of chloroethylsulfonate derivatives in an attempt to find compounds that would be capable of crosslinking DNA in the

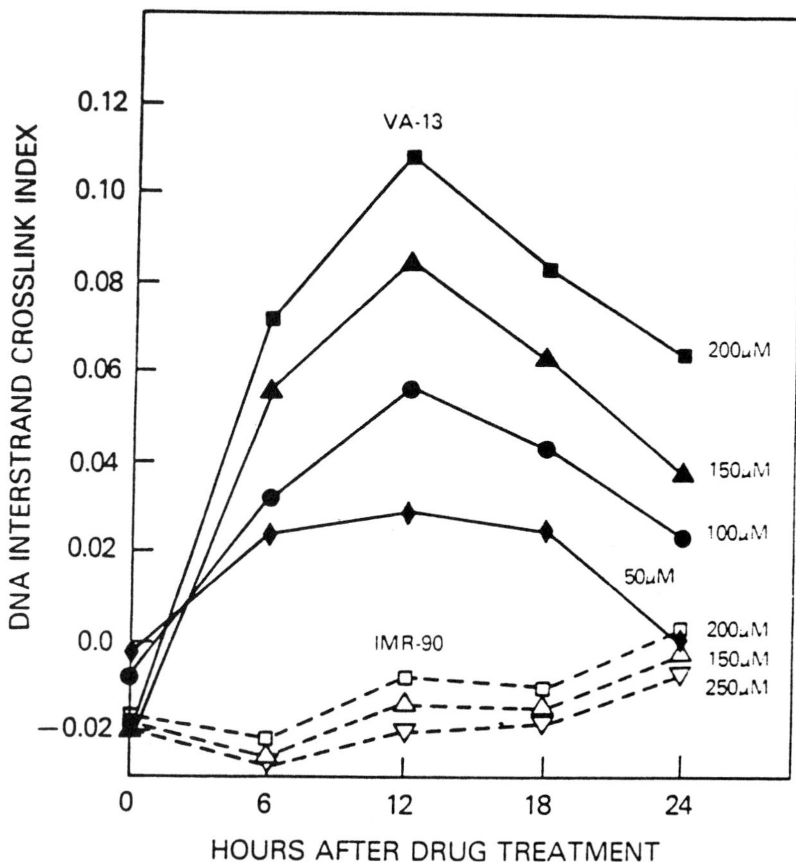

Figure 6. Difference in interstrand crosslinking responses between a normal human cell strain (IMR–90) and a transformed line (VA–13) that has become deficient in guanine-O6-alkyltransferase (designated Mer⁻ phenotype). The cells were treated with the indicated concentrations of clomesone for 2 hours and then incubated for various times in the absence of drug. (From Gibson et al. Cancer Res. 45:1674, 1985.)

same manner as chloroethylnitrosoureas, but that would not form extraneous types of alkylations or isocyanates. The best compound, 2-chloroethyl-(methanesulfonyl)methansulfonate (clomesone), was found to have activity comparable to chloroethylnitrosoureas against a broad spectrum of murine tumors, including intracranial tumors (J. Plowman, Developmental Therapeutics Program, NCI, personal communication). In accord with the chemical expectation, clomesone was found to produce 2-chloroethyl, but not 2-hydroxyethyl, adducts of guanine in DNA.[35]

Moreover, clomesone produced interstrand crosslinks in human Mer⁻ cells (Fig. 6),[34] and the crosslinking of DNA is suppressed by guanine-O6-alkyltransferase.[18] Thus, this compound meets the objective of producing a more restricted range of chemical reactions while retaining the alkyltransferase-related interstrand crosslinking and the high degree of antitumor activity.

This structure also lends itself to further chemical modification to optimize the chemical specificity and pharmacologic properties of the drug. Two types of structure modification would be of interest. First, the methyl group could be substituted to alter the DNA sequence selectivity of the alkylation, as discussed in the next section. Second, the chlorine could be replaced by a fluorine, which may further restrict the types of chemical reaction that occur, because only the most easily formed crosslinks would then be likely to be produced. (As already noted, the chemically analogous 2-fluoroethylnitrosoureas have been found to have antitumor activity at least equal to that of the 2-chloroethylnitrosoureas, but produce a much lower frequency of interstrand crosslinks.)

DNA Sequence Selectivity of Guanine Alkylations

It has been proposed that the effectiveness of alkylating agents may depend upon bifunctional reaction selectively at guanine-rich regions of the genome.[49,57] This possibility was strengthened by the finding that chloroethylnitrosoureas, as well as a variety of nitrogen mustards, react preferentially at guanines located within runs of successive guanines.[38] However, clomesone was found to be unusual in that it reacts at all guanines almost equally. Hence, it may be that the antitumor activity of clomesone is the net result of an enhanced effectiveness due to more restricted chemical reactions and a reduced effectiveness due to loss of selectivity of reaction within clusters of guanines.

The selectivity for reaction within clusters of guanines appears to be due to the strong electronegative potential in the DNA major groove in such sequence regions.[49] Most alkylating species derived from nitrogen mustards or chloroethylnitrosoureas bear a positive charge or the positive end of a strong dipole, and this may in part be the reason for the DNA sequence selectivity. Clomesone, however, is uncharged, and this may be why it fails to exhibit any sequence selectivity. However, derivatives of clomesone could be prepared that would have a cationic group attached to the molecule so as to restore the sequence selectivity. These considerations constitute a rational molecular approach for the development of drugs that could be highly effective in the treatment of certain types of tumors. However, further developments in this area will depend upon acceptance of this class of drugs for clinical investigation.

Identification of Potentially Sensitive Tumors

Human malignant glioma cell cultures derived from surgical tissue samples of grade III-IV tumors have been studied in order to determine whether significant differences exist in DNA crosslinking responses within this relatively homogeneous histologic group of tumors.[68] Substantial differences were found among the different cell strains, in regard to interstrand crosslinking by chloroethylnitrosoureas. Furthermore, the cell strains tended to exhibit individual patterns of sensitivities to different interstrand crosslinking drugs (Fig. 7).

These and the preceding findings suggest that further progress towards truly effective cancer chemotherapy may require appropriate biochemical characterization of the individual tumor in order to identify the types of drugs to which a tumor could respond. For the case of chloroethylnitrosoureas and clomesone, sensitive assays for guanine-O6-alkyltransferase levels in small tissue samples are available which may allow potentially sensitive tumors to be identified.[24,84,86]

Prospects

From what is known about the actions of the chloroethylnitrosoureas, it is clear that the potential effectiveness of these or related drugs in man has not been adequately investigated. What questions need to be explored? The high degree of effectiveness against a broad spectrum of rodent tumors shows that an action exists that is selective against certain types of neoplasms. We know that this is an alkylation reaction, probably involving the guanine-O6 position of DNA, and that differential cytotoxicity depends, at least in part, on the activity

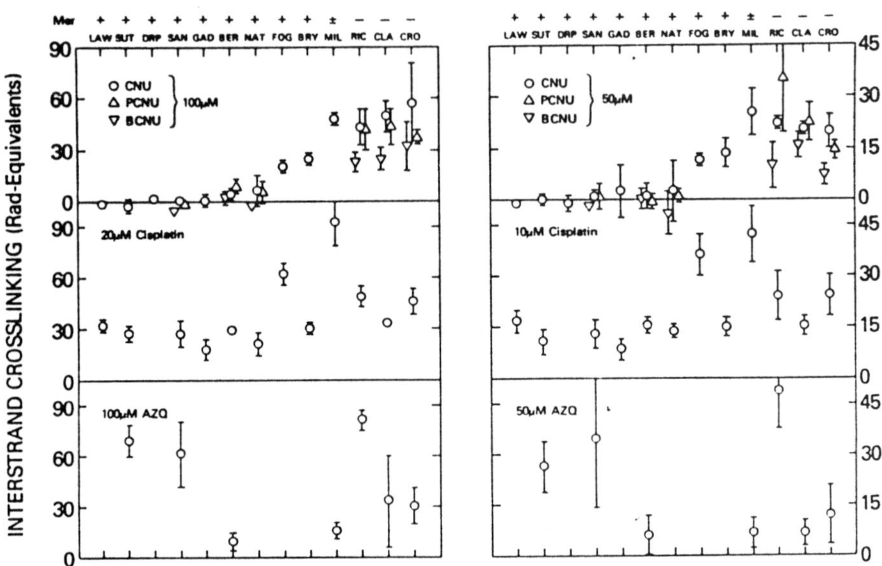

Figure 7. Interstrand crosslinking responses of a variety of human glioblastoma cell strains treated with chloroethylnitrosoureas, cisplatin or aziridinylbenzoquinone (AZQ). Cells were treated with the indicated concentrations of drugs for 1–2 hours and then incubated for 4–6 hours to allow full development of interstrand crosslinks. (From Sariban et al. 1987).

of repair mechanisms that remove this alkylation. We do not know why the drugs are only poorly effective in man, but it is possible to formulate questions, the exploration of which could lead to much more effective therapies.

To begin with, we must recognize that these drugs may only be effective against tumor cells having relatively low levels of DNA guanine-O6-alkyltransferase (cells having the Mer⁻ phenotype). Although approximately 25% of human tumor cell strains in culture possess this phenotype, it is still not clear how frequently it exists in clinical tumors. This is a crucial question which can now be explored using highly sensitive methods for assay of the enzyme on small tissue samples. The drugs might be effective only against those tumors that have low levels of the alkyltransferase, but such tumors could be identified and it may be possible to develop effective treatments for them. This goal might be accomplished by developing compounds whose main action is to produce crosslinking adducts at DNA guanine-O6 positions.

If the initial results are encouraging, we would then be in a position to ask whether effectiveness against alkyltransferase-deficient tumors could be enhanced by modifying the chemical structure of the drug so as to enhance the selectivity for alkylation at crosslinkable sites (5'-GG–3' or 5'-GC–3') in DNA. With the accumulation of more information at the molecular biology level, it may become possible to optimize effectiveness by the design of drugs that would react selectively in certain genomic locales.

As more immediate goals, the replacement of BCNU, CCNU, and MeCCNU by low-carbamoylating congeners should be considered, and the relationships between the effectiveness of various haloethylating agents and the levels of alkyltransferase in the tumors should be investigated.

Finally, in regard to tumors that are not deficient in alkyltransferase, haloethylating agents are probably not appropriate for these cases, since such tumors would not have the biochemical sensitivity characteristic needed for response to these drugs. It is important not to obscure a possibly good treatment of an identifiable minority of tumors by mixing the data with results on tumors that do not possess the biochemical drug sensitivity characteristics needed for response.

REFERENCES

1. Abelson HT, Karlan D, Penman S. A comparison of the effects of alkylating agents 1,3-bis(2-chloroethyl)-1-nitrosourea, 1-(2-chloroethyl)-3-cyclohexyl)-1-nitrosourea and nitrogen mustard on nuclear RNA synthesis and processing. Biochim Biophys Acta 1974; 349:389–401.
2. Ahmad T, Frischer H. Active site-specific inhibition by 1,3-bis(2-chloroethyl)-1-nitrosourea of two genetically homologous flavoenzymes: glutathione reductase and lipomamide dehydrogenase. J Lab Clin Med 1985; 105:464–471.
3. Aida T, Bodell WJ. Effect of caffeine on cytotoxicity and sister chromatid exchange induction in sensitive and resistant rat brain tumor cells treated with 1,3-bis(2-chloroethyl)-1-nitrosourea. Cancer Res 1987; 47:5052–5058.
4. Aida T, Cheitlin RA, Bodell WJ. Inhibition of O6-alkylguanine-DNA-alkyltransferase activity potentiates cytotoxicity and induction of SCEs in human glioma cells resistant to 1,3-bis(2-chloroethyl)-1-nitrosourea. Carcinogenesis 1987; 8:1219–1223.
5. Ali-Osman F, Giblin J, Berger M, Murphy MJ Jr, Rosenblum ML. Chemical structure of carbamoylating groups and their relationship to bone

marrow toxicity and antiglioma activity of bifunctionally alkylating and carbamoylating nitrosoureas. Cancer Res 1985; 45:4185–4191.

6. Babson JR, Abell NS, Reed DJ. Protective role of the glutathione redox cycle against adriamycin-mediated toxicity in isolated hepatocytes. Biochem Pharmacol 1981; 30:2299–2304.

7. Babson JR, Reed DJ. Inactivation of glutathione reductase by 2-chloroethylnitrosourea-derived isocyanates. Biochem Biophys Res Commun 1978; 83:754–762.

8. Babson JR, Reed DJ, Sinkey MA. Active site specific inactivation of chymotrypsin by cyclohexyl isocyanate formed during degradation of the carcinostatic 1-(2-chloroethyl)-3-cyclohexyl-1-nitrosourea. Biochemistry 1977; 16:1584–1589.

9. Bedford P, Berger MR, Eisenbrand G, Schmahl D. The level of DNA interstrand crosslinking in bone marrow parallels the extent of myelosuppression in mice treated with four chloroethylnitrosoureas. J Cancer Res Clin Oncol 1984; 108:141–147.

10. Bedford P, Eisenbrand G. DNA damage and repair in the bone marrow of rats treated with four chloroethylnitrosoureas. Cancer Res 1984; 44:514–518.

11. Bodell WJ, Aida T, Berger MS, Rosenblum ML. Increased repair of O6-alkylguanine DNA adducts in glioma-derived human cells resistant to the cytotoxic and cytogenetic effects of 1,3-bis(2-chloroethyl)-1-nitrosourea. Carcinogenesis 1986; 7:879–883.

12. Bodell WJ, Aida T, Berger MS, Rosenblum ML. Repair of 06-(2-chloroethyl)guanine mediates the biological effects of chloroethylnitrosoureas. 1985; Environ Health Perspect 62:119–126.

13. Bodell WJ, Gerosa M, Aida T, Berger MS, Rosenblum ML. Investigation of resistance to DNA cross-linking agents in 9L cell lines with different sensitivities to chloroethylnitrosoureas. Cancer Res 1985; 45:3460–3464.

14. Bodell WJ, Rupniak HT, Rasmussen J, Morgan WF, Rosenblum ML. Reduced level of DNA cross-links and sister chromatid exchanges in 1,3-bis(2-chloroethyl)-1-nitrosourea-resistant rat brain tumor cells. Cancer Res 1984; 44:3763–3767.

15. Brent TP. Suppression of cross-link formation in chloroethylnitrosourea-treated DNA by an activity in extracts of human leukemic lymphoblasts. Cancer Res 1984; 44:1887–1892.

16. Brent TP. Isolation and purification of O6-alkylguanine-DNA alkyltransferase from human leukemic cells. Prevention of chloroethylnitrosourea-induced cross-links by purified enzyme. Pharmacol Ther 1985; 31:121–140.

17. Brent TP, Houghton PJ, Houghton JA. O6-alkylguanine-DNA alkyltransferase activity correlates with the therapeutic response of human rhabdomyosarcoma xenografts to 1-(2-chloroethyl)-3-(trans-4-methylcyclohexyl)-1-nitrosourea. Proc Natl Acad Sci USA 1985; 82:2985–2989.

18. Brent TP, Lestrud SO, Smith DG, Remack JS. Formation of DNA interstrand cross-links by the novel chloroethylating agent 2-chloroethyl(methylsulfonyl)methanesulfonate: suppression by O6-alkylguanine-DNA alkyltransferase purified from human leukemic lymphoblasts. Cancer Res 1987; 47:3384–3387.

19. Brodie AE, Babson JR, Reed DJ. Inhibition of tubulin polymerization by nitrosourea-derived isocyanates. Biochem Pharmacol 1980; 29:652–654.

20. Day RS, Babich MA, Yarosh DB, Scudiero DA. The role of O6-methylguanine in human cell killing, sister chromatid exchange induction and mutagenesis: a review. J Cell Sci [Suppl] 1987; 6:333–353.

21. Day RS, Ziolkowski CH. MNNG-pretreatment of a human kidney carcinoma cell strain decreases its ability to repair MNNG-treated adenovirus 5. Carcinogenesis 1981; 2:213–218.

22. Day RS, Ziolkowski CH, Scudiero DA, Meyer SA, Mattern MR. Human tumor cell strains defective in the repair of alkylation damage. Carcinogenesis 1980; 1:21–32.

23. Dolan ME, Corsico CD, Pegg AE. Exposure of HELA cells to 0(6)-alkylguanines increases sensitivity to the cytotoxic effects of alkylating agents. Biochem Biophys Res Commun 1985; 132:178–185.

24. Dolan ME, Scicchitano D, Pegg AE. Use of oligodeoxynucleotides containing O6-alkylguanine for the assay of O6-alkylguanine-DNA-alkyltransferase activity. Cancer Res 1988; 48:1184–1188.

25. Dolan ME, Morimoto K, Pegg AE. Reduction of O6-alkylguanine-DNA alkyltransferase activity in hela cells treated with O6-alkylguanines Cancer Res 1985; 45:6413–6417.

26. Dolan ME, Young GS, Pegg AE. Effect of O6-alkylguanine pretreatment on the sensitivity of human colon tumor cells to the cytotoxic effects of chloroethylating agents. Cancer Res 1986; 46:4500–4504.

27. Eisenbrand G, Muller N, Schreiber J, Stahl W, Sterzel W, Berger MR, Zeller WJ, Fiebig H. Drug design: nitrosoureas. IARC Sci Publ 1986; 78:281–294.

28. Erickson LC, Bradley MO, Ducore JM, Ewig RA, Kohn KW. DNA cross-linking and cytotoxicity in normal and transformed human cells treated with antitumor nitrosoureas. Proc Natl Acad Sci USA 1980; 77:467–471.

29. Erickson LC, Bradley MO, Kohn KW. Differential inhibition of the rejoining of X-ray-induced DNA strand breaks in normal and transformed human fibroblasts treated with 1,3-bis(2-chloroethyl)-1-nitrosourea in vitro. Cancer Res 1978; 38:672–677.

30. Erickson LC, Laurent G, Sharkey NA, Kohn KW. DNA cross-linking and monoadduct repair in nitrosourea-treated human tumor cells. Nature (Lond) 1980; 288:727–729.

31. Ewig RA, Kohn KW. DNA-protein cross-linking and DNA interstrand cross-linking by haloethylnitrosoureas in L1210 cells. Cancer Res 1978; 38:3197–3203.

32. Fornace AJ, Kohn KW, Kann HE. Inhibition of the ligase step of excision repair by 2-chloroethyl isocyanate, a decomposition product of 1,3-bis(2-chloroethyl)-nitrosourea. Cancer Res 1978; 38:1064–1069.

33. Frischer H, Ahmad T. Severe generalized glutathione reductase deficiency after antitumor chemotherapy with BCNU[1,3-bis(chloroethyl)-1-nitrosourea]. J Lab Clin Med 1977; 89:1080–1091.

34. Gibson NW, Erickson LC, Kohn KW. DNA damage and differential cytotoxicity produced in human cells by 2-chloroethyl (methylsulfonyl)methanesulfonate (NSC 338947), a new DNA-chloroethylating agent. Cancer Res 1985; 45:1674–1679.

35. Gibson NW, Hartley JA, Strong JM, Kohn KW. 2-chloroethyl (methyl-sulfonyl)methanesulfonate (NSC-338947), a more selective DNA alkylating agent than the chloroethylnitrosoureas. Cancer Res 1986; 46:553–557.

36. Gombar CT, Tong WP, Ludlum DB. Mechanism of action of the nitrosoureas. IV. Reactions of bis-chloroethyl nitrosourea and chloroethyl cyclohexyl nitrosourea with deoxyribonucleic acid. Biochem Pharmacol 1980; 9:2639–2643.

37. Harrison SD Jr, Mann DM, Giles RC Jr. Effect of nitrosoureas on Calmodulin activity in vitro and in mouse intestine in vivo. Cancer Chemother Pharmacol 1985; 14:146–149.

38. Hartley JA, Gibson NW, Kohn KW, Mattes WB. DNA sequence selectivity of guanine-N7 alkylation by three antitumor chloroethylating agents. Cancer Res 1986; 46:1943–1947.

39. Kann HE, Kohn KW, Widerlite L, Gullion D. Effects of 1,3-bis(2-chloroethyl)-1-nitrosourea and related compounds on nuclear RNA metabolism. Cancer Res 1974; 34:1982–1988.

40. Kann HE, Blumenstein BA, Petkas A, Schott MA. Radiation synergism by repair-inhibiting nitrosoureas in L1210 cells. Cancer Res 1980; 40:771–775.

41. Kann HE, Kohn KW. Inhibition of DNA repair by the 1,3-bis(2-chloroethyl)-1-nitrosourea breakdown product, 2-chloroethyl isocyanate. Cancer Res 1974; 34:398–402.

42. Kann HE, Schott MA, Petkas A. Effects of structure and chemical activity on the ability of nitrosoureas to inhibit DNA repair. Cancer Res 1980; 40:50–55.

43. Kehrer JP, Paraidathathu T. Enhanced oxygen toxicity following treatment with 1,3-bis(2-chloroethyl)-1-nitrosourea. Fundam Appl Toxicol 1984; 4:760–767.

44. Kohn KW. Interstrand cross-linking of DNA by1,3-bis(2-chloroethyl)-1-nitrosourea and other 1-(2-chloroethyl)-1-nitrosoureas. Cancer Res 1977; 37:1450–1454.

45. Kohn KW. Mechanistic approaches to new nitrosourea development. Recent Results Cancer Res 1981; 76:141–152.

46. Kohn KW. Biological aspects of DNA damage by crosslinking agents. In: Molecular Aspects of Anticancer Drug Action. New York, MacMillan, 1983; pp. 315–361.

47. Kohn KW. DNA crosslinking agents. Prog Cancer Res Ther 1984; 28:181–188.

48. Kohn KW, Gibson NW. DNA cross-linking by chloroethylating agents. IARC Sci Publ 1986; 70:155–162.

49. Kohn KW, Hartley JA, Mattes WM. Mechanisms of DNA sequence selective alkylation of guanine-N7 positions by nitrogen mustards. Nucleic Acids Res 1987; 15:10531–10549.

50. Lown JW, Chauhan SM. Mechanism of action of (2-haloethyl)nitrosoureas on DNA. Isolation and reactions of postulated 2-(alkylimino)-3-nitrosooxazolidine intermediates in the decomposition of 1,3-bis(2-chloroethyl)-,1-(2-chloroethyl)-3-cyclohexyl-, and 1-(2-chloroe-

thyl)-3-(4'-trans methylcyclohexyl)-1-nitrosourea. J Med Chem 1981; 24:270–279.

51. Lown JW, Koganty RR, Bhat UG, Chauhan SM, Sapse AM, Allen EB. Isolation and characterization of electrophiles from 2-haloethylnitrosoureas forming cytotoxic DNA cross-links and cyclic nucleotide adducts and the analysis of base site-selectivity by AB initio calculations. IARC Sci Publ 1986; 70:129–136.

52. Lown JW, Koganty RR, Bhat UG, Sapse AM, Allen EB. Mechanism of interstrand cross-linking of DNA by anticancer 2-haloethylnitrosoureas. Drugs Exp Clin Res 1986; 12:463–473.

53. Lown JW, McLaughlin LW, Chang YM. Mechanism of action of 2-haloethylnitrosoureas on DNA and its relation to their antileukemic properties. Bioorg Chem 1978; 7:97–110.

54. Ludlum DB. Nature and biological significance of DNA modification by the haloethylnitrosoureas. IARC Sci Publ 1986; 78:71–81.

55. Ludlum DB. Formation of cyclic adducts in nucleic acids by the haloethylnitrosoureas. IARC Sci Publ 1986; 70:137–146.

56. Ludlum DB, Mehta JR, Tong WP. Cross-link formation in DNA by rat liver O6-alkylguanine-DNA alkyltransferase. Cancer Res 1986; 46:3353–3357.

57. Mattes WM, Hartley JA, Kohn KW. DNA sequence selectivity of guanine-N7 alkylation by nitrogen mustards. Nucleic Acids Res 1986; 14:2971–2987.

58. McKenna R, Ahmad T, Ts'ao CH, Frischer H. Glutathione reductase deficiency and platelet dysfunction induced by 1,3-bis(2-chloroethyl)-1-nitrosourea. J Lab Clin Med 1983; 102:102–115.

59. Mehta JR, Ludlum DB, Renard A, Verly WG. Repair of O(6)-ethylguanine in DNA by a chromatin reaction from rat liver: transfer of the ethyl group to an acceptor protein. Proc Natl Acad Sci USA 1981; 78:6766–6770.

60. Montgomery JA, McCaleb GS, Johnston TP, Mayo JG, Laster WR. Inhibition of solid tumors by nitrosoureas. I. Lewis lung carcinoma. J Med Chem 1977; 20:291–295.

61. Morten JE, Margison GP. Increased O6-alkylguanine alkyltransferase activity in Chinese hamster V79 cells following selection with chloroethylating agents. Carcinogenesis 1988; 9:45–49.

62. Parker S, Kirk MC, Ludlum DB. Synthesis and characterization of O6-(2-chloroethyl)guanine: a putative intermediate in the cytotoxic reaction of chloroethylnitrosoureas with DNA. Biochem Biophys Res Commun 1987; 148:1124–1128.

63. Parker S, Kirk MC, Ludlum DB, Koganty RR, Lown JW. Reaction of 1,3-bis(2-chloroethyl)-1-nitrosourea (BCNU) with guanosine: evidence for a new mechanism of DNA modification. Biochem Biophys Res Commun 1986; 139:31–36.

64. Pegg AE. Properties of the O6-alkylguanine-DNA repair system of mammalian cells. IARC Sci Publ 1984; 57:575–580.

65. Pegg AE. Factors affecting O6-alkylguanine-DNA-alkyltransferase activity. Banbury Rep 1986; 23:287–297.

66. Pegg AE, Scicchitano D, Morimoto K, Dolan ME. Specificity of O6-alkylguanine-DNA alkyltransferase. IARC Sci Publ 1987; 84:30–34.

67. Sariban E, Erickson LC, Kohn KW. Effects of carbamoylation on cell survival and DNA repair in normal human embryo cells (IMR-90) treated with various 1-(2-chloroethyl)-1-nitrosoureas. Cancer Res 1984; 44:1352–1357.
68. Sariban E, Kohn KW, Zlotogorski C, Laurent G, D'Incalci M, Day R, Smith BH, Kornblith PL, Erickson LC. DNA cross-linking responses of human malignant glioma cell strains to chloroethylnitrosoureas, cisplatin, and diaziquone. Cancer Res 1987; 47:3988–3994.
69. Scicchitano D, Jones RA, Kuzmich S, Gaffney B, Lasko DD, Essigmann JM, Pegg AE. Repair of oligodeoxynucleotides containing O6-methylguanine by O6-alkylguanine-DNA-alkyltransferase. Carcinogenesis 1986; 7:1383–1386.
70. Scudiero DA, Meyer SA, Clatterbuck BE, Mattern MR, Ziolkowski CH, Day RS. Sensitivity of human cell strains having different abilities to repair O6-methylguanine in DNA to inactivation by alkylating agents including chloroethylnitrosoureas. Cancer Res 1984; 44:2467–2474.
71. Shealy YF, Krauth CA, Laster WR Jr. 2-Chloroethyl(methylsulfonyl)-methanesulfonate and related (methylsulfonyl)methanesulfonates: antineoplastic activity in vitro. J Med Chem 1984; 27:664–670.
72. Singer B. Alkylation of the O6 of guanine is only one of many chemical events that may initiate carcinogenesis. Cancer Invest 1984; 2:233–238.
73. Singer B. In vivo formation and persistence of modified nucleosides resulting from alkylating agents. Environ Health Perspect 1985; 62:41–48.
74. Smith AC, Boyd MR. Preferential effects of 1,3-bis(2-chloroethyl)-1-nitrosourea (BCNU) on pulmonary glutathione reductase and glutathione/glutathione disulfide ratios: possible implications for lung toxicity. J Pharmacol Exp Ther 1984; 229:658–663.
75. Smith BH, Greenwood MA, Kornblith PL, Ellis J, Gibson C, Cummins CJ. Non-nuclear cytotoxic actions of DNA cross-linking and/or alkylating agents in glioma-derived cell lines. (meeting abstract) J. Neuro-oncol 1984; 2:268.
76. Tew KD, Kyle G, Johnson A, Wang AL. Carbamoylation of glutathione reductase and changes in cellular and chromosome morphology in a rat cell line resistant to nitrogen mustards but collaterally sensitive to nitrosoureas. Cancer Res 1985; 45:2326–2333.
77. Tew KD. Cytotoxic consequences of a carbamoylating nitrosourea in a nitrogen mustard resistant cell line. (meeting abstract) Proc Ann Meet Am Assoc Cancer Res 1985; 26:341.
78. Thomas CB, Osieka R, Kohn KW. DNA cross-linking by in vivo treatment with 1-(2-chloroethyl)-3-(4-methylcyclohexyl)-1-nitrosourea of sensitive and resistant human colon carcinoma xenografts in nude mice. Cancer Res 1978; 38:2448–2454.
79. Tong WP, Kirk MC, Ludlum DB. Molecular pharmacology of the haloethyl nitrosoureas: formation of 6-hydroxyethylguanine in DNA treated with BCNU (N,N(1)-bis[2-chloroethyl]-N-nitrosourea). Biochem Biophys Res Commun 1981; 100:351–357.
80. Tong WP, Kirk MC, Ludlum DB. Formation of the cross-link 1-[N(3)-deoxycytidyl],2-[N(1)-deoxyguanosinyl]ethane in DNA treated with N,N'-bis(2-chloroethyl)-N-nitrosourea. Cancer Res 1982; 42:3102–3105.

81. Tong WP, Kohn KW, Ludlum DB. Modifications of DNA by different haloethylnitrosoureas. Cancer Res 1982; 42:4460–4464.
82. Tong WP, Kirk MC, Ludlum DB. Mechanism of action of the nitrosoureas—V. formation of O6-(2-fluoroethyl)guanine and its probable role in the crosslinking of deoxyribonucleic acid. Biochem Pharmacol 1983; 32:2011–2015.
83. Wheeler GP, Johnston TP, Bowdon BJ, McCaleb GS, Hill DL, Montgomery JA. Comparison of the properties of metabolites of CCNU. Biochem Pharmacol 1977; 26:2331–2336.
84. Wu RS, Hurst-Calderone S, Kohn KW. Measurement of O6-alkylguanine-DNA alkyltransferase activity in human cells and tumor tissues by restriction endonuclease inhibition. Cancer Res 1987; 47:6229–6235.
85. Yagi T, Day RS. Differential sensitivities of transformed and untransformed murine cell lines to DNA cross-linking agents relative to repair of O6-methylguanine. Mutat Res 1987; 184:223–227.
86. Yarosh DB. Quantitation of DNA repair capacities of human tumor cells estimation of transfer of DNA adducts to repair proteins. Pharmacol Ther 1985; 31:141–151.
87. Yarosh DB, Hurst-Calderone S, Babich MA, Day RS. Inactivation of O6-methylguanine-DNA methyltransferase and sensitization of human tumor cells to killing by chloroethylnitrosourea by O6-methylguanine as a free base. Cancer Res 1986; 46:1663–1668.
88. Yarosh DB, Foote RS, Mitra S, Day RS. Repair of O(6)-methylguanine in DNA by demethylation is lacking in mer- human tumor cell strains. Carcinogenesis 1983; 4:199–205.
89. Yarosh DB, Rice M, Ziolkowski CHJ, Day RS. O6-methylguanine-DNA methyltransferase in human tumor cells. UCLA Symp Mol Cell Biol 1983; 11:261–270.
90. Yarosh DB, Rice M, Day RS, Foote RS, Mitra S. O6-methylguanine-DNA methyltransferase in human cells. Mutat Res 1984; 131:27–36.

20

Immunotherapy of Human Glioma with Lymphokine-Activated Killer Cells and Interleukin-2

Elizabeth Ann Grimm

Introduction

Immunotherapy of human cancer has always been attractive to tumor immunologists and oncologists. As new and promising immunotherapeutic modalities are devised, it is standard to apply them under adjuvant conditions to cancer patients who have failed all other standard therapies. Patients with malignant glioma currently have a very poor prognosis despite combined treatment with surgery, radiation, and/or chemotherapy.[1,2] Therefore, a number of studies attempting immunotherapy of glioma are currently in progress and have been the subject of several excellent review articles.[3-6] These include both systemic as well as intracerebral infusion of lymphokines, monoclonal antibodies, tumor vaccines, immunostimulatory bacterial extracts, and lymphocytes. Infusion of effector lymphoid cells intralesionally in humans[7-13] or systemically in animal models[14-16] appear especially promising for treatment of glioma. Through such attempts we have begun to learn a great deal concerning the immunologic state of the brain as well as the influence that tumors in the brain may have upon any form of immunotherapy.

From: Kornblith PL, Walker MD (editors). Advances in Neuro-Oncology. Futura Publishing Company, Inc., Mount Kisco, NY, © 1988.

As recently as 1948, Medawar[17] proposed that the brain was "privileged immunologically" due to the absence of rejection of foreign tissue implanted into experimental animal brains. While these initial experiments were interpreted to mean that the brain was totally devoid of immune response, we now know that this is not true. Modulation of the peripheral immune functions such as production or injection of T lymphocytes immunized against myelin basic protein resulted in severe brain damage in the form of experimental autoimmune encephalitis.[18-20] Further evidence that components from the systemic immune system could invade the brain come from studies in which brain tumors have been found to be surrounded by lymphocytes.[21-23] The current understanding of the blood-brain barrier is that it can be either circumvented or destroyed by components of the immune system, and that it is not necessarily intact in the areas of tumor vascularization. While the brain is very special immunologically, the teleologic reasons are speculative. Nevertheless, the unique circumstance of the brain provides a milieu of great interest to immunologists by providing a moderately isolated and contained system.

A number of problems have been identified which complicate immunotherapeutic attempts of brain tumors. Several major and consistent findings have been made. First, human brain tumors secrete a variety of immunosupressive substances which inhibit the generation of competent effector mechanisms.[24-26] Second, glioblastoma multiforme is extremely heterogenous in its in vivo state. As reported by Shapiro et al.,[27,28] a number of different phenotype and genotype expressing cells compose the original tumor, and bear little or no resemblance to eventual tissue cultured tumor lines. Third, it is most likely that glioma cells are not immunogenic as they appear to lack unique antigens recognized by the cellular immune system.[25,26,29] The expression of glioma antigens recently recognized serologically[30,31] and identified by monoclonal antibodies[32,33] would indicate that indeed unique molecular epitopes are expressed on the external surface of glioma tumor cells; however, these do not appear to be sufficiently immunogenic to stimulate the cellular immune system. Therefore, the lack of immunogenicity of brain tumors coupled with the absence of a classical lymphatic system provides a challenge to those who wish to explore immunotherapy of the brain.

In 1982, it was first reported that cancer patients' or normal persons' lymphocytes could be activated by in vitro incubation with interleukin–2 (IL-2) to a tumoricidal state.[34-36] The activation required at least 2 days in culture and was sensitive to inhibitors of proliferation. These lymphokine-activated killer cells (LAK) were profound in their ability to lyse autochthonous natural killer (NK) resistant fresh uncultured melanoma, sarcoma, and adenocarcinoma. More recently, Jacobs et al.[37] reported that LAK cells generated from glioma patients' peripheral blood lymphocytes kill autochthonous fresh glioma tumor targets in short-term cytotoxicity assays. These results combined with the previous reports of safe administration of lymphoid cells into the brain,[7-10] prompted us to initiate experiments designed to approach LAK cell therapy of brain tumors. Not only did we hope to determine whether LAK cells administered intraoperatively into the tumor site would manifest any beneficial results to the patient, we were also interested in the academic question of whether LAK cells would work in human systems in a relatively sequestered site. The purpose of this chapter is to describe general LAK cell characteristics and classification, to give specific results of the LAK cells applied to human and rat glioma tumor systems, and finally, to describe our initial clinical protocol results for treatment of glioma patients with LAK cells and/or interleukin-2.

General Characteristics of LAK

The LAK System is Distinct from NK and CTL.

The term *lymphokine-activated killer cell* (LAK) was coined to describe a novel lymphocytotoxic system with many apparent characteristics distinct from the previously accepted natural killer (NK) and cytotoxic T lymphocyte (CTL) cells.[34] LAKs are defined as interleukin-2 (IL-2) activated cytotoxic cells capable of lysing NK-resistant fresh human tumors. The rapid acceptance of this system by the immunologic community was due in part to its easily reproducible methodology, but also because of previously reported compelling evidence for existence of a third distinct lymphocytotoxic system. The prior unavailability of purified IL-2 combined with the widespread use of cultured tumor, rather than fresh tumor, unknowingly complicated a prior clearer understanding of such systems.

The current interest in the LAK system is due mainly to its tumor-killing ability, but secondarily to the current availability of purified recombinant interleukin-2 (rIL-2). IL-2 is a 15,000 dalton glycoprotein secreted by helper T lymphocytes in response to various im-

---

Table 1
Human LAK and Cell Lysis

Cells Sensitive to Lysis by Human LAK
    Fresh Tumors
        (Autologous and allogeneic)
        Melanoma
        Sarcoma, Osteo and Soft tissue
        Carcinoma
        Glioma
        Benign Schwannoma
    Cultured Tumors
        Placenta
        Fetal tissue (first trimester)
        EBV—transformed B cells
        TNP—modified PBL

Cells not Lysed by Human LAK
    LAK
    Bowel, fresh normal
    Colon, fresh normal
    Kidney, fresh normal
    Liver, fresh normal
    Pancreas, fresh normal
    Con A Lymphoblasts

---

munologic stimuli such as bacteria, alloantigens, and mitogenic lectins. The primary role for IL-2 is that of a growth factor (IL-2 was originally designated T-cell growth factor or TCGF), and is the obligatory second signal responsible for clonal expansion of antigen primed lymphocytes.

LAK are distinct based on a variety of characteristics including kinetics of activation, target cell specificity, stimulus responsible for activation, phenotype of precursor and effector cells, and specificty of lysis directed toward fresh autologous and allogeneic tumor cells (sarcoma, melanoma, adenocarcinoma, glioma, lymphoma) and for modified self (TNP-PBL) in short-term chromium 15 release assays (Table 1).

IL-2 Alone Directly Activates LAK

From the viewpoint of classical immunology, the characteristics of LAK activation are enigmatic. Naive lymphocytes respond directly

Table 2
Comparison of NK, LAK and CTL

	Lytic Activity		
Characteristic	*NK*	*LAK*	*CTL*
Development Kinetics	Spontaneous	by Day 2–3	by Day 5–7
Stimulus	None, IFN augments	IL-2, ± IFN^{-8}	Specific antigen
Specificity of cytotoxicity	Bone marrow; leukemia cells K562	Fresh solid tumors, (plus all NK targets) TNP-PBL	Specific antigen expressing cells
Precursor location	Intestinal mucosa TDL− PBL+ Spleen+	TDL+ Spleen+ PBL+ Tumor+ BM+ Cord Blood+ Intestinal mucosa+	TDL unknown PBL+
Serologic phenotype of effector	OKM1+ OKT3− OKT8− Leu 11+ Leu 7+	OKM1− OKT3+ OKT8+ Leu 1+ Leu 11− Tac+ 4F2+	OKM1− OKT3+ OKT8+ Leu 1+ Leu 11− Tac+ 4F2+
Serologic phenotype of precursor	unknown	OKM1− OKT3− OKT11± Leu 1− OKT9− OKT10− TAC− Leu 11±	OKM1− OKT3+ Leu 1+

to IL-2 in the absence of any known antigenic exposure.[36] Activation can be performed in serum-free medium and using lymphocytes from human cord blood, thoracic duct, or bone marrow. Activation is relatively rapid, requiring only 2 to 3 days in vitro, but it is clearly the result of differentiation and proliferation because of its sensitivity to either mitomycin C pretreatment or irradiation of the responder cells. LAK do not derive from previously primed (memory) CTL as shown by a different serologic phenotype (Table 2). Purified recombinant

IL-2 is sufficient for LAK activation; however, under some circumstances, interferon gamma can augment this activation.[39]

Autologous and Allogeneic Tumors are Lysed Comparably by LAK and LAK Clones

The hallmark of the LAK system is its extremely efficient and rapid ability to kill fresh tumor cells. It is generally accepted that classical NK cells do not kill fresh solid tumors to any significant degree, and that CTL generation to autologous human tumors is irreproducible using current methodology. While some fresh human tumors may be NK-sensitive (leukemias or some blood born metastases) and others may be antigenic and relatively lacking immunosuppressive factors so that they stimulate CTL production, these are likely to be rare and probably do not become clinically detectable. Because of an as yet undefined lytic potential, LAK kill all types of NK resistant tumors, but do not require any tumor present for activation. All fresh normal cells for which we could obtain single cell suspensions in vitro were all LAK-resistant. Because LAK have been infused intravenously,[40] or injected in various organs[12-14] directly in human and animals with no obvious deleterious effects, we conclude that LAKs recognize aspects of tumors that are absent on normal tissue.

III. Experimental Results of the LAK System Applied to Malignant Glioma

Presence of Glioma Tumor During LAK Activation Can Be Inhibitory

Injection of IL-2 directly into tumor sites has been shown in animal models to be successful to reducing tumor[41] and/or resulting in a state of immunity.[42-45] To determine whether LAK could be generated in such a milieu, we tested the effects of tumor presence on LAK activation as a function of IL-2 concentration. Table 3 indicates that with either cultured glioma or fresh human sarcoma tumors, LAK activation was considerably suppressed. Many human tumors are known to secrete immunosuppressive factors, which can inhibit

Table 3
LAK Activation Inhibited by Tumor Presence

| | % Lysis of fresh tumor after 6 days of culture | | | | | |
| | Units of IL-2 per ml | | | | | |
Tumor Cultured	*500*	*250*	*100*	*50*	*25*	*0*
A. Glioma cells/ml $\times 10^{-4}$						
0	63	64	65	45	35	0
1	29	23	28	24	3	1
10	12	13	6	10	6	3
50	5	17	9	8	2	0
100	0	1	0	0	0	0
200	0	0	0	0	0	0
B. Fresh Sarcoma $\times 10^{-4}$						
0	35	36	32	23	19	0
1	18	17	27	18	12	0
10	13	11	9	7	3	0
50	4	15	7	11	6	0
100	0	6	0	0	0	0
200	0	0	0	0	0	0

Tissue cultured glioma cells[27] or fresh sarcoma[14] were co-cultured with allogeneic normal PBL and IL-2 at the concentrations shown. After 6 days the culture contents were tested for LAK activity toward either the glioma in A, or sarcoma in B.

LAK activation. Even at 500 units per ml of IL-2, we were unable to generate optimal LAK at a 100:1 lymphocyte to tumor ratio with either type of tumor cell included in the culture. If LAK activation in vivo at the tumor site is to be considered as a therapeutic option, then the lymphocytes and IL-2 must be available in excessive quantities in relation to the number of tumor cells, or tumors must not be as immunosuppressive as those we tested. However, once activated, these LAK can be maintained in the presence of activation-suppressive tumor cells at very high tumor to LAK ratios as reported previously.

LAK Activation is Inhibited by Hydrocortisone, but not Cyclosporine

Because we have been successful in activating patients' PBL into LAK after extensive chemotherapy, it was of interest to us to define what effect known immunosuppressive drugs would cause. Our recent results showed that LAK activation is exquisitely sensitive to hydrocortisone, even at doses that have little or no effect on CTL activation (10^{-5} to 10^{-6} M).[46] Because glioma patients often receive dexamethasone, we purposefully tested the PBL from patients receiving up to 40 mg daily for LAK activation potential. Jacobs et al. reported that in all such patients, LAK were produced that significantly killed autologous as well as allogeneic fresh glioma.[37] Interestingly, cyclosporine A (CsA, Sandoz Pharmaceuticals) had no effect on LAK activation but totally prevented the activation of CTL.

LAK Recognition of Glioma Tumor Target Cells Requires a sensitive Protein

The susceptibility of human tumor cells to killing by LAK was found to be abrogated by treating tumor cells with proteolytic enzymes. Treatment of human glioma with either trypsin or chymotrypsin eliminated the ability of these tumor cells to be killed. Treated cells remain completely viable and regained their LAK sensitivity after culture for 24 hours under standard tissue culture conditions.[47,48] Glycosidases, neuraminidase, or periodate treatment of tumors had no effect on glioma lysis (Table 4). These results further indicate a role for a protein determinant in LAK recognition of glioma and other tumor target cells and provide the basis for our studies of LAK recognition currently in progress.

Therapeutic Potential of LAK for Human Glioma: Preliminary Clinical Trial Results

The unusual attributes of the LAK system point toward an unique antitumor effector mechanism that may well have application in cancer immunotherapy. Our approach to adoptive immunotherapy is the activation in vitro of lymphocytes from cancer patients by culture with IL-2 and then adoptively transferring these back to the cell donor. Initial studies have shown that such autochthonous cell infusion is feasible, both via intravenous and intratumor injection, without untoward effects. Infusion of activated cytotoxic lymphocytes has proven safe with some resulting stabilization and temporary regression of disease in melanoma and renal cell carcinoma.

Table 4

LAK Cell Killing of Allogeneic Glioma: Effect of Pretreating Glioma
with Various Enzymes

| | *% Killing of Tissue Culture Glioma Target Cells by LAK** | | |
| | *Glioma Derived From* | | |
Pretreatment of Human Glioma Cells	*Patient A*	*Patient C*	*Patient D*
None	43	43	32
Trypsin 1.0 mg/ml	−9	−2	14
Chymotrypsin 1.0 mg/ml	9	10	20
Glycosidase 1.0 mg/ml	40	59	34
Neuraminidase 0.05 units/ml	47	53	40
Periodate 2.5 millimolar	52	NT**	52

* Effector: Target = 100:1.
** NT = Not tested.

Other studies in which IL-2 was administered alone or in conjunction
with lymphocytes established the toxicity of IL-2 at high doses, and
clearly defined the safe limits when given systemically. In contrast
to the systemic toxicity of IL-2 found by Lotze,[49] we have found no
toxicity when escalating doses were administered intracerebrally
into the peritumor area of glioma patients during surgery. In our
view, IL-2 may be meant to act locally in tissue at sites of immune
responses, where it is not perceived as toxic, while in the peripheral
blood mechanisms it is rapidly eliminated. Evidence favoring this
view is the preliminary report by Pizza[50] that IL-2 administrated into
the bladder of bladder cancer patients resulted in notable tumor
regressions.

We have administered IL-2 and/or LAK cells in a total of 11 malignant glioma patients as a preliminary part of our phase I trial. The
absence of adverse side effects in our first nine patients permitted us
to continue into the potentially therapuetic part of this trial in which
autochthonous LAK (1×10^{10}) suspended in IL-2 (10^6 units) are injected intraoperatively after removal of the bulk of glioma tumor. To
date, two patients have received this combined therapy with no adverse effects. Specifically, escalating doses of LAK cells (10^8–10^{10}) or
recombinant IL-2 (10^4–10^6 units) were administered by direct injection into the brain tissue following operative tumor removal. IL-2 or

LAK were suspended in 5 cc of HBSS and injected at a rate of approximately 1 cc/minute through a 20 gauge blunt brain cannula via multiple intracerebral injections (five to eight, depending on the size of the tumor) evenly around the resection cavity. Prior to injection, an aliquot of the LAK cell suspension was sent for gram stain analysis and culture, and another aliquot was cryopreserved for later use in immunological testing. The specific details of patient selection, autochthonous LAK activation, trial design, and initial results were published in detail by Jacobs et al. [12,13]

The results were consistent in that none of the 11 patients treated with IL-2, LAK, or the combination exhibited signs of toxicity. Signs and symptoms of toxicity which were assessed included fever, chills, lethargy, malaise, skin reaction, weakness, nausea, diarrhea, frequency, urgency, hematuria and incontinence. There were no indications of skin reactions and the CBC and electrolyte patterns remained normal pre- and post-treatment. As reported,[13] CAT scans with contrast obtained on patients 7 to 10 days post-treatment were not different from scans obtained following uncomplicated craniotomy for tumor removal suggesting that intracerebral injection of IL-2 or LAK cells is not associated with radiographic changes. Compared to pre-treatment status, the neurological state of 10 of 11 patients has either remained the same or improved slightly. Our first patient, now surriving at 14 months, developed a left-sided hemisensory neglect which was evident on the first post operative day. This focal deficit was secondary to a stroke involving the right posterior thalamus as demonstrated by CAT scan. This stroke was most likely due to the surgical sacrifice of a small feeding arteriole in the course of removing a deep temporal lobe lesion. At 6 months follow-up, this patient's deficit had not significantly improved. Another patient became moderately lethargic the first postoperative day and CAT scan at that time demonstrated pneumocephalus. The pneumocephaly resolved and the patient became fully alert 24 hours following placement on 100 O_2. A third patient died 9 weeks post-surgery and injection of 10^6 units IL-2. The cause of death was progressive tumor growth as demonstrated by CAT scan.

As shown in Table 5, patient lymphocytes cultured without IL-2 did not lyse autologous or allogeneic glioma cells. However, when these cells were cultured with IL-2, LAK cells were generated which produced a significant lysis of autologous fresh glioma as well as both autologous and allogeneic tissue culture glioma. LAK cells did not

Table 5

In Vitro Killing of Glioblastoma by Brain Tumor Patient
Lymphocytes Cultured without IL-2 (PBL) or IL-2 (LAK)
% Killing Target Cells*

Patient	Effector Cells	Autologous Fresh Brain Tumor	Autologous Tissue Culture Brain Tumor	Autologous PBL	Allogeneic Tissue Culture Brain Tumor
1.	PBL	6.2	6.4	NT	NT
	LAK	37.2	60.6	NT	NT
2.	PBL	NT**	−1.8	5.5	−7.1
	LAK	NT	80.8	5.9	82.9
3.	PBL	NT	−1.4	−.10	−.7
	LAK	NT	57.7	6.2	61.1
4.	PBL	NT	−8.2	−1.20	−4.8
	LAK	NT	78.9	6.5	73.5
5.	PBL	6.8	3.4	4.2	−6.9
	LAK	5.3	49.5	4.9	52.7
6.	PBL	−.3	−7.8	3.7	−0.6
	LAK	55.5	71.4	3.1	55.5
7.	PBL	4.5	6.4	8.2	6.1
	LAK	24.7	84.2	11.1	62.3
8.	PBL	−6.4	1.1	−2.6	−4.9
	LAK	36.7	95.6	7.2	18.8

* Effector: Target = 100:1.
** NT = Not tested.

lyse autologous normal PBL. When the lymphocytes of patients involved in our phase I study were tested, LAK cells were generated which significantly lysed glioma.

Our current of in vitro activation and intraoperative infusion of LAK circumvents some potential problems associated with the immunosuppressive substances elaborated from glioma cells. By this method we are able to critically control the activation environment and optimize effector cell production. Certainly more patients and longer follow-up times are needed to assess any significant therapeutic effects; however, we are confident that our materials and procedures are relatively safe and should be studied further.

Summary

Lymphokine-activated killer cells (LAK) are the product of fresh lymphocytes incubated with interleukin-2 for at least 3 days. LAK are functionally distinct from all other lymphocyte classes, because they do not require antigen for activation, and kill nonimmunogenic tumor cells with marked efficiency. LAK kill fresh human tumor in vitro, and are currently being tested for therapeutic efficiacy. We can make LAK from the puiripheral blood lymphocytes of malignant glioma patients which kill the autologous as well as allogeneic tumor cells in vitro. Injection of LAK and IL-2 intraoperatively into the resection cavity of glioma patients can be performed safely and without toxicity.

REFERENCES

1. Walker MD, Alexander E jr, Hunt WE, MacCarty CS, Maholey MS, et al. Evaluation of BCNU and/or radiotherapy in the treatemnt of anaplastic gliomas. A cooperative clinical trial. J Neurosurg 1978; 49:333–343.
2. Walker MD, Green SB, Byar DP, Alexander E, Batzdorf U, et al. Randomized comparisons of radiotherapy and nitrosourea for the treatment of malignant glioma after surgery. N Engl J Med 1980; 303:1323–1329.
3. Brooks WH, Roszman TL. Cellular responsiveness of patients with primary intracranial tumors. In: Brain Tumours: Scientific Basis, Clinical Investigation, and Current Therapy, Thomas DGT, Graham DI, eds., London, Butterworths, 1980; pp. 121–132.
4. Apuzzo MLJ, Mitchell MS. Immunological aspects of intrinsic glial tumors. J Neurosurg 1981; 55:1–18.
5. Stavrou D, Bilzer TH, Hulten M, Zanker KS, Anzil AP, et al. Immunological aspects of experimental brain tumors. Anticancer Res 1982; 2:151–156.
6. Mahaley MS Jr, Gillespie GY. Immunotherapy of patients with glioma: fact, fancy, and future. In: Progress in Experimental Brain Tumor Research, Vol. 11, Basel, S. Karger, 1984.
7. Takakura K, Miki Y, Kubo O, et al. Adjuvant immunotherapy for malignant brain tumors. Jpn J Clin Oncol 1972; 12:109–120.
8. Takakura K, Miki Y, Kubo 0. Adjuvant immunotherapy for malignant brain tumors in infants and children. Childs Brain 1975; 1:141–147.
9. Young HF, Kaplan A. Immunotherapy of human gliomas. In: Waters H, ed., Immunotherapy: The Handbook of Cancer Immunology, Vol. 5, New York, Garland STPM Press, 1978; pp. 357–382.
10. Young HF, Kaplan A, Regelson W. Immunotherapy with autologous white cell infusions ("lymphocytes") in the treatment of recurrent glioblastoma multiforme. A preliminary report. Cancer 1977; 40:1037–1044.
11. Jacobs SK, Wilson DJ, Kornblith PL, Grimm EA. Studies on the im-

munotherapy of human gliomas using autologous lymphokine activated killer cells. Surg Forum 1985; 36:504–506.

12. Jacobs SK, Wilson DJ, Kornblith PL, Grimm EA. Interleukin–2 or autologous lymphokine activated killer cell treatment of malignant glioma: Phase I lymphokine activated killer (LAK) cells in the treatment of malilgnant glioma: preliminary report. J Neurosurg (in press).

14. Yamasaki T, Honda H, Yamashita J, Namba Y, Hanboka M. Characteristic immunological responses to an experimental mouse brain tumor. Cancer Res 1983; 43:4610–4617.

15. Yamasaki T, Honda H, Yamashita J, Watanabe Y, Namba Y, et al. Specific adoptive immunotherapy of malignant glioma with long-term cytotoxic T lymphocyte line expanded in T-cell growth factor. Neurosurg Rev 1984; 7:37–54.

16. Yamasaki T, Honda H, Yamashita J, Watanabe Y, Namba Y, et al. Specific adoptive immunotherapy with tumor-specific cytotoxic T-lymphocyte clone for murine malignant gliomas. Cancer Res 1984; 44:1776–1783. 17. Medawar PB. Immunity to homologous grafted skin. III. The fate of skin homografts transplanted to the brain, to subcutaneous tissue and to the anterior chamber of the eye. Br J Exp Pathol 1948; 29:58–69.

18. Paterson PY. Transfer of allergic encephalomyelitis in rats by means of lymph node cells. J Exp Med 1960; 111:119–136.

19. Paterson PY. Experimental autoimmune (allergic) encephalomyelitis. Induction, pathogenesis, and suppression. In: Miescher PA, Mueller-Eberhard HJ, eds., Textbook of Immunopathology, Vol. 1, ed 2, New York, Grune & Stratton, 1976; pp.179–213.

20. Traugott U, Stone SH, Raine CS. Experimental allergic encephalomyelitis: migration of early T-cells from the circulation into the central nervous system. J Neurol Sci 1978; 36:55–61.

21. Ridley A, Cavanaugh JB. Lymphocytic infiltration in gliomas evidence of possible host resistance. Brain 1971; 94:117–124.

22. Takeuchi J, Barnard RO. Perivascular lymphocytic cuffing in astrocytomas. Acta Neuropathol 1976; 35:265–271.

23. Palma L, Di Lorenzo N, Guidetti B. Lymphocytic infiltrates in primary glioblastomas and recidivous gliomas. Incidence, fate, and relevance to prognosis in 228 operated cases. J Neurosurg 1978; 49:854–861.

24. Fontana A, Hengartner H, deTribolet N, Weber E. Glioblastoma cells release interleukin–1 and factors inhibiting interleukin–2–mediated effects. J Immunol 1984; 132:1837–1844.

25. Gately MK, Glaser M, McCarron RM, Dick SJ, Dick MD, et al. Mechanisms by which human gliomas may escape cellular immune attack. Acta Neurochir 1982; 64:175–197.

26. Grimm EA, Jacobs SK, Lanza L, Roth JA, Wilson DJ. Is there a role for IL-2 activated cytotoxic lymphocytes (LAK) in cancer therapy? In: Frost P, Kripke M, eds., Immunology and Cancer, U of Texas Press, 1983.

27. Shapiro JR, Yung WKA, Shapiro WR. Clonal tumor cell heterogeneity. Prog Exp Tumor Res 1984; 27:49–66.

28. Shapiro JR, Yung WKA, Shapiro WR. Isolation, karyotype, and clonal growth of heterogeneous subpopulations of human malignant gliomas. Cancer Res 1981; 41:2349–2359.

29. Kumar S, Taylor G, Steward JK, et al. Cell-mediated immunity and blocking factors in patients with tumours of the central nervous system. Int J Cancer 1973; 12:194–205.
30. Kornblith PL, Dohan FC Jr, Wood WC, et al. Human astrocytoma: serum-mediated immunologic response. Cancer 1974; 33:1512–1519.
31. Kornblith PL, Pollock LA, Coakham HB, et al. Cytotoxic antibody responses in astrocytoma patients. J Neurosurg 1979; 51:47–52.
32. Sikora K, Alderson T, Philips J, Watson JV. Human hybridoma from malignant gliomas. Lancet 1982; 11–14.
33. Philips J, Alderson T, Sikora K, Watson JV. Localization of malignant glioma by a radiolabelled human monoclonal antibody. J Neurol Neurosurg Psychol 1983; 46:388–392.
34. Grimm EA, Mazumder A, Zhang HZ, Rosenberg SA. The lymphokine activated killer cell phenomenon: Lysis of NK-resistant fresh solid tumor cells by IL-2 activated autologous human peripheral blood lymphocytes. J Exp Med 1982; 155:1823–1841.
35. Grimm EA, Ramsey K, Mazumder A, Wilson DJ, Djeu J, et al. Lymphokine-activated killer cell phenomenon: II. The precursor phenotype is serologically distinct from peripheral T lymphocytes, memory CTL, and NK cells. J Exp Med 1983; 157:884–897.
36. Grimm EA, Robb RJ, Roth JA, Neckers LM, Lachman L, et al. The lymphokine activated killer cell phenomenon. III. Evidence that IL-2 alone is sufficient for direct activation of PBL into LAK. J Exp Med 1983; 158:1356–1361.
37. Jacobs SK, Wilson DJ, Kornblith PL, Grimm EA. In vitro killing of human glioblastoma by interleukin–2 activated autologous lymphocytes. J Neurosurg 1986; 64:114–117.
38. Rosenberg SA, Grimm EA, McGrogan N, Doyle M, Kawasaki E, et al. Biologic activity of recombinant human interleukin–2 produced in E. Coli. Science 1984; 223:1412–1415.
39. Itoh K, ShiibaK, Shimizo Y, Suzuki R, Kumagai K. Generation of activated killer cells by recombinant interleukin–2 in collaboration with interferon–2. J Immunol 1985; 134:3124.
40. Rosenberg SA, Rosenstein M, Grimm EA, Lotze M, Mazumder A. The use of lymphoid cells expanded in IL-2 for the adoptive immunotherapy of murine and human tumors. In: Thymic Hormones and Lymphokines, Goldstein AL, ed., New York, Plenum Press, 1984; p. 191.
41. Rosenberg, SA, Mule JJ, Spiess PJ, et al. Regression of established pulmonary metastases and subcutaneous tumor mediated by the systemic administration of high dose recombinant IL-2. J Exp Med 1985; 161:1169.
42. Conlon PJ, Hefeneider SH, Henney CS, Gillis S. The effects of interleukin–2 on primary in vivo immune responses in the potential role of T-cells in cancer therapy. Fefer A, Goldstein A, eds., New York, Raven Press, 1982; pp. 113–125.
43. Cheever MA, Greenberg PD, Fefer A, Gillis S. Augmentation of the anti-tumor therapeutic efficacy of long-term cultured T lymphocytes by in vivo administration of purified interleukin–2. J Exp Med 1982; 155:968–980.
44. Pretkau V, Mills GB, Bleackley RC. Enhancement of anti-tumor immune

responses with interleukin–2 in the potential role of T-cells in cancer therapy. Fefer A, Goldstein A, eds., New York, New York, 1982; pp. 147–159.

45. Forni G, Giovarelli M, Santoni A. Lymphokine-activated tumor inhibition in vivo. I. The local administration of interleukin–2 triggers nonreactive lymphocytes from tumor-bearing mice to inhibit tumor growth. J Immunol 1985; 134:1305–1311.

46. Grimm EA, Muul LM, Wilson DJ. Cyclosporine and hydrocortisone exert differential inhibitory effects on the activation of human cytotoxic lymphocytes by recombinant IL-2 versus allospecific CTL. Transplantation 1985; 39:537.

47. Jacobs SK, Melin G, Holcomb B, Parham CW, Kornblith PL, et al. Lymphokine activated killer (LAK) cell mediated lysis of murine glioma: trypsin-chymotrypsin sensitive glioma protein is responsible for tumor selective recognition by LAK cells. Brain Res (in press).

48. Jacobs SK, Parham CW, Holcomb B, Kornblith PL, Grimm EA. Lymphokine activated killer (LAK) cell mediated killing of human glioma: effect of pretreating glioma with various membrane modifying agents. J Neuro-Oncol (in press).

49. Lotze pn, Matory YL, Ettinghausen SE, Raynor AA, Sharrow SO, et al. In vivo administration of purified human Interleukin–2. II Half life, immunologic effects, and expansion of Peripheree lymphoid cells in vivo with interleukin 2. J Immunol 1985; 135:2865–2875.

50. Pizza G, Severini G, Mennite D, DeVinci C, Corrado F. Tumor regression after intralesional injection of interleukin 2 in bladder cancer. Preliminary report. Int J Cancer 1984; 34:359–367.

21

Immunotoxins: Potential Adjuncts in Tumor Cell Killing

John Zovickian

Introduction

Current therapy for malignant tumors of the central nervous system (CNS) is unsatisfactory.[56,60,72,73] Inability to direct conventional treatment modalities specifically to tumor produces unacceptable toxicity to normal tissues and limits therapeutic efficacy. The advent of monoclonal antibody technology has led to recognition of cell-surface antigens that are selectively expressed on neoplastic compared to normal tissues.[33] Such antigenic differences may be sufficient for therapeutic purposes.[5,27]

Immunotoxins comprise a new class of cell-type specific cytotoxic reagents which consist of a monoclonal antibody linked to a protein toxin. Such hybrid molecules are designed to combine the tumor cell-type selectivity of monoclonal antibodies with the extreme potency of protein toxins. Immunotoxins have displayed high orders of potency and cell-type specificity in vitro.[52,78] Results of in vivo studies, however, have been variable and, in general, less impressive,[78] due, at least in part, to inadequate access of immunotoxin to tumor tissue. Zovickian et al.[85] have proposed a role for properly designed immunotoxins in the treatment of compartmental CNS neo-

From: Kornblith PL, Walker MD (editors). Advances in Neuro-Oncology. Futura Publishing Company, Inc., Mount Kisco, NY, © 1988.
Acknowledgments: I am indebted to Dr. Richard J. Youle for his assistance in preparation of this chapter. I thank Ms. Doreen Quimby and Ms. Lynn Schofield for expert typing.

plastic disease. Specifically, immunotoxins may be particularly efficacious in treating CNS neoplasms involving compartments—intrathecal, intraventricular, or cystic—where access of immunotoxins to tumor would not rely upon transvascular delivery.

I will review the rationale and strategies for construction of immunotoxins. I will discuss the potential advantages and problems associated with use of immunotoxins to treat malignant tumors of the CNS. I will review results of recent in vitro studies demonstrating potent and specific killing of human glioblastoma and medulloblastoma cells by an anti-transferrin receptor-ricin immunotoxin, and I will discuss in vivo studies of immunotoxin efficacy in the treatment of leptomeningeal neoplasia in a guinea pig model. Finally, I will consider future directions in immunotoxin construction and application in the treatment of CNS neoplastic disease.

Rationale Underlying Construction of Immunotoxins

Many substances act to kill cells by disrupting membrane function, energy metabolism, or DNA, RNA, or protein synthesis. Lack of cell-type specificity, however, limits the clinical application of many of these agents. Most conventional anti-cancer drugs, for example, rely on the tendency of tumor cells to divide more rapidly than normal cells to achieve selective cytotoxicity. Unfortunately, because certain normal tissues (such as gastrointestinal epithelium and hematopoietic stem cells of bone marrow) contain many proliferating cells, the margin of selectivity between tumor cells and normal cells is usually too small for the drugs to be curative.

Other substances, such as hormones, growth factors, and antibodies, act on cells in a variably selective fashion, due to their specific interaction with receptors or antigens on the cell surface.

The rationale underlying the construction of immunotoxins, then, is to utilize the cell-type selectivity of antibodies—or other cell-type specific proteins—to direct various cytotoxic agents to defined groups of cells.

Paul Ehrlich postulated in 1906 that tissue-specific dyes could be coupled with toxic metals to generate a new class of tissue-specific reagents, and he synthesized a conjugate composed of Evan's blue dye and arsenic.[28] Mathé[38] in 1958 made the first antibody-drug conjugate, linking an antibody to the dihydrofolate reductase inhibitor methotrexate. Mathé conjugated methotrexate to the globulin fraction of hamster anti-mouse L1210 leukemia serum and reported prolonged survival of tumor-inoculated mice that had been treated with the methotrexate-linked antibody, as compared to mice treated with normal globulin bound to methotrexate or mice treated with methotrexate and antibody given separately. Mathé's experiments were extended by other investigators who studied different drugs for their suitability in antibody-drug complexes. Agents examined include the alkylating agent chlorambucil, p-phenylenediamine mustard, vindesine, cytosine arabinofuranoside, and the antibiotics daunomycin and adriamycin.[3]

These antibody-drug conjugates have shown a modestly selective cytotoxic effect. The critical shortcoming with this approach, however, is that conventional anti-cancer agents act stoichiometrically to kill cells. Accordingly, a very large number of molecules is required for cell killing. Chlorambucil, for example, requires more than 20,000 alkylations per cell to induce cell death and, in general, conventional chemotherapeutic drugs require more than 10^4–10^5 molecules per cell to achieve cell killing.[11] In contrast, tumor-selective antibodies generally bind 10^3–10^5 sites per cell, usually much less in vivo.[78] It is evident, then, that the number of molecules of drug required for cell killing may exceed the number of antibody-binding sites per cell, making it difficult to deliver a sufficiently large number of molecules of drug for cell killing. This problem pointed to the need for more potent cytotoxic agents to achieve successful antibody-mediated tumor cell killing.

The Toxins

Many protein toxins of plant or bacterial origin exist that act catalytically, rather than stoichiometrically, to kill cells. Because they act as enzymes, these toxic proteins are much more potent than chemotherapeutic drugs. For example, it has been demonstrated that, in vitro, a single molecule of diphtheria toxin[77] or ricin[12] in the cytosol is sufficient to kill a cell. More importantly, however, these toxins are able to kill cells with only 10–2,000 molecules bound per cell.[52] Accordingly, they possess the required potency to achieve antibody-mediated killing of tumor cells, which may not have a high density of tumor-associated antigens on their surface.

The successful construction of immunotoxins requires an under-

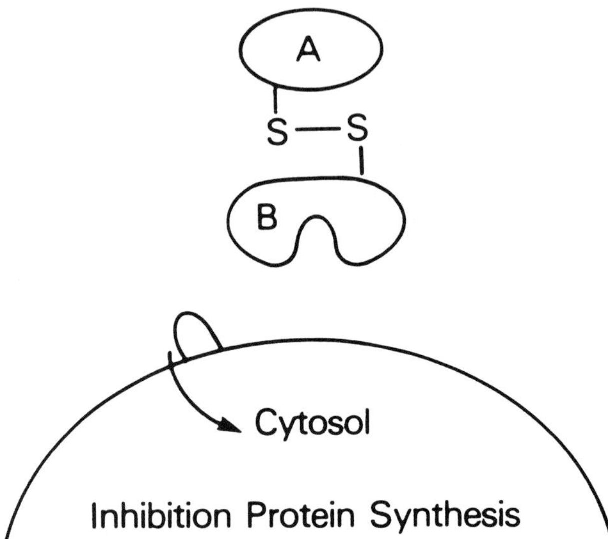

Figure 1. Schematic drawing depicting generalized structure of a hetero-dimeric protein toxin. The A-chain subunit is an enzyme which, once within the cytosol, blocks protein synthesis and kills the cell. The B-chain subunit binds the toxin to cell-surface receptors and facilitates translocation to the cytosol.

standing of the structural-functional relationships of the toxins from which the toxic component of the hybrid molecule is derived.

Diphtheria toxin and the plant proteins ricin, abrin, and modeccin all share a general structure which consists of two polypeptide chains. These chains, called the A and B chains, are linked by a disulfide bond and possess different activities. The A chain is an enzyme which, once within the cytosol, kills cells by catalytically inhibiting protein synthesis. Although highly active in cell-free systems, the A chain by itself is virtually nontoxic to cells and animals.[52] The B chain, while not toxic in cell-free systems, has two functions that are critical for cell killing. The B chain binds the toxin to cell-surface receptors, and it facilitates the passage of the A chain into the cytosol.[79,83] Because cell-surface receptors for the B chain of these toxins are present on the surface of most eukaryotic cells, the unmodified toxins have little cell-type specific toxicity. Figure 1 schematically depicts the structure of a protein toxin.

Diphtheria Toxin

Diphtheria toxin is a 60,000 molecular weight protein secreted by *Corynebacterium diphtheriae*. Proteolytic nicking at a particular arginine-rich site produces disulfide-linked A and B subunits. The A-chain subunit is an enzyme that catalyzes the transfer of ADP-ribose from NAD+ to a novel amino acid called "diphthamide" in elongation factor 2. The ADP-ribosylated elongation factor 2 is unable to catalyze the translocation reaction of peptidyl-t-RNA on ribosomes, thus blocking protein synthesis and killing the cell.[53] Diphtheria toxin B chain binds the toxin to specific cell-surface receptors and facilitates entry of A chain into the cytosol. The nature of the receptor for diphtheria toxin is not known.

Ricin

Ricin is a 62,000 molecular weight disulfide-linked heterodimer purified from castor bean seeds. It belongs to a group of plant proteins, including abrin and modeccin, which have similar structures and mechanisms of action (although extracted from unrelated plants).[51] This structure is similar to that of diphtheria toxin, but the A and B chains function differently.

The enzymatically active A chain, once within the cytosol, inactivates ribosomes by modifying specific nucleoside residues in 28 S ribosomal RNA, thus blocking protein synthesis and killing the cell.[13] The A-chain enzyme alone, while able to inactivate 1,500 ribosomes per minute in simple buffer solution,[52] has no toxic effect on intact cells.

The ricin B chain has two functions. It binds ricin to cell-surface oligosaccharides containing a terminal galactosyl residue, and it facilitates translocation of the toxic A chain into the cytosol.[79,83] Cytosol entry represents the rate-limiting step for immunotoxin activity,[84] and much attention has focused on the pathway by which toxins enter the cytosol. Youle and Colombatti[79] utilized monoclonal antibodies within hybridoma cells to localize ricin functionally en route to the cytosol. They found that the intracellular antibodies blocked ricin toxicity and concluded that ricin enters the cytosol not directly from endocytotic vesicles, but rather via the protein secretory apparatus. The authors further showed that the galactose-binding activity of the B chain is required in an intracellular compartment for translocation of A chain to the cytosol. As I will discuss later, this finding contains important implications for the design of optimal toxin conjugates.

Two concepts critical to the design of immunotoxins follow from this basic understanding of ricin subunit structure and function. First, the presence of galactose or lactose in the medium will block ricin's binding to cells in vitro by competing for the galactose-binding sites on the B chain. Secondly, antibody-toxin conjugates constructed with the intact ricin molecule can interact with cells via two potential binding sites. Intact toxin conjugates can bind via their antibody component specifically to antigen-positive target cells, and the conjugates can bind in non-cell-type specific fashion via the ricin B chain galactose-binding sites to receptors present on most eukaryotic cells.

Strategies for the Construction of Immunotoxins

Moolten and Cooperband[44] in 1970 reported construction of the first antibody-toxin conjugate. They coupled diphtheria toxin to the IgA fraction of guinea pig antiserum to mumps virus. The target cells were monkey kidney cells that were infected with mumps virus and thus expressed viral surface antigens. This first immunotoxin displayed high in vitro potency but only two-fold selectivity between antigen-positive and antigen-negative cells.

This retention of toxicity for nontarget cells led to a different approach to designing immunotoxins. Instead of adding a new binding moiety to the intact toxin, a new binding moiety was substituted for the B subunit. Thus, the enzymatically active A chain, nontoxic to cells by itself, would be directed by the new binding moiety to a specific cell population, as dictated by the substituted binding moiety (Fig. 2).

Chang and Neville[10] in 1977 linked the hormone human placental lactogen via a disulfide bond to diphtheria toxin A chain. Although they demonstrated that the binding function of the hormone and the enzymatic activity of the A chain were preserved, Chang and Neville could not demonstrate toxicity of the hormone-A chain conjugate. Several A-chain conjugates were subsequently constructed using other hormones as the substituted ligand. Cawley et al.[9] prepared an epidermal growth factor (EGF)-ricin A chain conjugate which displayed toxicity for 3T3 cells. The toxic effect could be blocked by excess EGF, and lactose did not affect the conjugate's cytotoxicity, indicating that its toxic effect was not due to traces of intact ricin.

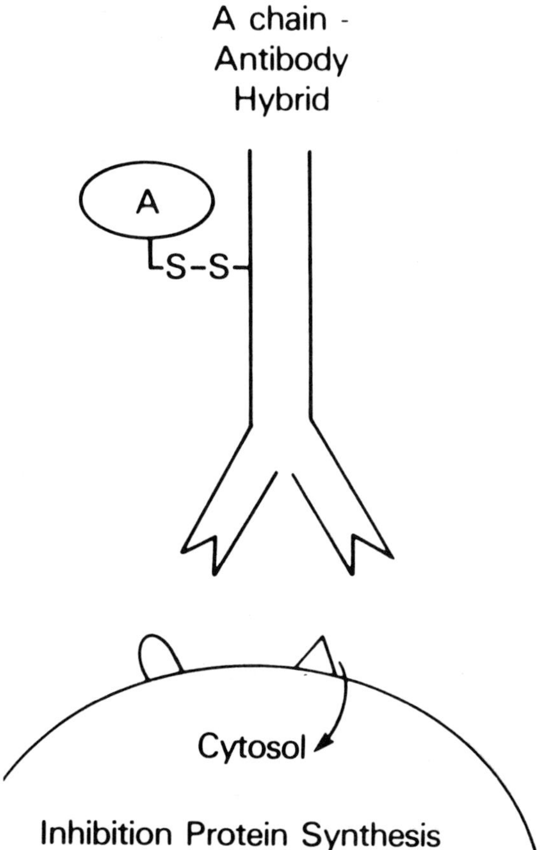

Figure 2. Schematic drawing of a toxin A-chain immunotoxin. The toxin B-chain is replaced by a cell-type specific antibody. A-chain toxicity is thus mediated by the antibody, but the B-chain entry activity is lost.

In contrast, an EGF-diphtheria A chain hybrid had no effect on 3T3 cells, despite preserved ADP-ribosylating activity of the diphtheria A-chain component and ability of the conjugate to compete with radiolabeled EGF for cell-surface receptors. Other hormone-A chain conjugates have been constructed using insulin and diphtheria A chain,[42] as well as the B subunit of human chorionic gonadotropin and ricin A chain.[48,49] Both of these conjugates exhibited relatively low in vitro potency. Finally, conjugates have been prepared using thyrotropin releasing hormone and diphtheria toxin-related peptides,[1] and using melanotropin.[23]

Similarly, conjugates have been constructed by linking polyclonal antibodies to the A chain of toxins through a disulfide bridge. In 1980, Krolick et al.[35] reported construction of an immunotoxin composed of ricin A chain linked to affinity-purified polyclonal antibodies which were directed against the idiotype of the cell-surface IgM of the mouse B-cell tumor BCL_1. This anti-idiotype antibody-ricin A chain hybrid killed 70% of BCL_1 tumor cells in vitro at 0.25 μg/ml but had minimal effect on antigen-negative cells. Because a B-cell tumor is of monoclonal origin, its cell-surface idiotype represents a clonally expressed and "tumor-specific" marker. Accordingly, Krolick et al. had prepared an immunotoxin that was directed against a truly tumor-specific antigen expressed by all cells of a tumor. A major difficulty with use of antisera against tumor cells, however, is obtaining enough antibody of sufficiently high specificity against cell-surface antigens.

Monoclonal antibody technology now allows production of large quantities of antibody of defined specificity. This technology initially raised hopes that hybridomas obtained against human tumors could produce monoclonal antibodies that would react with specific antigens not present on normal cells. With the exception of monoclonal antibodies directed against the idiotype of monoclonal tumors,[41] however, truly "tumor-specific antigens" have not been identified. Nevertheless, hybridomas have been isolated that produce antibodies highly specific for "tumor-associated antigens" and, while not absolutely specific for tumors, such antibodies may, in certain cases, possess sufficient specificity to be of therapeutic importance in the targeting of toxins to neoplastic tissue.

Gilliland et al.[19] in 1980 first reported construction of an immunotoxin using a monoclonal antibody directed against a tumor-associated antigen. They coupled the A chain of ricin and diphtheria via a disulfide bridge to a monoclonal antibody directed against a colorectal carcinoma tumor-associated antigen. Both the ricin A-chain and diphtheria A-chain conjugate killed 50% of colorectal carcinoma cells in culture at a concentration of about 10^{-9} molar after a 24-hour exposure but were not toxic for cells that lacked the antigen.

A number of immunotoxins have subsequently been prepared by linking monoclonal antibodies directed against tumor-associated antigens to the A-chain subunit of ricin or diphtheria toxin. Some of these conjugates have exhibited both a high degree of cell-type selectivity and a high degree of potency in vitro.[83] In general, however, the A-chain hybrids have displayed reduced potency relative to the parent (whole) toxin and, at best, their cytotoxicity has been variable and unpredictable. Gilliland et al.[19] for example, found that their anti-colorectal carcinoma monoclonal antibody-A chain conjugates were 1921,000 times less active than native diphtheria toxin.

The variable potency of ricin A chain immunotoxins led Youle et al.[80] in 1979 to propose that the B chain played a role in immunotoxin entry beyond that of binding to the cell surface. This hypothesis was supported by the finding that free ricin B chain increased the rate of cell killing by an A-chain immunotoxin by fivefold, without increasing the amount of the immunotoxin bound by cells.[83] Other investigators showed that ricin B chain increased toxicity of an A-chain immunotoxin at least 1,000-fold,[39] and that ricin B chain linked to antibody against target cell antigen,[70] or against A-chain immunotoxin itself,[71] can also potentiate cytotoxicity of ricin A-chain immunotoxins in vitro. Thus, the high degree of cell-type specificity achieved with conjugates between antibodies and toxin A-chain subunits occurred at the expense of much of the potency of the native toxin. Furthermore, this loss of potency could be attributed to a role of the B chain in facilitating immunotoxin entry into the cytosol.

Recognition of the B-chain entry function led to a new strategy in immunotoxin construction in which intact ricin toxin was linked to monoclonal antibodies, and antibody-mediated cell killing was achieved in vitro by addition of excess lactose or galactose in the culture media (Fig. 3). Immunotoxins constructed with intact ricin can bind to cells via either their antibody component or the ricin B subunit. Addition of lactose saturates the galactose-binding sites on the ricin B subunit and inhibits ricin from binding and killing cells via cell-surface galactose-containing receptors.

Youle and Neville [82] in 1980 reported construction of an intact ricin conjugate prepared with a monoclonal antibody directed against the Thy 1.2 antigen, expressed on the murine thymus cell surface. The anti-Thy 1.2-ricin conjugate in the presence of 100 millimolar lactose selectively killed antigen-positive target cells at concentrations that did not kill antigen-negative cells. This selectivity, expressed as the ratio of immunotoxin concentrations required to kill both (Thy 1.2-positive and Thy 1.2-negative) cell types, was 700-fold. In addition to this high degree of cell-type selectivity, the anti-Thy 1.2-ricin conjugate was equally as toxic as native ricin, and the con-

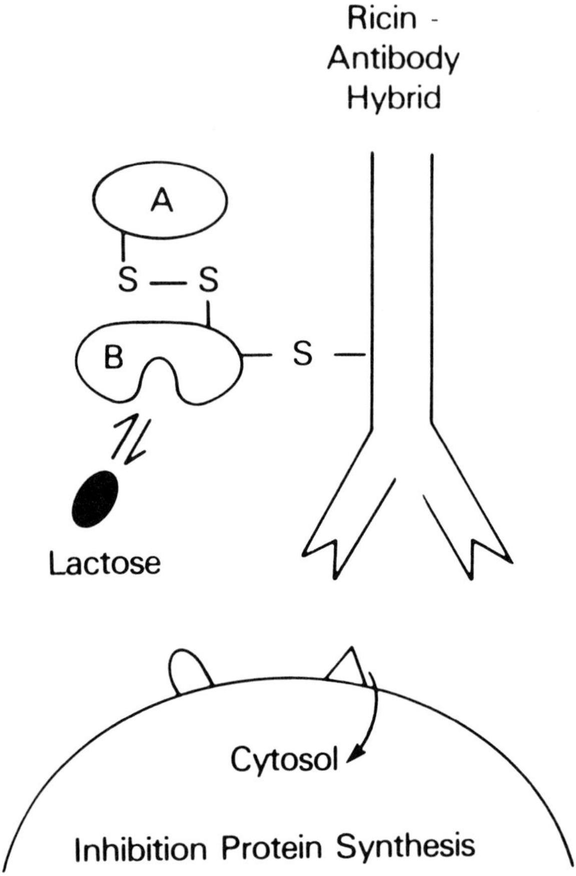

Figure 3. Schematic drawing of an intact ricin immunotoxin. The whole ricin molecule is linked to an antibody. Excess lactose blocks the galactose-binding sites on the B-chain subunit, so that binding is mediated by the cell-type specific antibody. The B-chain entry function is preserved.

jugate's toxicity was unchanged in the presence of lactose, whereas toxicity of native ricin was reduced 100-fold in the presence of lactose.

Using a much more sensitive clonogenic assay of cytotoxicity, Stong et al.[64] found that 1,000 ng/ml of T101-ricin in the presence of 100 millimolar lactose killed 5.1 logs of target CEM cells and less than 1 log of nontarget cells, for a specific log kill of 4.5 (>99.99%). In contrast, Casellas et al.,[8] using a similar assay with the same target

CEM cell line, found that T101-ricin A chain killed only 0.5 logs of CEM cells. These results reinforce the evidence for the extraordinary potency and cell-type selectivity that can be achieved with intact ricin immunotoxins in vitro, and they demonstrate again the higher potency of intact ricin conjugates compared to A-chain conjugates.

Clinical Application of Immunotoxins: Advantages and Disadvantages

Immunotoxins possess several properties that make them well suited for clinical tumor therapy. Their major advantage is the potential for extreme tumor cell selectivity, which depends largely upon the nature of the antibody-target antigen interaction. I have already noted that, in vitro, immunotoxins can kill 4.5 logs (>99.99%) of target cells without killing nontarget cells.[64] Furthermore, Thorpe et al.,[65] using an immunotoxin prepared with the plant toxin saporin in a nude mouse tumor model; and Gregg et al,[22] using an intact ricin immunotoxin as well as a recombinant ricin A-chain immunotoxin in a syngeneic guinea pig tumor model, both demonstrated a median 5 log (99.999%) kill of tumor cells in vivo. The extent to which such tumor cell selectivity can be achieved clinically, however, remains to be determined.

The extreme potency of immunotoxins means that they can kill target tumor cells at concentrations far below those required by conventional chemotherapeutic drugs. The alkylating agent BCNU, for example, can kill 50% of human glioblastoma-derived cells in culture at concentrations of 10^{-3} to 10^{-6} molar.[34,55] In contrast, Zovickian et al.,[85] using an intact ricin immunotoxin, reported 50% killing of glioblastoma cells in vitro at a concentration of 10^{-13} molar. While different assay conditions preclude exact comparisons, the numbers do convey the extraordinary potency of the immunotoxin, its potency exceeding that of BCNU's by 7–10 orders of magnitude, or 10 million- to 10 billion-fold.

Other potential advantages of immunotoxins in tumor therapy concern their mechanism of tumor cell killing. Because immunotoxins kill cells independently of DNA systhesis, unlike radiation therapy or conventional chemotherapeutic drugs, immunotoxins kill quiescent cells. Furthermore, their cytotoxicity is not affected by conditions of hypoxia, a factor responsible for resistance of tumor cells to radiation therapy[25] and chemotherapy.[40] Finally, combination chemotherapy, using regimens of drugs which act at different levels of DNA synthesis, is generally more effective than single agent therapy. Immunotoxins, which act by shutting down protein synthesis, may be highly effective when combined with conventional chemotherapeutic drugs, or even with radiation therapy.[16,17,69,74] Additionally, the side effects of immunotoxins and chemotherapeutic drugs or radiation therapy may not be cumulative.[16,17]

Certain properties of immunotoxins, however, present special problems in their application to tumor therapy. One potential problem already alluded to concerns the cell-type selectivity of those immunotoxins which are constructed with the whole ricin molecule. While intact ricin immunotoxins display much greater potency than immunotoxins prepared with the ricin A subunit, whole ricin conjugates require the presence of lactose to block endogenous binding of the ricin B chain to generate antibody-specific killing in vitro.[80] Theoretical considerations predict a similar problem in vivo; however, the results of Gregg et al.[22] (noted above), as well as those of Zovickian and Youle[86] (discussed below), suggest that careful dosage adjustment may minimize nontarget cell toxicity of intact ricin immunotoxins in vivo.

A second potential problem is the mounting of an immune response by the patient to administered mouse monoclonal antibodies[59] and to administered toxin.[15] The response to monoclonal antibody-toxin conjugates in humans, however, is not well defined,[36] and use of human monoclonal antibodies[62] or less immunogenic Fab or F(ab)₂ fragments[63] may reduce this potential problem. Additionally, patients who are immunosuppressed because of their underlying disease or because of chemotherapy or radiation therapy may mount an attenuated anti-immunotoxin immune response,[20,43] and the first dose of immunotoxin therapy—before patient antibodies arise—may have a significant therapeutic effect. Finally, to the extent that the CNS is partially an "immunologically privileged site,[58,75]" immunotoxins targeted to tumors within the CNS may be protected from a patient's immune response.

The greatest problem in applying immunotoxins to the clinical sphere concerns their access to tumor tissue, largely due to their large size, which limits diffusion out of the vascular system. Badger and Bernstein,[2] using a murine model, showed that saturation of binding sites in a subcutaneous tumor nodule required intravenous infusion of 160 mg/kg of monoclonal antibody. While feasible for monoclonal antibody therapy, such large amounts of immunotoxin would cause unacceptable toxicity. As I will discuss in the following section, the problem of tumor access may stand as an even greater obstacle in the treatment of parenchymal CNS tumors.

Application of Immunotoxins to the Treatment of CNS Neoplastic Disease

Tumors of the CNS pose special problems in the clinical application of immunotoxins. The marked biologic heterogeneity of malignant gliomas includes variable expression of antigens both among and within tumors and, possibly, with time.[4,7,76] Accordingly, although monoclonal antibodies have been raised against a spectrum of human neuroectodermal tumor- and human glioma-associated antigens,[5] the innate antigenic heterogeneity of malignant glial tumors compounds the problem of identifying "tumor-associated antigens" which would provide sufficient tumor specificity to be of operational importance in selectively targeting toxins to malignant tissue.

Zovickian et al.[85] exploited the selective distribution of transferrin receptors (TR) in certain malignant tumors to achieve selective killing of malignant brain tumor-derived cells in culture. The TR is a cell surface glycoprotein which mediates uptake of iron.[68] Many tumors selectively express very high levels of TR relative to normal tissues,[14,18,61] providing the possibility of using monoclonal antibodies against the human TR to target anti-TR immunotoxins to tumor tissue. The authors constructed an immunotoxin composed of a murine monoclonal antibody (5E9)[26] against the human TR coupled to intact ricin. The cytotoxic effect of the anti-TR-ricin immunotoxin was assayed as inhibition of protein synthesis in human glioblastoma-derived and human medulloblastoma-derived cell lines, and the presence of TR on these cell lines, as well as on surgical samples of glioblastoma, medulloblastoma, and normal brain, was assayed using solid phase radioimmunoassay techniques.

The anti-TR-ricin immunotoxin killed 50% and 90% of human glioblastoma cells in culture at concentrations of 2.5×10^{-12} molar and 3.8×10^{-11} molar, and 50% and 90% of human medulloblastoma cells in culture at 6.0×10^{-12} molar and 3.6×10^{-11} molar, respectively. Monensin, a carboxylic ionophore which facilitates delivery of immunotoxin to the cytosol, potentiated cytotoxicity of the immunotoxin 1,000 fold ($1C_{50} > 4.8 \times 10^{-13}$ molar) but did not affect cytotoxicity of ricin alone. Excess anti-TR monoclonal antibody, which competes for binding sites with the anti-TR-ricin immunotoxin and thus provides the clearest measure of antibody-specific cytotoxicity, blocked cytotoxicity by immunotoxin by 90% but had no effect on killing by ricin. Concentrations of immunotoxin more than 40 times greater than necessary to kill 60% of target tumor cells showed no reactivity against a cell line that lacked human TR.

Solid phase radioimmunoassay demonstrated the glioblastoma- and medulloblastoma-derived cell lines to express $> 1.6 \times 10^5$ TR sites per cell. Surgical samples of glioblastoma and medulloblastoma showed two- to four-fold greater reactivity with the anti-TR monoclonal antibody than with control (nonspecific) antibody, whereas normal brain had no detectable TR.

The anti-TR-ricin conjugate is the first anti-TR conjugate constructed with intact ricin. Its potency exceeds that of any other anti-TR immunotoxin described, and it is the first immunotoxin shown to be selectively toxic to human malignant brain tumor cells.

Immunotoxins directed against the human TR possess properties which make them especially attractive as potential clinical agents in the treatment of malignant CNS tumors. Most cells do not express detectable levels of TR,[18,31] and the results of this work suggest that normal brain expresses levels of TR significantly lower than present in malignant brain tumor tissue. Accordingly, in some cases, TR may be used as a marker to distinguish tumor cells from normal brain. Because iron is essential for tumor growth, it is not likely that tumor cells would escape anti-TR mediated cell killing via mechanisms of antigenic heterogeneity,[7] antigenic modulation,[50] or genetic loss[30] of TR. Additionally, because transferrin enters cells via receptor-mediated endocytosis,[32,47] the TR should facilitate internalization of bound anti-TR-toxin hybrid into the cell. TR are not shed into the circulation[67] and, thus, would not block anti-TR-mediated cell killing. Finally, although TR are expressed on some proliferating normal cells and on normal tissues with high iron requirements (such as placenta and maturing erythroid cells),[18] Trowbridge et al.[66] found no evidence of acute toxicity to normal tissues in mice with in vivo administration of a rat anti-mouse TR monoclonal antibody. Moreover, it has been demonstrated that early hematopoietic precursors and stem cells in murine bone marrow are relatively insensitive to an anti-TR-ricin A chain immunotoxin that was active against tumor cells in vitro.[37] These considerations, together with the in vitro results reviewed above, suggest that immunotoxins prepared with intact ricin and directed against the human TR may have a role in the treatment of malignant CNS tumors.

As in other systems, however, the chief problem in the clinical application of immunotoxins to the treatment of tumors of the CNS concerns their access to brain tumor tissue. In addition to the general problem of limited transvascular diffusion, the large size of immunotoxins presents a particularly difficult obstacle in parenchymal brain tumors in those areas where an intact blood-brain barrier may further exclude immunotoxins from target tissue.[24] Blood-brain barrier disruption may enhance immunotoxin delivery to intracerebral tumors,[6,46] but there is little information available describing accessibility of immunotoxins or antibodies to human intracerebral tumors.

Insofar as delivery stands as a potential obstacle to the use of immunotoxins in the treatment of parenchymal brain tumors, immunotoxins may be most effective in the therapy of CNS neoplastic disease confined to compartments—intrathecal, intraventricular, or cystic—where tumor access will not depend upon transvascular transport. To test this hypothesis, Zovickian and Youle[86] examined the efficacy of intrathecal immunotoxin therapy for a tumor of the cerebrospinal fluid (CSF) compartment. A syngeneic animal model of leptomeningeal neoplasia was developed in which percutaneous inoculation of L_2C leukemia cells into the cisterna magna of strain 2 guinea pigs produced disseminated leptomeningeal and intraventricular leukemia and death. Percutaneous intracisternal injection of an anti-idiotype monoclonal antibody (M6)-intact ricin immunotoxin 24 hours following intracisternal inoculation of 10^5 tumor cells (10,000 times the lethal dose) produced prolonged survival ($p<0.005$) in tumor-bearing animals, and 8% of animals survived long-term. The immunotoxin therapy caused no detectable toxicity. Intracisternal injection of either M6 monoclonal antibody alone or a nonspecific control immunotoxin had no therapeutic effect. The observed extension of survival in the immunotoxin-treated animals was shown, based on tumor doubling time as well as results of dose-response survival experiments, to correspond to a median 2—3 log (99.9%) and, in some animals, possibly a 5 log (99.999%) or greater kill of tumor cells. These results thus extend, for the first time, immunotoxin therapy to the CSF compartment, and they support a proposed role for immunotoxins in the regional treatment of CNS neoplastic disease.

Future Directions

Reid et al.[54] in 1978 reported the effect of diphtheria toxin on various human tumors in the athymic nude mouse. The mouse is much less sensitive to diphtheria toxin than are other species, including humans. The authors showed that human tumors grown subcutaneously in nude mice completely disappeared when the tumor-bearing animals were given a single intraperitoneal injection of diphtheria toxin one month after tumor implantation. Furthermore, of the different human tumors tested, the tumor found to be most sensitive to diphtheria toxin was a grade IV astrocytoma. This dramatic anti-tumor effect, of course, reflects the mouse's inherent resistance versus the human's inherent sensitivity to diphtheria toxin. The critical implication, however, is that given a large enough therapeutic window between toxicity for tumor compared to toxicity for normal tissues tumors can be cured using toxic proteins. The challenge is to design therapeutic agents which possess both the high order of potency and tumor cell-type specificity to achieve the necessary therapeutic window.

Elimination of the non-cell-type specific binding function of the toxin B chain, while preserving its entry function, would theoretically allow the preparation of a new class of monoclonal antibody-toxin conjugates which possess heretofore unrealized cell-type specific cytotoxicity (Fig. 4). Unfortunately, attempts to dissociate the binding

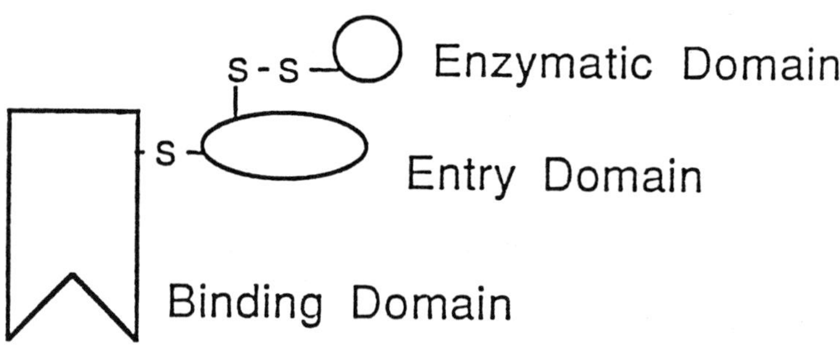

Figure 4. Schematic drawing depicting an immunotoxin containing the enzymatic domain of the toxin A-chain and the entry domain, but not the binding domain, of the toxin B-chain. Target cell specificity is thus determined fully by the antibody binding domain. This antibody-toxic protein conjugate combines the cell-type specificity of the antibody with the full potency of the protein toxin.

from the entry activity in ricin B chain by chemical modification[29,57,81] have not succeeded. Furthermore, since the galactose-binding site is required not only for toxin binding but also for translocation of toxin to the cytosol, dissociation of these activities in ricin may not be possible.[79]

However, Greenfield et al.[21] have now reported the identification of point mutations in the B chain of diphtheria toxin which block non-cell-type specific binding but preserve cytosol entry. The authors showed that linkage of the genetically altered toxins with a monoclonal antibody reconstituted full target cell toxicity indistinguishable from that of the native toxin linked to the same monoclonal antibody without restoring nontarget cell toxicity.

This discovery marks a new era whereby toxic proteins hopefully may be altered to produce clinical reagents which possess the therapeutic window necessary to achieve tumor cell killing without affecting normal cells.

REFERENCES

1. Bacha P, Murphy JR, Reichlin S. Thyrotropin releasing hormone-diphtheria toxin-related polypeptide conjugates: Potential role of the hydrophobic domain in toxin entry. J Biol Chem 1983; 258:1565–1570.
2. Badger CC, Bernstein ID. Therapy of murine leukemia with monoclonal antibody against a normal differentiation antigen. J Exp Med 1983; 157:828–842.
3. Baldwin RW, Embelton MJ, Gallego J, et al. Monoclonal antibody drug conjugates for cancer therapy. In Roth JA (ed): Monoclonal Antibodies in Cancer. Mount Kisco, NY: Futura Publishing Co, 1986; pp 215–257.
4. Bigner DD. Biology of gliomas: potential clinical implications of glioma cellular heterogeneity. Neurosurgery 1981; 9:320–326.
5. Bullard DE, Bigner DD. Applications of monoclonal antibodies in the diagnosis and treatment of primary brain tumors. J Neurosurg 1985; 63:2–16.
6. Bullard DE, Bourdon M, Bigner DD, et al. Comparison of various methods for delivering radiolabeled monoclonal antibody to normal rat brain. J Neurosurg 1984; 61:901–911.
7. Capone PM, Papsidero LD, Chu TM. Relationship between antigen density and immunotherapeutic response elicited by monoclonal antibodies against solid tumors. J Natl Cancer Inst 1984; 72:673–677.
8. Casellas P, Canat X, Fauser AA, et al. Optimal elimination of leukemic T-cells from human bone marrow with T101-ricin A chain immunotoxins. Blood 1985; 65:289–297.
9. Cawley DB, Herschman HR, Gilliland DG, et al. Epidermal growth factor-toxin-A-chain conjugates: EGF-ricin A is a potent toxin while EGF diphtheria fragment A is non-toxic. Cell 1980; 22:563–570.

10. Chang TM, Neville DM. Artificial hybrid protein containing a toxic protein fragment and a cell membrane receptor-binding moiety in a disulfide conjugate. I. Synthesis of diphtheria toxin fragment-A-S-S human placental lactogen with methyl–5–bromovalerimidate. J Biol Chem 1977; 252:1505–1514.

11. Crathorn AR, Roberts JJ. Mechanism of the cytotoxic action of alkylating agents in mammalian cells and evidence for the removal of alkylated groups from deoxyribonncleic acid. Nature 1966; 211:150–153.

12. Eikland K, Olsnes S, Pihl A. Entry of lethal doses of abrin, ricin, and modecin into the cytosol of HeLa cells. Exp Cell Res 1980; 126:321–326.

13. Endo Y, Mitsui K, Motizuki M. The mechanism of action of ricin and related toxic lectins on eukaryotic ribosomes. The site and the characteristics of the modification in 28S ribosomal RNA caused by the toxins. J Biol Chem 1987; 262:5908–5912.

14. Faulk WP, Hsi B, Stevens PJ. Transferrin and transferrin receptors in carcinoma of the breast. Lancet 1980; 2:390–392.

15. Fodstad O, Kvalheim G, Godal A, et al. Phase I study of the plant protein ricin. Cancer Res 1984; 44:862–865.

16. Fodstad O, Pihl A. Synergistic effect of adriamycin and ricin on L1210 leukemia cells in mice. Cancer Res 1980; 40:3735–3739.

17. Fodstad O, Pihl A. Synergistic effect of ricin in combination with daunorubicin, cis-dichlorodiammineplatinum (II), and vincristine in systemic L1210 leukemia. Cancer Res 1982; 42:2152–2158.

18. Gatter KC, Brown G, Trowbridge IS, et al. Transferrin receptors in human tissues: their distribution and possible clinical relevance. J Clin Pathol 1983; 36:539–545.

19. Gilliland DG, Steplewski Z, Collier RJ, et al. Antibody-directed cytotoxic agents: Use of monoclonal antibody to direct the action of toxin A-chains to colorectal carcinoma cells. Proc Natl Acad Sci USA 1980; 77:4539–4543.

20. Godal A, Fodstad O, Pihl A. Antibody formation against the cytotoxic proteins abrin and ricin in humans and mice. Int J Cancer 1983; 32:515–521.

21. Greenfield L, Johnson VG, Youle RJ. Point mutations in diphtheria toxin separate binding from entry and amplify immunotoxin selectivity. Science 1987; 238:536–539.

22. Gregg EO, Bridges SH, Youle RJ, et al. Whole ricin and recombinant ricin A chain idiotype-specific immunotoxins for therapy of the guinea pig L_2C B cell leukemia. J Immunol 1987; 138:4502–4508.

23. Griffin TW, Raso V, DeMartino HL. Inhibition of leucine incorporation in cultured melanoma cells by a conjugate of melanotropin and the toxic A-chain of ricin. Proc AACR Abstr. 1981; No. 838.

24. Groothius DR, Fischer JM, Vick NA, et al. Comparative permeability of different glioma models to horseradish peroxidase. Cancer Treat Rep 1981; 65:(Suppl 2):13–18.

25. Hall EJ. Welcome and overview. CROS conference on chemical modification—radiation and cytotoxic drugs. Int J Radiat Oncol Biol Phys 1982; 8:323–325.

26. Haynes BF, Hemler M, Cotner T, et al. Characterization of a monoclonal

antibody (5E9) that defines a human cell surface antigen of cell activation. J Immunol 1981; 127:347–351.

27. Hillstrom KE, Hillstrom I. Foreward, in Roth JA (ed): Monoclonal Antibodies in Cancer. Mount Kisco, NY: Futura Publishing Co, 1986; pp. ix-xiv.

28. Himmelweit F (ed): The Collected Papers of Paul Ehrlich. Vol 381. New York: Pergamon Press, 1980.

29. Houston LL. Inactivation of ricin using 4-azidophenyl-B-D-galacto-pyranoside and 4-diazophenyl B-D-galactopyranoside. J Biol Chem 1983; 258:7208–7212.

30. Hyman R, Cunningham K, Stallings V. Evidence for a genetic basis for the class A thy-1 defect. Immunogenetics 1980; 10:261–271.

31. Jefferies WA, Brandon MR, Hunt SV, et al. Transferrin receptor on endothelium of brain capillaries. Nature 1984; 312:162–163.

32. Klausner RD, Renswoude J, Ashwell G, et al. Receptor-mediated endocytosis of transferrin in K562 cells. J Biol Chem 1983; 258:4715–4724.

33. Kohler G, Milstein C.: Continuous culture of fused cells secreting antibodies of predefined specificity. Nature 1975; 256:495–497.

34. Kornblith PL, Szypko PE. Variations in response of human brain tumors to BCNU in vitro. J Neurosurg 1978; 48:580–586.

35. Krolick KA, Villemez C, Isakson P, et al. Selective killing of normal or neoplastic B cells by antibodies coupled to the A chain of ricin. Proc Natl Acad Sci USA 1980; 77:5419–5423.

36. Laurent G, Pris J, Farcet J, et al. Effects of therapy with T101-ricin A-chain immunotoxin in two leukemia patients. Blood 1986; 67:1680–1687.

37. Lesley J, Domingo DL, Schulte R, et al. Effect of an anti-murine transferrin receptor-ricin A conjugate on bone marrow stem and progenitor cells treated in vitro. Exp Cell Res 1984; 150:400–407.

38. Mathé G, Loc TB, Bernard J. Effet sur la leucemie L1210 de al souris d'une combinaison par diazotation d'A-methopterine et de gamma-globulines de hamsters porteurs de cette leucemie par heterogreffe. C.R. Acad Sci (Paris) 1958; 246:1626–1628.

39. McIntosh DP, Edwards DC, Cumber AJ, et al. Ricin B chain converts a non-cytotoxic antibody-ricin A-chain conjugate into a potent and specific cytotoxic agent. FEBS Lett 1983; 164;17–20.

40. McNally NJ. Enhancement of chemotherapy agents. Int J Radiat Oncol Biol Phys 1982; 8:593–598.

41. Miller RA, Maloney DG, Warnke R, et al. Treatment of B-cell lymphoma with monoclonal anti-idiotype antibody. N Engl J Med 1982; 306:517–522.

42. Miskimins WK, Shimuzu N. Synthesis of cytotoxic insulin cross-linked to diphtheria toxin fragment A capable of recognizing insulin receptors. Biochem Biophys Res Commun 1979; 91:143–151.

43. Moolten FL, Capparell NJ, Zajdel SH. Antitumor effects of antibody-diphtheria toxin conjugates. III. Cyclophosphamide-induced immune unresponsiveness to conjugates. J Natl Cancer Inst 1972; 49:1057–1062.

44. Moolten FL, Cooperband SR. Selective destruction of target cells by diphtheria toxin conjugated to antibody directed against antigens on the cells. Science 1970; 169:68–70.

45. Moyniham M, Pappenheimer AM. Kinetics of adenosine diphosphoribosylation of elongation factor 2 in cells exposed to diphtheria toxin. Infect Immunol 1981; 32:575–582.
46. Neuwelt EA, Frenkel EP, Diehl J, et al. Reversible osmotic blood-brain barrier disruption in humans: implications for the chemotherapy of malignant brain tumors. Neurosurgery 1980; 7:44–52.
47. Octave J, Scheider Y, Hoffmann p, et al. Transferrin uptake by cultured rat embryo fibroblasts. The influence of lysosomotropic agents, iron chelators and colchicine on the uptake of iron and transferrin. Eur J Biochem 1982; 123:235–240.
48. Oeltmann TN, Health EC. A hybrid protein containing the toxic subunit of ricin and the cell-specific subunit of human chorionic gonadotropin. I. Synthesis and characterization. J Biol Chem 1979a; 254:1002–1027.
49. Oeltmann TN, Heath EC.A hybrid protein containing the toxic subunit of ricin and the cell-specific subunit of human chorionic gonadotropin. II. Biological properties. J Biol Chem 1979b; 254:1028–1032.
50. Old LJ, Stockert E, Boyse EA.Antigenic modulation. Loss of TL antigen from cells exposed to TL antibody. Study of the phenomenon in vitro. J Exp Med 1968; 127:523–539.
51. Olsnes S, Pihl A. Toxic lectins and related proteins, in Cohen P, van Heyninger S (eds): The Molecular Actions of Toxins and Viruses. Amsterdam: Elsevier/North Holland; 1980.
52. Olsnes S, Pihl A. Chimeric toxins. Pharmacol Ther 1982; 15:355–381.
53. Pappenheimer AM. Diphtheria toxin. Ann Rev Biochcm 1977; 46:69–94.
54. Reid LM, Colburn P, Sato G, et al. Approaches to chemotherapy using the athymic nude mouse, in Houchens DP, Ovejera AA (eds): Proceedings of the Symposium on the Use of Athymic (Nude) Mice in Cancer Research, New York: Gustav Fischer. 1978; pp. 123–131.
55. Rosenblum ML, Gerosa MA, Wilson CB, et al. Stem cell studies of human malignant brain tumors. Part 1: Development of the stem cell assay and its potential. J Neurosurg 1983; 58:170–176.
56. Salcman M. The morbidity and mortality of brain tumors. Neurologic Clin 1985; 3:229–257.
57. Sandvig K, Olsnes S, Pihl A. Chemical modifications of the toxic lectins abrin and ricin. Eur J Biochem 1978; 84:323–331.
58. Scheinberg LC, Taylor JM. Immunological aspects of brain tumors, in Krayenbuhl H, Maspes PE, Sweet WH (eds): Progress in Neurological Surgery, vol. 2, Chicago: Year Book. 1968; pp. 267–291.
59. Sears HF, Mattis J, Herlyn D, et al. Phase-I clinical trial of monoclonal antibody in treatment of gastrointestinal tumors. Lancet 1982; 1:762–765.
60. Shapiro WR: Treatment of neuroectodermal brain tumors. Ann Neurol 1982; 12:231–237.
61. Shindelman JE, Ortmeyer AE, Sussman HH. Demonstration of the transferrin receptor in human breast cancer tissue. Potential marker for identifying dividing cells. Br J Cancer 1981; 27:329–334.
62. Sikora K, Alderson T, Phillips J, et al. Human hybridomas from malignant gliomas. Lancet 1982; I:11–14.
63. Smith TW, Lloyd BL, Spicer N, et al. Immunogenicity and kinetics of

distribution and elimination of sheep digoxin-specific IgG and Fab fragments in the rabbit and baboon. Clin Exp Immunol 1979; 36:384–396.

64. Stong RC, Youle RJ, Vallera DA. Elimination of clonogenic T-leukemic cells from human bone marrow using anti-Mr 65,000 protein immunotoxins. Cancer Res 1984; 44:3000–3006.

65. Thorpe PE, Brown ANF, Bremner JAG, et al. An immunotoxin composed of monoclonal anti-thy 1.1 antibody and a ribosome-inactivating protein from saponaria officinalis: Potent antitumor effects in vitro and in vivo. JNCI 1985; 75:151–159.

66. Trowbridge IS. Therapeutic potential of monoclonal antibodies that block biological function, in Boss BD, Langman R, Trowbridge I, et al (eds): Monoclonal Antibodies and Cancer. Orlando, Academic Press. 1983; pp. 53–61.

67. Trowbridge IS, Domingo DL. Anti-transferrin receptor monoclonal antibody and toxin-antibody conjugates affect growth of human tumour cells. Nature 1981; 294:171–173.

68. Trowbridge IS, Newman RA, Domingo DL, et al. Transferrin receptors: structure and function. Biochem Pharmacol 1984; 33:925–932.

69. Uckun FM, Stong RC, Youle RJ, et al. Combined ex vivo treatment with immunotoxins and mafosfamid: a novel immunochemotherapeutic approach for elimination of neoplastic T cells from autologous marrow grafts. J Immunol 1985; 134:3504–3515.

70. Vitetta ES, Cushley W, Uhr JW. Synergy of ricin A-chain-containing immunotoxins and ricin B-chain-containing immunotoxins in vitro killing of neoplastic human B cells. Proc Natl Acad Sci USA 1983; 80:6332–6335.

71. Vitetta ES, Fulton RJ, Uhr JW. Cytotoxicity of a cell-reactive immunotoxin containing ricin A chain is potentiated by an anti-immunotoxin containing ricin B chain. J Exp Med 1984; 160:341–346.

72. Walker MD, Alexander E, Hunt WE, et al. Evaluation of BCNU and/or radiotherapy in the treatment of anaplastic gliomas. J Neurosurg 1978; 49:333–343.

73. Walker MD, Green SB, Byar DP, et al. Randomized comparisons of radiotherapy and nitrosoureas for the treatment of malignant glioma after surgery. N Engl J Med 1980; 303:1323–1329.

74. Weil-Hillman G, Uckun FM, Manske JM, et al. Combined immunochemotherapy of human solid tumors in nude mice. Cancer Res 1987 (in press).

75. Wikstrand CJ, Bigner DD. Immunobiologic aspects of the brain and human gliomas. A review. Am J Pathol 1980; 98:517–567.

76. Wikstrand CJ, Bigner SH, Bigner DD. Demonstration of complex antigenic heterogeneity in a human glioma cell line and eight derived clones by specific monoclonal antibodies. Cancer Res 1983; 43:3327–3334.

77. Yamaizumi M, Makada E, Uchida T, et al. One molecule of diphtheria toxin fragment A introduced into a cell can kill the cell. Cell 1978; 15:245–250.

78. Youle RJ, Colombatti M. Immunotoxins: monoclonal antibodies linked to toxic proteins for bone marrow transplantation and cancer therapy. In Roth JA (ed): Monoclonal Antibodies in Cancer. Mount Kisco, NY, Futura Publishing Co, 1986; pp. 173–213.

79. Youle RJ, Colombatti M. Hybridoma cells containing intracellular anti-

ricin antibodies show ricin meets secretory antibody before entering the cytosol. J Biol Chem 1987; 262:4676–4682.

80. Youle RJ, Murray GJ, Neville DM. Ricin linked to monophosphopenta-mannose binds to fibroblast lysosomal hydrolase receptors, resulting in a cell-type specific toxin. Proc Natl Acad Sci USA 1979; 76:5559–5562.

81. Youle RJ, Murray GJ, Neville DM. Studies on the galactose-binding site of ricin and the hybrid toxin man 6P-ricin. Cell 1981; 23:551–559.

82. Youle RJ, Neville DM Jr. Anti-thy 1.2 monoclonal antibody linked to ricin is a potent cell-type-specific toxin. Proc Natl Acad Aci USA 1980; 77:5483–5486.

83. Youle RJ, Neville DM Jr. Kinetics of protein synthesis inactivation by ricin-anti-thy 1.1 monoclonal antibody hybrids. J Biol Chem 1982; 257:1598–1601.

84. Youle RJ, Neville DM. Role of endocytosis and receptor recycling in ligand-toxin and antibody-toxin conjugate activity, in Vogel CW (ed): Immunoconjugates; Antibody Conjugates in Radioimaging and Therapy of Cancer. New York, Oxford University Press. 1987 (in press).

85. Zovickian J, Johnson VG, Youle RJ. Potent and specific killing of human malignant brain tumor cells by an anti-transferrin receptor antibody-ricin immunotoxin. J Neurosurg 1987; 66:850–861.

86. Zovickian J, Youle RJ. Efficacy of intrathecal immunotoxin therapy in an animal model of leptomeningeal neoplasia. J Neurosurg 1988; 68:767-774.

Epilogue

There is perhaps no more challenging task than to defeat a cancer that resists all of our efforts so effectively.

Unfortunately, there are still many human cancers in this category. Malignant human brain tumors have remained a sub set of human cancers which have provoked fairly universal despair. Indeed there are few clinicians who see patients with these tumors who even recommend agressive therapy. At present the majority of patients receive at most a biopsy and radiotherapy and in a remarkable number of cases no therapy at all.

In the context of such therapeutic nihilism, among the most important goals of workers in this field are to offer hope to the patients and stimulation to the clinician to at least seek to treat these tumors vigorously. Only through such therapeutic vigor, coupled with scholarly evaluation of the data can we eventually make progress in this field.

The goal of this book has therefore been to assemble relevant data about the current status of clinical management to help encourage more vigorous clinical care and to present the many of the more intriguing new areas wherein new research offers insights as to the biology and potential therapeutic interactions to stimulate even more research efforts in this field.

Index

Pierre Dessureault

combien long jusqu'à chez nous...
how far back is home...

MCPC/CMCP 1995

Pierre Dessureault

combien long jusqu'à chez nous...
how far back is home...

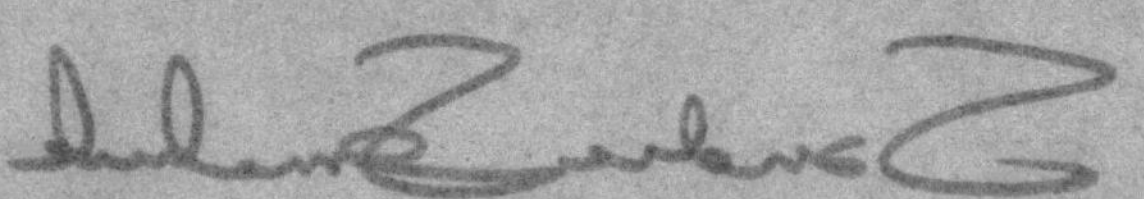

MCPC/CMCP 1995